Cardiac CT, PET and MR

Cardiac CT, PET and MR

Second Edition

EDITED BY

Vasken Dilsizian, MD, FACC, FAHA

Professor of Medicine and Radiology
Director, Cardiovascular Nuclear Medicine and PET Imaging
Chief, Division of Nuclear Medicine
University of Maryland School of Medicine
Baltimore, MD
USA

and

Gerald M. Pohost, MD, FACC, FAHA

Professor of Radiology, Keck School of Medicine
Professor of Electrical Engineering, Viterbi School of Engineering
University of Southern California
Los Angeles, CA;
Professor of Medicine, School of Medicine
Loma Linda University
Loma Linda, CA
USA;
Professor (Honorary), Xiamen University
Xiamen, Fujian
Peoples Republic of China

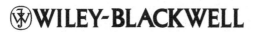

WILEY-BLACKWELL

A John Wiley & Sons, Ltd., Publication

This edition first published 2010, © 2010 by Blackwell Publishing Ltd

Blackwell Publishing was acquired by John Wiley & Sons in February 2007. Blackwell's publishing program has been merged with Wiley's global Scientific, Technical and Medical business to form Wiley-Blackwell.

Registered office: John Wiley & Sons Ltd, The Atrium, Southern Gate, Chichester, West Sussex, PO19 8SQ, UK

Editorial offices: 9600 Garsington Road, Oxford, OX4 2DQ, UK
The Atrium, Southern Gate, Chichester, West Sussex, PO19 8SQ, UK
111 River Street, Hoboken, NJ 07030-5774, USA

For details of our global editorial offices, for customer services and for information about how to apply for permission to reuse the copyright material in this book please see our website at www.wiley.com/wiley-blackwell

Library of Congress Cataloging-in-Publication Data

Cardiac CT, PET, and MR / edited by Vasken Dilsizian and Gerry Pohost. – 2nd ed.
p. ; cm.
Rev. ed. of: Cardiac CT, PET, and MRI / edited by Vasken Dilsizian and Gerald Pohost. 2006.
Includes bibliographical references and index.
ISBN 978-1-4051-8553-0
1. Cardiovascular system–Imaging.   2. Cardiovascular system–Tomography.   3. Cardiovascular system–Magnetic resonance imaging.   4. Tomography, Emission.   I. Dilsizian, Vasken.   II. Pohost, Gerald M.   III. Cardiac CT, PET, and MRI.
[DNLM: 1. Diagnostic Techniques, Cardiovascular.   2. Coronary Vessels–radionuclide imaging.
3. Diagnostic Imaging–methods.   4. Heart–radionuclide imaging. WG 141 C26456 2010]
RC683.5.I42C33 2010
616.1′0757–dc22   2010010793

ISBN: 9781405185530

A catalogue record for this book is available from the British Library.

Set in 9.5/12 pt. Minion by Aptara®, Inc., New Delhi, India

1   2010

Contents

List of Contributors

Stephen L. Bacharach, PhD
Adjunct Professor of Radiology
and Senior Tenured Research Scientist, NIH (ret)
Center for Molecular and Functional Imaging
University of California at San Francisco
San Francisco, CA
USA

Marcelo F. Di Carli, MD
Associate Professor of Radiology
Departments of Radiology and Medicine
Brigham and Women's Hospital
Harvard Medical School
Chief of Nuclear Medicine, Co-Director of
Cardiovascular Imaging
Boston, MA
USA

Timm-Michael L. Dickfeld, MD, PhD
Associate Professor of Medicine
Division of Cardiology
University of Maryland School of Medicine
Chief of Electrophysiology, VA Baltimore
Baltimore, MD
USA

Jane Francis, DCCR
Chief Cardiac MRI Radiographer
Department of Cardiovascular Medicine
University of Oxford
Oxford
UK

Richard T. George, MD
Assistant Professor of Medicine
Department of Medicine, Division of Cardiology
Johns Hopkins University
Baltimore, MD, USA

Robert J. Gropler, MD, FACC
Professor of Radiology, Medicine and Biomedical
Engineering
Lab Chief, Cardiovascular Imaging Laboratory
Mallinckrodt Institute of Radiology
Washington University School of Medicine
St. Louis, MO
USA

Udo Hoffmann, MD, MPH
Associate Professor of Radiology
Director, Cardiac MR PET CT Program
Massachusetts General Hospital
Harvard Medical School
Boston, MA
USA

Farouc A. Jaffer, MD, PhD
Assistant Professor of Medicine
Harvard Medical School, Boston, MA
Director of Vascular Imaging
Center for Molecular Imaging Research and Cardiovascular
Research Center, Attending Interventional Cardiologist
Massachusetts General Hospital
Boston, MA
USA

Subodh B. Joshi, MD, MPH
Research Fellow
Cardiac MR PET CT Program
Massachusetts General Hospital
Harvard Medical School
Boston, MA
USA

Hee-Won Kim, PhD
Assistant Professor of Radiology
USC/Keck School of Medicine
University of Southern California
Los Angeles, CA
USA

Joao A. C. Lima, MD, MBA
Professor of Medicine, Radiology and Epidemiology
Director of Cardiovascular Imaging
Johns Hopkins University
Baltimore, MD
USA

Jagat Narula, MD, PhD, FACC, FRCP
Professor of Medicine
Irvine School of Medicine
Chief, Division of Cardiology
Director, Memorial Heart & Vascular Institute
Medical Director

Edwards Lifesciences Center for Advanced Cardiovascular
  Technology
University of California
Irvine, CA
USA

Krishna S. Nayak, PhD
Associate Professor of Electrical Engineering, Biomedical
  Engineering, Medicine, and Radiology
Director, Magnetic Resonance Engineering Laboratory
Viterbi School of Engineering
Keck School of Medicine
University of Southern California
Los Angeles, CA
USA

Stephan G. Nekolla, PhD
Senior Physicist
Klinik für Nuklearmedizin
Technisch Universität München
Germany

Stefan Neubauer, MD
Professor of Cardiovascular Medicine
Department of Cardiovascular Medicine
University of Oxford
Oxford
UK

Patricia Nguyen, MD
Instructor, Department of Medicine
Division of Cardiovascular Medicine
Stanford University Medical Center
Stanford, CA
USA

Koen Nieman, MD, PhD, FESC
Resident in Cardiology
Department of Cardiology (Thoraxcenter) and Department
  of Radiology
Erasmus Medical Center
Rotterdam
The Netherlands

Ramdas G. Pai, MD , FACC, FRCP (Edin)
Professor of Medicine
Division of Cardiology
Loma Linda University Medical Center
Loma Linda, CA
USA

Linda R. Peterson, MD, FACC, FAHA
Associate Professor of Medicine and Radiology
Cardiovascular Division and Division of Geriatrics and
  Nutritional Sciences
Department of Medicine
Washington University School of Medicine
St. Louis, MO
USA

Matthew Robson, PhD
MRI Physicist
Department of Cardiovascular Medicine
University of Oxford
Oxford
UK

Ian S. Rogers, MD, MPH
First Year Clinical Fellow
Division of Cardiovascular Medicine
Stanford University Medical Center
Stanford, CA
USA

Antti Saraste, MD
Research Fellow
Nuklearmedizinische Klinik Technischen Universität
  München
Munich
Germany

Thomas H. Schindler, MD
Assistant Professor of Internal Medicine - Cardiology
Chief of Nuclear Cardiology and Cardiac PET
University Hospitals of Geneva
Geneva
Switzerland

Markus Schwaiger, MD
Director, Department of Nuclear Medicine
Nuklearmedizinische Klinik Technischen Universität
  München
Munich
Germany

**Joseph Selvanayagam, MBBS (Hons),
FRACP, DPhil, FCSANZ, FESC**
Professor of Cardiovascular Medicine
Flinders University of South Australia
Director Cardiac MR & CT
Flinders Medical Centre
Adelaide, SA
Australia

Hossam Sherif, MD
Research Fellow
Nuklearmedizinische Klinik Technischen
  Universität München
Munich
Germany

Eric M. Thorn, MD, MPH
Virginia Cardiovascular Associates, P.C.
Manassas, VA
USA

Quynh A. Truong, MD, MPH
Instructor in Radiology
Cardiac MR PET CT Program
Massachusetts General Hospital
Harvard Medical School
Boston, MA
USA

Ines Valenta, MD
Research Fellow
Nuclear Cardiology and Cardiac PET
University Hospitals of Geneva
Geneva
Switzerland

Padmini Varadarajan, MD, FACC
Associate Professor of Medicine
Division of Cardiology
Loma Linda University Medical Center
Loma Linda, CA
USA

Charles S. White, MD
Professor of Radiology and Medicine
University of Maryland School of Medicine
Chief of Thoracic Radiology
Department of Diagnostic Radiology
University of Maryland Medical Center
Baltimore, MD
USA

Raymond T. Yan, MD, MASc
Clinical and Research Fellow
Cardiac MR and CT Program
Division of Cardiology
Johns Hopkins Hospital
Baltimore, MD
USA

Phillip Yang, MD
Assistant Professor, Department of Medicine
Division of Cardiovascular Medicine
Stanford University Medical Center
Stanford, CA
USA

Foreword

Building upon several decades of technological development and clinical imaging experience, the field of cardiovascular imaging has made spectacular advances in recent years. The advanced imaging techniques—positron emission tomography (PET), cardiovascular magnetic resonance (CMR), and cardiac computed tomography (CT)—now deliver noninvasive coronary angiograms, new exquisitely detailed insights into the coronary artery wall, characterization of cardiac structure and function, and complementary functional data regarding perfusion, metabolism, and viability. These modalities challenge the existing paradigms for diagnosis and risk stratification while presenting uncertainties for the practitioner regarding their optimal clinical application relative to diagnostic angiography and standard stress testing. Against this rapidly evolving milieu, Drs Dilsizian and Pohost have produced a remarkably definitive and balanced text that captures the full scope, and the excitement, of current cardiovascular imaging knowledge. This new edition of *Cardiac CT, PET, and MR* is a timely, valuable resource for a wide range of readers including the researchers who continue to enrich the field, the imaging subspecialists (both beginner and expert) who refine the applications, and the clinicians who refer patients for diagnostic imaging procedures. The editors have recruited an internationally recognized and talented panel of expert authors, who are the leading authorities in their respective disciplines.

Cardiac CT, PET, and MR provides in-depth, comprehensive discussion of the technical characteristics and clinical applications of each of the advanced imaging modalities, including their comparative strengths and weaknesses. Essential reviews of imaging physics instrumentation and imaging protocols underlying PET, CMR, and CT technol-

ogy in the initial chapters provide the foundation for the broader discussion that follows of the many present and future applications of each of the imaging technologies. The rapidly accruing evidence base supporting the current state of the art is presented in detail in a well-balanced dialogue. The final chapters focus on the exciting new directions in fusion imaging with combined PET/CMR and PET/CT systems for concurrent assessment of anatomy and physiology, mapping applications to guide advanced cardiac electrophysiologic procedures, and the frontiers of noninvasive characterization of coronary plaque anatomy and pathobiology.

Noninvasive imaging methods are fundamental tools for all physicians involved in the diagnosis and treatment of patients with heart disease. PET, CMR, and CT have enormous potential to accelerate understanding of basic pathophysiologic processes in animals and humans while also providing the keys for early diagnosis and assessment of efficacy of new therapies. There is also great need for clinical trials and comparative effectiveness research to determine the right test for the right patient at the right time. An understanding of the current and future capabilities of noninvasive imaging is essential to fully achieve this potential. This new volume of *Cardiac CT, PET, and MR* itself has arrived at the right time to contribute importantly to this progress.

Robert O. Bonow, M.D.
Goldberg Distinguished Professor
Northwestern University Feinberg School
    of Medicine
Chief, Division of Cardiology
Northwestern Memorial Hospital
Chicago, Illinois

PART I

Instrumentation, Imaging Techniques, and Protocols

CHAPTER 1

Positron Emission Tomography

Stephen L. Bacharach
University of California, San Francisco, CA, USA

The goal of all cardiac nuclear imaging is to trace the fate of radioactively labeled biochemical compounds (tracers) within the body, usually in the myocardium or blood pool. One usually either makes a static image of the distribution of the radiotracer (e.g., ^{18}F-fluorodeoxyglucose (^{18}FDG) or thallium-201 (^{201}Tl)) or follows the uptake and clearance of the tracer with time. In the former case, static imaging is all that is required, while in the latter a series of images, acquired dynamically over time, is necessary. Positron emission tomography (PET) has these same goals. Although PET works in a manner very similar to conventional tomographic nuclear imaging techniques (e.g., single photon emission computed tomography or SPECT), there are some very significant differences. It is these differences that make PET of great potential value in nuclear cardiology, and it is these differences we will emphasize in this chapter.

Positron Decay

PET tracers, as their name implies, decay by emission of a positron. Except for their opposite charge, positrons are nearly identical to ordinary negatively charged electrons (which in fact are often called "negatrons"). They have the same mass and behave similarly when passing through the body. Positrons, however, are the "antimatter" of electrons. When a positron and an electron are in close proximity for more than the briefest interval, both will disappear (called "annihilation"), and their masses will be converted into energy

Cardiac CT, PET and MR, 2nd edition. Edited by Vasken Dilsizian and Gerry Pohost. © 2010 Blackwell Publishing Ltd.

in the form of two gamma rays traveling in almost exactly opposite directions. The energy of each photon is 0.511 meV (exactly the equivalent energy corresponding to the mass of the electron or positron). These photons are sometimes called "annihilation" photons. The two photons travel in nearly exactly opposite directions in order to conserve momentum. The entire process is illustrated in Figure 1.1. In this figure it is assumed that a positron emitter (in this case carbon-11 (^{11}C) is emitted by a tracer somewhere in the body (e.g., the myocardium). When the positron is emitted from the nucleus it is traveling at very high speed—nearly the speed of light. It moves through the tissue just as an electron would, bouncing off many of the atoms and losing energy as it does so. Eventually (typically within a millimeter or so, depending on the radionuclide) it slows down enough to spend a significant time near an electron. As soon as this happens the two annihilate and the two gamma rays (each with 0.511 meV) are emitted, as shown in Figure 1.1, each going in nearly the exact opposite direction. Although in Figure 1.1 the annihilation photons are shown traveling in exactly opposite directions, occasionally photons are emitted a few tenths of a degree more or less than *180°* apart.

PET scanners detect pairs of gamma rays resulting from annihilation. By determining where these two gamma rays (and all other pairs of gamma rays) originated, the PET scanner can produce an image showing the location in the body where the positrons have annihilated. However, if the positron has traveled far from its parent atom, the image will be inaccurate—the locus of the annihilating positron will not correspond to the locus of the radioactive atom. For this reason the initial speed

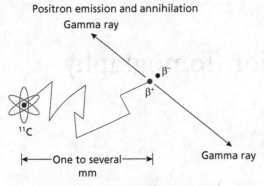

Positron emission and annihilation
Gamma ray

^{11}C

One to several
mm

Gamma ray

Figure 1.1 A positron is shown being emitted from the nucleus of ^{11}C. It is assumed that the ^{11}C atom is located in tissue. The positron is initially emitted at a speed which is a significant fraction of the speed of light. As it passes through the tissue, it gradually slows down, as it bounces off the atoms in the tissue. Eventually it slows down sufficiently so that it spends significant time near an atomic electron—its antimatter equivalent. When this happens the electron and the positron both annihilate—their mass being converted to energy in the form of two photons traveling in opposite directions, as shown.

(i.e., energy) of an emitted positron will affect the capacity of the PET scanner to accurately define the position of radioactive atoms within the myocardium. This in turn affects the ultimate spatial resolution of the images that can be obtained with a PET scanner.

There are many radioisotopes that emit positrons, and so would be suitable for use with a PET scanner. Several of the most important ones are listed in Table 1.1, along with their half-lives and some characteristics of the positron that is emitted

[1]. One of the reasons why PET has played such an important role in basic research is that several of the radioisotopes that are positron emitters (carbon, nitrogen, and oxygen) are the basic building blocks of all physiologically important biochemical compounds. This has permitted researchers to label amino acids, glucose, and a host of other biochemical compounds. Unlike the case with technetium-99m (^{99m}Tc), the labeling can often be done without making any alterations to the biochemical structure of the compound of interest. That is, a nonradioactive ^{12}C atom can be replaced with a ^{11}C atom, so that the resultant radiolabeled biochemical compound behaves just like the unlabeled one. The difficulty with ^{11}C, nitrogen-13 (^{13}N) and oxygen-15 (^{15}O) is that their half-lives are very short. This means they must be produced locally with an on-site cyclotron. It also means that the chemist in charge of labeling the biochemical compound of interest has very little time to do so. For these reasons (and others discussed below), the two most clinically important positron-emitting isotopes for cardiology are the last two on the list, fluorine-18 (^{18}F) and Rubidium-82 (^{82}Rb).

^{18}F has a 2-hour half-life. This is long enough to allow production at a site up to a few 100 km away. The recent dramatic increase in the use of ^{18}FDG for tumor imaging has resulted in a large number of such commercial production sites in the US (and to a lesser extent abroad). One can easily arrange for delivery of daily unit doses of ^{18}FDG. ^{18}FDG has proven very valuable in assessing myocardial viability [2]. Its use for this purpose has, in the past, been limited to large research institutions because

Table 1.1 Positron energies and ranges (in tissue).

Isotope	Maximum energy (meV)	Average energy (meV)	Average distance positrons travel (mm)	Maximum distance positrons travel (mm)
^{18}F	0.635	0.250	0.35	2.3
^{11}C	0.96	0.386	0.56	4.1
^{13}N	1.19	0.492	0.72	5.2
^{15}O	1.72	0.735	1.1	8.1
^{88}Ga	1.90	0.836	1.1	9.4
^{82}Rb[a]	3.35 (83%)	1.52	2.4	16.7

[a]Rb emits two different positrons. Eighty-three percent of the time it emits a 3.35-meV maximum energy positron and 12% of the time a 2.57-meV positron.

of the lack of availability of ^{18}FDG and a PET scanner. As mentioned, ^{18}FDG is now widely available commercially, and there are a huge number of new PET scanners which have been installed, the majority in nonresearch hospitals. Although most of these scanners were installed for oncology imaging, the machines are often suitable for cardiac imaging as well.

The other clinically important radiopharmaceutical in Table 1.1 is ^{82}Rb. This is a potassium analog and can be used to measure myocardial perfusion [3]. No labeling is required. Although it has a very short half-life (76 seconds), it can be produced from a longer lived ^{82}Sr generator, with a half-life of 25 days. At the moment such generators are fairly expensive, but the cost is expected to drop substantially if demand increases.

Aside from half-life, two other factors must be considered when determining the utility of a positron-emitting isotope. First, it is important that nearly all the decays are by positron emission, rather than by other forms of decay whose emissions cannot be imaged with a PET scanner. ^{11}C, ^{13}N, and ^{15}O all decay nearly 100% of the time by positron emission, and ^{82}Rb decays about 95% of the time by positron emission [4]. The remaining fraction of the decays is by electron capture—a process that produces radiation that cannot be imaged with a PET scanner. In addition, for ^{82}Rb a small fraction ($\sim$12%) of the positrons are accompanied by an additional high-energy gamma ray (0.778 meV) which can produce some interference with imaging the 0.511-meV annihilation photons and which increases radiation exposure slightly. There are other positron emitters (e.g., ^{94}Tc, ^{124}I, several isotopes of Cu, and many others) that have an even larger number of other emissions and other significant modes of decay. This often results in poorer dosimetry for the patient because these emissions may increase the patient's radiation exposure, but do not produce useful imaging information. Nonetheless, many of these isotopes have been used successfully in PET imaging.

The second factor one must consider when evaluating a radioisotope is the energy of the positron that is emitted. As mentioned above, this is important because what one images with a PET scanner is not the distribution of the radiotracer, but rather the distribution of the annihilation photons.

Positrons are not emitted with a single characteristic energy as are gamma rays. Instead they have a range of possible energies from 0 up to a characteristic maximum energy. Each positron-emitting radionuclide has its own characteristic maximum and average energy of positron emission, as shown in Table 1.1. Because of this, and because the path of the positron as it slows down is quite tortuous (e.g., Figure 1.1), not all the positrons emitted by a given type of atom travel the same distance—some travel quite far and others do not. Table 1.1 also shows the average distance from the parent atom each positron travels in tissue. The positrons emitted by ^{18}F have a very low energy. Thus, on average they travel only a very small distance away from the parent atom (about 0.35 mm). In contrast, ^{15}O emits positrons that are considerably more energetic and travel an average of 1.1 mm. Positrons from ^{82}Rb travel an average of 2.4 mm. Because the spatial resolution in a cardiac PET image can be as good as $\sim$5–7 mm, the extra blurring caused by the range of travel in tissue can be significant for isotopes such as ^{82}Rb, and to a lesser extent, ^{15}O.

Before we can further discuss the characteristics of PET scanners, it is necessary to understand how tomographic images are made and how they are "reconstructed" from the radioactivity seen by the ring of detectors surrounding the patient. Many treatises have been written dealing with the mathematical steps necessary to produce cross-sectional images with emission tomographs [5]. Here we will describe the reconstruction process in a physical, rather than in a mathematical, way.

To define the three-dimensional (3D) shape of an object, one must first be able to look at the object from all sides. This may be an evolutionary advantage of binocular vision (two eyes, not one). Each eye's slightly different view of the same object, when processed by the brain, allows formation of a 3D image of the object's surface. Because our eyes are not placed very far apart we cannot see all sides of an object at once, and so we must extrapolate (often incorrectly) using the information from the two angles we can see in order to visualize the object's full appearance. In a similar manner, a physician may wish to examine several planar ^{201}Tl scans, each taken at a different angle, in an effort to mentally reconstruct the 3D distribution of ^{201}Tl in

Need to know <u>Where</u> photons came from

<u>Extrinsic collimation</u>

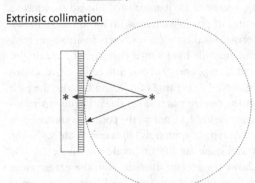

Collimator tells us where gamma ray came from

<u>Problem:</u> Collimators block about 999/1000 photons. *Very* low sensitivity device.

Figure 1.2 In single photon tomography (SPECT) a collimator is needed to tell the direction from which the gamma ray came. The camera must then rotate around the patient (the dashed line shows the rotation) in order to measure the projection images at every angle.

the myocardium. The situation in this case is more complex because nuclear medicine images portray not just the surface of an object, but its interior as well. That is, the object is transparent (except for attenuation) to its radiation.

Just as all sides of an object must be seen by the eye and brain to appreciate its 3D surface, many two-dimensional (2D) planar views, each taken at a different angle, are necessary to allow determination of the 3D interior activity concentration of an object. Each of these 2D views at a particular angle is referred to as a "projection." The reconstruction process (i.e., the method for producing tomographic slices) is based on acquiring these projections. PET, SPECT, and even computed tomography (CT) must all acquire projection images, and in fact all use a similar method for reconstructing the 2D projection images into tomographic slices. The only difference is in how each modality obtains its projection images. In SPECT these "projection" images are obtained by rotating a gamma camera around the object being imaged, as in Figure 1.2. In CT the views are obtained by rotating an X-ray tube around the patient and measuring how many photons are able to get through the body (so each projection is just a planar X-ray image—see Figure 1.3). We will see shortly how PET accomplishes the same thing—creating a planar image of the positron annihilation radiation at each angle.

In theory, an infinite number of projections are necessary to define the 3D distribution of activity in an object. In practice, cardiac SPECT images are

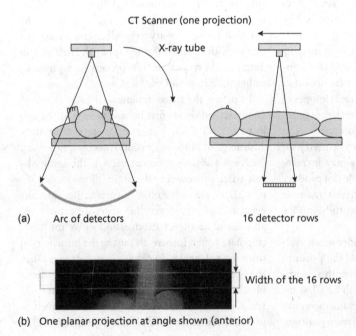

Figure 1.3 In X-ray computed tomography (CT) the X-ray tube must move around the body (a) to acquire projection images just as the gamma camera must move around the body in SPECT. Image (b) shows one planar projection. The tomographic image can be reconstructed from a set of these projections at all angles.

usually reconstructed from fewer than 100 angles, while several hundred different views, each at a different angle, are usually acquired for PET.

Once the PET (or SPECT or CT) scanner has collected data from all these projections, or views, several steps are necessary to create a tomographic slice. The details of these steps [5] are unimportant for understanding the rest of this chapter. They may be considered simply as mathematical operations that convert the many projection images into a single tomographic section or slice.

PET scanners can simultaneously obtain all the views necessary to reconstruct a tomographic image with the use of a ring (or multiple rings) containing hundreds or thousands of detectors that encircle the patient. The mechanical assembly holding all these detectors is called the "gantry." The means by which the ring of detectors acquires data for the many views required can be explained by first remembering the basic information that is needed to perform the reconstruction, i.e., the projection images. A projection image is made up of all the photons that came from a certain direction (projection angle). In the SPECT example of Figure 1.2 the camera is able to show from which direction the photons have come by using a collimator [6]. All photons that do not strike the camera perpendicular to its face are blocked by the collimator. So in Figure 1.2 the number of gamma rays detected at each point on the gamma-camera face must have come only from 270° (numbering angles clockwise, with 0 at the top). Unfortunately, blocking all the photons arriving from other angles is a very inefficient way to make a projection image. Many collimators block more than 999 out of every 1000 photons emitted by the radioactive atoms in the patient. Such a SPECT device would therefore waste over 99.9% of all the photons emitted by the patient. That is the price one pays for using a collimator to determine what direction the photons came from. PET can get the same information—how many photons were emitted and what direction they came from—without a collimator, potentially making PET far more sensitive than SPECT. How is this done? Consider Figure 1.4a, showing a ring of detectors surrounding the patient. Only four of the hundreds of detectors are shown (and those four are shown greatly enlarged for clarity). Imagine that a 511-keV photon has just struck detector 3, as in Figure 1.4a. If this were the

only piece of information that the PET scanner had, it would not be of any use. We would know that an annihilation had occurred, but we would not know from which direction it had come. It could have come from almost any direction. However, recall that for annihilation photons, there is always another photon traveling in the opposite direction. Therefore, if a 511-keV photon struck detector 3 and simultaneously (i.e., in "coincidence") another 511-keV photon struck detector 2, then the computer would realize that this pair of photons must come from a positron that annihilated somewhere along the line B connecting the two detectors (see Figure 1.4a). This is useful information—we know an annihilation occurred and we know from which direction the two photons came. This method of determining where the photons came from, without a collimator, is called "coincidence imaging" [7]. In reality the two photons may not be detected truly simultaneously. For example, the annihilation may occur closer to one of the detectors than the other, and so may reach that detector first (although the difference in time is usually on the order of a billionth of a second). One therefore usually accepts any pair of photons that occur within a narrow time interval as being in "coincidence." This window is called the "coincidence window" or "timing window" or the "resolving time" of the scanner, usually designated by the symbol τ. It is typically 5–20 ns wide, depending on the scanner.

The pairs of detectors in Figure 1.4b connected by solid lines (A-1, B-2, etc.) provide one "view" of the object at a given angle. Coincidences between A-2, B-3, C-4, etc. (dashed lines on Figure 1.4b) provide another view of the object, at a slightly different angle. The PET camera has electronic circuits that can distinguish coincidences from every possible pair of detectors in the field of view of the camera.

In Figure 1.4b, the solid lines comprising one "view" or projection are spaced rather far apart. To allow the PET scanner to distinguish small objects from one another, it is desirable that these lines be as close together as possible. This is accomplished by making the width of each detector small and placing the detectors as close together as possible. This decreases the spacing between lines and increases the number of possible angles (and therefore the number of views). Of course, increasing the total number of possible coincidences in this

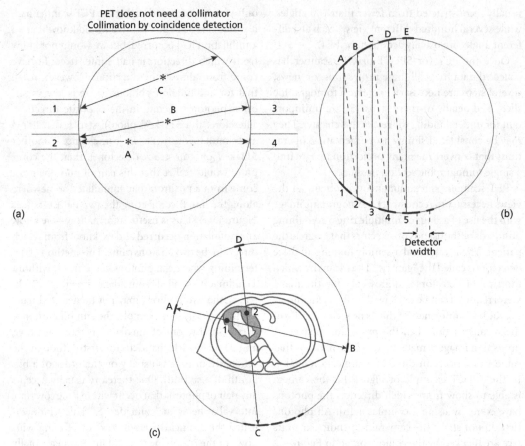

Figure 1.4 (a) Showing how the direction from which a photon came can be determined in positron emission tomography (PET) by use of coincidence detection. When detectors 2 and 3 both detect a photon at the same time, the computer deduces that the pair of photons must have come from an annihilation along the line connecting detectors 2 and 3, as shown. (b) Showing how groups of detector pairs can form a projection image at a particular angle. Two projection angles are shown—the solid line shows the anterior–posterior projection, while the dashed lines show a projection about 10° shifted. (c) Showing a schematic diagram of coincidence detection among crystals of one ring of detectors.

way increases the number of crystals, coincidence circuits, and other electronic components required, making the PET scanner more costly.

A factor that limits the number of crystals employed in a PET scanner is the number of photomultiplier tubes required. When a detector "detects" a gamma ray, it produces a small flash of light that is converted to an electronic pulse by a photomultiplier tube. Ideally each crystal would be attached to one photomultiplier tube, but the tubes cannot be made arbitrarily small and are quite expensive. Thus, manufacturers have devised schemes to allow one photomultiplier tube to share many crystals. A schematic diagram of coincidence detection among the crystals of one ring of detectors is shown in Figure 1.4c.

Most scanners for cardiac imaging use several rings of detectors, often separated by high atomic number shielding (e.g., lead, tungsten) called "septa," to acquire data for multiple slices. When a PET scanner is operated with septa between rings it is said to be operating in "2D" mode. This is a bit of a misnomer, since of course such a scanner still acquires 3D data. As will be discussed later, some scanners operate without the septa. Those scanners are said to be operating in "3D" mode [8–11]. To increase the number of slices, coincidences are often recorded between one detector in one ring, and an opposing detector in an adjacent ring. Such a slice would be called a "cross" slice. With three rings of detectors (numbered I, II, and III) five slices could be produced. The first would consist of all coincident events from opposing pairs of detectors in ring I (a direct slice); the second would be a cross slice consisting of all coincident events between one detector in ring I and an opposing detector in ring II (or vice versa); the third would be formed from events only in ring II, and so on. Some PET scanners have completely separate rings of detectors. With this design, what constitutes a cross slice and what constitutes a direct slice is obvious. Other scanners have crystals so close together in the Z-axis that the concept of physically separate rings no longer applies. What is important in any case is the final spatial resolution obtained (in all three directions) and the number of, and spacing between, slices.

Cardiac PET scanners reconstruct transaxial slices. The number and spacing of the slices is usually such that at least a 15-cm axial distance is encompassed by the slices—a quite adequate size for cardiac imaging—large enough to include the entire left ventricle in nearly all subjects. Depending on the scanner anywhere between 30 and 70 slices or more cover this ~15-cm axial field of view. It is often desirable to include some of the left atrium in the image also (even though it is not usually visualized well) to allow arterial blood concentrations of tracer to be measured. Some scanners permit a slight rotation and tilt of the gantry, but no scanner presently available can be positioned to yield true cardiac short-axis slices directly. Rather, one reformats the transaxial slices into short- or long-axis views.

It is important to understand the quantity being measured in the reconstructed image obtained from a PET scan. Each of the projections described previously measures simply the total number of coincidences seen by each detector pair at a given angle during a specific time period (the scan time). For example, in Figure 1.4b, one projection is formed by the solid lines A-1, B-2, etc. The quantity measured by each detector pair in this projection is the number of coincidences/second seen along the line, for example that formed by A-1. This "line" is not an infinitesimally thin line, but has a width, because the detector pair A and 1 both have finite width. The number of coincidences seen by the pair A and 1 are those produced by all the radioactive material lying in the volume between them. The units of the measurement are therefore "coincidences/second/volume." These projection data are reconstructed to determine the number of coincidences arising from each point in the final reconstructed image. Since each point in the image also represents a small volume in the object being imaged, the units are again coincidences/s/volume. Finally, it is assumed that the number of coincidences/second measured in a volume is directly proportional to the amount of radioactive material (usually measured in Bq (Bequerels) or Ci (Curies)) in that same volume. Providing all the corrections described below are made, this assumption is correct. The units of the PET scan can therefore be any of the following: coincidences/s/cc, Bq (or nCi)/cc, or grams of radiolabeled material/cc. Use of the last unit is possible because Bq can be easily converted to number of atoms or grams as long as the half-life is known.

Accidental Coincidences

Unfortunately, it is possible for two photons that did not come from the same annihilation event to be erroneously identified, quite by accident, as having occurred "simultaneously," that is, within the resolving time τ of the PET scanner.

Figure 1.5 illustrates such a case. Only one of the photons from annihilation A has reached a detector; the other missed the ring. At nearly the same time atom B decayed. Only one of its photons was detected, the other also missing the ring. If these two separate events happen to occur at nearly the same time within the resolving time of the PET scanner, they will be considered to be in coincidence. The PET scanner then will falsely treat the detection of the two photons as if they resulted from a single annihilation that took place along the line between the two detectors (the dashed line in Figure 1.5). Such false coincidence is called an accidental or random coincidence. Random coincidences produce background activity in the reconstructed image that varies slowly in magnitude at different positions over the image, depending on the radioisotope distribution.

Randoms

- Two single, unrelated photons are <u>accidentally</u> detected at same time
- # Randoms α (activity)^2

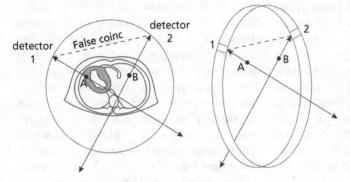

Figure 1.5 Illustrating how if by accident, two separate annihilation events (A and B) are detected at nearly the same time a false or "accidental" coincidence can occur. This accidental (or "random") coincidence causes the PET camera to erroneously think the annihilation occurred along the dashed line indicated.

Accidental coincidences between unrelated photons must be distinguished from "true" coincidences between pairs of annihilation photons. The probability that an accidental coincidence will occur depends on the duration of the resolving time interval, τ: if it is very long, it becomes much more likely for two unrelated photons to be accidentally in coincidence. The resolving time of a PET scanner is therefore an important parameter, defining how well the scanner will distinguish true coincidences from accidental ones.

A second factor influencing the number of accidental events recorded is the amount and location of activity detected by the PET scanner. If the activity within the patient is doubled, the number of true coincidences will of course double also. The number of accidental coincidences, however, will increase by a factor of 4, i.e., as the square of activity. This has important ramifications. At sufficiently high levels of activity (e.g., for ^{82}Rb scans [9,11,12]), the number of accidental coincidences may equal or even exceed true coincidences. With administration of excessive amounts of tracer, the patient may, therefore, be exposed to a higher radiation risk without a comparable increase in the amount of useful information obtained. The amount of activity constituting an excess varies with the machine used; it may be only a few millicuries in the field of view or as much as 50 or more mCi. Many manufacturers specify the concentration of activity that when placed in a specified phantom will produce equal numbers of true and accidental coincidences. This is useful to help evaluate the maximum activity that one might inject in a patient from the point of view of excessive randoms.

The reason that accidental events increase as the square of activity can be discerned from consideration of Figure 1.5. Suppose that detector one measures $S1$ (S refers to "singles") counts/second, independent of whether these counts were in coincidence with any other detector. The count rate observed by a single detector, as opposed to a coincident pair of detectors, is called the singles count rate of that detector. Suppose also that detector 2 measures a singles rate of $S2$/second. Consider that one photon has just struck detector 1. If an unrelated photon were to hit detector 2 within the next τ seconds or has already hit detector 2 within the previous τ seconds, it will be in accidental coincidence with the event recognized by detector 1. Because there are $S2$ events detected by detector 2 each second, the number of these that will occur during the τ seconds before or the τ seconds after the event in $S1$ is $S2 \times 2 \times \tau$. For every photon that strikes detector 1, there are therefore $2 \times \tau \times S2$ accidental coincidences/second. However, there are $S1$ photons striking detector 1 every second. Therefore the total number of accidental coincidences/second is:

$$\text{Accidental coincidences/second} = 2 \times \tau \times S1 \times S2$$

If the activity in the patient is doubled, the singles rate for every detector is also doubled, so both $S1$ and $S2$ double, giving a factor of 4 increase in accidental coincidences.

Consideration of the above equation suggests a way to correct for accidental coincidences. If the singles rate is measured at every detector, the number of accidental coincidences can be computed for every detector pair, and this number can be subtracted from the measured true events. Although measured singles rates include some counts from true coincidences, singles rates usually greatly exceed true coincidence rates. Thus, the error introduced by such a correction scheme is usually quite small.

Another approach to correction for random coincidences is the delayed coincidence method. Consider a single pair of opposing detectors in Figure 1.4. The output of detectors is split. One of the signals goes to the coincidence circuitry as usual. The other goes to a special circuit (or even a long length of wire) that causes a prolongation of travel time for the signal, perhaps of several 100 ns. This second wire is connected to the usual circuit, which determines whether the two pulses (one from the delayed signal from the second wire of one detector, and the second from the undelayed, first wire of the opposing detector) occurred within time τ of each other. If a true coincidence event occurs, the delayed signal traveling down the second wire will not register as a coincidence with the undelayed signal of the opposing detector. The signal traveling down the long wire would reach the coincidence electronics much later than the undelayed signal from the opposing detector. Any coincidences measured by this long wire would, therefore, only be accidental coincidences and not true coincidences. They could, therefore, be subtracted from the total number of coincidences measured with the undelayed standard short wires of both detectors to yield the number of true coincidences. The delayed coincidence method is quite accurate. However, it is limited by low signal-to-noise ratios because the number of randoms measured by the second delayed wire is often quite small, which may introduce additional noise into the final corrected image. On the other hand, use of the singles method discussed previously adds little noise to the image because the number of singles recorded by each detector is so high. However, the singles method has its own difficulties, and requires measurement of τ, which is subject to inaccuracies.

Attenuation Correction

If 511-keV annihilation gamma rays were made to travel through a substance with a very high atomic number, such as a lead brick, only a few of the photons would pass completely through the brick unaltered [13]. Most of the photons would interact with the atoms of lead. Of those that interacted, some would do so by a process called the photoelectric effect, which involves both an atomic electron and the nucleus of the lead atom. In this process, the photon completely disappears. It is totally absorbed or "stopped" by the lead, its energy transferred to the nucleus and a fast-moving atomic electron. Other gamma rays passing through the lead brick would interact by a process called scattering (or more properly Compton scattering, after A H Compton, its discoverer). In this process, the photon strikes one of the atomic electrons surrounding the atom, the gamma ray is deflected from its original direction and continues in a new direction with reduced energy. The bigger the angle of deflection, the more energy the gamma ray will have lost. A photon undergoing such a collision is said to have scattered. In lead, the two processes—complete absorption or stopping, and scattering—are both likely. In soft tissue, complete absorption almost never occurs. Instead, essentially all interactions result in the photon scattering. Even in bone, 511-keV photons are absorbed only rarely. Instead they most simply scatter.

Now consider photons emitted by a small region of myocardium. Some small fraction of the annihilation photons will be headed in a direction such that both photons would strike a detector in the ring. As these photons travel toward the detector, they must pass through the tissue of the body. If either of the photons scatters, it will no longer be headed toward the detector. In all probability it will miss the ring entirely, or on those occasions that it does not, its energy may be too reduced to be detected. A coincident event that would have occurred in the absence of intervening tissue, now does not occur. The photons emanating from this small section of the myocardium are said to have been attenuated, and the loss of detected events due to interactions with atoms of the intervening tissue is called attenuation. The number of photons that make it through unscathed decreases exponentially with the thickness (d) of interposed tissue:

Number of photons reaching the detector

= Number of photons headed for detector $\times\ e^{-\mu d}$

The constant μ is the attenuation coefficient and has a value of ~0.096 cm^{-1} for 511-keV photons in soft tissue. As can be seen by applying the equation above, only half of the photons will make it through 7.2 cm of tissue. Lower energy protons such as those emitted by ^{99m}Tc (140 keV) are attenuated more easily, because μ is higher at lower energies. It takes only 4.6 cm of tissue to stop half the photons of ^{99m}Tc from reaching their original destination. It would, therefore, seem that attenuation would be much more significant for SPECT scans than for PET scans, because the lower energy ^{99m}Tc photons used for SPECT scintigraphy are so much more easily attenuated. This presumption is, however, incorrect. In a PET scan, both photons in a pair must reach their respective detectors. As illustrated in Figure 1.6a, a photon headed toward detector D1 must travel through a thickness of tissue $X1$ without interaction, and the photon going in the opposite direction must travel through thickness $X2$ to reach detector D2. The total attenuation is then:

Number of coincidences

= (Number of photons headed for D1 and D2)

  $\times$ (probability photons gets to D1)

  $\times$ (probability photon gets to D2)

= (Number of photons headed for D1 and D2)

  $\times\ e^{-\mu(X1)} \times e^{-\mu(X2)}$

= (Number of photons headed for D1 and D2)

  $\times\ e^{-\mu(X1+X2)}$

= (Number of photons headed for detector)

  D1 and D2 $\times\ e^{-\mu D}$

where D is the total distance, $X1 + X2$, through the body.

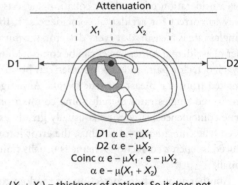

$$D1\ \alpha\ e - \mu X_1$$
$$D2\ \alpha\ e - \mu X_2$$
$$\text{Coinc}\ \alpha\ e - \mu X_1 \cdot e - \mu X_2$$
$$\alpha\ e - \mu(X_1 + X_2)$$

$(X_1 + X_2)$ = thickness of patient. So it does not
(a) matter how deep the tracer is in body!

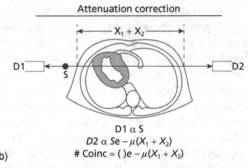

$$D1\ \alpha\ S$$
$$D2\ \alpha\ Se - \mu(X_1 + X_2)$$
(b) $\quad$ # Coinc = ( )e - $\mu(X_1 + X_2)$

Figure 1.6 (a) The attenuation suffered by the pair of photons does not depend on where in the body that pair of photons originated. No matter where they originate, together they have to traverse a thickness $X1 + X2$ of tissue. (b) Because of this, the same attenuation is experienced by a radioactive source placed outside the body, permitting the attenuation to be measured. One simply measures the number of pairs of photons detected without the patient and compares this to the number detected when the patient is present.

Therefore the attenuation of the pair of photons depends only on D, the total amount of tissue the pair of photons has to traverse. It does not depend on where in the body the annihilation occurred. One does not need to know $X1$ and $X2$, only the attenuation resulting from its sum, D. This is not the situation for SPECT, in which only one photon is detected. In the SPECT case one needs to know what depth (e.g., $X1$) the photon came from. This is a piece of information that is usually unknown and unmeasurable.

For typical chest thicknesses most of the photons will be attenuated. Often only ~10–30% will make it through the body. Photons traveling in other directions toward other detectors and those originating from other sections of the myocardium may be more or less extensively attenuated. In a 70-kg subject, attenuation by factors of 5–20 is not uncommon. Attenuation can be even greater in obese subjects. Obviously, attenuation has significant effects on the results of cardiac PET scans. Although this problem is serious with PET because both photons in a pair must survive intact, accurate attenuation correction is possible. In contrast, with methods such as SPECT in which only one photon is involved, such correction is not possible because the attenuation correction factor, $e^{-\mu(X1)}$, depends on measurement of the depth at which the isotope is located in tissue. This measurement cannot be made before imaging. The value necessary for attenuation correction of PET images, however, is $(X1 + X2)$. This quantity is independent of how deep the isotope is located in the body and depends only upon the attenuation through the total body thickness, which can be measured accurately. The most common method for making this measurement involves performance of a "blank" scan and an "attenuation" scan (often called a transmission scan). Figure 1.6b illustrates this approach for one detector pair [7,14]. Before the patient to be imaged is placed in the ring, a small positron-emitting source is placed at one side (as in Figure 1.6b) and the number of photons detected is recorded (just as in Figure 1.6b but without the patient). The position of the source is maintained, and the patient is positioned in the ring (before injection of the isotope) as in Figure 1.6b. Again, the number of photons are recorded. The difference in the

counts detected in the blank and transmission scans is of course caused by attenuation through the patient. For example, if S coincident counts were recorded by the detector pair shown in Figure 1.6b before the patient was in place, then $S \times e^{-\mu D}$ counts would be recorded by the same detector pair when the patient was interposed. The ratio of the counts without the patient (called the "blank" scan counts) to the counts with the patient in place (called the "transmission" scan counts) gives the factor $e^{+\mu D}$, which is the factor needed to correct for attenuation for this particular detector pair. Making the same measurement for all detector pairs permits complete attenuation correction.

In order to make the measurement of attenuation for all detector pairs, often a rod of activity is used with its long dimension oriented along the Z-axis (Figure 1.7). Such a rod is attached to a mechanism that rotates it at a fixed speed around the gantry. The rod is usually filled with a relatively long lived positron emitter (^{68}Ge which decays to ^{68}Ga). The rod is first made to rotate without the patient, giving the "blank" scan counts (Figure 1.7a). Then the patient is positioned and the measurement repeated (Figure 1.7b) giving the transmission scan. The ratio of the counts in the blank to the counts in the transmission for every detector pair gives the attenuation correction factor for that detector pair.

As the rod rotates, only those detectors that lie on the line formed by the detector, the rod, and the opposing detector can possibly be in coincidence. By turning on only the appropriate detectors as the rod rotates around the gantry, most accidental and scatter coincidences can be eliminated. With proper

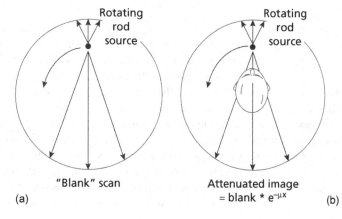

Figure 1.7 Illustrating [7] how the process described in Figure 1.6 can be implemented. In panel (a) the "blank" scan is taken with a source and no patient. In panel (b) the same source is used with the patient in place. For every possible pair of detectors the ratio of detected events with and without the patient is compared to compute the attenuation correction factor.

Rotating rod source

"Blank" scan

(a)

Rotating rod source

Attenuated image = blank * $e^{-\mu x}$

(b)

correction software, this also permits the transmission measurement to be made even after activity has been injected [15,16]. Some manufacturers use instead an isotope which emits only a single photon (e.g., ^{137}Cs). This makes it more difficult to remove scattered events, but in general both methods have been shown to work satisfactorily. Many modern PET scanners have been combined with a CT scanner, and in this case the CT scan (after suitable processing) can be used to perform attenuation correction. This will be discussed further later in this chapter.

A typical scanning sequence is: (1) obtain a blank scan (usually only done once per day or week); (2) for static FDG imaging, inject the patient, wait for uptake (typically 1 hour) then position the patient in the gantry and obtain a transmission scan either immediately prior or immediately following the emission scan. This minimizes motion between the transmission and emission scan. For dynamic scanning, the transmission scan must be taken prior to injection (or it can be done following the scan). As mentioned above, to perform the transmission scan after injection requires that hardware and software be available for correcting for emission activity present during the transmission scan. This is fairly straightforward when positron emitters (and coincidence detection) are used for the transmission source. It is often more difficult when single photon emitters are used for the transmission source. No matter what scheme is used, it is important to prevent patient motion between the transmission and emission scans. Such motion can produce appreciable errors in the uptake image [17].

Scatter

When annihilation photons pass through tissue, they frequently collide with electrons and scatter. The photon is deflected from its original direction and loses some fraction of its energy. The higher the angle of deflection, the greater the energy loss. The great majority of scattered photons never reach a detector, as illustrated in Figure 1.8. A small percentage of scattered photons, however, may still hit a detector in the ring and register coincidences, as shown in Figure 1.8. When this occurs, the PET camera erroneously computes the position of the radioactive atom (dotted line in Figure 1.8). Such

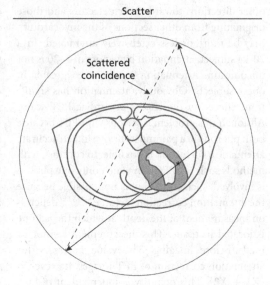

Scatter

Figure 1.8 Illustrating the effect of scattered radiation. If one of the pair of photons originating in the heart (shown as an asterisk in the free wall of the myocardium) scatters and is detected (as shown at about the 1-pm position in the detector ring), the PET scanner will erroneously think the positron was emitted along the dotted line. A "scattered coincidence" will have occurred.

mispositioning of events can cause false counts to appear in cold areas of an image when a hot region is nearby. In general, the phenomenon slightly blurs sources of radioactivity from hot regions into cold regions (even those a few cm away). This is of particular importance in cardiac imaging, since the observer is frequently trying to detect defects of uptake in segments of myocardium adjacent to normal regions (and perhaps adjacent to a hot liver).

Most PET scanners are designed to reduce the effects of scattered photons by rejecting those photons whose energy is below a certain threshold value. In most older, and some newer generation, scanners bismuth germinate (BGO) crystals are used. The energy resolution of these detectors is not very good, making it more difficult to reject scatter. Other crystal types (lutetium oxyorthosilicate (LSO) or gadolinium oxyorthosilicate (GSO)) in theory have better energy resolution, but in practice have yet to achieve much better scatter energy rejection than the new generation BGO scanners. In PET scanners with septa (2D scanners), scatter is usually fairly small anyway. However, as will be seen later, scanners without septa (3D mode) have several times higher scatter, and so the problem is more severe. If a scanner operates with an energy threshold of 360 keV, it can reject all photons that have been scattered by more than about 57°, but not those scattered less than this. Because photons are more likely to scatter at small angles, a large number of scattered photons will still be detected. Attempts to raise the energy threshold to, for example, 400 keV (as is being done in some of the scanners with LSO or especially GSO crystals) would result in the rejection of photons that had scattered by more than about 44°, but of course the higher one raises the threshold, the larger the fraction of unscattered photons that are rejected as well. Energy rejection can, therefore, be used to reduce large-angle scattering, but can only eliminate smaller angle scattering at the expense of eliminating unscattered photons as well. This situation will improve if the energy resolution of the scanner can be improved. Meanwhile, more empirical methods must be applied to correct for the remaining scatter. Most modern scanners have relatively sophisticated algorithms for correcting for this residual scatter [25]. However, especially for cardiac imaging (with its mixture of lungs and adjacent soft tissue) the algorithms are not perfect. The situation for septa-out (3D) imaging is more problematic, and for this and other reasons (as discussed further below), there is still discussion as to whether septa out imaging might be a poorer choice than 2D (septa-in) imaging for cardiac [9–12].

Deadtime

Quantitatively accurate PET studies require that the number of true coincidences be directly proportional to the concentration of radioactivity. In addition to physical phenomena such as scatter and accidental coincidences, a significant electronic effect in PET cameras can alter this relationship. Every time a photon produces a scintillation in a detector, a complex series of electronic events must occur: The light must be converted into an electronic pulse; the exact time of occurrence of the electronic pulse must be determined for use in timing coincidence; and the magnitude of the pulse must be computed to allow rejection of scattered events, etc. All of this takes time. If a second photon should arrive before the processing of the previous pulse is complete, the second pulse may be lost. There is, therefore, a time interval after a photon has interacted with a crystal during which the PET scanner electronics may be unable to process further pulses. Pulses that occur during this interval, termed the "deadtime," are lost. The higher the count rate, the larger will be the fraction of lost pulses. The number of coincidences/second at first increases linearly with activity, but at high activities it deviates from linearity due to this deadtime. Successive increases in activity produce successively smaller increases in coincidence rate.

The principal source of deadtime is often not the number of coincident events the machine must process per se, but rather the rate at which the system must process single photons (each one of which must be analyzed to see if it meets the energy requirements and to see if it is in temporal "coincidence" with another photon, etc.). The singles rate recorded by a detector is often one or more orders of magnitude greater than the coincident rate. Often the deadtime loss of a detector can be predicted quite accurately as a function of the singles rate measured by the detector. This relationship is the basis for one effective method for correcting for deadtime. The corrections can be quite large, especially with imaging techniques that require bolus injections of isotope (e.g., ^{82}Rb). It is probably best to limit the amount of activity injected so that the required deadtime correction during imaging will be less than a factor of 2. Activity levels greater than this will result in increased radiation exposure to the patient without a comparable increase in true coincidences. In addition, the accuracy of larger correction factors may be suspect.

In many circumstances cardiac PET studies are especially susceptible to the effects of deadtime, particularly with septa-out (3D) scanners. This is particularly true with dynamic cardiac studies that attempt to measure the wash-in or wash-out of activity from the myocardium, or to measure arterial activity as a function of time by monitoring the activity in the atrial or ventricular cavities. During a bolus injection or even during a 1-minute infusion of isotope, the PET camera field of view may contain a large fraction of the entire injected dose. This is in marked contrast to the 60 minutes postinjection static cardiac scans in which only a small percentage of the injected dose is in the field of view. The PET camera's deadtime characteristics (as well as random coincidences) may sometimes limit the amount of activity that can be administered. Again, the problem is far more severe when operating PET scanners in septa-out (3D) mode than in septa-in (2D) mode.

Resolution

The term "resolution" is one of many parameters used to characterize PET scanners. The term requires more careful definition. The spatial resolution of a PET scanner is a measure of how well the scanner can distinguish two small objects placed closely together. Certain standard measurements of resolution have been adopted. With one, a very small spot of radioactivity is placed in the scanner's field of view and is imaged. If the range of the positron is very small (e.g., that of a positron from an isotope such as ^{18}F embedded in plastic or aluminum), then comparison of the apparent size of the object in the image and the actual size of the object allows calculation of the scanner's resolution. However, very small point sources of radioactive material are hard to construct. Instead, often a thin rod of radioactive material, for example a long thin needle or capillary tube filled with ^{18}F, may be used. Steel prevents the positrons from leaving the needle. The needle or rod is placed in the scanner, with its long axis perpendicular to the plane of the ring as shown in Figure 1.9a. Data are acquired and the image is reconstructed as shown in Figure 1.9b. The top right of the figure shows a plot of the number of coincident events as a function of distance across the image. Typically such a plot follows a bell-shaped, approximately Gaussian curve. By convention, the width of this curve at half its maximum height (full width at half maximum, or FWHM) is used as a measure of spatial resolution. Since the initial measurement is obtained within one slice, or plane, it is called the "in-plane" resolution of the scanner. The in-plane resolution will usually be somewhat larger (perhaps a few millimeters or so, depending on the scanner) when the measurement is made at the edge of the field of view, rather than at the center. Because the free wall or apex of the myocardium may be 10 cm or more from the center of the field in a cardiac PET study, it is useful to know the PET scanner's resolution not just at the center, but also 10 or 15 cm from the center. In addition, at a given distance from the center of the scanner's field of view, the resolution in the anterior–posterior or Y direction may not be the same as that in the lateral, or X direction.

The scanner shown in Figure 1.9a is made up of crystals with a width, W length, L, in the axial or Z direction, and a depth, D. As pointed out previously the width, W, of the detectors influences the in-plane resolution. Similarly the length, L, of the detector in the Z direction determines, in part, the resolution of the scanner in the axial direction. To measure the resolution in this direction, a small "dot" of radioactive material, placed on the bed of the gantry, might be used. An image could be made of this dot of activity, the source could be moved through the gantry by 1 or 2 mm, and a second image made. Progressively moving the source of activity through the scanner in 1 or 2 mm steps, making an image at each location, would result in a series of images as a function of the Z-axis position of the source. Plotting the number of coincident events in each image as a function of the Z-axis position (clinically, the bed position), would produce a plot similar to those in Figure 1.9b. The FWHM resolution in the Z-axis direction is sometimes called the "slice thickness" because it is a measure of how far into the Z-axis the slice extends. A PET scanner, then, has at least two (possibly very different) spatial resolutions: The in-plane resolution (made up of the resolution in the anterior–posterior direction and the lateral directions,) and the Z-axis, or axial resolution.

The axial resolution, or slice thickness, should not be confused with the separation between slices. The spacing between slices may be greater or less than the "thickness" (i.e., FWHM in the axial direction) of each slice. If the spacing between slices is less than the thickness of the slice, then the slices may be considered to partially overlap. Even if the spacing between slices is greater than the slice thickness, some overlap will be present because the "edges" of a slice are not sharp but are Gaussian shaped.

The resolution of a PET image is determined by: The design of the machine (including crystal size and spacing, ring diameter, among other factors); physical factors such as the finite range of positrons

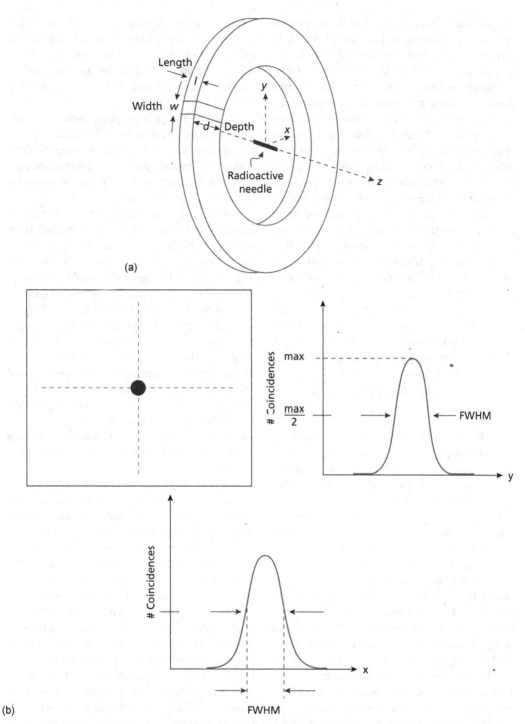

Figure 1.9 (a) Showing placement of rod source to measure in-plane resolution [7]. (b) Upper left: a transaxial image of the rod source. Upper right and lower left: profiles through the transaxial image.

in tissue and the deviation of annihilation photons from exact colinearity, and processing, including whatever smoothing is performed during or after reconstruction [19–23]. The effects of image processing are to some extent controllable. Positron range is of course a function of the isotope used. Its effects can be estimated as follows. If the number of positrons detected is plotted as a function of distance in tissue from the source, the number decreases almost exponentially with distance [20]. Some of the positrons therefore travel relatively far, altering the resolution curve from its usual Gaussian shape. The resolution curve produced by radioisotopes emitting very energetic positrons is a combination of the typical Gaussian curve illustrated in Figure 1.9b and the approximately exponential curve associated with positron penetration [21]. Therefore, the curve is roughly Gaussian in shape near the center, but exhibits a long, roughly exponential, tail. The amount of degradation in resolution that would occur with use of a positron with a relatively long range in tissue, such as ^{82}Rb, can be estimated as follows:

$$\text{Final resolution} = (R^2 + 1.89 \times (2 \times D)^2)^{0.5}$$

$$(1.1)$$

where R is the resolution of the scanner (including any smoothing) measured with a nearly zero-range positron source (e.g., when ^{18}F in a thin steel needle is used) and D is the average distance the positron travels, as shown in Table 1.1.

For example, with a scanner having 7-mm useable resolution as measured with ^{18}F, the resolution expected with the use of ^{82}Rb is based on the average distance an ^{82}Rb positron travels (D), 2.3 mm. The resolution of ^{82}Rb scan can be calculated from the equation above to yield a final resolution of approximately 9.4 mm FWHM—a significant increase compared with that of a lower energy positron emitter. The factor of 1.89 is entered into Equation (1.1) in consideration of the fact that the number of positrons decreases with distance in an exponential rather than a Gaussian manner. Because the resolution curve is not Gaussian with an isotope such as ^{82}Rb, specifying the FWHM does not tell the full story. The number of positrons decreases exponentially with distance from the source, so many positrons will travel much farther than the average. Some ^{82}Rb positrons will travel more than a centimeter before annihilating.

This produces an exponential tail on the resolution curve, in turn causing a small fraction of the counts in one part of an image to blur into other, distant parts of the image. To describe this effect, the full width at tenth maximum (FWTM) is measured in addition to FWHM.

To reduce the point-to-point random statistical fluctuations (called "noise") that are invariably present in a PET image, an image is often "smoothed" by averaging adjacent picture element (pixel) values together. Although this reduces image noise, it degrades resolution.

Various filters can be used at the time of reconstruction to facilitate smoothing. "Filtering" is the name given to the process of averaging neighboring pixels together [22] by replacing a pixel value with a weighted average of itself and its neighbors. For example, one commonly used filter replaces a pixel value with one-half times its own value plus one-eighth times each of its four nearest neighbors' values, so that the weighting factors for this filter would be 1/2 and 1/8. Such a filter will produce a less noisy image, but one with poorer spatial resolution. Filters are often given names (e.g., the "Hanning" and "Butterworth" filters). Despite their specialized names, all filters do nothing more than average neighboring pixels together; they differ only in their weighting factors, which may be positive or negative.

In addition to filters that reduce noise but worsen resolution, filters exist that improve resolution and exaggerate noise. Unfortunately, it is a consequence of the basic laws of physics that it is impossible to simultaneously reduce noise and improve resolution, and because of statistical fluctuations caused by the limited numbers of coincident events, PET images almost always must be filtered with a smoothing, rather than a resolution-improving, filter. Some 3D small animal PET scanners are the exceptions to this rule. In these scanners there are often plenty of coincident events, because the dose/gm injected is high (dosimetry is frequently not a limiting factor in animal imaging). Resolution recovery can then be used, at the expense of slightly worsening statistical fluctuations, to achieve the higher resolution often required for small animal imaging. Some resolution recovery techniques are most easily built-in to so-called "iterative reconstruction" programs.

Clinical PET scanner software usually gives the investigator a choice of which smoothing filter to use at the time of image reconstruction. It should be noted that iterative reconstruction techniques also have inherent "smoothing" (noise reduction combined with resolution worsening) built into them. In general, the more iterations (or iterations × subsets) the better the resolution and the worse the noise. In addition, some filtering is often applied post-reconstruction. It is important for the user of a PET scanner to be able to estimate the resolution of the final image, given the reconstruction parameters selected. Comparing two images reconstructed with different parameters can result in misleading clinical conclusions.

It is important to clarify the difference between resolution and the distance between pixels. Imagine a PET scanner with 7 mm in-plane resolution (i.e., 7 mm FWHM) and a 41 cm in-plane field of view. The reconstructed image could be stored in an array (i.e., a digitized image) of 256 × 256 pixels. Each pixel would be 41 cm/256 or 1.6 mm apart. The 7 mm FWHM would therefore correspond to about 4.4 pixels. If instead the reconstructed image were stored in a 512 × 512 matrix, each pixel would comprise 41 cm/512 or 0.8 mm. The resolution would remain 7 mm FWHM which, with this matrix size, would be represented by 8.8 pixels. Resolution is a function of the scanner and the reconstruction and filtering processes; it cannot be improved by increasing the number of pixels in the image matrix. Below a certain number of pixels/centimeter, however, the image will no longer be able to reflect the resolution inherent in the scanner. In general, with PET images acquired in vivo, at least three pixels should be available for every FWHM [3]. So for example, if the final resolution of the image is to be 9 mm, then the pixel size must be 3 mm or smaller.

Pixels are spaced a fixed distance apart in the x and y direction and so occupy an area. Nearly all scanners are of course multislice machines. A pixel, then, can also be thought of as occupying a volume in space, in which case it is referred to as a voxel.

Partial Volume Effect

Quantitative data are usually extracted from PET images with the aid of regions of interest (ROIs) drawn on the images. Analysis of the data contained in such regions yields either the total number of events/second occurring within the region (proportional to the total activity in the region), or

the mean number of events/second/voxel (proportional to the average concentration of activity in the region). Sometimes the maximum value within the ROI is also used. The resolution of the PET scanner, the size and placement of the region of interest, and the true anatomic size of the structure imaged all influence the accuracy of such measurements. Collectively, such influences are often described by a parameter called the partial volume effect [23,24].

To better understand what the partial volume effect is, assume that a "perfect" PET scanner exists, and it is used to image a 2-cm diameter cylinder of radioactivity. Assume further that after imaging for 100 seconds, 100,000 coincident events would be detected (therefore 1000 events/second) in a transaxial slice of the cylinder. The perfect scanner would produce an image like the one shown in Figure 1.10a. All pixels within the cylinder would have nearly the same value (apart from small statistical fluctuations which we will ignore), and all pixels outside it would have the value zero. Placing a 2-cm diameter region of interest around the image of the cylindrical object would give the total number of coincidences/second coming from the object (i.e., 1000 coincidences/second). All of the coincidences that were detected would occur within the region of interest.

If the same 2-cm diameter cylinder of radioactivity were imaged with an imperfect PET scanner (e.g., one with 7 mm FWHM resolution), the same 100,000 coincidences (or 1000/second) would be detected, but some of the coincidences would be blurred or spread outside the true dimensions of the cylinder (Figure 1.10b). Pixels near the center of the cylinder would not be affected as much because just as many counts would be blurred out as blurred into them from neighboring pixels, whereas pixels near the edge would be particularly affected. The same 2-cm diameter region of interest (shown as a dashed circle in Figure 1.10b) would now produce a value of only 785 events/second, the other 215 coincident events/second being spread out over pixels outside of the region of interest. The percentage of the counts retained in the region of interest is termed the "recovery coefficient": 785 of 1000 or 78.5% in this case.

The term "partial volume effect" describes this effect [23,24]. The poorer the resolution, the more blurred the data will be and the smaller the fraction of counts "recovered" within a given region

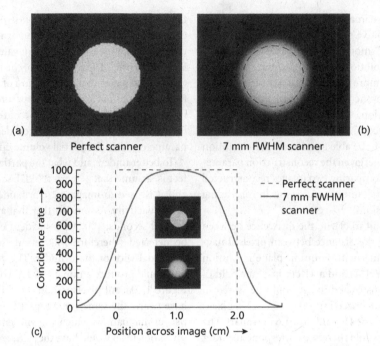

(a)

Perfect scanner

(b)

7 mm FWHM scanner

(c)

Figure 1.10 (a) A transaxial image of a 20-cm diameter uniform cylinder, taken with a "perfect" PET camera. (b) The same image taken with a real PET scanner, with 7 mm FWHM resolution. Note the blurry edges. (c) Line profile through the ideal image (dashed line) and through the real image (solid line). A region of interest (as shown in (b)) would recover only a portion of the activity in the image—the remaining activity would have blurred outside the region. The y-axis is a relative scale proportional to the counts/second at each pixel in the profile. FWHM, full width at half maximum.

of interest will be. As can be seen in Figure 1.10, a larger fraction of the total events can be recovered by enlarging the region of interest to more than the true 2 cm object size. If the region of interest were increased to 2.4 cm, 914 of the original total 1000 events/second would be recovered. If the region were sufficiently large, all the original events would be recovered. Unfortunately, in patients, the size of the region drawn may be limited by the presence of substantial amounts of activity in structures close to the organ being imaged.

In the discussion so far, it has been tacitly assumed that the only quantity of interest is the total activity in the region, or the total number of events/second occurring in the "organ" (in this case, the cylinder). More commonly, the average concentration of activity within a region is sought and so the counts/second/number of pixels in the ROI is measured. This is in fact the unit most commonly produced by PET scanners (usually converted to MBq/cc).

We must now reconsider what impact the partial volume effect will have on accuracy of measurements of average concentrations of activity within an ROI. Drawing "too large" a region in an effort to recover all the counts will actually have the opposite effect on mean activity concentration measurements. It will reduce the measured counts/second/pixel by increasing the total number of pixels. Again, consider the 2-cm diameter cylinder shown in Figure 1.10b. The "ideal" PET scanner might, for example, yield 1000 events/second total within the 2 cm diameter. Let us also suppose that this value could be converted to a concentration of activity of perhaps 5 nCi/mL. The ideal PET scanner would, therefore, yield a value of 5 nCi/mL at every pixel within the 2 cm diameter, and zero outside. The mean value within any region of interest of 2.0-cm diameter or smaller would give the same value of 5 nCi/mL. If the region were enlarged to more than the true size of the object, however, the measured nanocuries/milliliter would fall because the region of interest would begin to include some pixels with 0 nCi/mL. For the 7 mm FWHM PET scanner producing the image in Figure 1.10b, the 2.0-cm region of interest would yield too low a value for concentration of activity because events near the edge of the object would smear out to pixels outside the region. For the situation depicted in Figure 1.10, the drop would be from 5 to 3.9 nCi/mL, again with a recovery coefficient of 78.5%. If the region of interest were decreased in size, however, it would no longer include pixels near the edge and the concentration of activity would approximate the correct value of 5 nCi/mL. If the region of interest were 1.8 cm in diameter, the average counts/second/pixel would correspond to 4.3 nCi/mL (85% recovery), and if the region of interest were decreased still further to 1.6 cm, the value would be 4.5 nCi/mL (90% recovery). For measurements in nanocuries/milliliter or counts/second/pixel then, as the region of interest gets smaller, the average value within the region approaches the correct value.

Unfortunately, as the region of interest gets smaller, so does the total number of events contained in it, causing statistical fluctuations (the standard deviation) to increase. Conversely, if the region of interest is too large (larger than the object being imaged), the mean "nCi/mL" value drops. A rule of thumb is that if the edge of the region of interest is more than 2 FWHM interior to the object's anatomic borders, the influence of the partial volume effect will be small. Unfortunately, myocardial walls are typically no thicker than 1–2 cm (except in certain disease states), whereas FWHMs are typically no less than 0.7 cm. It will often be impossible to draw a region that is even one FWHM from both epi- and endocardial borders. Accordingly, myocardial PET images are significantly influenced by partial volume effects. In general, recovery coefficients are significantly less than 100%. Even worse, since the myocardial wall varies in thickness around the heart, the thinner regions will artifactually appear to have lower activity than thick regions, even when the true underlying concentration is homogeneous.

In summary: (1) To measure only the total activity within an organ, the region of interest should be drawn very generously around the whole organ being imaged. This can only be done if there are no nearby structures containing activity. Ideally, edges of the region of interest should be at least two FWHM larger than the true organ borders. This will lead to recovery of nearly all events that have "blurred out" of the organ; (2) To measure

radioactive concentrations within an organ rather than simply total activity: (a) the edges of the region should ideally be interior to the edges of the organ by two FWHM (this is of course often impossible); otherwise, recovery will be flawed, and (b) thin myocardial walls will in general give lower recovery than thick walls. The above discussion was focused on drawing regions within a slice. However, it should be remembered that partial volume effects occur in all three directions. The same considerations mentioned above for the x and y directions, also apply to the z direction.

It has been assumed that the activity concentration is uniform within the region of interest. If this is not the case, results should be interpreted with care because the mean value within a region of interest will depend on the position of the region within the heterogeneous structure.

It is possible to correct for the partial volume effect [24]. If the true anatomic dimensions of the object being imaged and the resolution of the PET scanner (and reconstruction process) producing the image are known, it is possible to calculate the recovery coefficients and use them to correct the data. Unfortunately, the effects of cardiac wall motion also come into play. Sections of myocardium may move into and out of a region of interest as the ventricle contracts. Wall motion therefore produces its own "blurring" which influences the partial volume effect in exactly the same way as does the "real" blurring (i.e., the resolution) of the scanner itself.

2D versus 3D PET scanners

The PET scanners described above consist of separate rings of detectors, each of which is separated by a thin strip of high atomic number material (e.g., lead, tungsten), called the septum, Figure 1.11a. The septa act as a sort of coarse collimator. The purpose of the lead septa between rings is to reduce the number of scattered photons seen by the detector, as shown in Figure 1.11a, line "D." In addition, the septa reduce the number of photons from out of the field of view (e.g., from the bladder) which can hit the detectors, Figure 1.11a, line "A." With the septa in place, only coincidences from crystals in the same ring (or a few adjacent rings) of detectors will be admitted. So the pair of annihilation photons "B" do not make it through the septa,

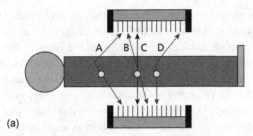

(a)

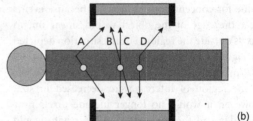

(b)

Figure 1.11 (a) Illustrating a multislice PET camera with septa (misleadingly called a "2D" scanner). The septa stop scattered photons, like (D), out of field photons like (A) as well as valid photons that happen not to produce coincidences within the crystals in a single ring (or nearby rings). Only photon pair (C), shown in black, is detected.

(b) The same scanner operating in "3D" mode, i.e., without the septa. Now both valid photons (B) and (C) are detected, increasing the sensitivity. However, this is at the expense of detecting lots of nonvalid photons such as the scattered pair (D) and the out of field photon (A). (figure re-drawn from Bacharach [26].)

while the annihilation pair of photons "C" do. As mentioned above, this mode of operation, with the septa in place, is called "2D" mode, or "septa-in" mode. The name "2D" is slightly misleading, since the data from a multislice PET scanner operating in 2D mode, is of course 3D. The nomenclature refers to the fact that the lead septa attempt to keep out any photons not originating from within a single detector ring (or a few adjacent rings). Together, the septa, combined with the limited energy discrimination, are able to reduce scatter in heart scans to about 10–15%—a quite clinically acceptable number. This remaining small scatter is easily, albeit approximately, corrected for by using software algorithms [25].

The interslice septa not only reduce scatter, but also reduce sensitivity. By restricting the coincidences to within a single ring or pair of adjacent rings, one has eliminated not only scattered photons, but also many of the photons that might have given valid coincidences between non-neighboring rings, for example line B in Figure 1.11a. Typically, by using the scatter reducing septa, sensitivity for coincident photons is reduced by about a factor of 3–7 (depending on scanner design) compared to the situation if the septa had not been present. This is not nearly as big a reduction as incurred in SPECT by using a collimator (typically a SPECT collimator might reduce sensitivity by a factor of 1000 or more). Therefore even with the lead septa between rings, PET is still very much more sensitive than SPECT. This is because SPECT requires a honeycomb of lead holes as its collimator, since the function of the SPECT collimator is to permit deter-

mination of the direction of the incident photons. PET uses coincidence detection to determine the location of the gamma rays, in principle requiring no collimator.

PET scanners with septa (i.e., 2D mode) actually work quite well for cardiac imaging. The sensitivity, despite the septa, is sufficient to obtain good quality images using 10–15 mCi FDG injections with 5–15 minutes of acquisition time. The septa keep random events and deadtime at acceptable levels, even for high-dose studies, such as 40–50 mCi ^{82}Rb injections (imaging 90 seconds postinjection), or 20 mCi ^{13}N-ammonia injections. This is true even for relatively slow crystals such as BGO. The septa are able to accomplish this because random events (and deadtime) are greatly affected by the number of "singles" events/second. That is random events are determined by the count rate for individual detectors, rather than by the coincident count rate. The presence of the septa greatly limits the number of singles events/second, making 2D imaging advantageous for high-activity studies. The use of septa, then, greatly reduces scatter, as well as random and deadtime corrections.

Despite the good performance of current generation 2D scanners for cardiac imaging, the need to perform whole-body oncology scans made manufacturers look for ways to increase sensitivity. Cardiac imaging would also benefit from a sensitivity increase, provided it could be accomplished without sacrificing other machine characteristics important to cardiac imaging. A gain in sensitivity would permit either shorter imaging time (less of an issue for cardiac imaging than for whole-body imaging), or increased total counts (useful for producing gated images), or better dosimetry, or some compromise between these factors.

Most new generation scanners have attempted to increase sensitivity by removing the septa, and operating in "3D" mode [26–29], Figure 1.11b. However, removing the septa greatly increases scatter, increases the effect of out of field activity, greatly increases randoms, and greatly increases the potential for deadtime. Comparing Figure 1.11a and Figure 1.11b illustrates why this is so. In 2D mode (Figure 1.11a) only one of the four photon pairs (the black one) was detected. In Figure 1.11b all four were detected. Only two of them (B and C) actually carry valuable information.

Typically, removal of the septa increases scatter in cardiac imaging to 50% or more for large subjects. Software to correct for scatter is available, but the accuracy of the correction is not nearly as good in 3D mode as in 2D mode for thoracic imaging, and of course the magnitude of the necessary correction is many times bigger for 3D mode than 2D. Scatter is especially important when imaging cold areas near hot regions, such as a defect surrounded by normal uptake tissue. In such situations, scatter artifactually increases the counts in the defect region. If the scatter correction algorithm is not perfect, the defect size and extent can be significantly biased. Scatter correction is thought to be slightly less important for hot spot tumor imaging, but of course even in this situation, scatter can result in inaccurate quantitation, or even artifacts. It was hoped that the better energy resolution of the newer crystal types (e.g., LSO and GSO) might greatly reduce the additional scatter caused by removing the septa. While these detectors have slightly improved the scatter problem, they have not yet proven to be the panacea originally hoped for. On the other hand, the faster response time of these new crystals was successful in reducing random events by roughly a factor of 1.5–2.

Despite the difficulties, the removal of the septa seems to have been clinically acceptable for oncology imaging—the reduced scan time compensating for a greater difficulty in quantifying uptake. For cardiac imaging much work is still being done to determine under what circumstances 3D imaging might be acceptable. Certainly it will be useful when dosimetry considerations dictate a low

injected dose (e.g., for multiple sequential studies), or if only limited amount of the tracer was available (e.g., for some hard to produce radiopharmaceuticals). For static FDG imaging it may well prove perfectly acceptable (providing scatter can be adequately corrected). For dynamic imaging (e.g., bolus injections of ^{82}Rb or ^{13}N-ammonia) 3D imaging is more problematic. Much work is needed to determine the optimum activity levels that will be acceptable for 3D scanners, and whether 2D or 3D imaging is better in such circumstances. This is very important work, because many current generation scanners can only function in 3D mode (i.e., the septa cannot be inserted or retracted at will).

An additional problem with removing the septa is that the axial sensitivity rapidly decreases from a maximum at the center of the axial field of view, to the end slices. This is because in 3D coincidences are allowed between many rings of detectors, as in Figure 1.11b. This is fine in the center of the field, but as one approaches the edge of the field of view, there are fewer and fewer adjacent rings, causing the sensitivity to drop. This loss of sensitivity at the edges means that the effective overall sensitivity is not as high as one might predict. For oncology studies it means that significant overlap must occur between the axial fields of view at each imaging location. For cardiac studies it simply means that the noise will increase rapidly for slices further from the center of the axial field of view.

PET Time of Flight Imaging

Recently machines have been introduced which incorporate "time-of-flight" information in the acquisition process. Time of flight refers to measuring the precise time difference between the times the two 511-keV annihilation photons are detected. In Figure 1.4 it is assumed that the photon that hits detector A also hits B "simultaneously," where by "simultaneously" we mean that the two events occur within the resolving time of the coincidence circuits. This resolving time is relatively coarse. Obviously, since detector A is closer to the origin of the photons than detector B, in theory detector A would see the photon slightly sooner than B. However, as the photons travel at the speed of light this time difference is much smaller than the resolving time of most current generation PET scanners. The co-incidence between A and B then only tells us that the annihilation (and therefore the radiotracer) lies somewhere along the line between A and B. It does not tell us where along that line the annihilation occurred. To determine where along the line the radiotracer lies, we need to examine all the coincidences from all detector pairs, and then reconstruct the data. If, however, one could measure this small time difference between when detector A was struck compared to when detector B was struck, it would be possible to determine exactly where along the line the photon originated, making reconstruction unnecessary. Unfortunately, current detector and instrumentation technology is not nearly good enough to achieve this accuracy of time measurement. Still, some new machines are able to roughly measure this time difference, and so pin down the approximate location of where the annihilation occurred along the coincidence line, at least within 10s of cm. Such approximate information unfortunately is insufficient for avoiding the reconstruction process. But by adding even such crude timing information, it should be possible to improve the statistical quality of the data (i.e., the noise), and perhaps in the future reduce scatter. Machines with this ability have only recently been introduced, so their clinical utility is at present unclear. Still, as electronics (and perhaps detectors) get faster, this approach may prove useful. It should be noted that the idea of adding "time-of-flight" information to PET scanners is actually quite old. But only recently has the idea been revisited.

Use of PET/CT in Cardiology

The vast majority of new PET scanners being sold today are combined with a CT scanner. The CT scan can be used to replace the much slower rotating ^{68}Ge rod source transmission scan thereby reducing scan time by 3–6 minutes/field of view. In addition the rotating rod transmission source, due to limited counts, introduced noise into the corrected PET images. The CT images are by comparison nearly noise free. The two scanners are physically located in the same gantry, but do not perform scans simultaneously. Instead one usually first acquires (for oncology) a rapid spiral CT scan (perhaps 20 seconds for a head to thigh scan) and then

the much slower PET scan (several minutes/bed position). With the rotating rod source method scans of 4–6 minutes/bed position were commonly used. This resulted in 24–36 minutes of extra scan time for a six-bed position oncology whole-body scan. With CT this is reduced to ~20 seconds. In addition it soon became clear that much valuable clinical information was present in the fused CT and PET images.

Transmission scan time is much less an issue with cardiac scans, because they are acquired at a single bed position. The reduced attenuation correction noise would, however, be beneficial. In addition, it is possible that combining CT cardiac data with PET metabolic or perfusion data, as obtained from PET/CT machines, will be of clinical value. There have been several reports in the past of the clinical utility of fusing coronary angiograms with SPECT perfusion data. Recently 64 slice CT scanners have begun to be marketed with PET scanners. Many of these scanners are fast enough to permit CT cardiac gating, and will even operate with commercially available CT coronary angiography software. Many of the other cardiac CT procedures (aside from angiography) that could be used with PET often still involve contrast media. For example, even with very low concentrations of contrast media in the blood, it is reasonably easy to identify the endo- and epicardial borders using gated CT images. Thus one could correct the PET data for any partial volume effects, for example caused by thinning of one part of the myocardium compared to another. In addition, while gated FDG PET is adequate for global measures of ventricular function [30–36], the gated CT would also allow measurement of myocardial thickening—a very useful adjunct to PET physiologic (metabolic or perfusion) imaging.

Unfortunately, there are at present some unresolved issues associated with using a high speed CT scan for attenuation correction of cardiac images. A few of these are discussed briefly below.

Use of CT Images for Attenuation Correction

As described above, when using a PET scanner, transmission related noise can be nearly eliminated by using the CT data to perform the attenuation correction. The physics of the process has been described in detail previously [37–40]. In short, a

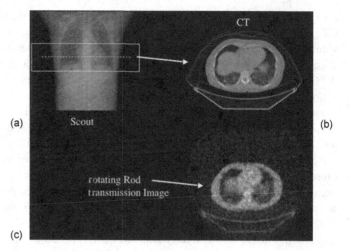

Figure 1.12 (a) Scout view (single planar projection) taken with the stationary X-ray tube of a CT scanner. A single PET field of view (the box) is selected in order to produce CT tomographic slices, one of which is shown in (b). (c) Shows a transmission image taken with a rotating ^{68}Ge rod source. Obviously the CT slice has much better statistics. CT, computed tomography.

CT scan is taken of the patient immediately prior to the PET scan. Usually a quick scout acquisition is first taken, and from this scan, one can accurately position both the axial CT scan, and the subsequent PET imaging, over the cardiac chambers. Typical images are shown in Figure 1.12. The CT scan is assumed to be aligned with the subsequent PET scan, just as the conventional transmission scan obtained with a ^{68}Ge rod source is assumed to be aligned. The CT scan, even at relatively low exposure settings (e.g., 140 kVp, 80 mA, 1.5 pitch, rotation speed of 0.8 seconds) has far less noise than does the typical ^{68}Ge rod source transmission scan (Figure 1.12). The CT scan is resampled to the same size as the PET data, is suitably blurred, and scaled [26] so as to convert the pixel values from Hounsfield units to the attenuation coefficients, which would be obtained at 511 keV. The scaled, resampled CT data is then used to correct the PET data prior to reconstruction.

This procedure works reasonably well for oncology whole-body imaging, although there are some difficulties. Some of these difficulties are potentially exacerbated when the process is applied to cardiac imaging. There is a small but growing body of literature concerning the accuracy and reliability of the CT attenuation correction for tumor imaging [37,41,42]. There is a growing body of corresponding data validating the method for cardiac imaging [39,43,44].

The two principal areas of concern for CT attenuation correction in cardiac PET are listed below:

1 Scaling the CT Hounsfield units to 511-keV attenuation coefficients.

The X-ray beam from the CT scanner is of much lower energy than the 511-keV photons being imaged. In addition, the X-ray beam produces a continuous spectrum of energies all the way up to the peak (kVp). The attenuation of these lower energy CT photons is therefore much greater than the attenuation experienced by the 511-keV annihilation photons. To correct for this the attenuation values produced by the CT scanner have to be converted to 511-keV attenuation values. This aspect of PET/CT has been well validated in oncology imaging, and has been shown to work quite well in general [37,41,42], with only a few caveats. The only potential difficulties that might occur during cardiac imaging are if contrast media has been used during or prior to the CT scan [42,45–49], or if metallic objects (e.g., clips, shoulder or arm prostheses) are in the plane of the cardiac images. When arms are not up (i.e., arms at the side), some artifacts and noise can be introduced into the CT scan. There may also be some small concern caused by the proximity of the myocardium to the ribs.

2 Misalignment between CT and emission data

Misalignment between the CT data and the PET data is a potential problem when using CT data to perform attenuation correction for PET. The misalignment can be inadvertent (i.e., patient motion between the time of the CT and emission acquisitions) or "effective" misalignment due to patient respiration and myocardial motion during the cardiac cycle. We assume here that the PET and CT portions of the machine itself have been previously determined to be in accurate mechanical alignment.

The effects of a misalignment between the attenuation scan and the emission scan have already been investigated for PET [17]. Prior to PET/CT the only cause of this misalignment was whatever inadvertent patient motion might have occurred between the two scans. Relatively small misalignments can cause a myocardium with uniform uptake to appear nonuniform. In PET/CT the misalignment comes not only from inadvertent patient motion, but also from the motion of the internal organs caused by respiration. The CT scan is usually acquired quite rapidly, perhaps taking less than 1 second/slice. The CT therefore captures the chest at one phase of the respiratory cycle. The PET emission data, on the other hand, is acquired over many minutes, and so is an average over many respiratory cycles. The two data sets therefore do not overlay each other. The problem is most severe at the boundaries between low and high attenuation regions. For oncology studies this is usually at the dome of the liver. For heart studies it is all regions of the myocardium surrounded by lungs. In addition, not only does the heart itself appear to move with respiration, so too does the liver. As the liver moves into or out of the cardiac slices, the attenuation for those slices can change substantially. Figure 1.13 illustrates the effect, showing a CT slice captured at normal tidal end-inspiration and normal tidal end-expiration.

Several studies have examined the effects of respiratory motion on PET/CT in oncology [50–55] and it is useful to consider how those findings might apply to cardiac imaging. In oncology applications, one of the most notable effects is at the dome of the liver, where respiratory motion is large and there is an air-tissue interface. In one study [55], nearly all (84%) subjects exhibited a cold artifact at the top of the liver, with 16% of the subjects having a defect categorized as moderate. The source of the defect was thought to be the incorrect attenuation correction, due to inconsistencies at the lung/liver interface in the CT compared to the emission PET. Similar effects occur with the free wall of the heart [43,56]. A tissue/lung interface exists, and there is indeed respiratory motion (as well as cardiac motion, depending on the speed of the CT scanner). The magnitude of such effects in the heart can be significant [43]. Previous results describing the effects of misalignment between attenuation and emission data are germane [17]. Much work remains to be done in using CT images to correct for attenuation. One solution would be to slow down the CT scan (using very slow rotations and low mA) so as to average a few respiratory cycles together [57,58]. While this may lengthen the scan unacceptably for multilevel oncology imaging, it should be quite practical for cardiac imaging. It can, however, produce artifacts in the CT data. Another excellent solution that has been put forth, is to acquire a very low dose CT cine of the heart over 1 or more respiratory cycles, and then average the cine frames together. This avoids the CT artifact problem. Still

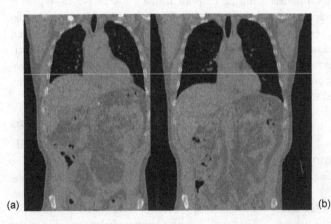

(a)   (b)

Figure 1.13 Two coronal CT views at exactly the same level: (a) taken at normal end-expiration; (b) at normal end-inspiration. Note movement of the dome of both the liver and the heart.

another solution would be to use respiratory gating or even 4D imaging [50]. All of these solutions at present may add considerable complexity to the acquisition, but manufacturers are rapidly realizing the necessity for making such corrections in a clinically feasible fashion.

It should be noted that many CT scanners routinely scan fast enough to capture only a portion of the cardiac cycle itself. Again, problems similar to those described above may occur. Here, however, the motion (and so potential misalignment) is presumably smaller. In addition only a minimal reduction in CT scan speed would average several cardiac cycles together.

In summary, combining CT with PET imaging is likely to prove even more valuable for cardiac imaging than for oncology imaging. The additional information associated with overlaying physiologic data (metabolism, blood flow, etc.) with CT angiographic data, coupled with wall thickness and thickening measurements would seem to portend significant advances in the field of cardiac imaging. However, the problems associated with respiratory motion are likely to be much worse for cardiac imaging than for oncology imaging. Considerable work has been done to address these problems, and cardiac PET/CT is rapidly achieving its full potential.

References

1. ICRP. *Radionuclide Transformations*. New York: Pergamon Press, 1983.
2. Dilsizian V. *Myocardial Viability: A Clinical and Scientific Treatise*. New York: Futura Publishing Company, Inc., 2000.
3. Bacharach SL, Bax JJ, Case J, *et al*. PET myocardial glucose metabolism and perfusion imaging: part I – guidelines for patient preparation and data acquisition. *J Nucl Cardiol*. 2003;10(5):545–556.
4. Lederer CM, Shirley VS. *Table of Isotopes*, 7th edition. New York: Wiley, 1978.
5. Parker J. *Image Reconstruction in Radiology*. Boca Raton: CRC Press, 1990.
6. Maass RE, Bacharach SL. Imaging Instrumentation. In: Iskandrian AE, Verani MS (eds). *Nuclear Cardiac Imaging: Principles and Applications*. New York: Oxford press, 2003, pp. 28–50.
7. Bacharach SL. The physics of positron emission tomography. In: Bergmann SR, Sobel BE (eds). *Positron Emis-*
8. Bacharach SL. The new generation PET/CT scanners: implications for cardiac imaging. *J Nucl Cardiol* 2004;11: 388–392.
9. Knesaurek K, Machac J, Krynyckyi BR, *et al*. Comparison of 2-dimensional and 3-dimensional Rb-82 myocardial perfusion PET imaging. *J Nucl Med*. 2003;44(8): 1350–1356.
10. Knesaurek K, Machac J, Krynyckyi BR, *et al*. Comparison of 2D and 3D myocardial PET imaging. *J Nucl Med*. 2001;42(5):170.
11. Machac J, Chen H, Almeida OD, *et al*. Comparison of 2D and high dose and low dose 3D gated myocardial Rb-82 PET imaging. *J Nucl Med*. 2002;43(5):777.
12. Votaw JR and White M. Comparison of 2-dimensional and 3-dimensional cardiac Rb-82 PET studies. *J Nucl Med*. 2001;42(5):701–706.
13. Murphy PH. Radiation Pysics and Radiation Safety. In: Iskandiran AE, Verani MS (eds). *Nuclear Cardiac Imaging: Principles and Applications*. New York: Oxford University Press, 2003, pp. 7–27.
14. Bacharach SL. Attenuation correction: practical considerations. In: Schwaiger M (ed.). *Cardiac Positron Emission Tomography*. Boston: Kluwer Academic Publishers, 1996, pp. 49–64.
15. Carson RE, Daubewitherspoon MF, Green MV. A method for postinjection pet transmission measurements with a rotating source. *J Nucl Med*. 1988;29(9): 1558–1567.
16. Thompson CJ, Ranger NT, and Evans AC, Simultaneous transmission and emission scans in positron emission tomography. *IEEE Trans Nucl Sci*. 1989;36(1):1011–1016.
17. McCord ME, Bacharach SL, Bonow RO, *et al*. Misalignment between pet transmission and emission scans – its effect on myocardial imaging. *J Nucl Med*. 1992;33(6): 1209–1214.
18. Bendriem B, Soussaline F, Campagnolo R, *et al*. A technique for the correction of scattered radiation in a pet system using time-of-flight information. *J Comput Assist Tomogr*. 1986;10(2):287–295.
19. Hoffman EJ, Phelps ME. Resolution limit for positron – imaging devices – reply. *J Nucl Med*. 1977;18(5):491–492.
20. Evans R. *The Atomic Nucleus*. New York: McGraw-Hill, 1955, pp. 625–629.
21. Phelps ME, Hoffman EJ, Huang SC, *et al*. Effect of positron range on spatial-resolution. *J Nucl Med*. 1975; 16(7):649–652.
22. Bacharach SL. Image analysis. In: Wagner HN, S Z, Buchanan JW (eds). *Principles of Nuclear Medicine*. Philadelphia: W.B. Saunders, 1995, pp. 393–404.

sion Tomography of the Heart. Mount Kisco, NY: Futura Publishing Co., 1992, pp. 13–44.

23. Hoffman EJ, Huang SC, Phelps ME. Quantitation in positron emission tomography: effect of object size. *J Comput Assist Tomogr*. 1979;3:299–308.

24. Soret M, Bacharach SL, Buvat I. Partial volume effect in PET tumor imaging. *J Nucl Med*. 2007;48:926–931.

25. Bergstrom M, Eriksson L, Bohm C, et al. Correction for scattered radiation in a ring detector positron camera by integral transformation of the projections. *J Comput Assist Tomogr*. 1983;7(1):42–50.

26. Bacharach SL. The new generation PET/CT scanners: implications for cardiac imaging. In: Zaret BL, Beller GA (eds). *Clinical Nuclear Cardiology: State of the Art and Future Directions*. Philadelphia: Mosby, 2005.

27. Muehllehner G, Karp JS, Surti S, Design considerations for PET scanners. *Q J Nucl Med*. 2002;46(1):16–23.

28. Alessio AM, Kinahan PE, Cheng PM, et al. PET/CT scanner instrumentation, challenges, and solutions. *Radiol Clin North Am*. 2004;42(6):1017.

29. Surti S, Karp JS, Kinahan PE. PET instrumentation. *Radiol Clin North Am*. 2004;42(6):1003.

30. Schaefer WM, Lipke CSA, Nowak B, et al. Validation of an evaluation routine for left ventricular volumes, ejection fraction and wall motion from gated cardiac FDG PET: a comparison with cardiac magnetic resonance imaging. *Eur J Nucl Med Mol Imaging*. 2003;30(4):545–553.

31. Rajappan K, Livieratos L, Camici PG, et al. Measurement of ventricular volumes and function: a comparison of gated PET and cardiovascular magnetic resonance. *J Nucl Med*. 2002;43(6):806–810.

32. Machac J, Mosci K, Almeida OD, et al. Gated rubidium-82 cardiac PET imaging: evaluation of left ventricular wall motion. *J Am Coll Cardiol*. 2002;39(5):393A–393A.

33. Khorsand A, Graf S, Pirich C, et al. Gated cardiac PET for assessment of LV volume and ejection fraction. *J Nucl Med*. 2001;42(5):741.

34. Block S, Schaefer W, Nowak B, et al. Comparison of left ventricular ejection fraction calculated by EGG-gated PET and contrast left ventriculography. *J Nucl Med*. 2001;42(5):734.

35. Willemsen AT, Siebelink HJ, Blanksma PK, et al. Left ventricle ejection fraction determination with gated (18)FDG-PET. *J Nucl Med*. 1999;40(5):166P–166P.

36. Cooke CD, Folks RD, Oshinski JN, et al. Determination of ejection fraction and myocardial volumes from gated FDG PET studies: a preliminary validation with gated MR. *J Nucl Med*. 1997;38(5):198–198.

37. Burger C, Goerres G, Schoenes S, et al. PET attenuation coefficients from CT images: experimental evaluation of the transformation of CT into PET 511-keV attenuation coefficients. *Eur J Nucl Med Mol Imaging*. 2002; 29(7):922–927.

38. Koepfli P, Wyss CA, Hany TF, et al. Evaluation of CT-transmission for attenuation correction in quantitative myocardial perfusion measurement using a combined PET-CT scanner: a pilot dose-finding study for different CT energies. *Circulation*. 2001;104(17):2778.

39. Koepfli P, Hany TF, Wyss CA, et al. CT Attenuation correction for myocardial perfusion quantification using a PET/CT hybrid scanner. *J Nucl Med*. 2004;45:537–542.

40. Kinahan PE, Hasegawa BH, Beyer T. X-ray-based attenuation correction for positron emission tomography/computed tomography scanners. *Semin Nucl Med*. 2003;33(3):166–179.

41. Nakamoto Y, Osman M, Cohade C, et al. PET/CT: comparison of quantitative tracer uptake between germanium and CT transmission attenuation-corrected images. *J Nucl Med*. 2002;43(9):1137–1143.

42. Visvikis D, Costa DC, Croasdale I, et al. CT-based attenuation correction in the calculation of semi-quantitative indices of F-18 FDG uptake in PET. *Eur J Nucl Med Mol Imaging*. 2003;30(3):344–353.

43. LeMeunier L, Maass-Moreno R, Carrasquillo JA, et al. PET/CT imaging: effect of respiratory motion on apparent myocardial uptake. *J Nucl Cardiol*. 2006;13:821–830.

44. Vass M, Sasaki K, Pan T. Investigation of heart motion with multi-slice cardiac CT for attenuation correction of PET emission data. *Radiology*. 2002;225:520–520.

45. Dizendorf E, Hany TF, Buck A, et al. Cause and magnitude of the error induced by oral CT contrast agent in CT-based attenuation correction of PET emission studies. *J Nucl Med*. 2003;44(5):732–738.

46. Nakamoto Y, Chin BB, Kraitchman DL, et al. Effects of nonionic intravenous contrast agents at PET/CT imaging: phantom and canine studies. *Radiology*. 2003; 227(3):817–824.

47. Cohade C, Osman M, Nakamoto Y, et al. Initial experience with oral contrast in PET/CT: phantom and clinical studies. *J Nucl Med*. 2003;44(3):412–416.

48. Burger CN, Dizendorf EV, Hany TF, et al. Impact of transient oral contrast agent on CT-based attenuation correction in combined PET/CT studies. *Radiology*. 2002;225:409–409.

49. Antoch G, Jentzen W, Stattaus J, et al. Effect of oral contrast agents on CT-based PET attenuation correction in dual-modality PET/CT tomography. *Radiology*. 2002; 225:423–424.

50. Pan T. Comparison of helical and cine acquisitions for 4D-CT imaging with multislice CT. *Med Phys*. 2005; 32(2):627–634.

51. Beyer T, Antoch G, Blodgett T, et al. Dual-modality PET/CT imaging: the effect of respiratory motion on combined image quality in clinical oncology. *Eur J Nucl Med Mol Imaging*. 2003;30(4):588–596.

52. Goerres G, Buehler TC, Burger C, et al. CT based attenuation correction using a combined PET/CT scanner:

influence of the respiration level on measured FDG concentration in normal tissues. *J Nucl Med.* 2002;43(5):887.

53. Goerres GW, Kamel E, Heidelberg TNH, *et al.* PET-CT image co-registration in the thorax: influence of respiration. *Eur J Nucl Med Mol Imaging.* 2002;29(3):351–360.

54. Goerres GW, Burger C, Kamel E, *et al.* Respiration-induced attenuation artifact at PET/CT: technical considerations. *Radiology.* 2003;226(3):906–910.

55. Osman MM, Cohade C, Nakamoto Y, *et al.* Respiratory motion artifacts on PET emission images obtained using CT attenuation correction on PET-CT. *Eur J Nucl Med Mol Imaging.* 2003;30(4):603–606.

56. Bacharach SL. PET/CT attenuation correction: breathing lessons. *J Nucl Med.* 2007;48:677–679.

57. Pan T, Mawlawi O, Nehmeh SA. Attenaution correction of PET images with respiration-averaged CT images in PET/CT. *J Nucl Med.* 2005;46:1481–1487.

58. Cook RAH, Carnes G, Lee TY, *et al.* Respiration-averaged CT for attenuation correction in canine cardiac PET/CT. *J Nucl Med.* 2007;48:811–818.

CHAPTER 2

Cardiovascular Magnetic Resonance: Basic Principles, Methods, and Techniques

Joseph Selvanayagam[1], Matthew Robson[2], Jane Francis[2] & Stefan Neubauer[2]

[1] Flinders University of South Australia *and* Flinders Medical Centre, Adelaide, SA, Australia
[2] University of Oxford, Oxford, UK

Introduction

Unlike the physics of X-ray imaging (attenuation of X-ray beam by tissue) or the physics of ultrasound imaging (reflection of ultrasound by tissue), the physics underlying magnetic resonance imaging (MRI) are substantially more complex. This technique has evolved over the past half-century through a number of landmark discoveries and investigations. In 1946, Bloch [1] and Purcell [2] independently discovered the phenomenon of *nuclear magnetic resonance,* or NMR (later shortened, although physically incorrect, to *magnetic resonance,* or MR), and both later shared the Nobel Price in Physics for this discovery. In 1973, Lauterbur [3] and Mansfield independently proposed that the spatial distribution of nuclear spins may be determined through local variation of field strength, i.e., by use of a magnetic field gradient; both received the 2003 Nobel price in Medicine for this discovery. In 1976, again working independently, Radda's [4] and Jacobus's [5] groups were the first to record an MR signal from heart, in the form of a ^{31}P-MR spectrum. Cardiac magnetic resonance spectroscopy (MRS) thus substantially preceded the development of cardiac magnetic resonance (CMR). In 1977, Damadian's group [4] reported whole-body

MRI, and soon thereafter, MRI of the brain and of other nonmoving or easily immobilized organs became ready for clinical prime time. The heart has long escaped high-resolution detection by MRI, because it is a constantly moving structure, posing a number of additional technical challenges to its detection by MR. CMR has come to fruition only since the mid 1990s, mainly due to major advances in hardware design (high-field, highly homogenous magnets), coil design (cardiac phased array, etc.), sequence development (TrueFISP) and computing power. The latter has been instrumental in speeding up image reconstruction and postprocessing, a previously critical bottleneck in CMR. In coming years, further major technical breakthroughs in CMR development are anticipated, e.g., in perfusion, coronary and atherosclerosis imaging and in MRS, and it is conceivable that, due to its unique versatility and noninvasive nature, CMR may become the primary diagnostic modality in cardiovascular medicine.

Physical Principles Underlying MRI

MRI views the water and fat in the human body by observing the hydrogen nuclei in these molecules. MR is sensitive to any nucleus that possesses a net "spin." Nuclear spin is a fundamental property of atomic nuclei that depends on the numbers of

Cardiac CT, PET and MR, 2nd edition. Edited by Vasken Dilsizian and Gerry Pohost. © 2010 Blackwell Publishing Ltd.

Table 2.1   Myocardial tissue concentrations and MR sensitivity of elements important for MR imaging/spectroscopy.

Nucleus	Natural abundance (%)	Relative MR sensitivity (%)	Myocardial tissue concentrations
^{1}H	99.98	100	H_2O 110 M; up to ~90 mM (CH_3-^{1}H of creatine)
^{13}C	1.1	1.6	Labeled compounds, several mM
^{23}Na	100	9.3	10 mM (intracellular); 140 mM (extracellular)
^{31}P	100	6.6	Up to ~18 mM (PCr)

MR, magnetic resonance.

neutrons and protons it contains, and so nuclei either have it (e.g., Hydrogen (^{1}H), Phosphorus (^{31}P), Sodium (^{23}Na)) or they do not (e.g., Helium (^{4}He), Carbon (^{12}C), Oxygen (^{16}O), see Table 2.1). Certain common elements occur as a mixture of different isotopes, and in this case some of the fraction may be visible (i.e., ^{3}He is visible but ^{4}He is not). The high concentration of hydrogen (^{1}H) nuclei in the human body (up to 110 M) coupled, with its high "relative MR sensitivity," makes it the nucleus most suitable for high-resolution MRI.

Nuclei possessing net spin will behave as tiny radio-frequency receivers and transmitters when placed in a strong magnetic field. The frequency and strength of the transmitter both increase with increasing magnetic field strength. Typical clinical MRI systems possess fields of 1.5 Tesla (the Tesla (T) is the unit of magnetic field strength, or more accurately magnetic flux density). Even at these high magnetic field strengths the signals obtained from biological tissues are still very small, and the size of this signal can limit the quality of the images resulting in noise (graininess) obscuring the structures of interest. The NMR phenomena on which MRI is based involve transmitting radio-frequency pulses to the nuclei, which elevates them to a different energy level, from which they subsequently re-emit a radio-frequency signal. We can receive and acquire this re-emitted signal, and by manipulating this basic process we can perform MR imaging.

General Physics of MR

One feature of MR is that the frequency at which signals are received and re-emitted (and known as the resonant frequency) is exquisitely sensitive to the exact magnetic field, for example hydrogen nuclei (lone protons) resonate at 42.575 MHz/T. So, if we were to have two regions where the magnetic field is different by a small amount (for example at 1.000 and 1.001 T), then the protons in one region will transmit at 42.575 MHz (the Larmor frequency for protons), and protons from the other region will transmit at 42.575 + 0.042 MHz. If we sample this transmitted signal it is possible to determine these two different frequencies in the same way that a musician can distinguish between two tones at different audible frequencies. Numerically this transformation from a sampled signal to the component frequencies is known as a Fourier transform (Figure 2.1).

Instead of using two discrete regions, in MRI we generally apply a linearly increasing magnetic field (lower at one side of the magnet and higher at the other side). As a result, each point in the body will have a discrete resonance frequency and hence the amplitude of the signal at a specific frequency will represent the number of protons at that specific location. The approach of using a magnetic field gradient while the data are sampled allows the patient to be "imaged" in a single dimension, and comprises part of standard imaging methods. The direction of this gradient is described as the "read-out" direction in the MR image. To extend acquisition to two or more dimensions, additional switched magnetic field gradients (generally known simply as "gradients") need to be applied in the directions perpendicular to the "read-out" direction. For two-dimensional (2D) imaging, the above process is repeated a large (typically 256) number of times with different "gradients" applied in the second dimension for short intervals prior to acquisition, and the position is encoded in the phase of the signal. Each of these steps is known as a "phase

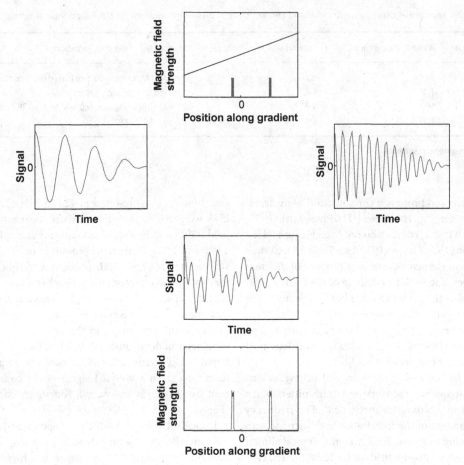

Figure 2.1 Two regions of protons are shown within a field gradient in the top figure. The signals from each of the two regions are shown (left and right), but in reality it is only the sum of these two signals that we can sample (center). By Fourier transforming the signal we can examine the sample.

encode" step and the number of these is generally[1] equal to the number of pixels in the phase-encode direction. The time required for each phase-encode step is known as the repetition time and signified as TR.

As we are interested in slices through the sample that are thin, rather than projections of the sample (as in an X-ray) we also use a process known as slice selection (Figure 2.2). This involves using a radio-frequency (RF) excitation pulse that only contains a narrow range of frequencies. By playing out such a pulse while a field gradient is applied we only ex-cite nuclei within a narrow slice. By applying the

above three mechanisms we can obtain a 2D image from a discrete slice of the sample. By modifying the frequency of the RF pulse, and by playing out the gradient pulses on more than one axis simulta-neously we can move the slice of interest freely. We are not limited to axial planes, and can acquire data with oblique or doubly oblique axes with complete flexibility.

Basic Imaging Sequences

The term "Pulse sequence" or "Imaging sequence" describes the way in which the scanner plays out RF pulse and gradient fields and how it acquires and reconstructs the resultant data to form an image. Different orders of these pulses have defined names (for example, FLASH, True-FISP, FSE) to

---

[1] This generalization is broken by partial Fourier and by the par-allel acquisition approaches (iPAT, SENSE, SMASH, etc.).

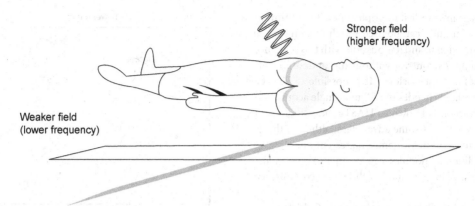

Figure 2.2 A schematic diagram illustrating the principles of slice/slab selection in cardiac magnetic resonance imaging. A slope or gradient in the magnetic field combined with a radio-frequency pulse containing only a narrow band of frequencies selects a slice or slab. Only where the frequencies contained in the r.f. pulse coincide with the resonant or Lamor frequency, do the nuclei get excited (slice/slab).

describe them. The details of the sequence required for its application will also need to include the exact timings (e.g., repetition time (TR)), the amplitude, duration and shapes of the gradient and RF pulses, the resolution parameters, and for cardiovascular applications these details will also include information on the cardiac gating strategy. This set of additional parameters is labeled the "protocol." Varying the protocol provides enormous flexibility for each imaging sequence.

In CMR we usually obtain 2D data acquired from a slice (for example 5 mm thick). Images can either be acquired in real-time or over a series of heartbeats. In the first case the spatial and temporal resolution will be limited by the available imaging time. In the second case we require that the breath is held[2] and so assume that the heart is perfectly periodic and a fraction of the phase-encoding steps of the image are acquired at the same relative phase of the cardiac cycle. The latter approach results in improved spatial and temporal resolution. If the assumption of periodicity is broken (e.g., in the case of arrhythmia, or failure to hold breath for long enough) then image artifacts[3] will result.

The basic imaging sequences used in cardiac MR are:

- FLASH (fast low angle shot). This plays out a small excitation RF pulse which is followed by a rapid readout and then spoiling (or removing) of the residual signal to prevent it appearing as an artifact in subsequent acquisitions. The process is repeated yielding a single phase-encode line per acquisition.

- TrueFISP (aka balanced FFE (balanced fast field echo)). This sequence is similar to FLASH but instead of spoiling the magnetization at the end of each acquisition it re-uses that signal. Compared to FLASH the benefit of this approach is that the images are of higher signal-to-noise, the disadvantages being increased sensitivity to artifacts, increased RF power deposition, and contrast that is more complex to interpret.

- FSE (fast spin echo, TSE (turbo spin echo)). This sequence acquires a number of phase-encode lines per acquisition by playing out a series of refocusing pulses after the initial excitation pulse. These refocusing pulses are a phenomenon of MR (not described here), which allow us to hold onto the signal created by the excitation pulse for longer so

---

[2] Breath-holding provides the most simple and robust method for cardiac imaging. Alternative approaches do exist that involve determining the phase of breathing either using external devices or using MRI-based measurements, and dynamically modify the scan accordingly, therefore, eliminating the requirement for breath-holding. The MRI-based (or navigator) methods allow for long scans where breath-holding is impossible.

---

[3] An artifact is an imperfection in the image that is not purely due to noise. Noise appears as a speckling of the image.

that we can sample it multiple times. The optimum excitation pulse can be used which maximizes the available signal, and it is possible with this sequence to obtain T_2 contrast without the undesirable effects of T_2^* (see below). It is possible to acquire all the phase encodes in FSE in a single acquisition (this variant is known as HASTE, and single-shot FSE), which has some advantages, although this is likely to result in low temporal resolution.

Additional modules can be included with the above sequences to modify the image contrast, for example:

● Black-blood pulses can be applied which effectively remove all the signal from material that moves quickly (e.g., blood). This is usually performed using double-inversion, which requires a delay prior to acquisition so is most compatible with FSE-based sequences.

● Inversion-recovery is a prepulse method that allows us to introduce T_1 contrast into an image. We can choose an inversion time that completely removes the signal from materials with a certain T_1. In practice this is often used when we want to see small changes in T_1 in late-enhancement type sequences (see Section Assessment of Myocardial Viability).

● Saturation-recovery is another prepulse method that allows us to introduce T_1 contrast into an image. By saturating the signal with an RF pulse we can see how quickly the signal recovers and has the benefit over inversion recovery that it does not require a long delay time. In practice this is often used when we want to see small changes in T_1 in cardiac perfusion scans (see Section Myocardial Perfusion).

● Fat-suppression (or water suppression) can be used to remove all the signal from either of these tissues, which may improve the delineation of the structures of interest.

The above acquisition approaches represent no more than the "tip-of-the-iceberg" regarding all possible MRI acquisition strategies, but will include 95% of all practical CMR applications.

Image Contrast

If all the nuclei behaved identically, then the above imaging methods would provide a map of the patient whereby the intensity at a pixel would depend purely on the concentration of that nucleus at that

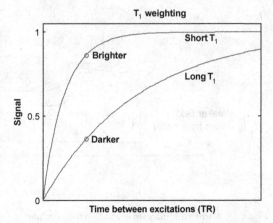

Figure 2.3 This oversimplified figure shows that the magnetization recovers quickly for tissues with a short T_1 but more slowly for tissues with a long T_1. By manipulating the repetition time (in this figure, but also the "flip angle") we can convert this difference in longitudinal magnetization into transverse magnetization and hence image intensity.

location in the body. However, several additional mechanisms affect this simple picture, which make MRI a considerably more powerful technique.

● Spin-lattice relaxation (T_1) relates to the time it takes for the signal to recover after an excitation pulse. This can simply be thought of as the time needed for the proton system to become active again, and so if we acquire separate phase-encodes rapidly (e.g., short TR), then tissues with a long T_1 will not recover quickly enough and will be darkened in the image (this effect is known as "saturation"), whereas tissues with a short T_1 will recover quicker and so will be brighter in the image (Figure 2.3). T_1 contrast can also be manipulated by changing the size of the excitation pulse (this parameter is known as the "flip angle"), as the spins will require more time to recover from the application of large flip angle than from a small one. Consequently, decreasing TR and increasing the flip angle will both increase the amount of T_1 weighting, whereas decreasing TR and the flip angle will decrease the amount of T_1 weighting.

● The spin–spin relaxation time (T_2) relates to the time that the signal is available for sampling after excitation. To benefit from this method we can excite the nucleus, and then wait a short period (e.g., 50 ms) before acquiring data. Tissues with a short T_2 (e.g., fast decay rate) will be darkened almost

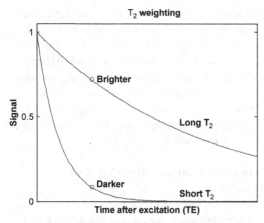

Figure 2.4 The transverse magnetization from the tissue with short T_2 decays rapidly after excitation, whereas this magnetization persists for the long T_2 species. These two tissues can be distinguished in an image by using a long echo time (as shown by the markers).

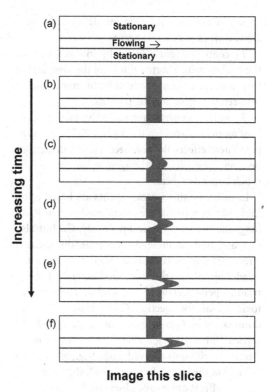

Image this slice

Figure 2.5 The above figures show the sample evolving with time. Initially (a) none of the sample is saturated. With the application of a slice selective saturation pulse a slab of signal is saturated (b). As time progresses unsaturated blood flows into the region that was previously saturated. If we select our slice thickness and imaging time correctly we can obtain an image that shows the blood without the stationary tissues

completely in the image, whereas tissue with a long T_2 (e.g., slow decay rate) will be darkened much less in the image (Figure 2.4). Fluid generally has a long T_2 and so T_2 weighted imaging is sensitive to edema. T_2 is used to refer specifically to the relaxation rate in fast spin-echo type sequences (e.g., the family of FSE sequences described above), and a different parameter T_2^* is used to describe the equivalent time for a gradient echo type sequence (e.g., FLASH). This is useful for example to look at iron overload where the T_2^* is shortened [6]. The echo time (TE) is the time between excitation and acquisition and determines the amount that the image is affected by the T_2^* and T_2 (known as the degree of T_2 weighting).

• In-flow—In the cardiovascular system the motion or flow of the protons will affect the image contrast in a similar way as the T_1. In this case spins may move from out of the imaging slice, where they are not affected by the flip-angle to a location where they become visible in our image. In this case the in-flowing spins will have additional brightness as they will not be subject to the signal attenuation due to the effect of T_1 saturation (described above). MR angiography utilizes this inflow to make blood in vessels (e.g., moving blood) bright, while suppressing the stationary signals (Figure 2.5)

Alternative methods exist to quantitatively examine flow velocities. These methods use the field gradients to encode the position of the blood and then decode this position at a later time. Stationary signal is unaffected by this encoding and decoding, but moving tissues accumulate a change in the phase of their signal which provides quantitative information on flow rates. This method is known as "phase-velocity," as the velocity is encoded in the phase of the signal [7].

Contrast Agents

Up until this point we have only been concerned with the indigenous contrast in the sample that is due to the molecular environment of the water and fat. Addition of even small amounts of certain molecules, called MR contrast agents, can massively change relaxation rates (i.e., T_1, T_2, and T_2^*) within the patient, which results in major changes in the appearance of an MR image. Fundamentally, there are two types of contrast agents:

- T_1 contrast agents, which by interaction with the nuclear spins shorten the T_1 of the sample. For this to operate there needs to be intimate contact between the agent and the protons.
- T_2 and T_2^* contrast agents. In this case the contrast agents will shorten the T_2 and T_2^* of the sample. These effects do not need close interactions between the nuclei and the agent as they occur over much larger distances.

In each case the contrast agents are based upon molecules or ions that are magnetically active. Paramagnetic moieties (typically, Fe, Dy, Gd but also O_2) are used as these demonstrate the greatest effects. The most commonly used nucleus is Gd (Gadolinium), and this is chelated (with diethylene-triaminepentaacetate, DTPA) so as to render it non-toxic and safe for injection. Gd compounds act predominantly as T_1 contrast agents in the blood and myocardium, although where the contrast cannot freely mix with the observed water (e.g., in the brain because of the blood–brain barrier), their small T_2 and T_2^* effects can also be observed. Gd-based contrast agents are approved for clinical use, but for historic reasons at the time of writing these are not yet approved for cardiac application in the US, although this will most likely be rectified in the near future. Iron oxide particles predominantly affect the T_2 and T_2^* of the sample. In MR images the regions where these particles accumulate will decrease the signals in T_2-weighted images. For both types of contrast agent the effects are regionally specific, i.e., compounds affect the contrast at the site of the contrast agent and by an amount that increases with contrast agent concentration. This can be used, for example, when looking at myocardial infarction when contrast agent remains within infarcted tissue at higher concentration than in surrounding normal tissue ~10–20 minutes after administration of an appropriate agent (see Assessment of Myocardial Viability). By adding MR contrast agents to compounds that can adhere to specific molecules (e.g., Fibrin) we can create "targeted contrast agents." This type of molecular imaging provides a promising approach for the future.

Contrast agents can be produced that remain within the vascular system, and are thus termed "intravascular." With an agent that decreases the T_1 it is possible to boost the signal in angiographic examinations, and hence improve the image quality. Presently Gd-DPTA is used in such angiographic examinations, but as it is not an "intravascular" agent the acquisition needs to occur when the Gd-DTPA is undergoing its first-pass through the vascular tree. "Intravascular" contrast agents would remove this restriction, enabling longer, and hence higher quality imaging. Presently no agents of this kind are approved for clinical use.

The CMR Scanner—How We Use the Physics

The physics and engineering of MRI is immensely complex, but much like a modern motorcar it is not essential to understand all the details to be able to use the machine.

To minimize the effects of electrical interference from the outside world (e.g., radio-transmitters, electronic devices) the MRI system is placed within an electrically shielded "box" (a Faraday cage), this is normally hidden in the walls of the scanning room. CMR scanners are a subset of MRI scanners, but with specific characteristics. Here MRI systems are described with special note to what is required for CMR.

The most important feature of the CMR scanner is the magnet. A strong homogeneous magnetic field can be obtained by building a solenoidal electromagnet from superconducting wires carrying large electrical currents at very low temperatures. These magnets are kept permanently at magnetic field. Some clinical systems operate at 0.5, 1.0 T and some new systems are available at 3.0 T, but the majority of MR systems operate at 1.5 T. Cardiac imaging at fields outside this range is more difficult although scientific results have been demonstrated. The field of the magnet is highest in the center of bore[4] of the magnet and this is where the organs of interest (i.e., the heart and vascular system) need to be positioned. The magnetic field also extends out from the magnet. Modern systems use "active-shielding" which minimizes this effect, but even with this technology the "fringe" field will extend to approximately 3–5 m (10–16 ft) or so in each direction around the magnet (including the floors above and below).

---

[4]The term "bore" is used to describe the hole through the middle of the magnet.

The equipment for transmitting RF pulses into the patient (the RF transmit coil) and for creating the linear magnetic field gradients (the gradient coil) are enclosed within the bore of the magnet and are not visible during operation. The gradient system on CMR machines needs to be particularly powerful as this component relates directly to the rate at which images can be acquired. The rapidly switching currents in the gradient coil interact with the magnetic field of the magnet, which results in forces being exerted on the gradient coil. The gradient coil is build strongly so as to resist these forces, but these small motions and distortions of the coil act like a speaker producing large amounts of audible noise when running fast-imaging sequences.

Additional RF reception coils are placed onto the patient, and may also be built into the patient bed, and these are used to receive the signals that are re-emitted by the nuclei. Smaller coils provide a higher signal to noise ratio than large coils, but also have a smaller region of sensitivity. RF coil manufacturers tailor their designs for specific parts of the body to optimize this trade-off, and frequently will use multiple coils within a single structure to maximize the signal while also maximizing the region of sensitivity. These complex coil combinations are known as "phased-array" coils and are standard for cardiac imaging.

The other visible component of an MRI system is the patient bed. This is required to position the patient accurately at the center of the MRI system. The MRI system is operated from away from the magnet itself via a computer allowing the operator to acquire and display images. An additional room is required to house the electronics, cooling, and other control hardware associated with the MRI system, this equipment is generally hidden. A typical layout of these components is shown in Figure 2.6 for a cardiovascular imaging system.

CMR Imaging Techniques

General Overview of the CMR Examination

Careful preparation of the patient is necessary in order to maximize diagnostic information from the CMR scan. This includes screening of the patient to exclude any contra-indication to the MR examination (see Section Safety and Contraindications), undressing and wearing clothes with no metallic

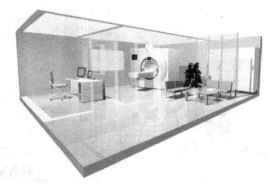

Figure 2.6 Computer generated diagram of a scanning suite. The internal walls are displayed semi-opaque so each part of the system is visible. Note the operator console, magnet and control hardware (image supplied courtesy of Siemens Medical Solutions).

fastenings, and adequate preparation of the chest prior to electrode positioning for electrocardiogram (ECG) gating. To ensure good contact it may be necessary to shave the chest to remove any excess hair, and/or use abrasive skin preparation to remove any dead skin cells and moisture. It is possible to double the amplitude of the signal with correct preparation and a simple, important rule is: "No trigger, no scan." If repeated breath-hold images are to be taken then it may be worthwhile training the patient outside the magnet of the breathing commands to be used.

Figure 2.7 demonstrates the use of a four-lead ECG configuration and electrode positioning placed both anteriorly and posteriorly. The benefits of anterior lead placement are larger amplitude and ease of repositioning, but there may be respiration-induced artifacts. Posterior lead placement can help counteract this at the expense of signal amplitude. Once the patient is ready then he/she is placed supine on the scanner table and an RF receiver coil is placed over the anterior chest wall. This is used in combination with elements of the spine array coil to ensure good signal from both the anterior and the posterior chest wall.

ECG Gating and Physiological Monitoring

Gating is described simply as the detection of the R-wave by the MR system and is used to "trigger" or synchronize the acquisition to the patient's heart rate. Correct gating relies on good R wave detection and a regular R-R interval. Deterrents to successful

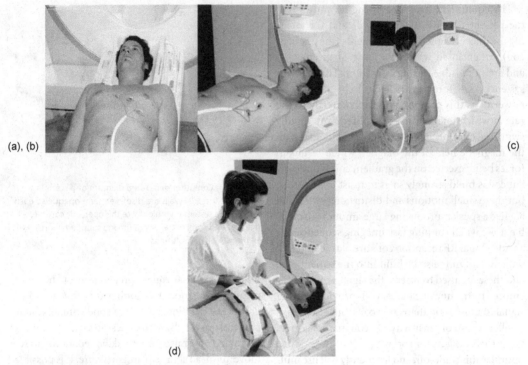

(a), (b)   (c)

(d)

Figure 2.7 Suitable sites on the anterior (a, b) or posterior (c) chest wall for optimal electrocardiographic detection; (d) demonstrates the correct positioning of the body flex array coil for cardiac magnetic resonance examination.

CMR imaging include poor R wave detection (Figure 2.8), an inadequate ECG, and the presence of tachyarrhythmias and/or ventricular ectopic beats. When using prospective cardiac gating, the MR system detects the R-wave and then begins the imaging sequence. However, as this method only uses 80–90% of the R-R interval, data are not acquired during end-diastole.

Retrospectively gated sequences are now widely available, whereby the sequence is continuously repeated, the R-R interval monitored and the data retrospectively fitted, allowing acquisition of the entire cardiac cycle. This method has the added benefit of compensating for some variation in the R-R interval during acquisition. A new feature of some CMR systems is arrhythmia detection, which

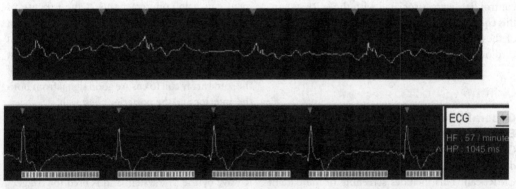

Figure 2.8 Top panel shows an example of poor R wave recognition in a patient positioned within the magnet bore. In contrast (bottom panel), there is accurate R wave detection during this prospectively gated cine acquisition. Cine frames are indicated by the green squares below the trace.

allows the R-R interval that is used for acquisition to be fixed by the operator, thus eliminating data obtained during ectopic beats. This approach may particularly aid data acquisition in patients with atrial fibrillation.

One important consideration is the effect of the magnetic field on the ECG waveform. Blood flow, particularly in the aorta, causes an additional electrical signal detected by the ECG leading to a magnetohydrodynamic effect. This is generally superimposed on the T wave and can make the analysis of the ECG within the magnetic field very difficult. The only diagnostic feature of the ECG that is reliable while a patient is inside the bore is the heart rate (provided QRS detection is good), whereas it is difficult to comment on changes in the P wave, the ST segment and the T wave. The development of techniques such as the vector ECG which uses 3D collection of ECG data and separates artifact from the true ECG signal have helped overcome some of the ECG problems associated with CMR and improve image quality and scan efficiency [8]. Another novel method of ECG synchronization is the self-gating approach where information regarding cardiac motion is extracted from the image data [9]. This method does not require an ECG to be obtained.

The other main cause of image degradation in CMR is respiration-artifact. Most patients are able to hold their breath during image acquisition, particularly with the recent introduction of parallel imaging techniques such as iPAT and SENSE which reduce breath-hold times considerably. However, especially in instances where the patients cannot hold their breath (e.g., older subjects, significant cardiac/respiratory disease), and/or in cases where longer acquisition times are unavoidable (e.g., coronary artery imaging), respiratory gating with MR navigators is essential for artifact free images. Navigator echo techniques are used for respiratory compensation, in conjunction with ECG gating. The navigator echo is combined with the imaging sequence and enables movement to be tracked throughout the respiratory cycle. It comprises of signal from a column perpendicular to the direction of movement. The usual placement for CMR is on the dome of the diaphragm, and the sequence only acquires when the diaphragm is in a predefined position with a small tolerance window. Although this might reduce scan efficiency and hence prolong imaging time, it does allow acquisition to take place with the patient breathing freely (Figure 2.9). Figure 2.10 shows some common artifacts encountered during CMR imaging.

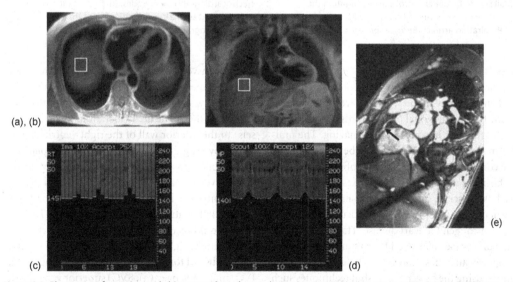

(a), (b)

(c)

(d)

(e)

Figure 2.9 Placement of a navigator (white square) on the right hemi-diaphragm in the transverse (a) and coronal (b) planes. (c) diaphragm position during the respiratory cycle (*y*-axis) against time (*x*-axis). (d) navigator trace during image acquisition set at 145 ± 8 mm. Acquisition takes place as indicated by white "bar"; (e) resulting short axis view showing the right coronary artery (RCA)—black arrow.

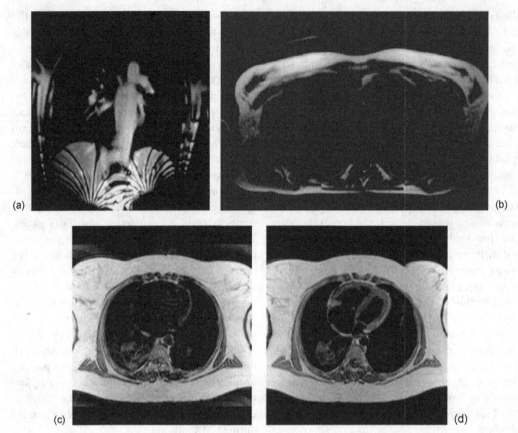

Figure 2.10 Common artifacts seen during cardiac magnetic resonance imaging: (a) Metal artifact from a small clip in the patient's trousers highlighting the importance of removing all clothing with metal fastenings. (b) Respiration artifact during a spin echo anatomical imaging sequence. (c) Poor definition of cardiac structures with spin echo sequence due to incorrect positioning of electrocardiographic electrodes. (d) Significant improvement seen after repositioning of the electrocardiographic electrodes.

Cardiac Anatomy

Cardiac anatomy can easily be demonstrated using MR imaging techniques, which are not confined to the three orthogonal planes (transverse, coronal, and sagittal) as in conventional imaging. The multiplanar capabilities of CMR can be used to define the conventional imaging planes of the heart, such as horizontal and vertical long axes, short axis, as well as prescribe any imaging plane specific to a particular pathology. This is particularly useful in cases of congenital heart disease. The three orthogonal planes (see Figure 2.11) remain important for diagnosis and these can be easily and quickly acquired using the newer single-shot techniques such as HASTE, where a stack of images can be obtained in a single breath-hold.

The transverse plane is useful for a good overview of size, shape and position of the cardiac chambers and great vessels and should be inclusive from of the top of the aortic arch (including the great vessels) to the inferior wall of the right ventricle, typically covering 20–24 slices. The coronal plane is useful for an assessment of the descending aorta, inferior vena cava (IVC), superior vena cava (SVC), both ventricles, left atrium and pulmonary veins and the left ventricular outflow tract (LVOT). The slices should reach from the descending aorta posteriorly to the right ventricle anteriorly. The sagittal plane is useful for visualizing the descending aorta, IVC (inferior vena cava), SVC (superior vena cava), and the right ventricle. In addition, the oblique sagittal view, which is planned from the transverse

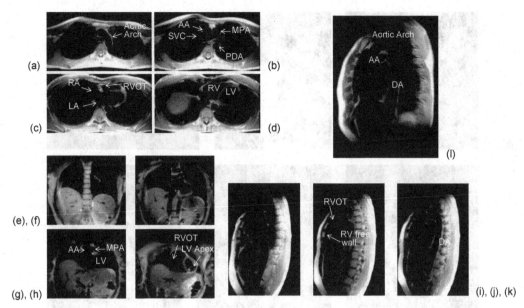

Figure 2.11 Anatomical images with a turbo spin echo sequence showing the heart and great vessels in a transverse (a–d), coronal (e–h) and sagittal (i–k) planes. (l) Shows an oblique sagittal view of the proximal ascending and descending aorta, the so-called "hockey stick" view. (AA, proximal ascending aorta; DA, descending aorta; LA, left atrium; LV, left ventricle; MPA, main pulmonary artery; PDA, proximal descending aorta; RA, right atrium; RV, right ventricle; RVOT, right ventricular outflow tract; SVC, superior vena cava)

multislice series can be a useful addition when assessing the aorta and gives the familiar "hockey-stick" view of the whole of the aorta.

Cardiac Function

CMR has rapidly become the imaging method of choice and the gold-standard in the assessment of cardiac function of both normal and abnormal ventricles [10–13]. With regard to measurement of global left ventricular (LV) function, given its 3D nature and order of magnitude greater signal-to-noise ratio, CMR is highly superior to 2D echocardiography [10]. This imaging is typically performed in, although not limited to, the conventional serial short-axis views and the three cardinal long-axis views. The ability of CMR to image in any plane without the need for optimal imaging windows allows for unprecedented flexibility for the interrogation of abnormal heart structures. This has allowed reductions of study sizes of 80–97% to achieve the same statistical power for demonstrating given changes of left ventricular volumes, ejection fraction, or cardiac mass [10]. It can be per-

formed quickly and easily, and can be incorporated into a comprehensive CMR examination.

The following method is employed at the authors' institution, and is a widely accepted approach to quantify left ventricular (LV) volumes, mass and function (Figures 2.12–2.14). The methods described may not be possible from all manufacturers, and variations from the described protocol may be necessary. After careful preparation of the patient and explanation of the importance of consistent breath-hold technique, multislice, multiplanar localizer images are performed in a single breath-hold. Prescribing a plane from the transverse plane using the mitral valve and the apex of the left ventricle as anatomical markers, localizer ("pilot") images are obtained in the vertical long axis (VLA). The resultant VLA pilot is then used to prescribe the horizontal long axis (HLA) pilot using the same anatomical landmarks.

It is important to accurately define the base of the heart when using this or a similar piloting method. As illustrated in figures, using the HLA and VLA pilots, three short-axis (SA) slices are acquired with the basal slice parallel to the atrioventricular (AV)

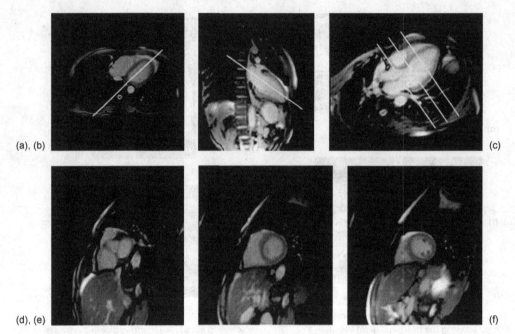

(a), (b)   (c)

(d), (e)   (f)

Figure 2.12 Sequence of images (a–f; g–k (Figure 2.13)) demonstrating the correct acquisition of the long axis and short axis planes for cine imaging. Initially, multiplanar localizer images are performed in a single breath-hold (a). Using the transverse localizer (a), in the plane indicated by the solid line in (a), pilot images are then performed in the vertical long axis (VLA) plane (b). The resultant VLA pilot is used to prescribe (as indicated by the solid line in (b)) the horizontal long axis (HLA) pilot (c) Using the HLA and VLA pilots, three short-axis (SA) slices (d–f) are next acquired with the basal slice parallel to the atrioventricular (AV) groove (indicated by three solid lines in (c)).

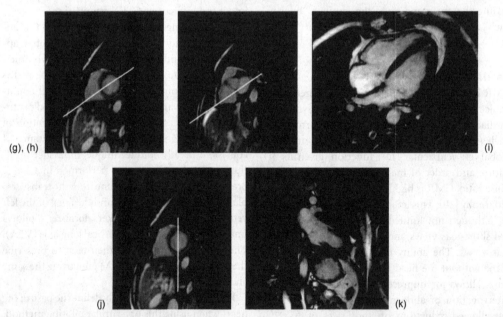

(g), (h)   (i)

(j)   (k)

Figure 2.13 To acquire the horizontal long axis cine (i) the mid ventricular short-axis pilot (g; e (Figure 2.12)) is used to position the slice through the maximum lateral dimensions of both ventricles and avoid the left ventricular outflow tract as illustrated by panels (g) and (h). To acquire the VLA cine (k), the mid ventricular short-axis pilot is again used and placed in the plane as indicated in panel (j).

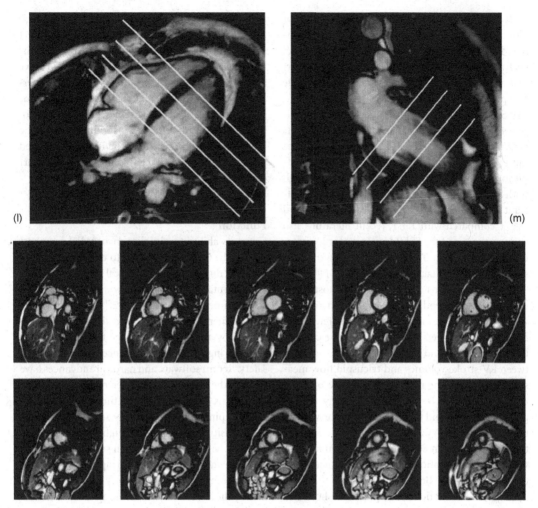

Figure 2.14 This figure demonstrates the resultant horizontal long axis (l), VLA (m) and short-axis cine stack from base to apex (bottom panel).

groove. The distance between the slices is chosen such that they encompass the basal, mid and apical regions of the left ventricle. These "scout" images can then be used to plan cine images in two long-axis (HLA, VLA), and LVOT views.

When acquiring the short axis volume stack from the two long-axis cines, the position of the basal slice is critical. Most errors in volume calculation are introduced here if this stage is not carefully planned. Using the end-diastolic frames from the VLA and HLA cines, the first slice is placed in the atrioventricular (AV) groove. Subsequent slices are placed parallel to this covering the entire left ventricle. Typically slice thickness is 7–8 mm with a 3 or 2 mm inter-slice gap. Imaging is usually performed in expiration as this generally produces a more consistent, reproducible breath-hold position.

Volume and mass data is calculated by drawing epicardial and endocardial regions of interest (ROI) at end-systole and end-diastole. Papillary muscles and trabeculae should be included in mass calculation and excluded from ventricular volumes. Various programs are available to aid calculation of these values, e.g., ARGUS® (Siemens Medical Solutions), and MASS®, (Medis, Netherlands). Normal, gender specific values for left and right ventricular volumes and mass in adults have been defined [13]. Earlier studies used a gradient echo approach, such as a turboFLASH sequence, which has inferior blood/myocardial contrast definition when compared to newer steady state acquisition techniques such as TrueFISP. Recent studies have provided normal volume and mass ranges using steady state free precession (SSFP) sequences [12]. These show that SSFP sequences produce larger ventricular volumes and smaller ventricular mass measurements (when compared to gradient echo sequences) in the same reference population due to the improved definition of the blood-endocardial border. Although both SSFP and turboFLASH sequences show significant SNR increases in the myocardium and blood at 3 T compared with 1.5 T, recent literature also support the use of the SSFP sequences for LV functional assessment at 3T (notwithstanding the possibility of more artifacts with SSFP at 3 T) [14].

CMR is also considered to be the most accurate imaging method for the evaluation of right ventricular (RV) volumes. CMR measurement of RV volumes has been validated with close correlation between RV and LV stroke volumes, and between RV stroke volumes and tricuspid flow measurements [15]. The inherent 3D nature of CMR makes it particularly well suited to study the RV given its complex and variable (even in normal volunteers) morphology [16]. CMR measurements of the RV volumes can either be acquired in a transverse (axial) orientation or in an axis aligned along the LV short axis. Both methods have their advantages and limitations. Using the LV short axis plane, only one data set is required for both LV and RV measurements. In addition, in the images acquired using the axial orientation, the partial volume effect of blood and myocardium on the inferior wall of the RV can make it difficult to identify the blood/myocardial boundary. However, assessment of the RV in the (LV) short axis orientation also has important limitations: the position of the pulmonary and tricuspid valves cannot be clearly identified and therefore, the basal boundary of the RV can be difficult to define. This can result in significant error because the basal slice has a large area. In a recent study that compared the two methods for RV volume measurements, Alfakih *et al.* found that the there were systematic differences between them, and that the axial orientation resulted in better inter- and intraobserver reproducibility [17]. An alternative method has been proposed by Strugnell

et al. (the "modified RV short axis series"), where the short axis slice is oriented to the outflow tract of the right ventricle [18]. This new method potentially improves visualization of the tricuspid valve and makes analysis easier and less prone to operator error than the current standard technique for CMR assessment of RV volumes. However, use of this method is more time consuming and may be limited to indications where the RV volumes need precise measurement (e.g., adult congenital heart disease).

Dynamic Measures of Left Ventricular Function

Given its ability to visualize myocardial segments accurately, CMR can be used to define ventricular function during pharmacological stress, principally with dobutamine (DMR). Although DMR imaging has been performed since 1992 [19], early studies to document inducible myocardial ischemia were limited by an inability to image the entire cardiac cycle during peak stress and concerns about patient safety. Recent software and hardware advances have enabled the investigators to overcome most of these limitations. Shorter repetition times, phase encoding grouping and phased array surface coils allow for acquisition of images with high temporal resolution and with spatial resolution sufficient to delineate the endocardial border during peak stress [20]. Earlier concerns of patient safety have been alleviated by the introduction of hemodynamic monitoring and wall motion display software that allows the physician to safely monitor patients during stress testing.

Practical Aspects of DMR Imaging

In preparation for a DMR study patients are instructed to refrain from taking any β-blockers and nitrates 24 hours prior to the examination. Short acting β-blocker (e.g., Esmolol 0.5 mg/kg) is used as an antidote and should be easily accessible during scanning. Table 2.2 details the monitoring requirements needed for stress MR imaging. As with its use in other cardiac imaging, severe arterial hypertension (>220/120 mmHg), recent acute coronary syndrome, significant aortic stenosis, complex cardiac arrhythmias, and significant hypertrophic obstructive cardiomyopathy are some of the contraindications to the use of dobutamine stress testing.

Table 2.2   Monitoring requirements needed for stress MR imaging.

Heart rate and rhythm	Continuously
Blood pressure	Every minute
Pulse oximetry	Continuously
Symptoms	Continuously
Wall motion abnormalities	Every dose increment

Scan protocol: All 17 segments of the heart can be covered by a combination of three SA and two long-axis views (HLA, VLA). The SA and 2 long-axis cines are performed at rest and are also repeated during stress at each dobutamine dose. Scans are terminated when the submaximal heart rate is reached, systolic blood pressure decreases >20 mmHg below baseline, blood pressure increases >240/120 mmHg, intractable symptoms, new or worsening wall motion abnormalities occur in at least two adjacent left ventricular segments, or in the presence of complex cardiac arrhythmias.

Image interpretation: Multiple cine loop display is recommended, showing at least four different stress levels for each slice simultaneously. The ventricle is analyzed by 17 segments per stress level [21]. Analysis is carried out visually according to the standards suggested by the American Society of Echocardiography. Segmental wall motion is classified as normokinetic, hypokinetic, akinetic, or dyskinetic and assigned one to four points, respectively. The sum of points is divided by the number of analyzed segments and yields the wall motion score. Normal contraction results in a wall motion score of one, a higher score is indicative of wall motion abnormalities. During dobutamine stress with increasing doses, a lack of increase in either wall motion or systolic wall thickening, a reduction of both, or significant changes in the rotational pattern of left ventricular myocardium ("tethering") are indicative of pathological findings. Nagel *et al.* compared DMR imaging to dobutamine stress echocardiography (DSE) in patients referred for diagnostic coronary angiography [22]. They showed that DMR imaging provided superior specificity (86% vs 70%) and sensitivity (89% vs 74%) in detecting coronary stenosis >50%, principally as the number of myocardial segments visualized as "good" or "very good" image quality was far greater

with DMR than with DSE. Among patients with regional wall motion defects at rest, DMR has been shown to have a sensitivity of 89% and specificity of 85% for identifying coronary artery stenosis greater than 50% [23]. Recently, prognostic and safety information has been published that compares this favorably with more established modalities [24].

Tissue Contractility
Beyond analysis of global and segmental function, MR offers techniques for assessment of regional and tissue contractility (Figure 2.15).

MR tagging: This method was first developed by Zerhouni and colleagues [25]. A radio-frequency tag is a region within the imaged tissue where the net magnetization has been altered with radio-frequency pulses. Each tag or "saturation grid" is created as a 3D plane that extends through the tissue, and it is seen as a tag line when imaged in an orthogonal view. Typical tagging schemes include stacks of parallel lines [26], grids [27], and radial stripes [28]. By tracking material points as a function of time, it is possible to compute the description of motion around a given point in the tissue as it traverses through time and space. Although the concept of radio-frequency tagging has been proposed over a decade ago, automated software to analyze the images has only recently become available [29,30], and the clinical use of the method remains to be determined.

Tissue velocity mapping and DENSE: The tissue phase mapping technique allows the determination of three-dimensional velocity tensors over the cardiac cycle, i.e., for rotation, radial and longitudinal movement, with a pixel-by-pixel spatial resolution nearing that of "conventional" cine MRI [31]. This has been investigated in clinical studies in both patients and volunteers, and newer navigator sequences (obviating the need for breath-holding, and hence with the potential for improving spatial resolution) have been developed [32]. Displacement encoded imaging using stimulated echoes (DENSE) can also provide information on myocardial displacement, velocity and strain [33].

Assessment of Myocardial Viability
Viability assessment can be defined practically as detecting myocardium that shows severe dysfunction at rest, but which will improve function,

either spontaneously with time (stunned) or following revascularization (hibernating). The identification of residual myocardial viability is critical to the management of patients with ischemic heart disease. Contrast-enhanced MRI (ceMRI) with gadolinium-DTPA was described in 1984 in a canine model of acute MI [34]. Injured myocardium demonstrates significantly greater T_1 shortening after contrast. These initial studies however, were hampered by insufficient image contrast between normal and injured myocardium due to technical (e.g., gradients, phased array) and sequence limitations.

Delayed Enhancement MRI

In recent years, a number of studies have demonstrated the effectiveness of a segmented inversion recovery fast gradient echo (seg IR-GE) sequence for differentiating irreversible injured from normal myocardium with signal intensity differences of nearly 500% [35]. This technique of delayed enhancement imaging (DE-MRI), pioneered by Simonetti, Kim, and Judd, has been shown in animal and human studies, to identify the presence, location, and extent of acute and chronic myocardial irreversible injury [36–39]. The development of the late gadolinium enhancement CMR technique (LGE-CMR) [35] has revolutionized the role of CMR in clinical and research practice and has potential roles in both diagnosis and prognosis of newly diagnosed coronary artery disease/heart failure patients. Specific patterns of fibrosis and scarring have been identified in many of the cardiomyopathy states [40–43]. Delayed enhancement MRI (DE-MRI), allows assessment of the transmural extent of irreversible injury, and is superior to SPECT for the identification of subendocardial myocardial infarction [44–46]. Furthermore, it permits quantification of even small areas of myocardial necrosis, both due to native coronary disease and, after percutaneous and surgical revascularization [47–49].

Practical Aspects of Delayed Enhancement Image Acquisition

Delayed enhancement imaging can be performed in a single brief examination, requiring only a peripheral intravenous line. It does not require pharmacological or physiological stress. Initially cine images are obtained to provide a matched assessment of left ventricular (LV) contractile function. A bolus of 0.10–0.20 mmol/kg intravenous gadolinium chelate is then given by hand injection. After a 10- to 15-minute delay (see below), high spatial resolution delayed enhancement images of the heart are obtained at the same imaging planes as the cine images using the seg IR-GE pulse sequence. Each delayed enhancement image is acquired during a 8- to 14-second breath-hold, and the imaging time for the entire examination (including cine imaging) is generally 30–40 minutes. Figure 2.16 demonstrates two patient examples.

Segmented Inversion Recovery Fast Gradient Echo Sequence

The timing diagram for the seg IR-GE pulse sequence is shown in Figure 2.17. Immediately after the onset of the R wave trigger, there is a delay period before a nonselective 180° inversion pulse is applied. Following this inversion pulse, a second variable wait period (usually referred to as the inversion time or TI), occurs corresponding to the time between the inversion pulse and the center of acquisition of k-space lines. The flip angle used for radio-frequency excitation for each k-space line is shallow (20–30°) to retain regional differences in magnetization that result from the inversion pulse and TI delay.

The following factors need to be considered when performing DE-MRI:

Dose: The dose of gadolinium given is usually 0.1–0.2 mmol/kg. Early validation studies used doses as high as 0.3 mmol/kg in animal models [50] and 0.2 mmol/kg in patients [38]. Sufficient time is required in order to allow the blood pool signal in the LV cavity to decline and provide discernment between LV cavity and hyperenhanced myocardium. This is particularly important in imaging small subendocardial infarcts, and when using a higher dose (i.e., 0.2 mmol/kg).

Gating factor: Image contrast is also optimized by applying the inversion pulse every other heartbeat in order to allow for adequate longitudinal relaxation between successive 180° inversion pulses. If there are limitations related to breath-hold duration and/or bradycardia, every heartbeat imaging may have to be performed. In this situation there may be

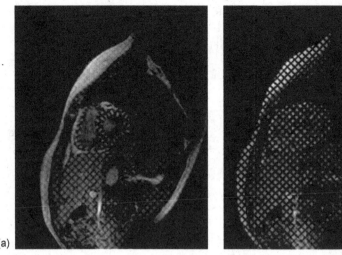

(a)

(b)

Figure 2.15 Cardiac tagging short axis images obtained in a normal heart using a complementary spatial modulation of magnetization (CSPAMM) technique. The initial rectangular tagging grid at end-diastole (a) is distorted by cardiac contraction, as seen in the end-systolic image (b).

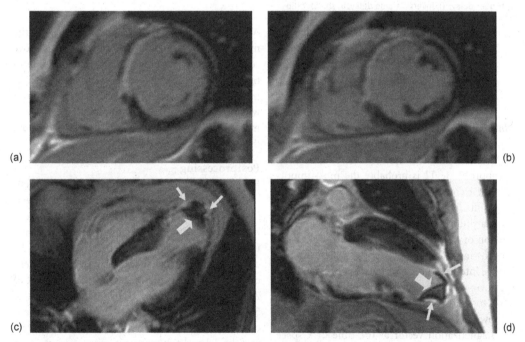

(a)

(b)

(c)

(d)

Figure 2.16 Two patient examples of delayed hyperenhancement (DHE) imaged with a segmented inversion recovery gradient echo sequence at 10 minutes post Gd-DTPA injection (0.1 mmol/kg). Panels (a) and (b) demonstrate anteroseptal DHE in a patient presenting with 2-week-old anterior myocardial infarction and proximal left anterior descending artery (LAD) occlusion. Panels (c) and (d) are from a patient with history of apical myocardial infarction 12 months prior and mid LAD occlusion, showing thinned apical wall with fully transmural DHE (small arrows). Coexistent apical thrombus is also seen in this patient (block arrows).

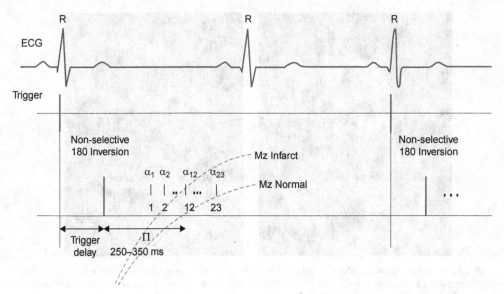

Figure 2.17 Timing diagram of two-dimensional segmented inversion-recovery fast gradient echo pulse sequence. (ECG, electrocardiogram; RF, radio frequency; TD, trigger delay; TI, inversion time delay; α, shallow flip angle excitation) See text for further details. (Reproduced from Simonetti *et al.* [35], with permission from the publishers.)

incomplete relaxation of normal myocardium. Incomplete relaxation will result in not only an artificially shorter "effective" TI needed to null normal myocardium, but may also lead to a reduction in the image intensity differences between infarcted and normal myocardium.

Inversion time (TI): This is defined as the time between the 180° pulse and the center of acquisition of the *k*-space lines. Selecting the appropriate TI is probably the most important element in obtaining accurate imaging results. The TI is chosen to "null" normal myocardium, the time at which the magnetization of normal myocardium reaches the zero crossing (Figure 2.17). This is when the image intensity difference between infarcted and normal myocardium is maximized. If the TI is too short, normal myocardium will be below the zero crossing and will have a negative magnetization vector at the time of *k*-space data acquisition. Since the image intensity corresponds to the magnitude of the magnetization vector, the image intensity of normal myocardium will increase as the TI becomes shorter and shorter, whereas the image intensity of infarcted myocardium will decrease until it reaches its own zero crossing.

At the other extreme, if the TI is set too long, the magnetization of normal myocardium will be above zero and will appear gray. Although areas of infarction will have high image intensity, the relative contrast between infarcted and normal myocardium will be reduced. All CMR platforms now have automated TI finding sequences can help is establishing the optimal inversion time.

Postprocessing

For routine clinical reporting, the 17-segment model recommended by the American Heart Association can be used [21]. The extent of hyperenhanced tissue within each segment is graded visually using a 5-point scale in which a score of 0 indicates no hyperenhancement; 1, hyperenhancement of 1–25% of the segment; 2, hyperenhancement of 26–50% of the segment; 3, hyperenhancement of 51–75% of the segment; and 4, hyperenhancement of 76–100% of the segment. It is advisable to interpret the delayed enhancement images with the cine images immediately adjacent which provide a reference of the diastolic wall thickness of each region.

Myocardial Perfusion

Contrast agents based on paramagnetism (e.g., gadolinium) or superparamagnetism (e.g., Fe^{2+}) can be tracked as they traverse the myocardium after intravenous injection to assess myocardial perfusion at rest and with a vasodilator (e.g., adenosine). Quantitative results have been achieved in animal studies with an intravascular agent such as a macromolecular blood pool marker, although such compounds are not yet licensed for use in humans. At the same time, semi-quantitative/quantitative approaches are feasible in humans with a conventional extra-cellular MR contrast agent (Gd-DTPA).

First Pass Imaging

CMR perfusion imaging during first pass injection of a Gadolinium chelate contrast agent bolus was introduced in early 1990s [1,2]. CMR first pass perfusion has rapidly grown since its introduction with further advances in the image acquisition and analysis of the acquired data. The main advantages of MR first pass myocardial perfusion are the high spatial resolution and lack of radiation exposure allowing repeated studies. The spatial resolution is high enough to appreciate perfusion changes in the subendocardial region which is most sensitive to early changes in myocardial blood flow.

In first pass imaging a bolus of contrast agent is injected directly into a peripheral vein and a sequence of images is then obtained to show the dynamic passage of the tracer through the heart (Figure 2.18). Previous studies evaluating the utility of perfusion CMR in evaluating CAD have found moderate–high diagnostic accuracy [51,52]. A recent meta-analysis by Nandalur et al. showed overall sensitivity of 91% and specificity of 0.81% for CMR perfusion imaging in the diagnosis of CAD compared to quantitative coronary angiography [26]. Recent work has also shown that diagnostic accuracy from first pass CMR perfusion imaging can be further augmented by using a higher field strength (increased signal to noise, increased sensitivity) [53] and/or by combining perfusion with late gadolinium enhancement (reduced misreads due to artifact, increased specificity) [54].

MR Sequences & Contrast Agents

The most significant parameter that a perfusion sequence must optimize is the temporal resolution as the contrast agent only spends a relatively short period of time passing through the myocardium. During this time the required data must be obtained at a sufficient rate so that the reconstructed images provide a measure of the change in contrast agent concentration over time. For a complete perfusion study, up-to three to five separate short axis slices need to be simultaneously obtained to achieve sufficient coverage of the myocardium. The most commonly used perfusion sequences are turboFLASH, SSFP, multishot echo planar (EPI), and hybrid EPI-gradient echo (GRE) sequences. Fast T_1 weighted imaging sequences such as spoiled gradient-echo imaging with TRs as short as 2 ms and a magnetization preparation (either inversion recovery or saturation recovery) for T_1 weighting are applied to image the contrast enhancement during the first pass of contrast agent.

The most common compound bolus used is an extra-cellular MR contrast agent such as Gd-DTPA. Rapid contrast injection is crucial as this improves the sensitivity for detecting changes in myocardial perfusion [55]. The goal is to assure that the primary bottleneck to the rate of contrast enhancement is the rate of transport of the contrast through the myocardial tissue and not the rate at which the contrast agent is injected. The regional image intensity contrast enhancement should ideally be proportional to the contrast agent concentration. Such an approximate linear relationship between regional signal intensity and contrast agent concentration is only observed at lower contrast agent dosages-typically, <0.05 mol/kg of Gd-DTPA for fast IR-prepared gradient echo sequences (TR <3 ms; TE < 2 ms) [56].

Vasodilator Stress

A complete discussion on the effects of adenosine/diapyridamole is beyond the scope of this chapter. Briefly, vasodilation with dipyridamole or adenosine induces an increase of blood flow in myocardial areas supplied by normal coronary arteries ("coronary steal"), whereas no (or only minimal) change is found in areas supplied by stenotic coronary arteries. With adenosine a maximal coronary vasodilation can be achieved safely with an intravenous infusion at a rate of 140 µg/kg/min. For cardiac imaging 4–6 minutes of infusion are recommended. The vasodilatory effect of adenosine may result in a mild-to-moderate reduction in systolic, diastolic and mean arterial blood pressure (<10 mmHg) with a reflex increase in heart

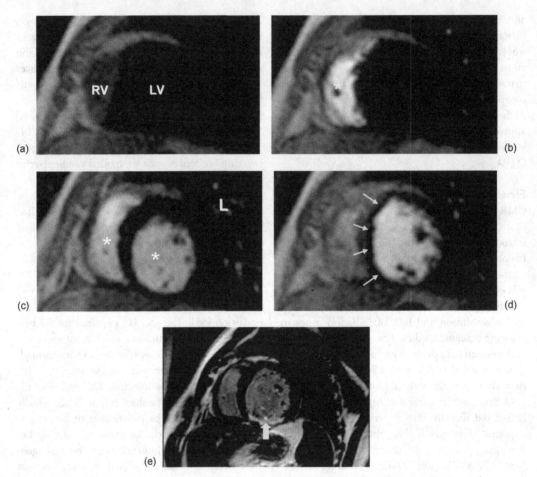

Figure 2.18 Example of cardiac magnetic resonance perfusion images obtained with a turboFLASH sequence during first pass rapid injection of an extra-cellular contrast agent (Gd-DTPA). Images were acquired in a basal short-axis view, and show (a) before contrast injection, (b) the contrast agent first in the right ventricle, (c) contrast agent then the lungs and left ventricle and (d) agent in the left ventricle cavity and myocardium. Perfusion defect is seen in the antero-septum, infero-septum, and inferior wall (arrows). Corresponding "delayed enhancement" image (e) is shown at the same slice position, demonstrating inferior wall delayed hyperenhancement (block arrow). Patient had evidence of significant left anterior descending artery (LAD) and right coronary artery (RCA) disease. L, lungs; LV, left ventricle; RV, right ventricle; single asterisk (*), contrast agent.

rate. Although some patients may complain about anginal chest pain or dyspnea, these effects respond promptly to discontinuation of the drug and usually do not require medical intervention. Studies in over 10,000 patients during thallium radionuclide imaging, echocardiography, SPECT and MRI have shown that pharmacological stress testing with adenosine presents a safe method of acquiring stress imaging data [51,57]. However, adenosine should be used with caution in patients with pre-existing atrioventricular (AV) block or bundle branch block and should be avoided in patients with high-grade AV block, sinus node dysfunction or reversible airways obstruction (e.g., asthma).

Practical Aspects of Image Acquisition

An intravenous line should be started before the examination for administration of the contrast agent. A16G or 18G peripheral needle is usually sufficient together with a power injector at a rate of 5–10 mL/second. Contrast administration needs to be followed without delay by an injection of physiologic saline solution to assure that the entire contrast agent dose is injected into the vein.

Monitoring of the patients' blood pressure, heart rate, and, preferably, also the arterial oxygen saturation is recommended.

Practical tips that aid successful perfusion imaging:

1 The recommended contrast agent dose varies from 0.02 mmol/kg to 0.1 mmol/kg Gd-DTPA depending on the sequence used and the type of assessment needed (quantitative versus qualitative).

2 Double oblique slices that give a short axis view of the heart are recommended. For multislice acquisitions the interslice gap should be 30–50% of the chosen slice thickness. Slice positions are customarily chosen to cover the location of wall motion defects that are detected on the cine imaging usually performed before hand.

3 Minimize the field of view without causing aliasing ("wrap around") artifacts. It is our practice to perform a test image (without contrast) to determine any wrap artifact and adjust the slice position accordingly. Choosing the read-out direction parallel to the chest wall often reduces the likelihood of aliasing and other artifacts.

4 Perform the scan with the patient holding their breath in inspiration. Begin the scan as soon as the patient starts the breath-hold, and the contrast agent injection can be started after acquisition of 3–5 "baseline" images.

Qualitative Analysis and Visualization

Most recent literature (both single [53,54] and multicenter studies [58]) evaluating the diagnostic accuracy of first pass perfusion methods has been published using visual assessment: experience is required to reach an acceptable standard. The main artifacts occurring during the initial passage of the contrast bolus are due to susceptibility at the endocardium blood–pool interface, sometimes making diagnosis of subendocardial perfusion deficits difficult. The trabeculae of the papillary muscles are especially prone to susceptibility artifacts and such findings should not be interpreted as evidence of a regional ischemic perfusion abnormality.

Semi-quantitative Analysis

Here the endo- and epicardial contours of left ventricular myocardium are traced and corrected manually for changes of diaphragmatic position due to breathing or diaphragmatic drift. The myocardium is then divided into 6–8 equiangular segments per slice, and an additional region of interest is placed within the cavity of the left ventricle excluding the myocardial segments and the papillary muscles (Figures 2.19 and 2.20). Images acquired after premature ventricular beats or insufficient cardiac triggering need to be excluded from the analysis to guarantee steady-state conditions. Signal intensity is determined for all dynamics and segments. The upslope of the resulting signal intensity time curve is determined by the use of a linear fit. To correct for possible differences of the input function, the results of the myocardial segments are corrected by dividing the upslope of each myocardial segment by the upslope of the left ventricular signal intensity curve. Perfusion reserve index is calculated by dividing the results of stress imaging by the results obtained at rest.

Quantitative Analysis

In recent years, first pass CMR perfusion techniques have been shown to measure myocardial blood flow quantitatively and has been validated against microspheres in animal models [15,16] In assessment of quantitative myocardial blood flow number of tracer kinetic models has been used which includes models such as Fermi Function model [14,18] and Kety-Schmidt model [19,20]. However these models have varying complexity and assumptions to calculate the myocardial blood flow from the measured data. This raises the question of which model is appropriate in which situation since all the assumptions may not hold true in all situations. Recently Jerosch-Herold *et al.* proposed a model independent deconvolution method to quantify myocardial perfusion from first pass CMR and validated this against perfusion with radioisotope labeled microspheres [15]. Theoretical basis for the model-independent deconvolution comes from central volume principal which was originally introduced by Zierler [21,22]. So far, only one study has compared quantitative CMR perfusion against positron emission tomography (PET) in the clinical setting [17]. In this study, in healthy human volunteers, there was a significant correlation for both dipyridamole-induced flow and myocardial perfusion reserve (MPR) between CMR and PET. However, there was a systematic bias, such that CMR provided lower MPR values compared to PET (2.5

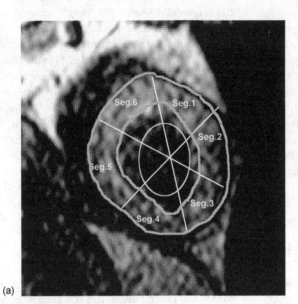

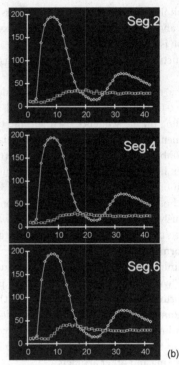

Figure 2.19 A T_1-weighted gradient-echo image in the short-axis view is shown with user-traced endo- and epicardial contours, and region of interest in the center of the left ventricle (LV) cavity. The LV wall was subdivided into six transmural myocardial segments that are arranged in circumferential order, starting at the anterior junction of the right ventricle and LV, which serves here as an anatomical landmark (a). SI in each segment is compared with SI curves of left ventricular cavity (b). SI is given in arbitrary units. (Reproduced from Al-Saadi et al., Circulation 2000;101:1379, with permission from the publishers.)

± 1.0 vs 4.3 ± 1.8). More clinical studies are currently underway to compare CMR absolute perfusion with the established gold standard-positron emission tomography—at both 1.5 T and 3 T.

Some researchers have also used double bolus technique for first pass CMR perfusion rather than single bolus for quatitative analysis of perfusion. It is suggested that double bolus technique provides less distortions of the LV cavity signal intensity and thereby allowing accurate depiction of the arterial input function [23]. Quantitative myocardial perfusion using double bolus first pass CMR perfusion has been validated in animal model against microspheres [23] and shown to differentiate hyperemic blood flow in healthy human subjects [24].

Noncontrast Perfusion and BOLD Sequences

Spin labeling techniques exploit the labeling of the nuclear magnetization of water protons, either by direct preparation of inflowing spins or by specific preparation of the imaging slice. In both cases, water is used a free diffusible contrast agent. Although easily repeatable, arterial spin labeling techniques applied at 1.5-T yield only a relatively small signal difference between normal and under-perfused myocardium (44% in a recent study by Wacker et al. [59]), but these techniques may become more practical when applied at higher field.

Blood oxygenation level–dependent (BOLD) MRI may overcome the tracer kinetic limitations of first pass perfusion imaging by observing changes in tissue oxygenation directly. BOLD utilizes the T_2^* effect, that is the incoherence in the phase behavior due to local inhomogenities in the magnetic field. Wacker and colleagues were the first to show that dipyridamole was associated with an increase of T_2^* in healthy volunteers but with a T_2^* decrease in patients with stenotic coronary arteries [60]. Although significant progress is being made

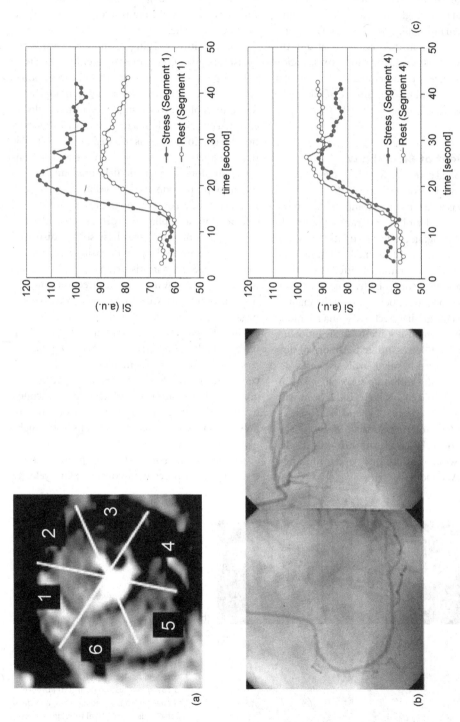

Figure 2.20 Segmentation of the myocardium into six equiangular segments per slice, starting clockwise from the anterior septal insertion point of the right ventricle (a). Coronary angiogram of the patient showing critical right coronary artery stenosis (b). In the normally perfused anterior segment, there is a clear increase of the upslope after adenosine (●) when compared with rest (○), whereas in the inferior segment of the same slice there is no change of the upslope after vasodilation (c). (Reproduced from Nagel et al. [51], with permission from the publishers.)

[59,61], BOLD imaging is not yet ready for clinical application to the heart as it is currently only possible to analyze single slices and the T_2^* signal differences remain small. The arrival of 3T systems hold much promise in this regard, as at 3 T the blood T_2 is much more sensitive to its oxygenation level than it is at 1.5 T, consequently intravascular contrast (a significant mechanism for BOLD in the myocardium) will be increased at 3 T.

Measurement of Blood Flow

Velocity-encoded cine (VENC) MR imaging allows accurate estimation of velocity profiles across a valve or any vascular structure, comparable to those provided by Doppler ultrasonography [62,63]. In addition, MR imaging is able to quantify flow volumes and does not have the same limitations with respect to acoustic penetration of different portions of the heart and therefore is better able to demonstrate distribution and velocity of flow throughout the heart. On cine gradient-echo MR images, blood has bright signal intensity due to fresh inflowing blood that has not been saturated. Abnormal flow patterns encountered in valvular disease cause dephasing of the spins within a voxel and result in signal loss (flow void). This flow void is seen with either stenosis or regurgitation and is caused by high-velocity flow and turbulence [64]. Its appearance depends on technical factors including display parameters (window width and level), flip angle and TE [65]. With long-TE sequences (12 ms), the

flow void is well demonstrated, whereas with short-TE sequences (<7 ms), it tends to be smaller. These variables must be taken into account when evaluating flow anomalies.

Flow-sensitive imaging techniques permit the measurement of flow expressed as either velocity or volume per unit of time. Currently, the most popular flow-sensitive cine MR imaging technique is referred to as phase-contrast, phase-shift, or velocity encoded (VENC) MR imaging. As described in Section Image Contrast, this is based on the principle that the phase of flowing spins relative to stationary spins along a magnetic field gradient changes in direct proportion to flow velocity. Magnitude images can be reconstructed to provide anatomical information, and phase images can provide flow velocity information. The phase shift is displayed as variations in pixel signal intensity on the phase map image. Stationary tissue appears gray on this image, whereas flow in a positive direction along the flow-encoding axis will appear bright and flow in a negative direction will appear dark (Figure 2.21). As a result, it is possible to differentiate antegrade from retrograde flow. Furthermore, as with Doppler ultrasonography, the phase map image can be color-coded to reinforce the differentiation between antegrade and retrograde flow. Velocity can be encoded in planes that are perpendicular to the direction of flow by using section-selective direction (through-plane velocity measurement), in planes that are parallel to the direction of flow by using phase-encoded or frequency-encoded directions (in-plane velocity

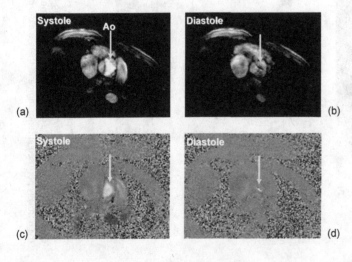

(a)

(b)

(c)

(d)

Figure 2.21 Transverse velocity encoded magnetic resonance magnitude (a and b) and phase (c and d) images centered on the aortic valve in a patient with severe aortic regurgitation. In systole (a and c), the leaflets are open and bright signal, indicating anterograde flow (arrows). In diastole (b and d) absence of coaptation is demonstrated, and dark signal indicates central retrograde flow. In this image (d), there is also adjoining lighter area due to aliasing effects.

measurement), or, more recently, in 3D. However, VENC MR imaging also has certain limitations and potential sources of error [66]. Because of the cyclic nature of phase, aliasing may appear if more than one cycle of phase shift occurs. To avoid aliasing, which occurs when the chosen velocity range is lower than the predicted maximum velocity, the velocity threshold must be correctly selected prior to acquisition.

VEC MR imaging can be used to calculate absolute velocity at any given time during the cardiac cycle at specified locations in the plane of data acquisition. Velocity can be measured for each pixel within a region of interest encircling all or part of the cross-sectional vessel area or across a valve annulus. The product of cross-sectional area (as determined from the magnitude image) and spatial mean velocity (i.e., the average velocity for all pixels in the cross-sectional area on the phase image) yields the instantaneous flow volume for each time frame during the cardiac cycle. Integration of all instantaneous flow volumes throughout the cardiac cycle yields the flow volume per heartbeat. This technique has been evaluated in vitro as well as in vivo by several authors and allows accurate measurement of aortic and pulmonary arterial flow, which represent the stroke volumes of the left and right ventricles, respectively [67]. It has also been used to calculate the ratio of pulmonary to systemic flow, thereby allowing noninvasive quantification of left-to-right shunts [68] and separate measurement of right and left pulmonary flows [69]. Moreover, these measurements can be used in the evaluation and quantitative assessment of valvular regurgitation and stenosis.

MR Angiographic Techniques

In recent years there has been considerable interest in magnetic resonance angiography (MRA) in which images of blood vessels are produced without detail from surrounding stationary tissue. MRA techniques fall into three broad categories: time of flight (TOF), phase contrast, and contrast-enhanced MRA. These have applications in imaging various vessels, particularly the aorta, carotids, renals, and peripheral arteries.

Time of Flight MRA (TOF MRA): Time of Flight MRA relies on the flow of fully relaxed material into the imaged volume for image contrast (see earlier section on image contrast). Fast gradient echo imaging is commonly used to perform 2D or 3D TOF MRA. In the former, thin slices are acquired one at a time, while in the latter, a volume is excited by the radio-frequency (RF) pulse.

Phase Contrast MRA: Phase contrast MRA relies on changes in the phase of the transverse magnetization induced by the application of a bipolar, flow sensitized gradient, which generate a phase difference between the stationary tissues and the moving blood. Phase contrast angiography has effective background suppression and provides quantitative flow measurements, but the acquisition time is long and the technique is only sensitive to a certain range of blood velocities.

Contrast-enhanced MRA (CE-MRA): This has become an increasingly popular angiographic technique over recently as it can be acquired during a single breath-hold, and hence has particular advantages in imaging areas of major respiratory motion such as the thorax and abdomen. The appropriate intravenous injection of Gd-DTPA leads to substantial local blood signal enhancement due to the shortening of the T_1 relaxation time of blood. Timing of the scan with respect to the intravenous bolus is critical for data collection. Consequently, it is good practice to administer a "test bolus" to estimate the contrast arrival time at the targeted vessel. Contrast-enhanced MRA is the preferred MRA technique for the evaluation of aortic aneurysms, pulmonary arterial disease, peripheral arterial disease, and renal disease. Renal CE-MRA is indicated in patients with hypertension to exclude vascular causes, and in patients with worsening renal function to exclude bilateral renal artery stenosis.

Coronary and Bypass Graft Imaging

The epicardial coronary arteries are small structures demanding images of high spatial resolution. For such high resolution imaging the need for high signal to noise (SNR) and contrast to noise (CNR) ratios often means prolonged imaging time. However, longer imaging time makes the image vulnerable to motion-related blurring, artifact and image degradation. Hence, adequate cardiac and respiratory motion suppression (see earlier section) is imperative for artifact free coronary imaging.

The principal sequences used for coronary imaging (summarized below) utilize the "time of flight" angiography principle that was mentioned above. "Black blood" coronary MRA takes advantage of the negative contrast between flowing coronary blood and surrounding tissues. "Black blood" methods may be particularly useful for patients with bypass grafts or intracoronary stents, as they are less sensitive to metallic implant susceptibility artifacts than gradient echo ("bright blood") imaging.

Contrast to noise ratio can also be improved by the use of MR contrast agents. Gadolinium based agents considerably reduce the T_1 relaxation time of blood resulting in an improved differentiation between coronary blood and the adjoining myocardium. Imaging can be done using saturation recovery or inversion recovery prepulses. Extracellular agents appear best suited to first pass breath-hold approaches, whereas intravascular contrast agents may be best for longer navigator/free-breathing CMRA.

Proximal coronary artery visualization has been the main aim of CMRA since initial studies were performed more than 10 years ago [70,71]. This showed that visualization is possible of proximal segments in a majority of motivated volunteers and patients. Two most commonly used techniques for CMRA performed at various CMR centers are briefly described below (Figure 2.22). A full discus-

sion of all the available techniques is beyond the scope of this chapter, but is available elsewhere.

3D segmented k-space gradient echo CMRA: First described by Li [70] and Botnar [72], this technique takes advantage of superior SNR and post processing capabilities of 3D imaging and provides high spatial resolution. As the data acquisition period is long, exceeding standard breath-hold duration, navigators are needed for respiratory gating. The use of T_2 preparatory pulses are also needed to enhance CNR and facilitate better identification of the coronary arteries from underlying tissue.

3D segmented k-space Echoplanar CMRA: Fast breath-hold or free-breathing 3D EPI coronary MRA, two to four excitation pulses are followed by a short EPI readout train [73,74]. This takes the advantage of the EPI speed while keeping the echo and acquisition time short to minimize blood flow and motion related artifacts.

Bypass Grafts: Early CMR studies for bypass graft assessment used nonrespiratory compensated, ECG triggered 2D spin echo and gradient echo techniques. Current approaches (often used in combination) can be broadly divided into techniques that assess patency, such as turbo spin echo (e.g., HASTE) and MR angiography, and those that assess graft flow reserve which can give information

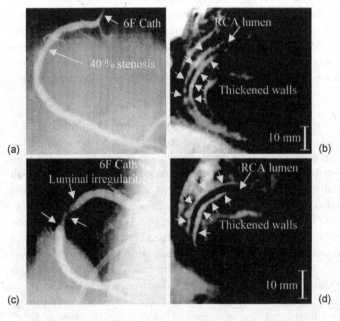

Figure 2.22 Black-blood 3D cardiac magnetic resonance vessel wall scans (b and d) demonstrate an irregularly thickened right coronary artery (RCA) wall (>2 mm) indicative of an increased atherosclerotic plaque burden. The inner and outer RCA walls are indicated by the yellow dotted arrows. Comparison is made with the corresponding diagnostic X-ray angiographic images (a and c). (Reproduced from Kim *et al.*, *Circulation* 2002;106:296, with permission from the publishers.)

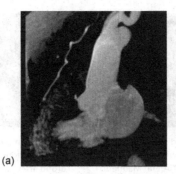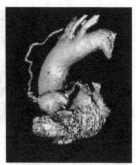

Figure 2.23 Contrast-enhanced MR angiogram of a patent LIMA graft 6 months post surgery. Acquisition of a 3D data set allows postprocessing with multiplanar reformation and maximum intensity projection (a). Surface rendered image is shown on panel (b) (images courtesy of Drs O. Mohrs and T. Voigtlaender, Frankfurt/Main, Germany).　(a)

(b)

about graft stenosis. 3D MR angiography using rapid contrast injection (after initially performing a timing sequence to determine the onset of peak Gadolinium-DTPA enhancement) is the preferred technique for assessing graft patency. Acquisition of a 3D data set allows postprocessing with multiplanar reformation and maximum intensity projection to identify grafts. Surface rendering of this 3D data set is also possible (see Figure 2.23).

Despite recent advances in technique development, MR coronary angiography at 1.5 T produces (at best) in-plane resolution of around 0.7 mm, which is inferior to that obtained with invasive X-ray coronary angiography (around 0.3 mm). As such, currently, it cannot replace the latter for routine clinical use.

Atherosclerosis Imaging

High-resolution MR has emerged as the leading in vivo imaging modality for atherosclerotic plaque characterization given the inherent advantages of noninvasiveness and high spatial resolution. MR differentiates plaque components on the basis of biophysical and biochemical parameters such as chemical composition and concentration, water content, physical state, molecular motion, or diffusion.

Since detected MR signals rely on the relaxation times T_1 and T_2 and on proton density, the MR images can be "weighted" to the T_1, T_2, or proton density values through adaptation of the imaging parameters (such as repetition time and echo time). For example, in a T_1-weighted (T1w) image, tissues with lower T_1 values will produce pixels with high signal intensity. Conversely, tissues with a longer T_2 relaxation time will appear hyperintense in a T_2-weighted (T2w) image. In a proton

density-weighted (PDW) image the contrast relies mainly on the differences in density of water and fat protons within the tissue. This contrast is also referred to as intermediate-weighted, as it represents a combination of T_1 and T_2 contrast. Applying these different "weightings," one can produce maps with varying contrast of the same object [75]. This makes the MR method uniquely suitable for the assessment of the vascular wall [76]. Improvements in MR technology, including the development of high-sensitivity coils and faster imaging protocols, have allowed the study of atherosclerotic plaques using multicontrast (T1w, T2w, and PDw) MR imaging [77]. MR imaging has been used for the study of atherosclerotic plaque in the human aorta [78], carotid arteries (Figure 2.24) [79,80], and in peripheral arteries [81]. Successful MR imaging of the coronary artery wall has been performed (Figure 2.25) [82], but is technically demanding due to the small size and highly tortuous course of the coronaries. Additionally, to obtain artifact-free images, cardiac and respiratory motion must be reliably suppressed. Use of navigator echoes accounts for any cardiac or diaphragmatic motion and allows to visualize the coronary wall in a time-efficient way without the need for breath-holding [83].

Studies on Human Atherosclerosis

Carotid artery

In vivo images of advanced lesions in carotid arteries were initially performed in patients referred for endarterectomy [84]. As the carotid arteries are superficial and less mobile they pose a less of a technical challenge for imaging than do the aorta or coronary arteries. Some of the MR studies of carotid arterial plaques include the imaging and

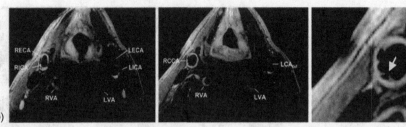

(a), (b)   (c)

Figure 2.24 Example of in vivo Carotid plaque imaging in a 61-year-old smoker who presented with recent anterior circulation transient ischemic attack (TIA). (a) Magnetic resonance T_2-weighted turbo-spin-echo images in a transverse plane showing increased wall thickness of the carotid and vertebral arteries, (b) Significantly thickened vessel wall in the left carotid bifurcation (LCA). Also shown are two arteriosclerotic lesions in the right common carotid artery (RCCA) with dark lipid core and thin fibrous cap (c). Close-up of right common carotid artery suggestive of plaque rupture (arrow). (Reproduced from Wiesmann *et al.* [80], with permission from the publishers)

characterization of normal and pathological arterial walls, the quantification of plaque size, and the detection of fibrous cap "integrity." Typically the images are acquired with resolution of $0.4 \times 0.4 \times 3$ mm^3 using a carotid phased-array coil. Most of the in vivo MR plaque imaging and characterization have been performed using a multicontrast approach with high-resolution black-blood spin echo—and fast spin echo—based MR sequences. The signal from the blood flow is rendered black by the use of preparatory pulses (e.g., radio-frequency spatial saturation or inversion recovery pulses) to better visualize the adjacent vessel wall.

MR angiography (MRA) and high-resolution black-blood imaging of the vessel wall can be combined. MRA demonstrates the severity of stenotic lesions and their spatial distribution, whereas the high-resolution black-blood wall characterization technique may show the composition of the plaques and may facilitate the risk stratification and selection of the treatment modality. Improvements in spatial resolution ($<250 \mu$m) have been possible with the design of new phased-array coils tailored for carotid imaging [85] and new imaging sequences such as long echo train fast-spin-echo imaging with "velocity-selective" flow suppression or double-inversion recovery preparatory pulses (black-blood imaging).

Aorta

In vivo black-blood MR atherosclerotic plaque characterization of the human aorta has been reported recently. Fayad *et al.* [78] assessed thoracic aorta plaque composition and size using T1W, T2W, and PDW images. The acquired images had a resolution of $0.8 \times 0.8 \times 5$ mm^3 using a torso

(a), (b)   (c)

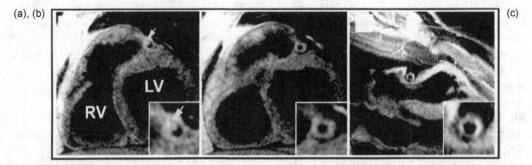

Figure 2.25 Human in vivo MR black-blood cross-sectional images that demonstrate a plaque with (presumed) deposition of fat (arrow, a) and a concentric fibrotic lesion (b) in the left anterior descending artery, and an ectatic, but atherosclerotic, right coronary artery (c). (Reproduced from Fayad *et al.*, *Circulation* 2002;106:2026, with permission from the publishers.)

phased-array coil. Rapid high-resolution imaging was performed with a fast spin echo sequence in conjunction with velocity-selective flow suppression preparatory pulses. Matched cross-sectional aortic imaging with MR and TEE showed a strong correlation for plaque composition and mean maximum plaque thickness.

Cardiac Magnetic Resonance Spectroscopy

Cardiac MRI uses the ^{1}H nucleus in water and fat molecules as it is the only signal source. In contrast, MRS allows the study of many additional nuclei with a net nuclear spin, i.e., with an uneven number of protons, neutrons or both. Importantly, MRS is the only available method for the noninvasive study of cardiac metabolism without external radioactive tracers (as used, for example, in positron emission tomography). Table 2.1 lists the nuclei most frequently used in cardiac MRS: ^{1}H (protons from metabolites other than water and fat), ^{13}C, ^{23}Na, and ^{31}P. Cardiac MRS is a fascinating method but has one major limitation: Low spatial and temporal resolution. The nuclei studied with MRS have a much lower MR sensitivity than ^{1}H and are present in much lower concentrations than those of ^{1}H nuclei of water and fat (Table 2.1). Therefore, the resolution of MRS is several orders of magnitude lower than that of MRI.

Basic Principles of MRS

The most extensively studied nucleus in cardiac MRS is phosphorus (^{31}P), and the basic principles of MRS, relevant for all nuclei, are best derived from a ^{31}P-MRS study of the most widely used animal model, the isolated buffer-perfused rodent heart [86]. MRS is performed using an MR spectrometer, which consists of a high-field (up to 18 T) superconducting magnet with a bore size ranging between ~5 cm and ~1 m. The magnet bore holds the nucleus-specific probe head with the radio-frequency (RF) coils, which are used for MR excitation and signal reception. The magnet is interfaced with a control computer, a magnetic field gradient system, and an RF transmitter and receiver. The magnetic field requires homogenization with shim gradients, as MRS demands high

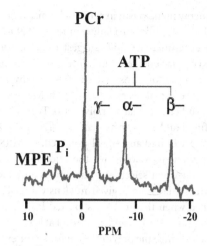

Figure 2.26 ^{31}P-MR spectrum of an isolated, buffer-perfused rat heart obtained within 5 minutes at 7 T.

magnetic field homogeneity. A radio-frequency impulse is sent into the RF coils for spin excitation. The resulting MR signal, the free induction decay (FID) is then recorded. The FID is subjected to Fourier transformation, which results in an MR spectrum.

A typical ^{31}P-MR spectrum from an isolated, beating rat heart, obtained in 5 minutes at 7 T is shown in Figure 2.26. A ^{31}P-spectrum shows six resonances, corresponding to the three ^{31}P-atoms of ATP, phosphocreatine (PCr), inorganic phosphate (Pi), and monophosphate esters (MPE). Different metabolites resonate at distinct frequencies, and this is termed the chemical shift phenomenon (quantified relative to the B_0 field in ppm = parts per million): different positions in the molecule lead to subtle differences in the local magnetic field strength, spreading the resonance frequencies of ^{31}P-metabolites over a range of ~30 ppm. From the fully relaxed state, the area under each ^{31}P-resonance is proportional to the amount of each ^{31}P-nucleus in the sample, and metabolite resonances are quantified by measuring peak areas. Relative metabolite levels are calculated directly (such as the phosphocreatine/ATP ratio), and absolute metabolite concentrations are calculated by comparing tissue resonance areas to those of an external ^{31}P-reference standard (e.g., phenylphosphonate) [87–89]. ^{31}P-MRS has been used extensively to study the relationships between cardiac function and energy metabolism in acute ischemia/ reperfusion and in chronic heart failure models [86,90–92]. These experimental studies suggest a crucial role of altered cardiac energetics in injured myocardium.

Due to the low sensitivity of MRS, many FIDs have to be signal-averaged to obtain MR spectra with a sufficient signal-to-noise ratio. Typically, for a perfused rat heart experiment at 7–12 T, 100–200 FIDs are acquired and signal-averaged. In MRS, it is important to account for the effects of partial saturation when selecting pulse angles and TR: a full MR signal from a given nucleus can only be obtained when the nucleus is excited from a fully relaxed spin state, i.e., when a time of at least $5 \times T_1$ has passed since the previous excitation (for example, T_1 of phosphocreatine at 1.5 T $\sim$ 4.4 seconds requiring TR of 22 seconds); "fully relaxed" spectra can therefore only be obtained with long TRs, leading to prohibitively long acquisition times. In practice, shorter TRs are used, but these yield spectra where a part of the signal is lost due to saturation effects ("partially saturated"). Since the T_1s of ^{31}P-metabolites such as phosphocreatine and ATP are different (T_1 of phosphocreatine is approximately twice as long as T_1 of ATP), the extent of saturation also varies for different ^{31}P-resonances. Thus, when quantifying partially saturated spectra, "saturation factors" need to be used for correction. These factors are determined for each metabolite by comparing fully relaxed and saturated spectra.

^{1}H has the highest MR sensitivity of all MR-detectable nuclei and very high natural abundance (Table 2.1). Many metabolites can be detected by ^{1}H-MRS, such as creatine, lactate, carnitine, taurine, and –CH_3 and –CH_2 resonances of lipids [93–95]. Particularly promising is the noninvasive measurement of total creatine [96,97]. Furthermore, tissue oxygenation can be followed noninvasively by ^{1}H-MRS using the oxymyoglobin and deoxymyoglobin resonances [98]. However, ^{1}H-MRS is technically demanding, as we need to suppress the strong ^{1}H signal from water which is 1,000,000 times more intense than the metabolite signals. Furthermore, the complex ^{1}H spectra show overlapping resonances, many of which remain to be characterized. Cardiac ^{1}H-MRS is only in its infancy, but the technique has enormous potential for clinical application.

The ^{13}C nucleus has a low natural abundance ($\sim$1%), and for a ^{13}C-MRS experiment, the heart has to be loaded with ^{13}C-labeled compounds such as 1–^{13}C-glucose. Typically, these are added to perfusion media or infused into a coronary artery during a defined study protocol. Substrate utilization by the heart [99,100] may then be investigated, or the activities of key enzymes or entire metabolic pathways can be quantified, e.g., citric acid cycle flux, pyruvate dehydrogenase flux, and beta-oxidation of fatty acids [101–103]. Clinical applications have yet to be reported for the heart, because MR-sensitivity and concentrations of ^{13}C nuclei are too low for spatially resolved detection in human heart within an acceptable acquisition time.

^{23}Na-MRS is the only noninvasive method for evaluation of changes in intra- and extracellular ^{23}Na during cardiac injury [104]. Maintenance of the sarcolemmal ^{23}Na concentration gradient (extracellular/intracellular concentration gradient $\sim$14:1) is a requirement for normal cardiac function. A cardiac ^{23}Na spectrum yields a single peak representing all ^{23}Na in the heart (the total Na^+ signal), and for discrimination of intra- and extracellular ^{23}Na pools paramagnetic shift reagents, e.g., $[TmDOTP]^{5-}$, have to be added to the perfusate. These high molecular weight chelate complexes are distributed in the extracellular space only, and ^{23}Na in the close vicinity of shift reagents undergoes a downfield chemical shift of its resonance frequency, so that extracellular and intracellular ^{23}Na peaks can be discriminated. This method is being used experimentally to examine the mechanisms of intracellular Na^+ accumulation in ischemia-reperfusion injury [105]. Unfortunately, ^{23}Na-MR shift reagents for clinical use are currently not yet available, so that only imaging of the total Na signal is feasible, as first demonstrated by DeLayre et al. [106]. However, even the total ^{23}Na signal holds biologically important information: In acute ischemia, the total myocardial ^{23}Na MRI signal increases due to breakdown of ion homeostasis and intra- and extracellular edema formation [107]. Furthermore, the total Na signal remains significantly elevated during chronic scar formation, as we have demonstrated in an experimental model [108], because of the expansion of the extracellular space in scar (Figure 2.27). In contrast, ^{23}Na content is not elevated in akinetic, but stunned or hibernating myocardium [90]. For

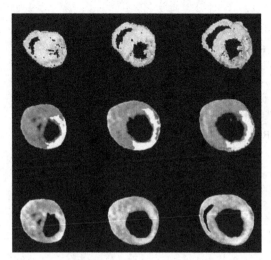

Figure 2.27 Bottom row: three adjacent slices of a 3D
^{23}Na-MRI data set in an isolated rat heart 4 weeks post-MI
after segmentation. Middle row: the region with signal
elevation of double standard deviation over mean in the
^{23}Na image is delineated in white, and is chosen for infarct
size measurement. Top row: corresponding histological
slices with stained infarcted area. The area of increased
^{23}Na signal intensity closely matches the histologic scar
area ($r = 0.91$; $p < 0.0001$). (Reproduced from Horn et al.
[90], with permission from Wiley & Sons, New York.)

these reasons, ^{23}Na MRI may allow detection of myocardial viability based on intrinsic tissue contrast.

Clinical Cardiac MRS Methods

Almost all human cardiac MRS studies have so far
been confined to the ^{31}P nucleus. Clinical cardiac
spectroscopy is a complex technique. There are
hardware requirements that usually do not come
with a standard CMR system: The RF generator
has to be able to produce frequencies other than
^{1}H ("broadband capability"), and a specific ^{31}P-
cardiac surface coil is needed, typically with a loop
diameter of 10–15 cm. The low resolution of MRS
cannot simply be offset by increasing imaging time,
which, for practical reasons, is limited to 60–90
minutes. ECG gating is required, but, given the
large voxel sizes and the already extended acquisition time, respiration gating is currently not employed. Field strength of clinical MRS systems is
much lower than that of experimental systems, i.e.,
typically 1.5 T, although 3 T systems have recently
become available. The cardiac muscle lies behind
the chest wall skeletal muscle, whose ^{31}P-signal re-

quires suppression by means of spectroscopic localization techniques. Localization methods used
for cardiac MRS include DRESS (depth-resolved
surface coil spectroscopy), rotating frame, 1D-CSI
(chemical shift imaging), ISIS (image-selected in
vivo spectroscopy), and 3D-CSI; some details are
given in Figure 2.28, for a full description of localization methods see review by Bottomley [109].
Although less comfortable for the patient, it is currently recommended to perform MRS studies in
prone position rather than supine, as this reduces
motion artifacts and brings the heart closer to the
surface coil, thus improving sensitivity. ^{1}H scout
images are first obtained to select the spectroscopic
voxel(s), followed by ^{31}P-acquisition for 20–50 minutes. Given the low sensitivity, ^{31}P-MRS voxel sizes
have been large, typically ~30 mL. A typical ^{31}P-MR
spectrum of a healthy volunteer is shown in Figure
2.29. Compared to the rat heart spectrum, two additional resonances are seen: 2,3-diphosphoglycerate
(2,3-DPG), arising from the presence of blood (ery-
throcytes) in the voxel, and phosphodiesters (PDE),
a signal due to membrane as well as serum phos-
pholipids. The 2,3-diphosphoglycerate resonances
overlap with the inorganic phosphate peak, which
therefore cannot be detected in most human ^{31}P-
MR spectra. For relative quantification of human
^{31}P-spectra, the phosphocreatine/ATP and phos-
phodiester/ATP peak area ratios are calculated. The
phosphocreatine/ATP ratio is a powerful indicator
of the energetic state of the heart. The meaning
of the phosphodiester/ATP ratio remains poorly
understood, and this ratio may not change with
cardiac disease. Human ^{31}P-resonances require correction for the effects of partial saturation according to the principles described for experimental
MRS. In addition, to account for saturation, either adiabatic pulses (creating identical flip angles across the entire sample volume) or B_1 field
characterization (taking into account variations in
flip angle) are required. ^{31}P-spectra should also
be corrected for blood contamination: Blood con-
tributes signal to the ATP-, 2,3-diphosphoglycerate-
and phosphodiester-resonances of a cardiac ^{31}P-
spectrum. As human blood spectra show an
ATP/2,3-diphosphoglycerate area ratio of ~0.11
and a phosphodiester/2,3-diphosphoglycerate area
ratio of ~0.19, for blood correction, the ATP
resonance area of cardiac spectra is reduced by 11%

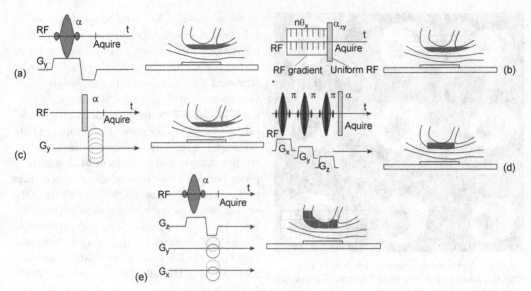

Figure 2.28 Basic pulse sequences for localized cardiac spectroscopy with surface coils. (a) "depth-resolved surface coil spectroscopy." A single section parallel to the plane of the surface coil is selected by applying an MR imaging gradient G in the presence of a modulated radio-frequency excitation pulse of flip angle. (b) The "rotating frame" MR method uses the gradient inherent in a surface coil to simultaneously spatially encode spectra from multiple sections parallel to the surface coil by means of application of a flip angle pulse, which is stepped in subsequent applications of the sequence. (c) The "one-dimensional chemical shift imaging" method similarly encodes multiple sections but uses an MR imaging gradient whose amplitude is stepped. (d) The "image-selected in vivo spectroscopy" method localizes to a single volume with selective inversion pulses applied with G_x, G_y, and G_z MR imaging gradients. All eight combinations of the three pulses must be applied and the resultant signals added and subtracted. (e) A section-selective "three-dimensional chemical shift imaging" sequence employs MR imaging section selection in one dimension and phase encoding in two dimensions. (Reproduced from Bottomley [109], with permission from the Radiological Society of North America.)

of the 2,3-diphosphoglycerate resonance area, and the phosphodiester resonance area is reduced by 19% of the 2,3-diphosphoglycerate resonance area [108].

Absolute quantification of phosphocreatine and ATP is difficult, but is an essential step for further development of clinical cardiac MRS, as the phosphocreatine/ATP ratio cannot detect simultaneous decreases of phosphocreatine and ATP, which have been demonstrated, for example, in the failing [110] or in the infarcted nonviable myocardium [111]. Quantification of absolute ^{31}P-metabolite levels is possible by obtaining simultaneous signal from a ^{31}P-standard and estimates of myocardial mass based on MR imaging [112]. An alternative strategy [113] is to use simultaneous acquisition of a ^{1}H-spectrum and to calibrate the ^{31}P-signal to the tissue water proton content. Probably the most advanced technique in this respect is SLOOP (spectral localization with optimum pointspread func-

tion), which allows interrogation of curved regions of interest matching the shape of the heart, and absolute quantification with high accuracy [114]. SLOOP requires a ^{31}P reference standard, flip angle calibration, B_1 field mapping and measurement of myocardial mass.

It has previously been impossible to interrogate the posterior wall of the human heart, due to its distance from the ^{31}P-surface coil. Pohmann and von Kienlin [115], have recently implemented acquisition-weighted ^{31}P-chemical shift imaging, which reduces the signal contamination between adjacent voxels, and, for the first time, ^{31}P-spectra from the posterior wall could be obtained. Acquisition-weighting should thus be implemented for all cardiac MRS protocols (Figure 2.30).

Methods for Clinical ^{23}Na-MRI

Although this is considered in this spectroscopy section ^{23}Na acquisition is strictly speaking an imaging

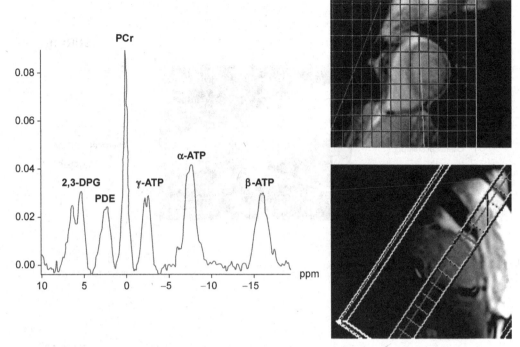

Figure 2.29 31P-MR spectrum from a healthy human volunteer, 3D-CSI technique. Voxel size 25 mm × 27 mm × 30 mm (20 mL). 2, 3-DPG, 2,3-Diphosphoglycerate; PDE, phosphodiesters; PCr, phosphocreatine; g-, a-, b-ATP, the three phosphorus atoms of adenosinetriphosphate. The right panels show short axis and vertical long axis proton scout images. The entire voxel grid of the 3D-CSI localization is shown in green, and the voxel corresponding to the 31P-spectrum is shown in blue.

technique, as there is a single frequency. Human sodium imaging requires specialist-built RF coils. Images are gated to the end-diastolic phase of the cardiac cycle but are acquired without respiratory gating due to the long duration of the scans Figure 2.31). The sodium nucleus is a spin-3/2 system, which in practical terms means that the decay is bi-exponential giving rise to two T_2 values. To completely characterize the signal, both components need to be obtained, and as the short T_2 is around 1 ms, specialist acquisition approaches are required for this. A number of such approaches have been developed [116,117]. One benefit arising from the properties of the sodium nucleus is that T_1 is very short and hence it is possible to use short repetition times, so that a large number of signal averages can be acquired to improve the SNR. The high concentration of sodium in the blood pool seriously hampers detection of epicardial infarction using present methods. Developments such as advanced coil designs, higher field strengths and the use of navigated acquisitions should improve the quality of human cardiac sodium imaging.

Perspective on MRS

Human cardiac MRS is feasible, but it is clear that a major technical development effort is still required to allow MRS to enter clinical practice. Major advances should be achievable in coil and sequence design, and through implementation of MRS at higher field strength [118]. Standardization of cardiac MRS approaches used at different centers is also an important issue. Until that time, MRS will remain a fascinating clinical research tool, allowing insight into cardiac metabolism in various forms of human heart disease.

Safety and Contraindications

As an MR system consists of a large, static magnetic field in which RF energy is periodically released during imaging, there are possible hazards associated

acquisition-weighted CSI:

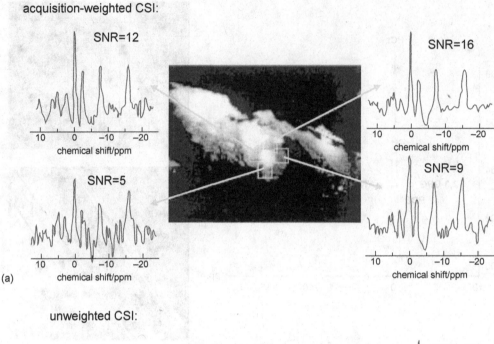

unweighted CSI:

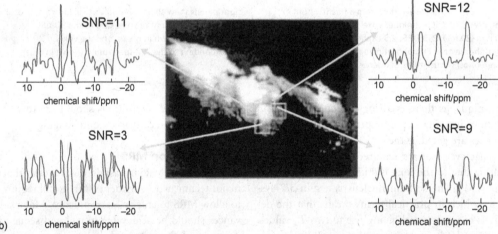

Figure 2.30 Results of (a) acquisition-weighted and (b) unweighted ^{31}P-Chemical shift imaging (CSI) experiment of a healthy volunteer. For both experiments, four spectra from the same voxel positions are shown. Nominal voxel size was 2.5 cm × 2.5 cm × 4.0 cm, and each experiment consisted of 2048 scans synchronized to the heartbeat. The spectra obtained with acquisition weighting show a considerably higher phosphocreatine/ATP ratio and a higher SNR for the phosphocreatine and ATP signals. Also, high-resolution spectra from the posterior wall can be obtained. (SNR, signal-to-noise ratio) (Reproduced from Pohmann and von Kienlin [115], with permission from Wiley & Sons, New York.)

with its use. In general, the potential hazard of implants or devices is dependent on such factors as its degree of ferromagnetism, geometry, location in the body, as well as the gradient and field strength of the imaging magnet.

In assessing whether a particular patient should be subjected to a CMR scan, the main rule, as with other investigations in medicine, is to determine the risk-benefit ratio to the patient of the proposed study. It is absolutely essential to carefully

Sodium (^{23}Na) images   Proton (^{1}H) images

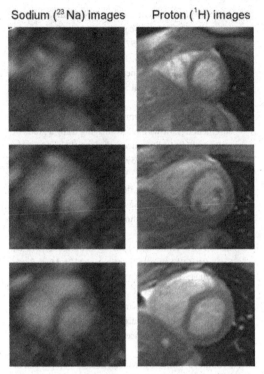

Figure 2.31 Here three slices from a 3D sodium data set show the concentration of the T_2 long in the tissue. Proton slices acquired during the same imaging session are shown for comparison. Sodium acquisition was cardiac gated and required a 22-minute acquisition using our ultra-short TE CSI approach. The image quality shown here is typical for all the acquisition methods at 1.5 T.

interview a patient prior to an MRI examination, and most centers would require a safety questionnaire to be completed. Whenever there is a concern about the safety of a patient with an implant, the CMR examination should be deferred until the device and the issues associated with it are clarified. Reference texts [119] and web-based information (www.MRIsafety.com) on the safety of specific devices are available.

Older cerebral aneurysm clips are ferromagnetic and there are a number of reports of fatal cerebral hemorrhage after MR examinations in this setting. Although modern aneurysm clips are nonferromagnetic, the type of clip should be established with certainty prior to performing the examination. Previous history of eye injury with metallic shards should also be sought and an X-ray performed of the orbit if there is doubt that the metallic fragment

has not been removed. Electronic devices such as cochlear implants, nerve stimulation units and a number of modern implants can be damaged or malfunction as a result of being in a magnetic field and are best avoided. Sternal wires and vascular clips are not contraindicated, although they do produce artifacts.

Pacemakers and cardioverter defibrillators (ICDs): Despite early reports [120] and a recent large study [121] of nonpacemaker dependent patients being safely scanned in a high field system, *a pacemaker-dependent patient is generally considered as an absolute contraindication to CMR scanning.* Cardiac pacemakers and ICDs present potential problems to patients undergoing MR procedures from several mechanisms including (1) movement of the device (e.g., the pulse generator and/or leads) due to the magnetic field of the MR system; (2) MR-related heating of leads by the time-varying magnetic fields; (3) inhibition or modification of the function of the device by the electromagnetic fields used for MR procedures; and (4) inappropriate or rapid pacing due to the pulsed gradient magnetic fields and/or pulsed radio-frequency (RF) fields (i.e., electromagnetic interference with the lead acting as an antenna) [122–124]. These problems may result in serious injuries or lethal consequences for patients, as well as device malfunctions or damage [124].

Stents: Every year approximately 457,000 metallic coronary artery stents are placed in the US alone [125]. In patients with coronary stents, MRI is believed to be safe once endothelialization [126] has occurred, because this presumably opposes possible dislodgement [119]. Therefore, manufacturers of stents [127] and professional associations of cardiologists [125] have traditionally recommended postponing elective MRI examinations for 4–8 weeks after stent placement. However, in vitro and animal studies [128–130] have shown that ferromagneticity and stent migration are absent or minimal with MRI of currently available stents. Early clinical studies on the outcome of patients who undergo MRI early after coronary stent placement also indicated that CMR at 1.5 T was safe in patients early after stent implantation [131,132]. Recently, a retrospective review of 111 patients who underwent MRI at 1.5 T (39% head/neck, 27% spine, 9% chest) less than 8 weeks after stent placement (and treated with aspirin and thienopyridine) showed that the risk of cardiac death, MI, or need for repeat revascularization due to associated stent thrombosis was very low [133]. Although the study did not have 30-day angiographic follow-up, the results are consistent with the 30-day cardiac event rates (0.5–1.9%) after coronary stent placement with contemporary anti-platelet therapy in patients not undergoing MRI [134]. These findings indicate that postponing CMR until after 8 weeks following coronary stenting does not seem necessary. This has been supported by a recent statement from the American Heart Association [135]. Stent safety has also been established for 3 T. An up-to date list can be found at mrisafety.com.

Valvular prostheses: Heart valve prostheses are all safe for CMR. These most recent recommendations supersede earlier suggestions that pre-6000 series Starr–Edwards valves might cause problems during MR. Studies at 1.5–2.35 T static magnetic fields have shown that there is no hazardous deflection during exposure of the magnetic field [119,136].

Claustrophobia: Despite the development of shorter magnets, and more open designs up to 10% of patients may experience varying degrees of claustrophobia. In our experience, the number is nearer to 5% [48], which can be reduced even further to about 2% of patients by the use of explanation, reassurance, and when necessary, light sedation [137].

Acknowledgement

The authors thank Drs Frank Wiesmann, Saul Myerson, and Damian Tyler for critical review of various subsections of this chapter.

References

1. Bloch F. Nuclear induction. *Phys Review (Physics)*. 1946;1(70):460–473.
2. Purcell E, Torrey H, Pound R. Resonance absorption by nuclear magnetic moments in a solid. *Phys Rev (Physics)*. 1946;1(69):37–38.
3. Lauterbur P. Image formation by induced local interactions: examples employing nuclear magnetic resonance. *Nature*. 1973;242:190–191.
4. Garlick PB, Radda GK, Seeley PJ. Phosphorus NMR studies on perfused heart. *Biochem Biophys Res Commun*. 1977;74(3):1256–1262.
5. Jacobus WE, Taylor GJt, Hollis DP, Nunnally RL. Phosphorus nuclear magnetic resonance of perfused working rat hearts. *Nature*. 1977;265(5596):756–758.
6. Anderson LJ, Holden S, Davis B, *et al.* Cardiovascular T2-star (T2*) magnetic resonance for the early diagnosis of myocardial iron overload. *Eur Heart J*. 2001;22(23):2171–2179.
7. Bryant DJ, Payne JA, Firmin DN, Longmore DB. Measurement of flow with NMR imaging using a gradient pulse and phase difference technique. *J Comput Assist Tomogr*. 1984;8(4):588–593.
8. Chia JM, Fischer SE, Wickline SA, Lorenz CH. Performance of QRS detection for cardiac magnetic resonance imaging with a novel vectorcardiographic triggering method. *J Magn Reson Imaging*. 2000;12(5):678–688.
9. Larson AC, White RD, Laub G, McVeigh ER, Li D, Simonetti OP. Self-gated cardiac cine MRI. *Magn Reson Med*. 2004;51(1):93–102.
10. Bellenger NG, Davies LC, Francis JM, Coats AJ, Pennell DJ. Reduction in sample size for studies of remodeling in heart failure by the use of cardiovascular magnetic resonance. *J Cardiovasc Magn Reson*. 2000;2(4):271–278.
11. Grothues F, Smith GC, Moon JC, *et al.* Comparison of interstudy reproducibility of cardiovascular magnetic resonance with two-dimensional echocardiography in normal subjects and in patients with heart failure or left ventricular hypertrophy. *Am J Cardiol*. 2002;90(1):29–34.
12. Alfakih K, Plein S, Thiele H, Jones T, Ridgway JP, Sivananthan MU. Normal human left and right ventricular dimensions for MRI as assessed by turbo gradient echo and steady-state free precession imaging sequences. *J Magn Reson Imaging*. 2003;17(3):323–329.
13. Lorenz CH, Walker ES, Morgan VL, Klein SS, Graham TP, Jr. Normal human right and left ventricular mass, systolic function, and gender differences by cine magnetic resonance imaging. *J Cardiovasc Magn Reson*. 1999;1(1):7–21.
14. Hudsmith LE, Petersen SE, Tyler DJ, *et al.* Determination of cardiac volumes and mass with FLASH and SSFP cine sequences at 1.5 vs. 3 Tesla: a validation study. *J Magn Reson Imaging*. 2006;24(2):312–318.
15. Helbing WA, Rebergen SA, Maliepaard C, *et al.* Quantification of right ventricular function with magnetic resonance imaging in children with normal hearts and with congenital heart disease. *Am Heart J*. 1995;130(4):828–837.
16. Helbing WA, Bosch HG, Maliepaard C, *et al.* Comparison of echocardiographic methods with magnetic resonance imaging for assessment of right ventricular function in children. *Am J Cardiol*. 1995;76(8):589–594.

17. Alfakih K, Plein S, Bloomer T, Jones T, Ridgway J, Sivananthan M. Comparison of right ventricular volume measurements between axial and short axis orientation using steady-state free precession magnetic resonance imaging. *J Magn Reson Imaging.* 2003;18(1):25–32.

18. Strugnell WE, Slaughter RE, Riley RA, Trotter AJ, Bartlett H. Modified RV short axis series–a new method for cardiac MRI measurement of right ventricular volumes. *J Cardiovasc Magn Reson.* 2005;7(5):769–774.

19. Pennell DJ, Underwood SR, Manzara CC, *et al.* Magnetic resonance imaging during dobutamine stress in coronary artery disease. *Am J Cardiol.* 1992;70(1):34–40.

20. Fayad ZA, Connick TJ, Axel L. An improved quadrature or phased-array coil for MR cardiac imaging. *Magn Reson Med.* 1995;34(2):186–193.

21. Cerqueira MD, Weissman NJ, Dilsizian V, *et al.* Standardized myocardial segmentation and nomenclature for tomographic imaging of the heart. A statement for healthcare professionals from the Cardiac Imaging Committee of the Council on Cliniical Cardiology of the American Heart Association. *Int J Cardiovasc Imaging.* 2002;18(1):539–542.

22. Nagel E, Lehmkuhl HB, Bocksch W, *et al.* Noninvasive diagnosis of ischemia-induced wall motion abnormalities with the use of high-dose dobutamine stress MRI: comparison with dobutamine stress echocardiography. *Circulation.* 1999;99(6):763–770.

23. Wahl A RS, Paetsch I, Gollesch A, *et al.* High dose dobutamine stress MRI for follow up after coronary revascularization procedures in patients with wall motion abnormalities at rest. *J Cardiovasc Magn Reson.* 2002;4:22–23.

24. Jahnke C, Nagel E, Gebker R, *et al.* Prognostic value of cardiac magnetic resonance stress tests: adenosine stress perfusion and dobutamine stress wall motion imaging. *Circulation.* 2007;115(13):1769–1776.

25. Zerhouni EA, Parish DM, Rogers WJ, Yang A, Shapiro EP. Human heart: tagging with MR imaging–a method for noninvasive assessment of myocardial motion. *Radiology.* 1988;169(1):59–63.

26. Mosher TJ, Smith MB. A DANTE tagging sequence for the evaluation of translational sample motion. *Magn Reson Med.* 1990;15(2):334–339.

27. Axel L, Dougherty L. Heart wall motion: improved method of spatial modulation of magnetization for MR imaging. *Radiology.* 1989;172(2):349–350.

28. Bolster BD, Jr., McVeigh ER, Zerhouni EA. Myocardial tagging in polar coordinates with use of striped tags. *Radiology.* 1990;177(3):769–772.

29. Ryf S, Spiegel MA, Gerber M, Boesiger P. Myocardial tagging with 3D-CSPAMM. *J Magn Reson Imaging.* 2002;16(3):320–325.

30. Croisille P, Guttman MA, Atalar E, McVeigh ER, Zerhouni EA. Precision of myocardial contour estimation from tagged MR images with a "black-blood" technique. *Acad Radiol.* 1998;5(2):93–100.

31. Hennig J, Schneider B, Peschl S, Markl M, Krause T, Laubenberger J. Analysis of myocardial motion based on velocity measurements with a black blood prepared segmented gradient-echo sequence: methodology and applications to normal volunteers and patients. *J Magn Reson Imaging.* 1998;8(4):868–877.

32. Petersen SE, Jung BA, Wiesmann F, *et al.* Myocardial tissue phase mapping with cine phase-contrast MR imaging: regional wall motion analysis in healthy volunteers. *Radiology.* 2006;238(3):816–826.

33. Gilson WD, Yang Z, French BA, Epstein FH. Measurement of myocardial mechanics in mice before and after infarction using multislice displacement-encoded MRI with 3D motion encoding. *Am J Physiol Heart Circ Physiol.* 2005;288(3):H1491–H1497.

34. Wesbey G, Higgins C, McNamara M, *et al.* Effect of gadolinium-DTPA on the magnetic relaxation times of normal and infarcted myocardium. *Radiology.* 1984;153(1):165–169.

35. Simonetti OP, Kim RJ, Fieno DS, *et al.* An improved MR imaging technique for the visualization of myocardial infarction. *Radiology.* 2001;218(1):215–223.

36. Sandstede JJ, Pabst T, Beer M, *et al.* Assessment of myocardial infarction in humans with (23)Na MR imaging: comparison with cine MR imaging and delayed contrast enhancement. *Radiology.* 2001;221(1):222–228.

37. Kim RJ, Fieno DS, Parrish TB, *et al.* Relationship of MRI delayed contrast enhancement to irreversible injury, infarct age, and contractile function. *Circulation.* 1999;100(19):1992–2002.

38. Choi KM, Kim RJ, Gubernikoff G, Vargas JD, Parker M, Judd RM. Transmural extent of acute myocardial infarction predicts long-term improvement in contractile function. *Circulation.* 2001;104(10):1101–1107.

39. Selvanayagam JB, Kardos A, Francis JM, *et al.* Value of delayed-enhancement cardiovascular magnetic resonance imaging in predicting myocardial viability after surgical revascularization. *Circulation.* 2004;110(12):1535–1541.

40. Mahrholdt H, Wagner A, Judd RM, Sechtem U, Kim RJ. Delayed enhancement cardiovascular magnetic resonance assessment of non-ischaemic cardiomyopathies. *Eur Heart J.* 2005;26(15):1461–1474.

41. Moon JC, McKenna WJ, McCrohon JA, Elliott PM, Smith GC, Pennell DJ. Toward clinical risk assessment

in hypertrophic cardiomyopathy with gadolinium car-diovascular magnetic resonance. *J Am Coll Cardiol.* 2003;41(9):1561–1567.

42. McCrohon JA, Moon JC, Prasad SK, *et al.* Differentiation of heart failure related to dilated cardiomyopathy and coronary artery disease using gadolinium-enhanced cardiovascular magnetic resonance. *Circulation.* 2003;108(1):54–59.

43. Moon JCC, Sachdev B, Elkington AG, *et al.* Gadolinium enhanced cardiovascular magnetic resonance in Anderson-Fabry disease1: evidence for a disease specific abnormality of the myocardial interstitium. *Eur Heart J.* 2003;24(23):2151–2155.

44. Wu E, Judd RM, Vargas JD, Klocke FJ, Bonow RO, Kim RJ. Visualisation of presence, location, and transmural extent of healed Q-wave and non-Q-wave myocardial infarction. *Lancet.* 2001;357(9249):21–28.

45. Wagner A, Mahrholdt H, Holly TA, *et al.* Contrast-enhanced MRI and routine single photon emission computed tomography (SPECT) perfusion imaging for detection of subendocardial myocardial infarcts: an imaging study. *Lancet.* 2003;361(9355):374–379.

46. Wu KC, Zerhouni EA, Judd RM, *et al.* Prognostic significance of microvascular obstruction by magnetic resonance imaging in patients with acute myocardial infarction. *Circulation.* 1998;97(8):765–772.

47. Wu KC, Kim RJ, Bluemke DA, *et al.* Quantification and time course of microvascular obstruction by contrast-enhanced echocardiography and magnetic resonance imaging following acute myocardial infarction and reperfusion. *J Am Coll Cardiol.* 1998;32(6):1756–1764.

48. Selvanayagam JB, Petersen SE, Francis JM, *et al.* Effects of off-pump versus on-pump coronary surgery on reversible and irreversible myocardial injury: a randomized trial using cardiovascular magnetic resonance imaging and biochemical markers. *Circulation.* 2004;109(3):345–350.

49. Selvanayagam JB, Porto I, Channon K, *et al.* Troponin elevation following percutaneous coronary intervention directly represents the extent of irreversible myocardial injury: insights from cardiovascular magnetic resonance imaging. *Circulation.* 2005;111(8):1027–1032.

50. Kim RJ, Wu E, Rafael A, *et al.* The use of contrast-enhanced magnetic resonance imaging to identify reversible myocardial dysfunction. *N Engl J Med.* 2000;343(20):1445–1453.

51. Nagel E, Klein C, Paetsch I, *et al.* Magnetic resonance perfusion measurements for the noninvasive detection of coronary artery disease. *Circulation.* 2003;108(4):432–437.

52. Schwitter J, Nanz D, Kneifel S, *et al.* Assessment of myocardial perfusion in coronary artery disease by mag-netic resonance: a comparison with positron emission tomography and coronary angiography. *Circulation.* 2001;103(18):2230–2235.

53. Cheng AS, Pegg TJ, Karamitsos TD, *et al.* Cardiovascular magnetic resonance perfusion imaging at 3-Tesla for the detection of coronary artery disease: a comparison with 1.5-Tesla. *J Am Coll Cardiol.* 2007;49(25):2440–2449.

54. Klem I, Heitner JF, Shah DJ, *et al.* Improved detection of coronary artery disease by stress perfusion cardiovascular magnetic resonance with the use of delayed enhancement infarction imaging. *J Am Coll Cardiol.* 2006;47(8):1630–1638.

55. Wilke N, Jerosch-Herold M, Stillman AE, *et al.* Concepts of myocardial perfusion imaging in magnetic resonance imaging. *Magn Reson Q.* 1994;10(4):249–286.

56. Jerosch-Herold M, Wilke N, Stillman AE. Magnetic resonance quantification of the myocardial perfusion reserve with a Fermi function model for constrained deconvolution. *Med Phys.* 1998;25(1):73–84.

57. Cerqueira MD, Verani MS, Schwaiger M, Heo J, Iskandrian AS. Safety profile of adenosine stress perfusion imaging: results from the Adenoscan Multicenter Trial Registry. *J Am Coll Cardiol.* 1994;23(2):384–389.

58. Schwitter J, Wacker CM, van Rossum AC, *et al.* MR-IMPACT: comparison of perfusion-cardiac magnetic resonance with single-photon emission computed tomography for the detection of coronary artery disease in a multicentre, multivendor, randomized trial. *Eur Heart J.* 2008;29(4):480–489.

59. Wacker CM, Hartlep AW, Pfleger S, *et al.* Susceptibility-sensitive magnetic resonance imaging detects human myocardium supplied by a stenotic coronary artery without a contrast agent. *J Am Coll Cardiol.* 2003;41(5):834–840.

60. Wacker CM, Bock M, Hartlep AW, *et al.* Changes in myocardial oxygenation and perfusion under pharmacological stress with dipyridamole: assessment using T*2 and T1 measurements. *Magn Reson Med.* 1999;41(4):686–695.

61. Friedrich MG, Niendorf T, Schulz-Menger J, Gross CM, Dietz R. Blood oxygen level-dependent magnetic resonance imaging in patients with stress-induced angina. *Circulation.* 2003;108(18):2219–2223.

62. Mostbeck GH, Caputo GR, Higgins CB. MR measurement of blood flow in the cardiovascular system. *AJR Am J Roentgenol.* 1992;159(3):453–461.

63. Rebergen SA, Van Der Wall EE, Doornbos J, de Roos A. Magnetic resonance measurement of velocity and flow: technique, validation, and cardiovascular applications. *Am Heart J.* 1993;126(6):1439–1456.

64. Didier D, Ratib O, Friedli B, et al. Cine gradient-echo MR imaging in the evaluation of cardiovascular diseases. *Radiographics.* 1993;13(3):561–573.

65. Suzuki J, Caputo GR, Kondo C, Higgins CB. Cine MR imaging of valvular heart disease: display and imaging parameters affect the size of the signal void caused by valvular regurgitation. *AJR Am J Roentgenol.* 1990;155(4):723–727.

66. Mohiaddin RH, Pennell DJ. MR blood flow measurement. Clinical application in the heart and circulation. *Cardiol Clin.* 1998;16(2):161–187.

67. Kondo C, Caputo GR, Semelka R, Foster E, Shimakawa A, Higgins CB. Right and left ventricular stroke volume measurements with velocity-encoded cine MR imaging: in vitro and in vivo validation. *AJR Am J Roentgenol.* 1991;157(1):9–16.

68. Hundley WG, Li HF, Lange RA, et al. Assessment of left-to-right intracardiac shunting by velocity-encoded, phase-difference magnetic resonance imaging. A comparison with oximetric and indicator dilution techniques. *Circulation.* 1995;91(12):2955–2960.

69. Caputo GR, Kondo C, Masui T, et al. Right and left lung perfusion: in vitro and in vivo validation with oblique-angle, velocity-encoded cine MR imaging. *Radiology.* 1991;180(3):693–698.

70. Li D, Paschal CB, Haacke EM, Adler LP. Coronary arteries: three-dimensional MR imaging with fat saturation and magnetization transfer contrast. *Radiology.* 1993;187(2):401–406.

71. Manning WJ, Li W, Boyle NG, Edelman RR. Fat-suppressed breath-hold magnetic resonance coronary angiography. *Circulation.* 1993;87(1):94–104.

72. Botnar RM, Stuber M, Danias PG, Kissinger KV, Manning WJ. Improved coronary artery definition with T2-weighted, free-breathing, three-dimensional coronary MRA. *Circulation.* 1999;99(24):3139–3148.

73. Wielopolski PA, Manning WJ, Edelman RR. Single breath-hold volumetric imaging of the heart using magnetization-prepared 3-dimensional segmented echo planar imaging. *J Magn Reson Imaging.* 1995;5(4): 403–409.

74. Slavin GS, Riederer SJ, Ehman RL. Two-dimensional multishot echo-planar coronary MR angiography. *Magn Reson Med.* 1998;40(6):883–889.

75. Fayad ZA, Fuster V. Clinical imaging of the high-risk or vulnerable atherosclerotic plaque. *Circ Res.* 2001;89(4):305–316.

76. Herfkens RJ, Higgins CB, Hricak H, et al. Nuclear magnetic resonance imaging of atherosclerotic disease. *Radiology.* 1983;148(1):161–166.

77. Fayad ZA, Fuster V. Characterization of atherosclerotic plaques by magnetic resonance imaging. *Ann N Y Acad Sci.* 2000;902:173–186.

78. Fayad ZA, Nahar T, Fallon JT, et al. In vivo magnetic resonance evaluation of atherosclerotic plaques in the human thoracic aorta: a comparison with transesophageal echocardiography. *Circulation.* 2000;101(21):2503–2509.

79. Yuan C, Beach KW, Smith LH, Jr., Hatsukami TS. Measurement of atherosclerotic carotid plaque size in vivo using high resolution magnetic resonance imaging. *Circulation.* 1998;98(24):2666–2671.

80. Wiesmann F, Robson MD, Francis JM, et al. Visualization of the ruptured plaque by magnetic resonance imaging. *Circulation.* 2003;108:2542.

81. Coulden RA, Moss H, Graves MJ, Lomas DJ, Appleton DS, Weissberg PL. High resolution magnetic resonance imaging of atherosclerosis and the response to balloon angioplasty. *Heart.* 2000;83(2):188–191.

82. Fayad ZA, Fuster V, Fallon JT, et al. Noninvasive in vivo human coronary artery lumen and wall imaging using black-blood magnetic resonance imaging. *Circulation.* 2000;102(5):506–510.

83. Botnar RM, Kim WY, Bornert P, Stuber M, Spuentrup E, Manning WJ. 3D coronary vessel wall imaging utilizing a local inversion technique with spiral image acquisition. *Magn Reson Med.* 2001;46(5):848–854.

84. Toussaint JF, LaMuraglia GM, Southern JF, Fuster V, Kantor HL. Magnetic resonance images lipid, fibrous, calcified, hemorrhagic, and thrombotic components of human atherosclerosis in vivo. *Circulation.* 1996;94(5):932–938.

85. Hayes CE, Mathis CM, Yuan C. Surface coil phased arrays for high-resolution imaging of the carotid arteries. *J Magn Reson Imaging.* 1996;6(1):109–112.

86. Neubauer S, Ingwall JS. Verapamil attenuates ATP depletion during hypoxia: 31P NMR studies of the isolated rat heart. *J Mol Cell Cardiol.* 1989;21(11):1163–1178.

87. Ingwall JS. Phosphorus nuclear magnetic resonance spectroscopy of cardiac and skeletal muscles. *Am J Physiol.* 1982;242(5):H729–744.

88. Neubauer S, Ertl G, Krahe T, et al. Experimental and clinical possibilities of MR spectroscopy of the heart. *Z Kardiol.* 1991;80(1):25–36.

89. Clarke K, Stewart LC, Neubauer S, et al. Extracellular volume and transsarcolemmal proton movement during ischemia and reperfusion: a 31P NMR spectroscopic study of the isovolumic rat heart. *NMR Biomed.* 1993;6(4):278–286.

90. Horn M, Weidensteiner C, Scheffer H, et al. Detection of myocardial viability based on measurement of sodium content: A (23)Na-NMR study. *Magn Reson Med.* 2001;45(5):756–764.

91. Liao R, Nascimben L, Friedrich J, Gwathmey JK, Ingwall JS. Decreased energy reserve in an animal model of dilated cardiomyopathy. Relationship to contractile performance. *Circ Res.* 1996;78(5):893–902.

92. Zhang J, Wilke N, Wang Y, *et al.* Functional and bioenergetic consequences of postinfarction left ventricular remodeling in a new porcine model. MRI and 31 P-MRS study. *Circulation.* 1996;94(5):1089–1100.

93. Ugurbil K, Petein M, Madian R, Michurski S, Cohn JN, From AH. High resolution proton NMR studies of perfused rat hearts. *FEBS Lett.* 1984;167:73–78.

94. Balschi JA, Hetherington HP, Bradley EL, Jr., Pohost GM. Water-suppressed one-dimensional 1H NMR chemical shift imaging of the heart before and after regional ischemia. *NMR Biomed.* 1995;8(2):79–86.

95. Balschi JA, Hai JO, Wolkowicz PE, *et al.* 1H NMR measurement of triacylglycerol accumulation in the postischemic canine heart after transient increase of plasma lipids. *J Mol Cell Cardiol.* 1997;29(2):471–480.

96. Bottomley PA, Weiss RG. Noninvasive localized MR quantification of creatine kinase metabolites in normal and infarcted canine myocardium. *Radiology.* 2001;219(2):411–418.

97. Schneider J, Fekete E, Weisser A, Neubauer S, von Kienlin M. Reduced (1)H-NMR visibility of creatine in isolated rat hearts. *Magn Reson Med.* 2000;43(4):497–502.

98. Kreutzer U, Mekhamer Y, Chung Y, Jue T. Oxygen supply and oxidative phosphorylation limitation in rat myocardium in situ. *Am J Physiol Heart Circ Physiol.* 2001;280(5):H2030–H2037.

99. Solomon MA, Jeffrey FM, Storey CJ, Sherry AD, Malloy GR. Substrate selection early after reperfusion of ischemic regions in the working rabbit heart. *Magn Reson Med.* 1996;35(6):820–826.

100. Malloy CR, Jones JG, Jeffrey FM, Jessen ME, Sherry AD. Contribution of various substrates to total citric acid cycle flux and anaplerosis as determined by 13C isotopomer analysis and O2 consumption in the heart. *Magma.* 1996;4(1):35–46.

101. Lewandowski ED. Cardiac carbon 13 magnetic resonance spectroscopy: on the horizon or over the rainbow? *J Nucl Cardiol.* 2002;9(4):419–428.

102. Burgess SC, Babcock EE, Jeffrey FM, Sherry AD, Malloy CR. NMR indirect detection of glutamate to measure citric acid cycle flux in the isolated perfused mouse heart. *FEBS Lett.* 2001;505(1):163–167.

103. Weiss RG. 13C-NMR for the study of intermediary metabolism. *Magma.* 1998;6(2–3):132.

104. Kohler SJ, Perry SB, Stewart LC, Atkinson DE, Clarke K, Ingwall JS. Analysis of 23Na NMR spectra from isolated perfused hearts. *Magn Reson Med.* 1991;18(1):15–27.

105. Clarke K, Cross HR, Keon CA, Radda GK, Ingwall JS. Cation MR spectroscopy (7Li, 23Na, 39K and 87Rb). *Magma.* 1998;6(2–3):105–106.

106. DeLayre JL, Ingwall JS, Malloy C, Fossel ET. Gated sodium-23 nuclear magnetic resonance images of an isolated perfused working rat heart. *Science.* 1981;212(4497):935–936.

107. Kim RJ, Lima JAC, Chen EL, *et al.* Fast 23Na magnetic resonance imaging of acute reperfused myocardial infarction. Potential to assess myocardial viability. *Circulation.* 1997;95:1877–1885.

108. Neubauer S, Krahe T, Schindler R, *et al.* 31P magnetic resonance spectroscopy in dilated cardiomyopathy and coronary artery disease. Altered cardiac high-energy phosphate metabolism in heart failure. *Circulation.* 1992;86(6):1810–1818.

109. Bottomley PA. MR spectroscopy of the human heart: the status and the challenges. *Radiology.* 1994;191(3):593–612.

110. Shen W, Asai K, Uechi M, *et al.* Progressive loss of myocardial ATP due to a loss of total purines during the development of heart failure in dogs: a compensatory role for the parallel loss of creatine. *Circulation.* 1999;100(20):2113–2118.

111. Yabe T, Mitsunami K, Inubushi T, Kinoshita M. Quantitative measurements of cardiac phosphorus metabolites in coronary artery disease by 31P magnetic resonance spectroscopy [see comments]. *Circulation.* 1995;92(1):15–23.

112. Bottomley PA, Hardy CJ, Roemer PB. Phosphate metabolite imaging and concentration measurements in human heart by nuclear magnetic resonance. *Magn Reson Med.* 1990;14(3):425–434.

113. Bottomley PA, Atalar E, Weiss RG. Human cardiac high-energy phosphate metabolite concentrations by 1D-resolved NMR spectroscopy. *Magn Reson Med.* 1996;35(5):664–670.

114. Meininger M, Landschutz W, Beer M, *et al.* Concentrations of human cardiac phosphorus metabolites determined by SLOOP 31P NMR spectroscopy. *Magn Reson Med.* 1999;41(4):657–663.

115. Pohmann R, von Kienlin M. Accurate phosphorus metabolite images of the human heart by 3D acquisition-weighted CSI. *Magn Reson Med.* 2001;45(5):817–826.

116. Boada FE, Gillen JS, Shen GX, Chang SY, Thulborn KR. Fast three dimensional sodium imaging. *Magn Reson Med.* 1997;37(5):706–715.

117. Pabst T, Sandstede J, Beer M, *et al.* Optimization of ECG-triggered 3D (23)Na MRI of the human heart. *Magn Reson Med.* 2001;45(1):164–166.

118. Lee RF, Giaquinto R, Constantinides C, Souza S, Weiss RG, Bottomley PA. A broadband phased-array system

for direct phosphorus and sodium metabolic MRI on a clinical scanner. *Magn Reson Med.* 2000;43(2):269–277.

119. Shellock FG. *Guide to MR Procedures and Mettallic Objects:Update 2001*, 7th edition. Philadelphia: Lippincott, Williams and Wilkins Healthcare, 2001.

120. Vahlhaus C, Sommer T, Lewalter T, *et al.* Interference with cardiac pacemakers by magnetic resonance imaging: are there irreversible changes at 0.5 Tesla? *Pacing Clin Electrophysiol.* 2001;24(4 Pt 1):489–495.

121. Martin ET, Coman JA, Owen W, Shellock FG. Cardiac pacemakers and MRI: safe evaluation of 47 patients using a 1.5 Tesla MR system without altering pacemaker or imaging parameters. *JACC. J Am Coll Cardiol.* 2004;43(7):1315–1324.

122. Achenbach S, Moshage W, Diem B, Bieberle T, Schibgilla V, Bachmann K. Effects of magnetic resonance imaging on cardiac pacemakers and electrodes. *Am Heart J.* 1997;134(3):467–473.

123. Duru F, Luechinger R, Candinas R. MR imaging in patients with cardiac pacemakers. *Radiology.* 2001;219(3):856–858.

124. Shellock FG, Tkach JA, Ruggieri PM, Masaryk TJ. Cardiac pacemakers, ICDs, and loop recorder: evaluation of translational attraction using conventional ("long-bore") and "short-bore" 1.5- and 3.0-Tesla MR systems. *J Cardiovasc Magn Reson.* 2003;5(2):387–397.

125. American Heart Association. *2002 Heart and Stroke Statistical Update.* Dallas, TX: American Heart Association, 2001, pp. 31–32.

126. Roubin GS, Robinson KA, King SB, 3rd, *et al.* Early and late results of intracoronary arterial stenting after coronary angioplasty in dogs. *Circulation.* 1987;76(4):891–897.

127. Corporation G. Instructions for use: coronary stent system. Available at: http://www.guidant.com/products/ultra_ifu.shtml. Accessed 27th December, 2003.

128. Hug J, Nagel E, Bornstedt A, Schnackenburg B, Oswald H, Fleck E. Coronary arterial stents: safety and artifacts during MR imaging. *Radiology.* 2000;216(3):781–787.

129. Scott NA, Pettigrew RI. Absence of movement of coronary stents after placement in a magnetic resonance imaging field. *Am J Cardiol.* 1994;73(12):900–901.

130. Strohm O, Kivelitz D, Gross W, *et al.* Safety of implantable coronary stents during 1H-magnetic resonance imaging at 1.0 and 1.5 T. *J Cardiovasc Magn Reson.* 1999;1(3):239–245.

131. Schroeder AP, Houlind K, Pedersen EM, Thuesen L, Nielsen TT, Egeblad H. Magnetic resonance imaging seems safe in patients with intracoronary stents. *J Cardiovasc Magn Reson.* 2000;2(1):43–49.

132. Kramer CM, Rogers WJ, Jr, Pakstis DL. Absence of adverse outcomes after magnetic resonance imaging early after stent placement for acute myocardial infarction: a preliminary study. *J Cardiovasc Magn Reson.* 2000;2(4):257–261.

133. Gerber TC, Fasseas P, Lennon RJ, *et al.* Clinical safety of magnetic resonance imaging early after coronary artery stent placement. *J Am Coll Cardiol.* 2003;42(7):1295–1298.

134. Orford JL, Lennon R, Melby S, *et al.* Frequency and correlates of coronary stent thrombosis in the modern era: analysis of a single center registry. *J Am Coll Cardiol.* 2002;40(9):1567–1572.

135. Levine GN, Gomes AS, Arai AE, *et al.* Safety of magnetic resonance imaging in patients with cardiovascular devices: an American Heart Association scientific statement from the Committee on Diagnostic and Interventional Cardiac Catheterization, Council on Clinical Cardiology, and the Council on Cardiovascular Radiology and Intervention: endorsed by the American College of Cardiology Foundation, the North American Society for Cardiac Imaging, and the Society for Cardiovascular Magnetic Resonance. *Circulation.* 2007;116(24):2878–2891.

136. Soulen RL, Budinger TF, Higgins CB. Magnetic resonance imaging of prosthetic heart valves. *Radiology.* 1985;154(3):705–707.

137. Francis JM, Pennell DJ. Treatment of claustrophobia for cardiovascular magnetic resonance: use and effectiveness of mild sedation. *J Cardiovasc Magn Reson.* 2000;2(2):139–141.

CHAPTER 3

Cardiac Computed Tomography

Ian S. Rogers[1], Quynh A. Truong[2], Subodh B. Joshi[2] &
Udo Hoffmann[2]

[1]Stanford University Medical Center, Stanford, CA, USA
[2]Massachusetts General Hospital, Harvard Medical School, Boston, MA, USA

Introduction

The field of cardiac computed tomography (CCT) imaging has made profound strides over the past decade due mostly to dramatic technical advances in computed tomography (CT) technology. Scanners with four detector rows and spatial resolutions of over a 1 mm that required breath-holds of 30 seconds or more have been replaced by scanners that boast as many as 320 detector rows, spatial resolutions approaching that of invasive angiography, or breath-holds of 2 seconds or less. Cardiologists and radiologists are collaborating on clinical care, education, and critical trials to advance our understanding of both the strengths and the limitations of this relatively new but groundbreaking technology. Given the rapid pace of development, some are concerned about the potential for entrepreneurship and inappropriate use of CT for indications that have not yet been validated. With appropriate checks and balances in place, CT stands to revolutionize the manner in which cardiovascular disease is diagnosed.

CT Fundamentals

As CT scanning uses X-ray absorption to create images, natural contrast will depend on physical density and the abundance of atoms with differing atomic numbers. Individual pixels are assigned a value that is the equivalent of the linear transfor-

mation of the X-ray attenuation coefficient as referenced to the value of water, called a "Hounsfield unit" (HU). Pixels with higher CT attenuation than water will appear brighter or whiter, while those with lower CT attenuation will appear darker or blacker than water, allowing for tissue and contrast differentiation of anatomic structures. Iodine and calcium have high atomic numbers and will appear bright in CT images. Hydrogen, which is abundant in fat, has a low atomic number and appears dark gray. Blood and soft tissue have similar attenuation and consist of similar proportions of the same atoms (hydrogen, oxygen, carbon) and thus appear light gray. Lung contains air which is of very low physical density and appears black. Noncontrast CT, therefore, can distinguish noniodinated blood from air, fat, and bone but not from muscle or other soft tissue. This distinction of blood and soft tissue requires mixing of an intravenously injected contrast agent with a high atomic number, typically iodine with blood, in order to distinguish blood from soft tissue. The accentuated absorption of X-rays by elements of high atomic number such as calcium and iodine allows excellent visualization of small amounts of arterial calcium as well as differentiation between the contrast-enhanced lumina of arteries and their intima-lined walls.

Instrumentation

Scanner Fundamentals

CCT studies have traditionally been conducted on two distinct types of scanners, electron beam computed tomography (EBCT) scanners and

Cardiac CT, PET and MR, 2nd edition. Edited by Vasken Dilsizian and Gerry Pohost. © 2010 Blackwell Publishing Ltd.

multidetector computed tomography (MDCT) scanners. CT technology has advanced rapidly over the past decade, particularly since the introduction of the MDCT in the late 1990s. In 1998, the 4-slice MDCT became commercially available, allowing for simultaneous acquisition of four slices of images and with a gantry rotation of 500 ms, enabled full volumetric coverage of the heart over multiple heartbeats but with a single breath-hold of approximately 30 seconds. When the 64-slice MDCT scanners became available in 2004, the rise in use of CCT became significant, enabled full heart coverage with fewer heartbeats and in a single breath-hold of approximately 10–15 seconds. As MDCT scanners represent the vast majority of scanners currently in clinical use, this chapter will refer to MDCT as "CT," unless otherwise stated.

CT scanners consist of four main components, which include the table on which the patient lays, the tube that emits an X-ray beam through the patient, the detector array, and the gantry that rotates the tube and detector array around the patient. A detector array contains a number of detector rows, each with a particular slice width. The number of detector rows in the z-axis is commonly referred to as the number of "slices" that the scanner possesses. For instance, the standard "64-slice" scanner scans 64 detector rows in the z-axis with each rotation. As such, if the detectors are 0.625 mm wide, one rotation provides 64 detector rows × 0.625 mm wide, or 4 cm of volume coverage.

The patient is positioned on the table in the center of the scanner and once the scan is initiated, the table moves the patient through the imaging plane at a predetermined speed, referred to as the pitch. The pitch is defined as the table movement per rotation/single-slice width. X-rays are projected by one or more tubes through the anatomic area being imaged as the gantry rotates and the table is advanced. Scanners utilize a slip-ring interconnect, which allows the X-ray tube(s) and detector rows to rotate continuously during image acquisition. The X-rays are attenuated to different degrees as they pass through varying tissues in the body and received by the detectors on the opposite side, 180° from the tube. Data acquired on the detector arrays are digitalized as gray-scale pixels to produce a cross-sectional image slice made up of a pixel matrix in the X-Y plane (typically 512 × 512 pixels). Although the gantry does rotate a full 360° around the patient, a commonly used technique called "half-scan reconstruction" necessitates only 180° of data to reconstruct one image. Multiple two-dimensional cross-sectional image slices are then added in series in the Z-direction (or longitudinal direction) to create three-dimensional (3D) reconstructed images. The average volume needed to cover an entire heart in the Z-direction is approximately 12–16 cm, thus to obtain full coverage of the entire heart most scanners require summation of data over several heartbeats.

Temporal and Spatial Resolution

As the most challenging aspect of imaging of the heart is its inherent motion, tremendous value is placed on the temporal resolution of cardiac scanners. The temporal resolution is most dependent on the speed of the gantry rotation, defined as the time it takes the gantry to make one complete 360° rotation. As the temporal resolution improves, the CT scanner is able to acquire motion-free images at higher heart rates. Most 64-slice scanners have a gantry rotation time of approximately 330 ms. This results in a temporal resolution of 165 ms, given that "half-scan reconstruction" necessitates only 180° of data to reconstruct one image. An effective temporal resolution of 83 ms can be achieved when multisegment reconstruction is utilized.

Temporal resolution improved to a true 83 ms when the first dual-source 64-slice scanner was introduced and both gantry speed and temporal resolution were improved to 280 ms and 75 ms, respectively, when the first dual-source 128-slice scanner was introduced. In contrast to the single-source 64-slice CT scanners that have one X-ray tube source and one detector array located on opposite ends making cross-sectional images for each 180° rotation, dual-source CT scanners have two X-ray tube sources and detector arrays, aligned approximately 90° apart from each other (Figure 3.1). With two X-ray tube and detector arrays positioned at right angles to each other, instead of a full 180° rotation only 90° of data is needed for image acquisition. Although the temporal resolution of CT continues to improve, it remains significantly inferior to that of invasive angiography. At least

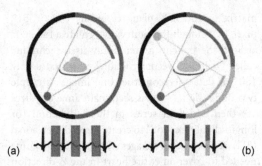

(a) (b)

Figure 3.1 Schematic depicting single-source 64-slice CT with half-scan reconstruction resulting in temporal resolution of 165 ms (a) and dual-source 64-slice CT with half-scan reconstruction resulting in temporal resolution of 83 ms (b).

one vendor has sought to obviate the relevance of temporal resolution by adding enough detector rows (currently as many as 320 detector rows) to cover the entire length of the heart, thus permitting image acquisition in one heartbeat.

Spatial resolution, defined as the minimum distance between two objects at which the objects are still discernible from each other, is also an important consideration in CCT acquisition. The spatial resolution of CT is composed of the X-Y pixel size in the imaging plane as well as the Z-plane, which creates a "voxel," the 3D volume counterpart for a pixel. Factors that can affect spatial resolution include slice collimation width, power of the X-ray source (both the tube current and the voltage), and reconstruction algorithm kernels. As the spatial resolution improves, the CT scanner is able to detect smaller size objects. Coronary arteries often start proximally with a modest diameter of approximately 3.5 mm and progressively taper to 1 mm or smaller distally, with submillimeter braches. High spatial resolution is critical in assessing these small vessels, particularly when atherosclerotic plaque narrows the lumen or intracoronary stents need to be examined for evidence of in-stent restenosis. Spatial resolution has progressively improved from 1.25 mm on 4-slice scanners to 1 mm on 16-slice scanners to 0.4–0.6 mm on 64-slice scanners. As of the time of preparation of this text, one vendor has marketed a scanner reporting spatial resolution up to 0.23 mm. If realized, such a spatial resolution would approach the 0.20–0.25 mm spatial resolution of invasive angiography.

Gating

The key distinctions between CCT studies and routine contrast-enhanced CT scans of the thorax include the timing of the contrast bolus to maximally opacify the coronary arteries and left heart, focus of the scan area on the heart and proximal great vessels, and the use of electrocardiographic (ECG) gating. Scans of the thorax acquired without ECG gating suffer from significant motion artifact in the rapidly moving heart. Therefore, ECG gating is almost always used in cardiac imaging, which synchronizes image acquisition to the cardiac cycle and reduces or effectively eliminates motion artifact. Depending on the detector width, summation of the images from multiple consecutive heartbeats would yield a 3D image of the heart.

ECG-gating can be either prospectively triggered or retrospectively gated. Most cardiac scan protocols have traditionally utilized retrospective ECG gating, in which images are acquired in the helical mode of operation, acquiring several simultaneous channels of data during continuous advancement of the CT table. The relationship of the scan coverage to the table speed is called the scan pitch and is properly defined as the ratio of the table increment over the detector collimation. The low scan pitch traditionally employed during cardiac acquisition in the helical mode (0.2–0.4) produces overlapping of the scanned area, which ensures contiguous sampling with no gap in coverage.

Tube current is delivered throughout the cardiac cycle when retrospective ECG gating is utilized, which can permit data set reconstruction at multiple points in the cardiac cycle (e.g., 35, 65, and 70% of the R-R interval), as opposed to the fixed 65 or 70% point of acquisition used with most prospectively triggered gating protocols. In addition, since the motion of different coronary arteries is not synchronous and the motion of the coronary arteries throughout diastole can be accentuated by diastolic dysfunction, using multiple points in the cardiac cycle allows improved image quality of all segments of the three coronary arteries. As such, this mode of acquisition is more forgiving if heart rate variability occurs. Moreover, tube current delivery throughout the cardiac cycle also permits reconstruction of a cine data set from images at 5 or 10% increments over the cycle (Figure 3.2). Unfortunately, these benefits come at the cost of increased

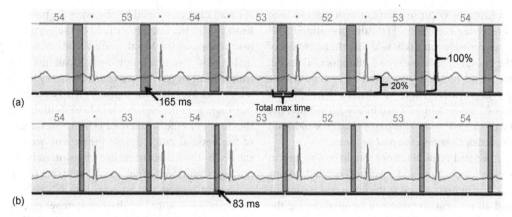

Figure 3.2 ECG tracings recorded during scan acquisition on a single-source 64-slice CT scanner (a) and on a dual-source 64-slice CT scanner (b) utilizing ECG tube modulation. Tube current is turned down to 20% of maximum during systole to minimize dose and increased to 100% during a predetermined period in diastole. The total maximum time window at 100% can be determined prior to acquisition and includes time for the tube(s) to "ramp up" to 100% and "ramp down" to 20%. The darker blue bars indicate the period of image reconstruction, the width of which is equal to the temporal resolution, 165 ms for the single-source scanner, and 83 ms for the dual-source scanner.

and often unnecessary radiation exposure to the patient.

Prospective ECG triggering, also sometimes known as the "step and shoot" mode of acquisition, acquires axial images only at fixed points in the R-R interval, such as at 65% of the R-R interval. After acquiring an axial image at one level, the table is advanced over the next heartbeat, permitting axial acquisition in a narrow window of the cardiac cycle every other heartbeat. This is analogous to the axial acquisition employed by EBCT scanners and is the mode used for coronary artery calcium scoring. The primary benefit of prospective-triggered scans is the reduction in radiation dose, as the X-ray tube is only "on" during that one phase of the cardiac cycle when the images are being acquired. The disadvantage of a prospective-triggered scan is that functional assessment, including determinations of left ventricular ejection fraction and aortic valve area, is not possible as only one phase is acquired and available for analysis. In addition, image quality may be compromised with misregistration and slab artifacts or breath-hold may be prolonged if ectopic beats, arrhythmias, or heart rate variability occurs during the CT acquisition. Thus, the heart rate should ideally be regular and slow (<65 beats/minute) with a prospectively triggered scan. While this technique minimizes radiation exposure to the patient significantly, some scanners are cur-

rently unable to adjust quickly if a sudden change in heart rate or an extrasystole occurs, which can result in non-imaged scan length.

Patient Preparation

CCT scans are generally very well tolerated and require little preparation on the part of most patients. To preclude substance-induced increases in heart rate, most institutions request that patients not ingest coffee, tea, or other caffeinated beverages for 12 hours prior to the exam and some institutions recommend abstaining from nicotine products for at least 4 hours prior to the exam. Abstinence from caffeine-containing beverages also avoids dehydration as a result of their diuretic properties. Some institutions further advise fasting for 2 or more hours prior to the exam due to the rare side effect of nausea from intravenous contrast agents, as fasting would help to ensure an empty stomach should a patient vomit. However, this side effect is rare enough with current contrast agents that many agree that fasting is not an absolute requirement for preparation.

Patients should be instructed to take most medications on the day of the scan that they would normally take, with the general exceptions of metformin and phosphodiesterase type 5 inhibitors. Metformin is generally held the day of and 48 hours following the scan due to the rare but serious risk of lactic acidosis, should contrast-induced nephropathy occur in a patient with diabetes who is receiving metformin [1]. Administration of nitroglycerin is contraindicated with the recent use of the phosphodiesterase type 5 inhibitors, sildenafil, vardenafil, and tadalafil, as these agents potentiate the hypotensive effect of nitrates. Nitroglycerin should not be administered to any patient that has taken tadalafil within the past 48 hours or sildenafil or vardenafil within the past 24 hours.

A focused medical history should be obtained to screen for absolute and relative contraindications to the scan itself as well as the intravenous contrast and all medications that will be used during the exam. History should include assessment for past contrast reactions, potential for pregnancy, renal insufficiency, or other chronic renal conditions, reversible obstructive pulmonary disease, valvular heart disease, and hypertrophic cardiomyopathy. Institutional policy and absolute need for the exam usually dictate the degree of renal insufficiency that is deemed acceptable. The focused history should also elicit the symptoms or conditions that have prompted the exam and confirm whether the patient has a history of coronary stent placement or coronary artery bypass surgery, as these factors may impact image acquisition and/or data reconstruction.

Intravenous catheter placement is most ideal with an 18-gauge catheter in the right antecubital fossa. Right-sided injections are preferred over left sided injections as left-sided injections may lead to streak artifact in the superior field of view from the transit of the contrast bolus across the left brachiocephalic vein. Twenty-gauge catheters and/or alternate sites may be used, provided that test injections of saline into the catheter support a fast injection rate.

Administration of beta-blocker prior to the scan, e.g., with either i.v. metoprolol (often given in 5 mg increments every 5 minutes up to a total dose of 25 mg immediately prior to the scan) or oral metoprolol (often given as 50 mg the evening prior to the scan and 50 mg 1 hour prior to the scan), is recommended when a patient's prescan heart rate is greater than 65 beats/minute. Intravenous diltiazem is used at some centers if a contraindication to beta blockade exists or if maximal beta blockade has not achieved adequate heart rate reduction. A useful assessment of the expected heart rate during the scan can be obtained by observing the patient's heart rate in the inspiratory hold of the breathing instructions, as the Valsalva effect tends to reduce and steady the heart rate by a small but not insignificant degree. Some clinicians nevertheless administer 5 mg of i.v. metoprolol even if a patient's heart rate is in the high 50s and low 60s to reduce the chance of a sudden increase in heart rate outside of the optimal range should the patient become startled by the sudden warmth of the contrast bolus during acquisition. Trial results and anecdotal experience suggest that prescan beta blockade is generally not required for diagnostic image quality when a scanner with a temporal resolution of less than 100 ms will be used [2]. Some institutions also administer i.v. lidocaine if premature ventricular contractions are noted prior to the scan; however, this practice has not been demonstrated to be significantly beneficial and may impart more risk than benefit, particularly in settings where experience with administering i.v. lidocaine is limited.

Following verification of a dependable ECG tracing and heart rate optimization, review of the scan procedure with the patient is important, particularly a discussion of the contrast administration and the breathing instructions. Patients should be advised of the symptoms that they are likely to feel with contrast administration (often described by patients as a "hot flash") to minimize the chance of them becoming startled by these symptoms, which can lead to an increase in heart rate and/or failure to adhere to the breathing instructions. A trial of the actual sequence of breathing instructions that the patient should expect, including a prolonged breath-hold, is very valuable as it provides the clinician the opportunity to gauge whether the patient will be able to comply with the breath-hold as well as the opportunity to stress the importance of holding still and following the instructions on the overall image quality.

Administration of sublingual nitroglycerin should be immediately prior to the scan, after all prescan instructions have been given, as the vasodilatory effects generally typically become noticeable 1 minute following administration and reach maximal efficacy 3 minutes following administration [3]. Nitroglycerin can be administered as 400–800 µg of a sublingual tablet or sublingual spray. In addition to the contraindication of

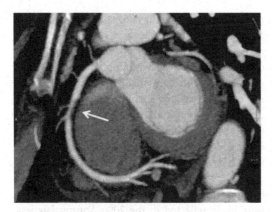

Figure 3.3 Maximal intensity projection of the right coronary artery, demonstrating significant stenosis from noncalcified plaque (white arrow) in a 52-year-old woman with atypical angina.

presence and extent of coronary artery disease (CAD) (Figure 3.3). Most acquisition protocols to maximize opacification of the coronary arteries and left heart consist of two to three stages. The first stage is acquisition of the topogram, or scout image, which is a low-dose projectional image of the chest that is similar to an anterior-posterior chest radiograph. This localizes the intended scan length and clarifies alignment, with most protocols imaging from the level of the carina to the level of the diaphragm. Protocols that include a supplemental calcium scoring data set perform this acquisition at this time, prior to proceeding with contrast administration.

administration with recent phosphodiesterase type 5 inhibitor use mentioned previously, caution should be used when considering nitroglycerin use in patients that are relatively hypotensive and/or volume depleted or if they have a known hypertrophic cardiomyopathy, restrictive cardiomyopathy, constrictive pericarditis, or severe aortic or mitral stenosis. Patients should be instructed that they may develop a headache following the use of nitroglycerin, this headache should abate after a few hours, and this headache may be reduced with mild analgesics.

Next, most protocols utilize a "test bolus" to determine the optimal time to image the contrast-enhanced heart. While protocols vary, a common test bolus involves the administration of a 20-mL intravenous bolus of contrast agent at a rate of 5 mL/second followed by 40 mL of saline injected intravenously at 5 mL/second. Sequential axial scans are then obtained at the level of the proximal ascending aorta at 2-second intervals beginning 8 or 10 seconds after contrast administration. Peak opacification time for the proximal ascending aorta is recorded in a region of interest and serves as the trigger time for initiating scan acquisition (Figure 3.4). To determine the total contrast volume to be infused for the actual acquisition, the time to peak opacification in the proximal ascending aorta is added to the time required to cover the scan length and this value is multiplied by the infusion rate (e.g., 5 mL/second).

Contrast-Enhanced Protocols

Protocol: Coronaries and Left Heart

The principal use of contrast-enhanced CCT remains the noninvasive direct assessment for the

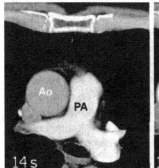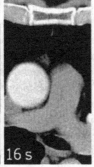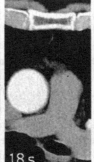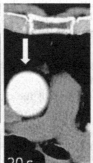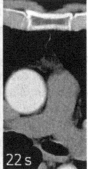

Figure 3.4 Sequential axial scans at the level of the proximal ascending aorta recorded during test bolus acquisition. Peak opacification time for the proximal ascending aorta is 20 seconds (arrow), which serves as the trigger time for initiating scan acquisition. Ao, aorta; PA, pulmonary artery.

Preparation for the actual contrast-enhanced acquisition is then finalized by selecting the scan length on the topogram, selecting the mode (i.e., retrospective vs. prospective) of acquisition, selecting the tube current and voltage, selection of dose reduction strategies (e.g., tube modulation), and entry of the trigger delay time into the scanner. To lower radiation exposure, we use a kVp of 100 for subjects with a BMI < 30 and a kVp of 120 for subjects with a BMI ≥ 30, as well as aggressive tube current modulation, attenuation adaptation, and adaptive pitch selection whenever feasible. After the contrast delivery volume and rate is ensured, the scanner and contrast delivery unit are simultaneously activated to begin acquisition.

Some institutions do not use a "test bolus" stage and instead rely on automated detection of contrast opacification in the proximal ascending aorta, a technique often known as "bolus tracking." With this technique, following the topogram stage, a single axial slice is acquired at the level of the proximal ascending aorta and a region of interest is then placed in the proximal ascending aorta. Once a predefined attenuation value of about 110–150 HU is reached, the breath-hold instruction is given (~4–6 seconds) and the CT scanner automatically initiates image acquisition with contrast enhancement increased to the desired level of enhancement. Using this technique, the CT technologist needs to pay close attention and manually override and initiate image acquisition should the CT scanner not automatically start acquiring images. We prefer the test bolus scan because it gives the patient a practice opportunity with their breath-hold, allows us to see how the contrast affects the heart rate (which may require us to give more beta-blocker), and also reassures us that the IV is working properly with the high power contrast injector.

Protocol Considerations: Assessment of Bypass Grafts

While luminal assessment of the native coronaries is often limited by dense coronary calcification in patients who have had previous coronary artery bypass grafting surgery, imaging of the grafts is typically quite feasible. Both arterial and venous grafts are less susceptible to motion than the native vessels [4] and the venous grafts are larger in diameter than the native coronaries, facilitating their assess-

ment. A caveat is that the native segments that serve as distal runoff from the grafts can be challenging to assess given their small size and vulnerability to calcification and cardiac motion.

A general principle is that if a referring physician seeks only to exclude significant graft disease, CT can often do so very accurately. However, if the referring physician requires assessment of the native coronaries, direct referral for invasive angiography is likely to more helpful given the higher rate of native segments that are unevaluable due to calcification with current technology. These limitations were likely reflected in the 2006 Appropriateness Criteria for CCT and cardiac magnetic resonance (CMR), which rated the use of CCT as "uncertain" for the evaluation of bypass grafts and coronary anatomy in symptomatic patients and as "inappropriate" in asymptomatic patients.

When scanning a patient with known coronary disease, the importance of heart rate control is amplified to minimize beam-hardening artifacts from the combination of coronary calcification and coronary motion. A heart rate goal of less than 60 beats/minute should be used, even when a scanner with a high temporal resolution is to be utilized. The scan length should extend from the lung apices to the level of the diaphragm to ensure complete visualization to the level of the anastomosis of the internal mammary arteries with the subclavian arteries, as stenosis can occur at the level of these anastomoses, leading to compromised distal flow.

Scan acquisition in the caudal–cranial direction is typically advised, as the diagnostic accuracy of a scan stands to be less compromised should a patient not be able to maintain a complete breath-hold during the prolonged scan time often required (typically 20 seconds on single-source 64-slice scanners). Respiratory motion artifact hampers assessments of the grafts (later in the scan during a caudal to cranial acquisition) less than it hampers assessment of the native coronaries and distal runoff vessels (later in the scan during a cranial to caudal acquisition). Additionally, an initial deceleration in heartbeat caused by the Valsalva-induced vagal response often takes place after the start of the breath-hold period; however, this phenomenon fades as the scan approaches 20 seconds [5], which can affect image quality if heart rate begins to accelerate at the level of the coronary ostia during a cranial to caudal acquisition [6].

Unlike the case with standard CCT, where 3D volume rendered reconstructions are rarely useful for more than demonstration purposes, 3D reconstructions can be helpful in cases scanned for bypass graft assessment as they facilitate identification of the origin, course, and distal anastomosis of grafts as well as their relation to other cardiac structures (Figure 3.5). This can be especially useful if a report of the operative bypass procedure is not available. While proximal venous graft occlusions can usually be readily identified on 3D reconstructions, caution should be exercised not to rely on 3D reconstructions alone for luminal assessment of the grafts or the native vessels, as changes in the window-level settings can cause vessels to appear both falsely patent and falsely stenotic. Instead, axial and multiplanar images should be used for luminal assessment. Review of reconstructions performed at multiple points in the cardiac cycle (e.g., 35, 65, and 75% of the R-R interval) can be helpful in improving assessment despite artifact from calcification and metallic surgical clips, as can reconstructing the data set with a sharp kernel.

Protocol Considerations: Assessment of the Pulmonary Veins

CCT is increasingly used prior to invasive catheter procedures that are used to treat arrhythmias. The anatomical information CT provides aids patient selection, can improve procedural efficiency, and can reduce complications. Atrial fibrillation ablation is a catheter-based procedure that involves electrically isolating regions of the left atrium by creating radio-frequency burns. The regions of the left atrium usually targeted in this procedure are the pulmonary vein ostia (Figure 3.6). CT can provide a 3D model of the left atrium and the pulmonary veins that can then be imported into an electroanatomic map. Incorporation of the CT data in such a way has been shown to reduce fluoroscopy times and reduce recurrence of atrial fibrillation [7].

CCT may also be helpful in reducing complications resulting from atrial fibrillation ablation. Accessory pulmonary veins are not uncommon, and their recognition preprocedure is desirable [8] to avoid trauma. A rare but lethal complication of atrial fibrillation ablation is an atrio-esophageal fistula [9] caused by burns to the esophagus through the left atrial wall. CCT may reduce the risk of this complication by defining the relationship between the esophagus and left atrial structures preoperatively [10]. After atrial fibrillation ablation, CCT is an ideal technique by which to evaluate for pulmonary venous stenosis [11]. The imaging protocol for the left atrium and pulmonary veins is almost identical to that for the coronary vessels other than the acquisition being initiated slightly earlier.

As the pulmonary veins and left atrial anatomy are large objects, detailed submillimeter spatial resolution is not a requirement for assessment of these structures. The protocol is similar whether a pulmonary vein study is performed for preatrial fibrillation ablation or for evaluation of postprocedural complication, such as pulmonary vein stenosis. Due to the limitations on ECG tube modulation when patients are in atrial fibrillation, nongated CT

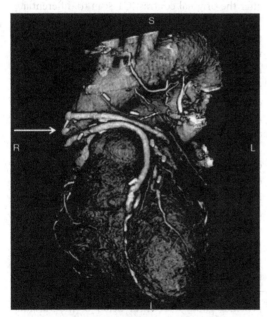

Figure 3.5 Volume rendered reconstruction from a 67-year-old patient who underwent cardiac computed tomography for atypical chest pain 3 year status-post coronary artery bypass graft (CABG) surgery. Although three sapheneous vein grafts (SVG) were originally implanted into the ascending aorta, proximal occlusion of one graft can be visualized (white arrow). The volume rendered image also suggests significant stenosis just distal to the anastomosis of an SVG with the left anterior descending artery (black arrow).

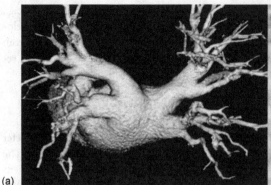
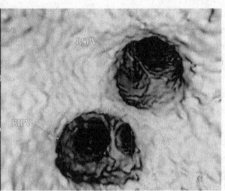

(a)   (b)

Figure 3.6 Volume rendered image of left atrium demonstrating four distinct pulmonary veins in their expected position (a) and endoluminal view of left atrium (b). The ostia of the right superior pulmonary vein (RSPV) and right inferior pulmonary vein (RIPV) can be easily visualized.

should be considered for a pulmonary vein study in these patients. Alternatively, a retrospectively ECG-gated CT could be performed with reconstruction performed during systole, although beta-blockers should be given to slow the heart rate to as close as 60 bpm with 64-slice CT and less than 100 bpm with dual-source CT.

As the contrast enhancement of the left atrium and pulmonary veins occurs slightly earlier than the opacification of the ascending aorta, arterial phase imaging similar to that of a left heart and coronary artery study can be used. Nitroglycerin is not necessary unless the coronary arteries are also in question. Beta-blockers can be given if necessary to optimize the heart rate. For preablation patients, because of the potential risk of atrio-esophageal fistula during the ablation procedure, a teaspoon of oral barium can be given prior to the CT scan to coat the esophagus to localize its relationship to the left atrium and pulmonary veins [10,12]. Oral barium is not necessary if the CT exam is to evaluate exclusively for pulmonary vein stenosis. To optimize coregistration with the electroanatomical mapping where the ablation procedure is performed with free-breathing, CT image acquisition should be obtained with an expiration breath-hold.

Either a test bolus or bolus tracking technique can be utilized after the topogram. Scan coverage should include the aortic arch vessels to the level of the bottom of the diaphragm. Caudo-cranial acquisition minimizes the interference of contrast flux in the superior vena cava. During the CT contrast scan acquisition, inspection of the left atrial appendage for a potential filling defect is recommended with immediate reconstruction of one data set for closer evaluation. If a filling defect is suspected, then an additional noncontrast-enhanced delayed CT scan should be performed within 30 seconds to 1 minute after the original contrast CT scan to differentiate between a left atrial thrombus (which will remain as a persistent filling defect) versus slow flow (which will "fill in" with resolution of the filling defect). To minimize the patient's radiation dose, the delayed scan should be prospectively triggered and image acquisition set at the level of the aortic arch to the middle of the ventricle just to target the left atrial appendage region.

Image reconstruction is typically performed during systole when the left atrium is largest using either fixed distance after the QRS duration (i.e., 250 ms) or a percentage phase reconstruction (i.e., 35%). For measuring luminal diameters, double-obliques of the myocardial perfusion reserve could provide true short-axis diameters. For anatomical description, evaluation of the pulmonary veins from the axial images and the longitudinal plane with maximum intensity projection reconstruction provides good anatomical detail of the variants of pulmonary veins, the number of aortic arch vessel, and location of the esophagus in relation to the left atrium. Volume-rendered techniques are additionally helpful for the electrophysiologist. The 3D volume rendering technique (3D-VRT) can isolate just the left atrium with pulmonary veins and aorta, while the "fly-through" or endoluminal view can provide intraluminal images of each of the pulmonary veins. The data from the contrast-enhanced CT can then be sent to the electrophysiologist for "merging" and coregistration for electroanatomical mapping using specialized software.

Protocol Considerations: Assessment of the Coronary Veins

Cardiac resynchronization therapy (CRT.), or biventricular pacing, is a treatment for congestive heart failure that involves placing a lead through the coronary sinus to pace the left ventricle. Pacing leads are also placed in the right ventricle allowing coordination of the timing of ventricular contraction. CT can be used to identify the coronary sinus and the coronary venous system into which the left ventricular lead can be placed [13]. With there being a wide variance in coronary venous anatomy, pre-procedure CT imaging allows locating the optimal venous structure (usually the posterolateral branch) to reduce the odds of suboptimal lead placement. The protocol for coronary venous imaging requires later image acquisition relative to coronary artery studies to allow time for venous filling. It is hoped that preprocedural evaluation of the coronary venous anatomy will improve both patient selection and clinical outcome.

The coronary sinus and venous tree with its tributaries can be visualized and can be defined preprocedurally by CT [14]. The CT imaging protocol is similar to that used for a standard coronary CT angiography with several important exceptions. For coronary venous imaging, inspiratory breath-hold is similar to that from a coronary artery study. Nitroglycerin is not needed as dilation of the coronary arteries may interfere with the evaluation of the cardiac veins, which course in similar directions as the coronary arteries. Depending on the type of CT scanner, the use of beta-blockers to achieve optimal heart rate may be considered. An ECG-gated CT could be performed with dual-source CT and beta-blockers to decrease the heart rate to as close to 60 bpm as possible. We do not recommend scanning atrial fibrillation patients with standard 64-slice or less CT due to its limited temporal resolution.

Caudo-cranial image acquisition is also preferred given that the coronary sinus is inferiorly positioned in the heart, although there does not appear to be much difference in our experience when cranio-caudal acquisition is performed. After the scout image, a test bolus protocol is preferred over bolus tracking to calculate the contrast agent transit time. For patients with severe left ventricular dysfunction, inform them that the test bolus scan is the longest of the image acquisitions and may take up to 30 seconds for the breath-hold. This is due to the poor cardiac output and prolonged transit time from the antecubital vein to the ascending or descending aorta. However, the subsequent CT venography breath-hold should be less than 15 seconds and is based on the scan range volume coverage of the heart. Scan coverage should be from the carina bifurcation to the diaphragm, similar to that of a coronary artery scan.

For optimal enhancement of the coronary venous system, the most notable distinction is that venous phase imaging is desired. An empiric 5- to 10-second delay should be added to the contrast agent transit time so that image acquisition will be performed during the venous and not arterial phase. We reserve an 8- to 10-second delay for patients with severely impaired left ventricular function. Whatever additional delay time used for venous phase imaging should be added to the volume of contrast, although this additional volume could be given at a slower rate (i.e., 2–3 mL/second) to minimize the contrast load. In our experience, the typical delay time to set on the CT scanner (using either the Siemens 64-slice CT or dual-source CT scanners) for CT venography is anticipated to be 40 seconds or longer for the CRT population, though this time may be variable depending on vendors.

With image reconstruction, quick review of all the phases obtained from the multiphase reconstructions would give guidance to which phase provides the best image. Typically, a systolic percentage phase of either 35 or 45% yields good visualization of the cardiac venous system. However, occasionally a small cardiac vein may appear at a diastolic phase, thus, close review of each of the phases is recommended. Evaluation of the coronary sinus, the presence of a Thebesian valve, and the cardiac veins that supply the posterolateral wall of the heart are of particular relevance to electrophysiologists. 3D-VRT images can be reconstructed to provide images of the heart and cardiac veins that electrophysiologists can easily identify and correlate to invasive coronary venography.

Protocol Considerations: Assessment of Valves

Cardiac ultrasound, with its very high temporal resolution and Doppler capabilities, is deservedly the first line test for valvular dysfunction. The necessary data for valvular imaging is acquired as part of a routine coronary CT study and therefore is considered useful added information; rarely would assessment of valvular function be the primary focus of a CT examination. One useful feature of CCT is the ability to reconstruct images in any plane. This can be helpful in valvular disease when specific views of a valve are crucial for accurate diagnosis, such as for defining valvular anatomy in patients being considered for percutaneous aortic valve replacement and mitral valve repair.

Aortic valve morphology can be reliably assessed by CCT. An en face view of the valve makes a bicuspid, unicuspid or quadracuspid aortic valve easy to identify [15] (Figure 3.7). Often the first clue of aortic valve disease on CT is valvular calcification, the degree of calcification correlating with the severity of stenosis [16]. Aortic stenosis can be quantified by planimetry of the valve orifice [17,18]. For this technique to be accurate the greatest valve orifice must be measured at the tips of the valve leaflets at the time of maximal opening in systole. Recent data has demonstrated that 50–100 ms after the R

wave on the electrocardiogram is the optimal time for measurement [19]. Quantification of aortic regurgitation by CT is more challenging. Planimetry of the regurgitant orifice has been validated against echocardiography but further research is awaited before this technique can be considered for routine clinical use [20].

Mitral valve morphology can also be assessed by CCT. Mitral annular calcification, while particularly striking, is not usually associated with hemodynamically significant valvular stenosis. Deposition of calcium in the leaflets themselves is less common but more likely to be a consequence of rheumatic heart disease and associated with significant stenosis. By allowing selection of the optimal image, planimetry of the mitral valve orifice is reliable [21]. Initial experience suggests that some quantification of mitral regurgitation may also be possible [22]. It is noteworthy that because of the relatively low temporal resolution, CCT may be less sensitive than echocardiography for the detection of mobile valvular vegetations. For patients with confirmed endocarditis, however, CT may be helpful for the identification of paravalvular abscesses. Perhaps the most useful application of CCT in patients with endocarditis, as in with patients with other valvular disease, is the exclusion of other coronary disease thus potentially avoiding invasive angiography prior to surgery [23,24].

Protocol Considerations: Assessment of the Thoracic Aorta

CT is an extremely useful modality to image the thoracic aorta, particularly in the evaluation of aortic aneurysms, aortic dissections, and in both blunt and penetrating thoracic trauma [25]. Contrast-enhanced CT can rapidly identify aortic tears, intramural hematoma, and dissection. In addition, the presence of mediastinal hematoma and other associated injuries can be assessed. However, as the aortic root is directly connected to the left ventricle and moves in concert with it, motion artifacts can create the appearance of a dissection flap and lead to concern for Stanford type A aortic dissection [26] in a not insignificant percentage of cases [27]. Motion can also preclude accurate aortic root measurement for potential sinus of Valsalva aneuryms. ECG gating can effectively control this motion and significantly reduce the incidence of motion

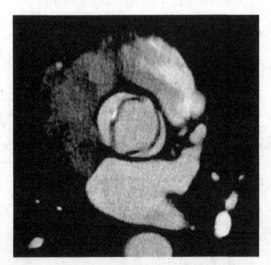

Figure 3.7 En face view of a bicuscpid aortic valve orifice in systole. Only two leaflets are visible resulting in the characteristic "fish-mouth" opening.

artifacts. As such, some experts have recommended that "ECG gating should be mandatory for thoracic aortic CT angiograms performed to detect potential aortic dissection" [28]. We agree that ECG gating should be utilized when evaluation of the aortic root and proximal ascending aorta is needed.

The protocol to provide full evaluation of the thoracic aorta differs from that focused to evaluate the coronary arteries principally in extending the field of view and increasing the contrast volume to sufficiently opacify the vessel, similar to the evaluation of coronary artery bypass grafts. The scan length should extend from the lung apices to the level of the diaphragm to ensure complete visualization of the arch vessels. Some bolus tracking techniques differ in that the trigger region of interest is placed in the descending thoracic aorta rather than in the proximal ascending aorta with the goal of maximizing the homogeneity of opacification within the aorta. If the coronary arteries will also be examined, scan acquisition in the caudal–cranial direction is typically advised. Nitroglycerin is not necessary if the coronary arteries will not be examined for luminal stenosis and should be withheld as clinically appropriate in the face of hemodynamic instability.

When the aorta is being evaluated for acute aortic injury (e.g., hematoma and dissection), most institutions perform a noncontrast-enhanced scan from the lung apices to the level of the diaphragm prior to any administration of contrast to increase the sensitivity of the examination for the detection of intramural hematoma. In cases where the scan length is planned to extend into the abdomen and pelvis for evaluation of the entire aorta, care should be taken to link an ECG-gated thoracic scan with a nonECG-gated scan of the abdomen and pelvis if possible, as continuing an ECG-gated scan into the abdomen and pelvis does not typically provide any additional diagnostic benefit but does significantly increase radiation exposure.

While these exams may be performed in critically ill patients who may require mechanical ventilation, invasive monitoring, and intravenous infusions pumps, most CT suites can easily accommodate life support equipment, which can remain in the room and operational throughout acquisition. Although magnetic resonance imaging (MRI) and transesophageal echocardiography (TEE) can provide unique information, MRI requires a long acquisition time and is frequently impractical in critically ill patients, while TEE is invasive, requires highly trained physicians to be available for acquisition, and has a known "blind spot" in the mid to distal ascending aorta. MRI may be a more optimal exam for serial measurements of aortic dilation over time, however, as ECG-gated CT exams can result in considerable exposure to radiation, particularly if retrospective gating is employed. In patients who are not candidates for MRI, prospective ECG gating can help to reduce the cumulative exposure from serial CT exams.

Protocol Considerations: Comprehensive Cardiothoracic CT—the "Triple Rule Out"

Recent technical developments now permit acquisition of high-quality images of the coronary arteries, thoracic aorta, and pulmonary arterial system in a single comprehensive cardiothoracic CT scan. Colloquially know as the "triple rule out," the goal of this protocol is to simultaneously exclude CAD, pulmonary embolism, and aortic dissection. The protocol may offer an attractive option to rapidly evaluate patients with undifferentiated chest pain in whom any of the three dedicated CT scans may be performed as standard of care, followed by diagnostic testing for one or more of the alternative pathologies. The prototypical case example is that of a patient with undifferentiated dyspnea and chest pain that extends to the back, who might otherwise receive CT angiography of the thoracic and abdominal aorta, a serum D-dimer assay (potentially followed by CT angiography of the pulmonary arteries), and a rest-stress nuclear myocardial perfusion study after prolonged observation and serial cardiac enzymes.

Initial data suggest that the protocol is feasible and that extracardiac findings (such as pneumonia and fractures) will be detected in some patients, which will change management [29,30]. Optimal image quality using the comprehensive protocol is challenged by the fact that patients experiencing acute chest pain and/or dyspnea often have higher heart rates and administration of intravenous beta-blockers is relatively contraindicated if pulmonary embolus is in the differential diagnosis. Moreover, radiation exposure can be high as the comprehensive protocol represents an ECG-gated scan of the

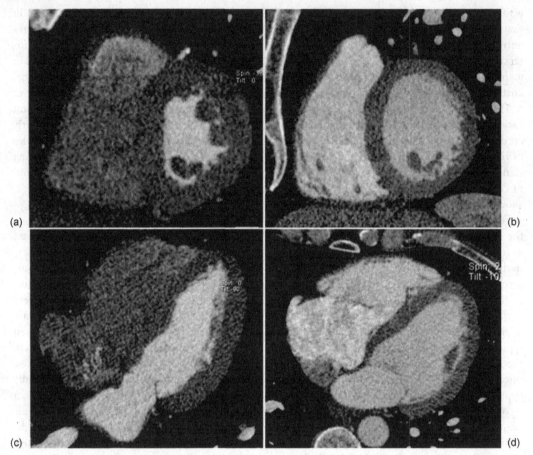

Figure 3.8 Short-axis and four-chamber views from a study protocoled to opacify the left heart and coronaries (a and c) and from a study protocoled to concomitantly opacify the pulmonary circuit and right heart (b and d).

entire thorax. The recent introduction of scanners with higher temporal resolution may help to overcome the limitations of higher heart rates and preclude the need for beta blockade.

The most straightforward comprehensive cardiothoracic protocol can be accomplished by extending the scan length to scan from the level of the diaphragm to the lung apices in a caudal to cranial direction and by adding a sufficient volume of contrast to concomitantly opacify the pulmonary circuit and right heart (Figure 3.8). This can be accomplished via a "test bolus" based protocol, such as 20 mL intravenous bolus of contrast agent at a rate of 5 mL/second followed by 40 mL of saline injected intravenously at 5 mL/second. Sequential axial scans are then obtained at the common level of the main pulmonary artery and proximal ascending aorta at 2-second intervals beginning 2–4 seconds after contrast administration. Note that this time is shorter for this protocol than for a standard coronary protocol (8–10 seconds) as contrast reaches the pulmonary arterial system earlier in patients with normal anatomy.

To determine the total contrast volume to be infused, the difference between time to peak opacification in the main pulmonary artery and time to peak opacification in the aorta is added to the time required to cover the scan length and this value is multiplied by the infusion rate (5 mL/second). Time to peak opacification in the aortic root remains the trigger time for initiating scan acquisition. Given that transit time through the pulmonary circuit is 8–10 seconds in many patients, a bolus tracking technique with 10 extra seconds of contrast beyond that required for a left heart scan could conceivably produce diagnostic opacification in many patients with current scanners if manual determination of the transit time is undesirable in a given clinical setting.

To lower radiation exposure, we use a kVp of 100 for subjects with a BMI <30 and a kVp of 120 for subjects with a BMI ≥30. Further dose-reduction techniques, such as aggressive tube current modulation, attenuation adaptation, and/or adaptive pitch selection, should be considered whenever possible. Overall, more research is needed to identify the patients in whom a comprehensive scan would be expected to be most helpful as well as to identify further means to reduce the higher radiation exposure inherent with such as protocol. As such, the 2006 Appropriateness Criteria for CCT and CMR concludes that the usefulness of "triple rule out" protocols is uncertain. This sentiment of uncertainty regarding the relative value of "triple rule out" protocols has been subsequently voiced by other experts, who caution that the widespread routine use of this protocol should be avoided at this time [31–33].

Coronary Artery Calcium Scoring

Risk stratification is an important element of CAD management. Because death or myocardial infarction is the first manifestation of CAD in approximately 50% of cases [34,35] there remains a need for primary prevention and in order to maximize the benefit, it is generally accepted that the intensity of intervention should reflect the degree of risk [36]. Traditionally, risk stratification has been based on the presence of risk factors such as smoking, hypertension, diabetes, in conjunction with age and sex. However, using traditional risk factors alone may underestimate the prevalence of subclinical CAD, [37]. This is particularly an issue in groups generally considered low risk [38]. There is evidence that less than half of the patients who suffer their first myocardial infarction would have qualified for primary preventative drug therapy based on clinical parameters alone [39]. The efficacy of HMG-CoAse reductase inhibitors ("statins") in reducing mortality and morbidity makes the early identification of CAD and effective risk stratification of enormous clinical importance.

Coronary artery calcium scoring uses noncontrast CT scanning to detect calcification in epicardial coronary vessels. Coronary artery calcification is pathognomic of atherosclerosis [40–42]. In patients with established CAD, coronary calcification is almost invariably present [43,44]. Calcification may be part of the healing process following plaque rupture and so be a marker of stability for a given plaque [45,46]. However, patients with extensive calcification are more likely to have other plaques at risk of rupture or rapid disease progression. Therefore, when used to assess the risk for the patient, as opposed to the risk related to a given atherosclerotic plaque, there is a sound rationale for the prognostic utility of coronary calcium scoring.

Technique

Calcium scoring can be performed on one of two types of CT scanners, electron beam CT (EBCT) on which the technique was first developed, or the newer multidetector CT. Although the validation and prognostic data for calcium scoring has been derived from EBCT, multidetector scanners are more readily available and for clinical purposes give equivalent results [47]. Standard protocols involve acquiring high-resolution axial noncontrast images which are then reconstructed at a slice thickness of 3 mm. A threshold of 130 HU is typically set and dedicated software then identifies calcification if contiguous pixels exceed this level.

The most widely used measure of coronary calcium is the Agatston score [48]. This value is obtained by multiplying the area of calcification by a weighting factor of 1–4 dependent on the intensity, in Hounsfield units, of that lesion. Although other methods of quantification such as the mass and volume scoring systems have greater reproducibility, virtually all prognostic data has been based on the Agatston score and therefore it remains the standard clinical measure (Figure 3.9).

Interpretation and Clinical Utility

There is now abundant evidence of the prognostic power of coronary artery calcium scoring. Compared with patients with an Agatston score of zero, patients with a score >400 have a 10-fold increased risk of cardiac events [49]. A dose–response relationship has been established with increasing calcium score being associated with increasing adverse cardiovascular events. This relationship has been confirmed in different population subsets, such as

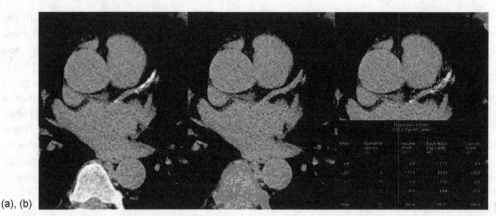

(a), (b)   (c)

Figure 3.9 Coronary artery calcium scoring.
(a) Noncontrast-enhanced axial CT image with calcification evident in left anterior descending coronary artery.
(b) Software automatically identifies structures with Hounsfield units exceeding threshold (pink), typically set between 130 and 200 HU. (c) User verifies identified structures as coronary calcium (depicted in this example in the LAD) and excludes noncoronary structures such as valvular calcification and vertebrae. The software then generates a calcium score based on the area and density of the identified coronary calcium.

the elderly, and in asymptomatic low risk populations [50,51]. Coronary calcification is affected by race; however, within a given racial group the relationship between calcium score and cardiovascular events remains strong. Importantly, calcium scoring adds incremental prognostic value to conventional risk factors, with increasing coronary calcification being associated with more adverse events within each clinically defined stratum of risk [52].

Calcium scoring, as a means of identifying asymptomatic individuals at increased risk of cardiovascular events, is best interpreted in the context of other traditional risk factors [53]. In a young patient at low risk, any coronary calcification is highly significant and predictive of later events. In contrast, a small quantity of coronary calcification in the elderly confers little increased risk above that which is already expected. There are a number of different systems by which background risk can be incorporated into the calcium score. One approach is to state where a given patient's calcium score lies in an age and sex matched normal distribution (http://www.mesa-nhlbi.org/Calcium/input.aspx). While easy to interpret, and available for different racial groups, a percentile rank gives no information regarding absolute risk of cardiovascular events. Indeed, being at the fiftieth percentile in a group at extremely high risk, or in the midst of a CAD epidemic, should hardly be considered reassuring.

Another approach derived from the Multi-ethnic Study of Atherosclerosis uses a convenient online tool to adjust the Framingham risk score according to the calcium score. The calcium score is used to calculate a new "arterial age" which is then entered into the Framingham risk score to give an absolute 10-year risk of cardiovascular events (http://www.mesa-nhlbi.org/Calcium/arterialage.aspx). While elegant, the arterial age adjustment is less well validated than alternative approaches. Arguably, the most robust interpretation of the calcium score is a binary one—either a patient has or does not have coronary calcification. As such, coronary calcium scoring is simply used as a means of identifying subclinical atherosclerosis.

The appropriate changes to patient management after coronary calcium scoring obviously depend on individual clinical characteristics; however, a number of general principles can be applied. Improvements in diet and exercise are advisable for everyone, and there is evidence that patient visualization of coronary calcium does result in positive lifestyle modification [54]. Current guidelines do not offer specific recommendations regarding preventative drug therapy based on coronary calcium scoring. The National Cholesterol Education Program (NCEP) III guidelines advise statin therapy in patients with CAD "equivalents," a standard which calcific coronary disease clearly meets. The unequivocal benefit of statins in patients with established macrovascular disease irrespective of baseline lipid levels [55] means the initiation of drug therapy is reasonable based on an elevated calcium score alone. There is evidence that clinicians respond to the detection of any coronary calcium in just such a manner initiating statins even in otherwise low risk populations [56]. Importantly, the potential harm done by withholding therapy means that the absence of coronary calcium should not lead to the cessation of statins in those that would otherwise qualify. A strategy trial assessing a coronary calcium guided approach would answer these questions but has yet to be performed.

The identification of coronary stenoses with a view to revascularization has been a central tenet of CAD management and calcium scoring has been used as a noninvasive means of predicting obstructive coronary disease. Calcium scores correlate well with atherosclerotic burden on a per patient basis [57–59] and higher calcium scores are more likely to be occur in patients with obstructive CAD [60,61]. However, marked calcification does not necessarily imply a hemodynamically significant stenosis. There is only a modest correlation between the degree of calcification and the degree of luminal narrowing for a given lesion [62]. This phenomenon may lead to the coronary calcification on CT being deemed a false positive when in fact it is due to the limitations of invasive angiography.

Luminal narrowing is heavily dependent on the extent of outward expansion of the vessel to compensate for the plaque, effectively preserving the vessel lumen, a process known as positive remodeling [63]. Early reports suggested that the absence of coronary calcification was sufficient to exclude obstructive coronary disease, and in the elderly a calcium score of zero does have a high negative predictive value [64]. Unfortunately, 8–10% of obstructive plaques are noncalcified, which makes exclusion of CAD based on the absence of calcium unreliable, particularly in younger patients.

Coronary calcium scoring has evolved into a robust technique for risk stratification. Although other uses have been suggested, its main role is to identify subclinical atherosclerosis. Calcium scoring is of greatest benefit in patients at low or intermediate risk for coronary disease in that it may identify patients who stand to benefit from preventative medical therapy who previously may not have been eligible.

Appropriate Use of CCT

The rapid increase in the use of cardiovascular CT, and cardiac imaging in general, has lead to a call for more careful patient selection [65]. A major step forward in this process has been the publication of appropriateness criteria formulated between multiple professional societies [66]. For most clinical indications there are alternative diagnostic modalities to CT. Deciding when CT is the most appropriate test therefore depends on the merits, and availability, of the alternative noninvasive imaging modalities. Each of the major imaging modalities has its own considerations.

CT requires the administration of iodinated contrast and is therefore needs to be used with caution in patients with renal insufficiency. Although reducing rapidly with new technology, the current radiation exposure from many CCT protocols remains significant. It is important to recognize that the risk of radiation-induced malignancy is highly dependent on age [1]. While it is less likely that the effects of radiation will manifest as a malignancy in patients scanned in their later decades of life, alternatives to CT should be considered in young patients. A major advantage of CCT is its efficiency and rapid image acquisition. Despite the short scan time, the ability to breath-hold remains a prerequisite for high quality images and very obese patients continue to pose a challenge. Although there are many clinical indications for CCT, its role in the evaluation of patients with acute chest pain is particularly important and deserves special attention.

Cardiac MRI is the other more recent imaging modality that has a still-evolving role. Its great strengths lie in tissue characterization and extraordinary breadth of information that can be obtained with different imaging sequences, all without any ionizing radiation. MRI is contraindicated in patients with certain metallic implants and not currently performed at most hospitals in patients with implanted cardiac pacemakers or defibrillators. Claustrophobia remains a concern given that the scan time can be an hour or more for some indications. For some imaging sequences, particularly delayed hyperenhancement imaging, gadolinium contrast is required, the use of which may be limited in patients with renal impairment. Patient cooperation and the ability to breath-hold are also crucial for image quality. Perhaps surprisingly, MRI image quality is not adversely affected by obesity; however, very large patients may not be accommodated by the diameter of the magnet bore or become very claustrophobic once inside. The greatest limitation of cardiac MRI remains the expertise required and lack of availability of scanners.

Echocardiography remains the first line imaging modality for most noncoronary indications. It involves no radiation, no contrast, and is portable. It is a particularly good choice in unstable patients as it can be performed at the bedside and requires little patient coordination or respiratory control. The temporal resolution of echocardiography is unsurpassed making it ideal for examining rapidly moving objects such as vegetations. The hemodynamic data obtained makes it an invaluable tool. Its chief limitation is spatial resolution and overall image quality. Some patients have poor acoustic windows leading to substantial degradation of image quality. At present, coronary imaging is not possible with echocardiography.

The strength of nuclear scintigraphy derives from its availability, ease of use, and unrivalled prognostic data. Studies combined with exercise stress can provide clinicians very useful information regarding patients' functional capacity. However, the radiation exposure from rest-stress SPECT is comparable to the exposure from CT, and the duration of time required for each scan and the relatively poor spatial resolution are significant drawbacks. False positive studies from attenuation artifacts in obese patients and women with significant breast tissue remain a limitation.

In conclusion, the greatest clinical role for CT remains in the rapid exclusion of coronary disease in symptomatic patients at low to intermediate risk for CAD. CCT is not considered appropriate for patients who will almost certainly need invasive intervention. That is, patients with a very high pretest probability of disease or those with acute chest pain and confirmatory EKG changes or troponin elevation should proceed directly to cardiac catheterization rather than undergoing CT. Further technical advances are likely to result in a broader range of indications for which CT is appropriate. Until that time, and as evidence of clinical benefit is gathered, judicious use of CCT, reserved for the indications for which it is deemed appropriate, is in the interests of patients and physicians alike.

References

1. Barrett BJ, Parfrey PS. Preventing nephropathy induced by contrast medium. *N Engl J Med*. 2006;354:379–386.
2. Ropers U, Ropers D, Pflederer T, *et al*. Influence of heart rate on the diagnostic accuracy of dual-source computed tomography coronary angiography. *J Am Coll Cardiol*. 2007;50:2393–2398.
3. Nyberg G, Holmberg B. Haemodynamic, anti-anginal and anti-ischaemic effects of sublingual nitroglycerin: dose-response, duration and time of onset of action. *Eur J Clin Pharmacol*. 1988;34:561–567.
4. Desbiolles L, Leschka S, Plass A, *et al*. Evaluation of temporal windows for coronary artery bypass graft imaging with 64-slice CT. *Eur Radiol*. 2007;17(11):2819–2828.
5. Nieman K, Rensing BJ, van Geuns RJ, *et al*. Noninvasive coronary angiography with multislice spiral computed tomography: impact of heart rate. *Heart*. 2002;88:470–474.
6. Hazirolan T, Turkbey B, Karcaaltincaba M, *et al*. Impact of scanning direction on heart rate at certain levels of heart in electrocardiogram-gated 16-multidetector computed tomography angiography of coronary artery bypass grafts. *J Comput Assist Tomogr*. 2007;31-1:5–8.
7. Kistler PM, Rajappan K, Jahngir M, *et al*. The impact of CT image integration into an electroanatomic mapping system on clinical outcomes of catheter ablation of atrial fibrillation. *J Cardiovasc Electrophysiol*. 2006;17(10):1093–1101.
8. Kaseno K, Tada H, Koyama K, *et al*. Prevalence and characterization of pulmonary vein variants in patients with atrial fibrillation determined using 3-dimensional computed tomography. *Am J Cardiol*. 2008;101(11):1638–1642.
9. Pappone C, Oral H, Santinelli V, *et al*. Atrioesophageal fistula as a complication of percutaneous transcatheter ablation of atrial fibrillation. *Circulation*. 2004;109(22):2724–2726.
10. Cury RC, Abbara S, Schmidt S, *et al*. Relationship of the esophagus and aorta to the left atrium and pulmonary veins: implications for catheter ablation of atrial fibrillation. *Heart Rhythm*. 2005;2(12):1317–1323.
11. Saad EB, Marrouche NF, Saad CP, *et al*. Pulmonary vein stenosis after catheter ablation of atrial fibrillation: emergence of a new clinical syndrome. *Ann Intern Med*. 2003;138(8):634–638.
12. Tsao HM, Wu MH, Higa S, *et al*. Anatomic relationship of the esophagus and left atrium: implication for catheter ablation of atrial fibrillation. *Chest*. 2005;128:2581–2587.

13. Abbara S, Cury RC, Nieman K, *et al.* Noninvasive evaluation of cardiac veins with 16-MDCT angiography. *AJR Am J Roentgenol.* 2005;185(4):1001–1006.

14. Van de Veire NR, Schuijf JD, De Sutter J, *et al.* Non-invasive visualization of the cardiac venous system in coronary artery disease patients using 64-slice computed tomography. *J Am Coll Cardiol.* 2006;48: 1832–1838.

15. Bouvier E, Logeart D, Sablayrolles JL, *et al.* Diagnosis of aortic valvular stenosis by multislice cardiac computed tomography. *Eur Heart J.* 2006;27(24):3033–3038.

16. Koos R, Kühl HP, Mühlenbruch G, Wildberger JE, Günther RW, Mahnken AH. Prevalence and clinical importance of aortic valve calcification detected incidentally on CT scans: comparison with echocardiography. *Radiology.* 2006;241(1):76–82.

17. Alkadhi H, Wildermuth S, Plass A, *et al.* Aortic stenosis: comparative evaluation of 16-detector row CT and echocardiography. *Radiology.* 2006;240(1):47–55.

18. Feuchtner GM, Dichtl W, Friedrich GJ, *et al.* Multislice computed tomography for detection of patients with aortic valve stenosis and quantification of severity. *J Am Coll Cardiol.* 2006;47(7):1410–1417.

19. Abbara S, Pena AJ, Maurovich-Horvat P, *et al.* Feasibility and optimization of aortic valve planimetry with MDCT. *AJR Am J Roentgenol.* 2007;188(2):356–360.

20. Feuchtner GM, Dichtl W, Schachner T, *et al.* Diagnostic performance of MDCT for detecting aortic valve regurgitation. *AJR Am J Roentgenol.* 2006;186(6):1676–1681.

21. Messika-Zeitoun D, Serfaty JM, Laissy JP, *et al.* Assessment of the mitral valve area in patients with mitral stenosis by multislice computed tomography. *J Am Coll Cardiol.* 2006;48(2):411–413.

22. Alkadhi H, Wildermuth S, Bettex DA, *et al.* Mitral regurgitation: quantification with 16-detector row CT–initial experience. *Radiology.* 2006;238(2):454–463.

23. Kim RJ, Weinsaft JW, Callister TQ, Min JK. Evaluation of prosthetic valve endocarditis by 64-row multidetector computed tomography. *Int J Cardiol.* 2007;120(2):e27–29.

24. Scheffel H, Leschka S, Plass A, *et al.* Accuracy of 64-slice computed tomography for the preoperative detection of coronary artery disease in patients with chronic aortic regurgitation. *Am J Cardiol.* 2007;100(4):701–706.

25. Fishman JE. Imaging of blunt aortic and great vessel trauma. *J Thorac Imaging.* 2000;15:97–103.

26. Qanadli SD, El Hajjam M, Mesurolle B, *et al.* Motion artifacts of the aorta simulating aortic dissection on spiral CT. *J Comput Assist Tomogr.* 1999;23:1–6.

27. Ko SF, Hsieh MJ, Chen MC, *et al.* Effects of heart rate on motion artifacts of the aorta on non-ECG-assisted 0.5-sec thoracic MDCT. *Am J Roentgenol.* 2005;184:1225–1230.

28. Cheong B, Flamm SD. Use of electrocardiographic gating in computed tomography angiography of the ascending thoracic aorta. *J Am Coll Cardiol.* 2007;49(16):1751.

29. White CS, Kuo D, Kelemen M, *et al.* Chest pain evaluation in the emergency department: can MDCT provide a comprehensive evaluation? *AJR Am J Roentgenol.* 2005;185:533–540.

30. Frauenfelder T, Appenzeller P, Karlo C, *et al.* Triple rule-out CT in the emergency department: protocols and spectrum of imaging findings. *Eur Radiol.* 2009;19(4):789–799.

31. Van Der Wall EE, Schuijf JD, Bax JJ. Triple rule-out CT coronary angiography: three of a kind? *Int J Cardiovasc Imaging.* 2009;25(3):327–330.

32. Stillman AE, Oudkerk M, Ackerman M, *et al.* Use of multidetector computed tomography for the assessment of acute chest pain: a consensus statement of the North American society of cardiac imaging and the European society of cardiac radiology. *Eur Radiol.* 2007;17:2196–2207.

33. Gallagher MJ, Raff GL. Use of multislice CT for the evaluation of emergency room patients with chest pain: the so-called "triple rule-out". *Catheter Cardiovasc Interv.* 2008;71(1):92–99.

34. Kannel WB, Schatzkin A. Sudden death: lessons from subsets in population studies. *J Am Coll Cardiol.* 1985;5(Suppl. 6):141B–149B.

35. Rosamond W, Flegal K, Furie K. Heart disease and stroke statistics–2008 update: a report from the American Heart Association Statistics Committee and Stroke Statistics Subcommittee. *Circulation.* 2008;117(4):e25–146.

36. Greenland P, Bonow RO, Brundage BH, *et al.* ACCF/AHA 2007 clinical expert consensus document on coronary artery calcium scoring by computed tomography in global cardiovascular risk assessment and in evaluation of patients with chest pain: a report of the American College of Cardiology Foundation Clinical Expert Consensus Task Force (ACCF/AHA Writing Committee to Update the 2000 Expert Consensus Document on Electron Beam Computed Tomography) developed in collaboration with the Society of Atherosclerosis Imaging and Prevention and the Society of Cardiovascular Computed Tomography. *J Am Coll Cardiol.* 2007;49(3): 378–402.

37. Hecht HS, Superko HR. Electron beam tomography and National Cholesterol Education Program guidelines in asymptomatic women. *J Am Coll Cardiol.* 2001;37(6):1506–1511.

38. Taylor AJ, Feuerstein I, Wong H, Barko W, Brazaitis M, O'Malley PG. Do conventional risk factors predict subclinical coronary artery disease? Results from the Prospective Army Coronary Calcium Project. *Am Heart J.* 2001;141(3):463–468.

39. Akosah KO, Schaper A, Cogbill C, Schoenfeld P. Preventing myocardial infarction in the young adult in the first place: how do the National Cholesterol Education Panel III guidelines perform? *J Am Coll Cardiol.* 2003;41(9):1475–1479.

40. Rifkin RD, Parisi AF, Folland E. Coronary calcification in the diagnosis of coronary artery disease. *Am J Cardiol.* 1979;44(1):141–147.

41. McCarthy JH, Palmer FJ. Incidence and significance of coronary artery calcification. *Br Heart J.* 1974;36(5):499–506.

42. Frink RJ, Achor RW, Brown AL Jr, Kincaid OW, Brandenburg RO. Significance of calcification of the coronary arteries. *Am J Cardiol.* 1970;26(3):241–247.

43. Budoff MJ, Diamond GA, Raggi P, et al. Continuous probabilistic prediction of angiographically significant coronary artery disease using electron beam tomography. *Circulation.* 2002;105(15):1791–1796.

44. Budoff MJ, Georgiou D, Brody A, et al. Ultrafast computed tomography as a diagnostic modality in the detection of coronary artery disease: a multicenter study. *Circulation.* 1996;93(5):898–904.

45. Huang H, Virmani R, Younis H, Burke AP, Kamm RD, Lee RT. The impact of calcification on the biomechanical stability of atherosclerotic plaques. *Circulation.* 2001;103(8):1051–1056.

46. Ambrose JA, Tannenbaum MA, Alexopoulos D, et al. Angiographic progression of coronary artery disease and the development of myocardial infarction. *J Am Coll Cardiol.* 1988;12(1):56–62.

47. Horiguchi J, Yamamoto H, Akiyama Y, Marukawa K, Hirai N, Ito K. Coronary artery calcium scoring using 16-MDCT and a retrospective ECG-gating reconstruction algorithm. *AJR Am J Roentgenol.* 2004;183(1):103–108.

48. Agatston AS, Janowitz WR, Hildner FJ, Zusmer NR, Viamonte M Jr, Detrano R. Quantification of coronary artery calcium using ultrafast computed tomography. *J Am Coll Cardiol.* 1990;15(4):827–832.

49. Pletcher MJ, Tice JA, Pignone M. Use of coronary calcification scores to predict coronary heart disease. *JAMA.* 2004;291(15):1831–1832. [author reply 1832–1833]

50. Vliegenthart R, Oudkerk M, Hofman A, et al. Coronary calcification improves cardiovascular risk prediction in the elderly. *Circulation.* 2005;112(4):572–577.

51. Taylor AJ, Bindeman J, Feuerstein I, Cao F, Brazaitis M, O'Malley PG. Coronary calcium independently predicts incident premature coronary heart disease over measured cardiovascular risk factors: mean three-year outcomes in the Prospective Army Coronary Calcium (PACC) project. *J Am Coll Cardiol.* 2005;46(5):807–814.

52. Greenland P, LaBree L, Azen SP, Doherty TM, Detrano RC. Coronary artery calcium score combined with Framingham score for risk prediction in asymptomatic individuals. *JAMA.* 2004;291(2):210–215.

53. Expert Panel on Detection, Evaluation, and Treatment of High Blood Cholesterol in Adults. Executive Summary of The Third Report of The National Cholesterol Education Program (NCEP) Expert Panel on Detection, Evaluation, And Treatment of High Blood Cholesterol In Adults (Adult Treatment Panel III). *JAMA.* 2001;285(19):2486–2497.

54. Orakzai RH, Nasir K, Orakzai SH, et al. Effect of patient visualization of coronary calcium by electron beam computed tomography on changes in beneficial lifestyle behaviors. *Am J Cardiol.* 2008;101(7):999–1002.

55. Heart Protection Study Collaborative Group. MRC(BHF Heart Protection Study of cholesterol lowering with simvastatin in 20,536 high-risk individuals: a randomised placebo-controlled trial. *Lancet.* 2002;360(9326):7–22.

56. Taylor AJ, Bindeman J, Feuerstein I, et al. Community-based provision of statin and aspirin after the detection of coronary artery calcium within a community-based screening cohort. *J Am Coll Cardiol.* 2008;51(14):1337–1341.

57. Rumberger JA, Schwartz RS, Simons DB, Sheedy PF 3rd, Edwards WD, Fitzpatrick LA. Relation of coronary calcium determined by electron beam computed tomography and lumen narrowing determined by autopsy. *Am J Cardiol.* 1994;73(16):1169–1173.

58. Rumberger JA, Simons DB, Fitzpatrick LA, Sheedy PF, Schwartz RS. Coronary artery calcium area by electron-beam computed tomography and coronary atherosclerotic plaque area. A histopathologic correlative study. *Circulation.* 1995;92(8):2157–2162.

59. Mintz GS, Pichard AD, Popma JJ, et al. Determinants and correlates of target lesion calcium in coronary artery disease: a clinical, angiographic and intravascular ultrasound study. *J Am Coll Cardiol.* 1997;29(2):268–274.

60. Rumberger JA, Sheedy PF, Breen JF, Schwartz RS. Electron beam computed tomographic coronary calcium score cutpoints and severity of associated angiographic lumen stenosis. *J Am Coll Cardiol.* 1997;29(7):1542–1548.

61. Shavelle DM, Budoff MJ, LaMont DH, Shavelle RM, Kennedy JM, Brundage BH. Exercise testing and electron beam computed tomography in the evaluation of coronary artery disease. *J Am Coll Cardiol.* 2000;36(1):32–38.

62. Simons DB, Schwartz RS, Edwards WD, Sheedy PF, Breen JF, Rumberger JA. Noninvasive definition of anatomic coronary artery disease by ultrafast computed tomographic scanning: a quantitative pathologic comparison study. *J Am Coll Cardiol.* 1992;20(5):1118–1126.

63. Glagov S, Weisenberg E, Zarins CK, Stankunavicius R, Kolettis GJ. Compensatory enlargement of human atherosclerotic coronary arteries. *N Engl J Med*. 1987;316(22):1371–1375.

64. Haberl R, Becker A, Leber A, *et al*. Correlation of coronary calcification and angiographically documented stenoses in patients with suspected coronary artery disease: results of 1,764 patients. *J Am Coll Cardiol*. 2001;37(2):451–457.

65. Gibbons RJ, Leading the elephant out of the corner: the future of health care: presidential address at the American Heart Association 2006 scientific sessions. *Circulation*. 2007;115(16):2221–2230.

66. Hendel RC, Patel MR, Kramer CM, *et al*. ACCF (ACR(SCCT(SCMR(ASNC(NASCI(SCAI(SIR 2006 appropriateness criteria for cardiac computed tomography and cardiac magnetic resonance imaging: a report of the American College of Cardiology Foundation Quality Strategic Directions Committee Appropriateness Criteria Working Group, American College of Radiology, Society of Cardiovascular Computed Tomography, Society for Cardiovascular Magnetic Resonance, American Society of Nuclear Cardiology, North American Society for Cardiac Imaging, Society for Cardiovascular Angiography and Interventions, and Society of Interventional Radiology. *J Am Coll Cardiol*, 2006;48(7):1475–1497.

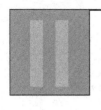

PART II
Clinical Applications

CHAPTER 4

PET Assessment of Myocardial Perfusion

Thomas H. Schindler[1], Ines Valenta[1] & Vasken Dilsizian[2]

[1]University Hospitals of Geneva, Geneva, Switzerland
[2]University of Maryland School of Medicine, Baltimore, MD, USA

Introduction

The advent of positron emission tomography (PET) in the 1980s dramatically changed the clinical utility of radiotracer techniques for the assessment of myocardial perfusion. While the basic principles of PET are similar to those of single photon emission computed tomography (SPECT), PET has several technical advantages over gamma-technique SPECT such as higher counting sensitivity, higher spatial resolution, and routine use of more accurate attenuation correction. In addition, most clinical PET scanners are full-ring devices that simultaneously measure projections at all angles, whereas conventional SPECT cameras require time to rotate the detector heads about the patient. The latter distinction between the cameras is significant because it enables PET to image rapidly changing processes, which, in turn, allows the possibility to quantify such things as myocardial perfusion in absolute as opposed to relative terms. Consequently, PET allows the possibility for quantification of local tracer activity concentration in (MBq/mL) and myocardial blood flow (MBF) in absolute units (mL/min/g tissue). However, with the introduction of high-speed SPECT cameras that use a bank of independently controlled detector columns with large-hole collimators, quantification of local tracer activity concentration of SPECT tracers may also be possible in the future [1].

Similar to SPECT, PET utilizes radionuclide tracer techniques that produce images of the *in vivo* radionuclide distribution using measurements made with an external detector system. Like CT, the resulting images represent cross-sectional slices through the patient. However, unlike CT, the image intensity acquired with SPECT and PET reflects organ function rather than anatomy. The functional information depicted in SPECT and PET images depends upon the radiopharmaceutical employed for that particular study. SPECT allows for the noninvasive evaluation of myocardial perfusion by extractable tracers such as thallium-201 and technetium-99m (Tc-99m) labeled perfusion tracers. PET, on the other hand, allows for the noninvasive assessment of regional MBF using physiological substrates prepared with positron-emitting isotopes such as oxygen, nitrogen, and rubidium. These isotopes have half-lives that are considerably shorter than those used in SPECT and typically must be produced in close proximity to the scanner, using a cyclotron or a generator.

The principle PET radiopharmaceuticals used for myocardial perfusion imaging include ^{82}Rubidium, ^{13}N-ammonia, or ^{15}O-water, each having their own unique properties that may make one preferable over another in certain applications (Table 4.1). In the clinical setting, however, ^{13}N-ammonia and ^{82}Rubidium are the only PET perfusion tracers that have received US Food and Drug Administration approval.

This chapter aims to review the role of PET myocardial perfusion imaging for the (1) identification

Cardiac CT, PET and MR, 2nd edition. Edited by Vasken Dilsizian and Gerry Pohost. © 2010 Blackwell Publishing Ltd.

Table 4.1 PET tracers of myocardial blood flow.

Tracer	Half-life	Method	Mechanism
O-15-water	2.4 minutes	Cyclotron	Freely diffusible, metabolically inert
N-13-ammonia	9.8 minutes	Cyclotron	Soluble, microsphere-like, metabolically trapped
Rubidium-82	75 seconds	Generator	Soluble, microsphere-like

and characterization of flow-limiting epicardial as well as subclinical coronary artery disease (CAD); (2) evaluation of the responses of MBF to physiologic and pharmacologic stimuli and their relationship to coronary circulatory function and coronary pathophysiology; and (3) assessment of the incremental value of absolute MBF measurements for the delineation of cardiovascular risk, patient outcome, and monitoring responses to therapeutic intervention.

Clinical Application of Myocardial Perfusion Imaging

The conventional assessment of relative myocardial distribution of the radiotracer in the left ventricle during exercise, pharmacologic vasodilation, or at rest, allows the identification of stress-induced myocardial perfusion defects and, thus, the presence of hemodynamically obstructive coronary lesions. Similar to SPECT [2,3], the identification of stress-induced scintigraphic perfusion defects by PET imaging provides important diagnostic and prognostic information [4–6]. However, un-like SPECT imaging, soft tissue attenuation correction with PET imaging is reliable and accurate. This accurate attenuation correction in concert with the higher spatial resolution may explain a 10% higher diagnostic accuracy of PET when compared to conventional SPECT imaging for the detection of flow-limiting coronary artery lesions (Table 4.2) [7,8]. Advantages of PET imaging, however, pertain not only to the high spatial and depth-independent resolution but also to the ability to quantify the radiotracer uptake in the myocardial tissue and to assess rapid alterations of radiotracer activity concentrations in the arterial blood and myocardium owing to a high temporal resolution in seconds. The latter advantages of PET imaging combined with tracer kinetic compartment models afford the noninvasive assessment of MBF in absolute terms.

In clinical practice, stress myocardial perfusion studies with SPECT or PET, are usually interpreted visually and in "relative" terms. That is, myocardial regions with the highest myocardial radiotracer uptake are assumed to be supplied by normal or nonobstructive epicardial coronary arteries. On the other hand, myocardial regions with

Table 4.2 Detection of flow limiting coronary artery lesions by PET.

Year	Author	Radiotracer	Prior MI (%)	Sensitivity (%)	Specificity (%)
1992	Marwick et al.	[82]Rubidium	49	90 (63/70)	100 (4/4)
1992	Grover-McKay et al.	[82]Rubidium	13	100 (16/16)	73 (11/15)
1991	Stewart et al.	[82]Rubidium	42	83 (50/60)	86 (18/21)
1990	Go et al.	[82]Rubidium	47	93 (142/152)	78 (39/50)
1989	Demer et al.	[82]Rubidium, ^{13}N-ammonia	34	83 (126/152)	95 (39/41)
1988	Tamaki et al.	^{13}N-ammonia	75	98 (47/48)	100 (3/3)
1986	Gould et al.	[82]Rubidium, ^{13}N-ammonia	Not reported	95 (21/22)	100 (9/9)
1982	Schelbert et al.	^{13}N-ammonia	0	97 (31/32)	100 (11/11)
	Total			92	92

decreased radiotracer uptake during stress are interpreted as being supplied by hemodynamically obstructive or flow-limiting epicardial coronary arteries. By applying quantitative tracer-kinetic modeling, PET permits quantification of regional MBF in absolute terms both in the visually normal and in the abnormal regions. Such quantification of MBF at rest and its response to vasomotor stress allows the computation of the regional myocardial flow reserve (MFR) and, thereby expand the scope of conventional scintigraphic myocardial perfusion imaging from identifying "end-stage" epicardial coronary artery narrowing to "earlier" identification and characterization of abnormalities in coronary artery circulatory function, perhaps subclinical stages of CAD [9–12]. The identification and characterization of such functional abnormalities of the coronary circulation, that may precede or accompany CAD-related structural alterations of the arterial wall, entails important predictive information for the development and/or progression of the CAD, and future cardiovascular events [13–15]. Beyond detection of CAD, abnormal MFR during pharmacologic vasomotor stress or during sympathetic stress with cold pressor testing (CPT) could provide insights into functional and/or structural alterations in individuals without hemodynamically obstructive epicardial lesions such as hypertrophic, dilated or Chagas cardiomyopathy.

Diagnostic Accuracy of PET for Identifying Flow-Limiting Epicardial Coronary Artery Lesions

The clinical utility of ^{13}N-ammonia or ^{82}Rubidium PET for identifying hemodynamically significant or flow-limiting epicardial coronary artery lesions is well established (Table 4.2). Regional myocardial perfusion is usually assessed at rest and during hyperemic flows, commonly with pharmacologic vasodilation. The average sensitivity and specificity of myocardial perfusion PET for detecting >50% luminal narrowing on coronary angiography is reported to be 91 and 89%, respectively [16].

The higher sensitivities and specificities achieved with PET when compared to SPECT myocardial perfusion imaging is likely related to the high spatial and contrast resolution of photon attenuation free PET images and to the superior properties of PET perfusion tracers. Since PET perfusion images are free of photon attenuation-related artifacts, PET is specifically suited for the detection of CAD in women with breast attenuation artifact, men with diaphragmatic attenuation artifact, and in subjects with large body habitus [17]. The higher diagnostic accuracy of PET for detecting flow-limiting coronary artery lesions was recently reproduced when CT attenuation rather than conventional rotating rod sources of germanium-68 (Ge-68)/gallium-68 (Ga-68) or Cesium-137 (Cs-137) were applied to acquire a transmission scan for attenuation correction. In a special population study consisting of women and obese subjects, the average sensitivity and specificity of ^{82}Rubidium PET acquired with an integrated PET-CT system for detecting ≥70% luminal narrowing on coronary angiography was 93 and 83%, respectively, with a diagnostic accuracy of 87% [17].

Limitations of Qualitative Assessment of Regional Myocardial Tracer Uptake

An important limitation of qualitative or semiquantitative evaluation of the myocardial radiotracer uptake of the left ventricle during pharmacologic stress is that balanced reduction in blood flow in all three vascular territories may go undetected due to the "relatively" homogenous appearing tracer uptake throughout the left ventricle. In this regard, the concurrent and unique ability of PET to assess MBF in *mL/min/g tissue* by means of radiotracer kinetic modeling may overcome the limitation of underestimating CAD in the reference region or balanced reduction of radiotracer uptake. By evaluating absolute MBF at rest and during stress, MFR, which represents the ratio between vasodilator stress (hyperaemic) and rest MBF, can be computed in all three vascular territories. In addition, PET imaging allows the evaluation of left ventricular ejection fraction (LVEF) during hyperemic stress-state rather than during poststress conditions, where MBF has returned back to its baseline rest-state, as is routinely performed for gated SPECT imaging.

Advantages of Quantitative Assessment of MBF and Flow Reserve

Quantitative assessment of regional MBF and MFR may identify not only flow-limiting isolated epi-cardial lesions but also the downstream functional outcome of anatomically mild, sequential coronary artery lesions or continuous tapering of coronary artery vessel due to diffuse atherosclerosis [18,19]' (Figure 4.1a–c). Thus, assessment of MBF and MFR in quantitative terms may unravel small

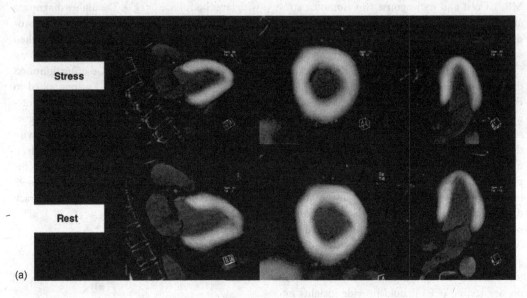

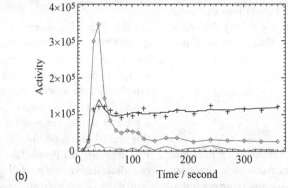

Figure 4.1 (a) Integrated PET/CT images (vertical, short, and horizontal axis): Normal myocardial perfusion as denoted on ^{13}N-ammonia PET images during hyperemic flow stimulation with dipyridamole and at rest accurately co-registered on the CT images of the PET/CT scanner. (b) Arterial radiotracer input function and myocardial tissue response: From regions of interest (ROI) assigned to the left ventricular blood pool and the left ventricular myocardium on the serially acquired images, time–activity curves are derived that describe the changes in radiotracer activity in arterial blood (counts per pixel per second) *(red curve)* and in myocardium (counts per pixel per second) *(white curve)* as a function of time. Through fitting of the time–activity curves with the operational equation formulated from the tracer kinetic model, estimates of myocardial blood flow (MBF) in units of milliliter of blood per minute per gram of myocardium (mL/g/min) are obtained. (c) Polar-map display of regional MBF quantification in mL/g/min with ^{13}N-ammonia PET during stress with dipyridamole stimulation, at rest, and its difference *(upper panel)* (Munich Heart Program software package, S. Nekolla). Regional MBF values of the left anterior descending artery (LAD), right coronary artery (RCA), and left circumflex artery (LCX) *(middle panel)*. The summarized quantitative data *(lower panel)*, indicate a normal myocardial flow reserve (MFR ≥ 2.5) in all three coronary territories indicative of normal hyperemic coronary flow increases and coronary circulatory function.

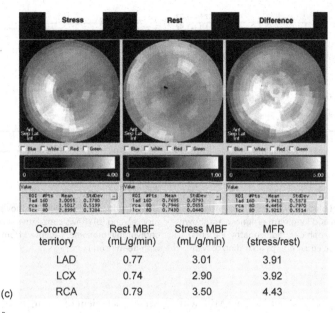

Coronary territory	Rest MBF (mL/g/min)	Stress MBF (mL/g/min)	MFR (stress/rest)
LAD	0.77	3.01	3.91
LCX	0.74	2.90	3.92
RCA	0.79	3.50	4.43

(c)

Figure 4.1 (*Continued*)

differences in regional hyperemic MBF increases and, thereby, identify functional abnormalities of the coronary circulation as early precursor of the CAD process [9,11,12,20,21]. These functional abnormalities may not only accompany structural alterations of the arterial wall but may also precede the morphological manifestation of the CAD process [22,23]. PET imaging, therefore, may identify early functional abnormalities of the coronary circulation before structural alteration of the arterial wall ensue, and hence provide important diagnostic and prognostic information [13–15]. Such abnormalities are often undetected on stress myocardial perfusion SPECT images alone [24]. While semi-quantitative assessment of relative myocardial perfusion detects with SPECT identifies the culprit or most significantly narrowed epicardial coronary artery lesion, PET quantification of MFR in each of the coronary artery vascular territories provides additional important information regarding the regulation and modulation of MBF in the normal and/or preclinical diseased coronary vascular state.

A previous angiographic investigation compared the intracoronary Doppler ultrasound measured coronary flow reserve with [201]thallium myocardial perfusion imaging in 55 patients with 67 stenotic coronary arteries, which were mostly intermediate in severity (mean stenosis was 59 ± 12%; ranging between 40 and 70%) [25]. As it was observed, a coronary flow reserve of less than 1.7 accurately predicted the presence of a stress [201]thallium scintigraphic defect with an agreement of 84% between both modalities. This magnitude of reduced coronary flow reserve in areas of scintigraphic perfusion defects following hyperemic flow increases widely agrees with other investigation [25,26], indicating that reduced MFR in the defect areas are indeed related to flow-limiting effects of focal epicardial artery lesions. More recently, among patients with CAD who underwent both SPECT and PET myocardial perfusion studies, 72% of the myocardial regions subtended with >50% coronary artery stenosis appeared normal on conventional SPECT perfusion imaging, while MFR, as determined by ^{15}O-water PET, was abnormally decreased (mean 2.22 ± 0.87 mL/min/g *tissue*) [24]. It remains unresolved, however, whether an abnormal MFR in myocardial territories subtended by >50% epicardial coronary artery narrowing but without stress-induced scintigraphic myocardial perfusion defects reflects true downstream consequences of epicardial lesions and/or coronary circulatory dysfunction.

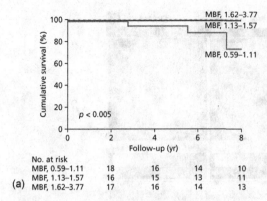

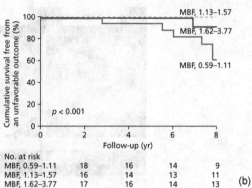

Figure 4.2 Myocardial blood flow (MBF) values after dipyridamole infusion and long term prognosis are shown in patients with hypertrophic cardiomyopathy. Patients were divided into three equal groups according to MBF after dipyridamole infusion. (a) Shows overall cumulative survival, and (b) shows cumulative survival free from an unfavorable outcome. (Adapted from Cecchi et al. [27], with permission.)

Quantitative approaches that measure MBF with PET identify multivessel CAD and offer the opportunity to monitor responses to risk factor modification and to therapeutic interventions. Recent studies have shown that diminished MFR by PET was also predictive of future cardiovascular outcome in patents without underlying CAD [27–29]. Among 51 patients with hypertrophic cardiomyopathy, who underwent MBF PET studies and were followed for an average of 8 years, 16 (31%) had cardiovascular events [27]. The overall accumulative survival (Figure 4.2, (a)) and cumulative survival free from an unfavorable outcome (Figure 4.2, (b)) were associated with the level of hyperemic MBF achieved during pharmacologic vasodilation. These findings suggest that the degree of microvascular dysfunction of the coronary microcirculation (as reflected by the diminished blood flow observed on PET) was predictive of future cardiovascular outcome. Similar results were attained among patients with idiopathic dilated cardiomyopathy [28,29]. Twenty-six patients with dilated cardiomyopathy, of whom 24 had angiographically normal coronary arteries, underwent MBF PET studies and were followed for approximately 3 years [28]. Nine (35%) patients died during the follow-up period. The overall accumulative 3-year survival was strongly associated with the spatial heterogeneity of myocardial perfusion derived from the coefficient of variance of absolute regional MBF. The probability of 3-year survival was 33% in subjects whose coefficient of variance was above the median compared with 90% in subjects whose coefficient of variance was below the median ($p < 0.01$). In a similar study of 67 patients with dilated cardiomyopathy who underwent MBF PET studies and were followed for a mean of 3–4 years, 24 (36%) patients had major cardiac events: 8 cardiac deaths and 16 progression of heart failure [29]. Impaired MBF reserve on PET was associated with an increase in relative risk of death or progression of heart failure of 3.5 times over other more common clinical and functional variables (Figure 4.3).

While assessment of myocardial perfusion with PET has become an indispensable tool in cardiac research, it remains underutilized in clinical practice. The main drawback for the technology is its cost. Not only are the PET cameras expensive, but radiotracers, which require either a cyclotron or an expensive generator for isotope production, are quite expensive to maintain unless maintenance costs are shared with other subspecialties such as oncology. As PET equipment becomes more widely utilized in cardiovascular disorders, it is expected that the additional clinical benefit of myocardial perfusion PET will be realized.

PET Myocardial Blood Flow Tracers

PET approaches for the measurement of regional MBF in absolute terms entail intravenous administration of positron-emitting perfusion tracers,

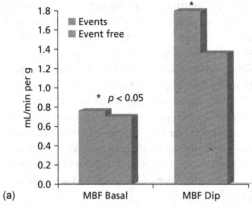

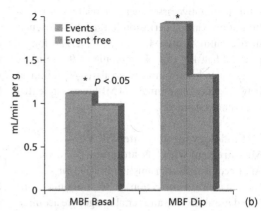

Figure 4.3 Mean values of myocardial blood flow (MBF) at rest and during dipyridamole vasodilation (MBF Dip) are shown for patients with dilated cardiomyopathy (a) and hypertrophic cardiomyopathy (b). Patients with unfavorable outcome (events) over the ensuing years exhibited impaired MBF with dipyridamole PET when compared to patients with favorable outcome (event free survival). (Adapted from Cecchi et al. [27] and Neglia et al. [29], with permission.)

such as ^{13}N-ammonia, ^{15}O-water, or [82]Rubidium (Table 4.1) and imaging transit time of the radiotracer through the central circulatory system to its extraction and retention in the left ventricular myocardium. ^{13}N-ammonia and ^{15}O-water are cyclotron-produced radiotracers, with relatively short physical half-lives of 9.8 and 2.4 minutes, respectively. Absolute MBF obtained with ^{13}N-ammonia and ^{15}O-water have been widely validated against independent microsphere blood flow measurements in animals and have yielded highly reproducible values over a range of 0.5–5.0 mL/g/min [30,31]. Similarly, measurements of MBF with ^{13}N-ammonia and ^{15}O-water in humans yield comparable estimates over a wide range of flow [32,33]. Although assessment of absolute MBF with ^{13}N-ammonia and ^{15}O-water are well established in the literature, their dependency on an on-site cyclotron limits their widespread clinical application. On the other hand, [82]Rubidium, with an ultra-short 75 seconds physical half-life, is available through a Strontium-82/Rubidium-82 generator system with a 4- to 5-week shelf life, and therefore more widely available for clinical use. However, quantification of absolute MBF with [82]Rubidium is rather challenging. In animal studies, using 2-compartment tracer kinetic model, quantification of MBF with [82]Rubidium was highly variable during hyperemic flow, generally underestimating MBF, but precise when quantifying MBF at rest [34,35]. Recent clinical investigations report more promising results for [82]Rubidium MBF quantification [36–38].

[13]N-Ammonia

[13]N-Ammonia consists of neutral ammonia (NH_3) in equilibrium with its charged ammonium ($^+NH_4$) ion. The neutral NH_3 molecule readily diffuses across plasma and cell membranes. As the capillary membrane presents no significant barrier to the exchange of NH_3 molecule, its first pass extraction into the myocardium approaches 100%. After NH_3 exchanges across the capillary membrane and accesses the interstitial space, it re-equilibrates with its ammonium form, which is trapped in glutamine via the enzyme glutamine synthase. Following cellular uptake and trapping of ^{13}N-ammonia in the myocardial cells, it competes with back diffusion of the tracer into the vascular space and blood. This competition causes a progressive decline in retention fraction with increasing blood flow. Thus, while the first-pass trapping of ^{13}N-ammonia at rest is high, because of the aforementioned tracer kinetic model, there is flow-dependent decline of the radiotracer "retention" fraction [39–41]. ^{13}N-ammonia localizes in the myocardium and does not persist in the cardiac blood pool. These properties of ^{13}N-ammonia make it a favorable MBF agent both for quantification of regional MBF as well as for acquiring statistically high count PET images, ideal for visual and

semi-quantitative assessment of relative distribution of myocardial perfusion in the left ventricular myocardium (Figure 4.1) [10,17,42]. The longer physical half-life of ^{13}N-ammonia of 9.8 minutes necessitates longer time intervals (≈45 minutes) between repeat assessments of MBF, e.g., sequential stress and rest studies.

Methodology for Absolute MBF Measurement with ^{13}N-ammonia

After acquiring a transmission image (for soft tissue attenuation correction), ^{13}N-ammonia is injected intravenously and serial images are acquired in order to capture the initial transit of the tracer through the central circulation and its extraction into the myocardium. The sequence of serially acquired dynamic images for ^{13}N-ammonia typically consists of 12 frames of 10 seconds each, followed by 2 frames of 30 seconds each, 1 frame of 60 seconds and at the end by a 1 frame of 900 seconds, accumulating to a total acquisition time of 19 minutes [30]. The final, 900-second transaxial image data set or so-called "static image" is then reformatted into short-axis and long-axis myocardial slices and assembled into polar maps [20]. The static image denotes the relative distribution of the radiotracer uptake in the myocardium. Once the static image set is assembled into polar map displays, it permits the semi-quantitative assessment of the extent and severity of regional perfusion defects (Figures 4.1 and 4.4). This is followed by assignment of regions of interest (ROI) to the three major coronary artery vascular territories, according to the polar map display, and a 25 mm^2 ROI is positioned in the left ventricular blood pool on a short-axis slice. ROIs are then copied to the serially acquired transaxial image data sets of the initial 2 minutes of data acquired after the injection of the radiotracer and time–activity curves are generated from the arterial radiotracer input function and the myocardial response to it (Figure 4.1b). A 2-compartment tracer kinetic model that mathematically describes the time-dependent exchange of ^{13}N-ammonia between the blood and myocardium is then fitted to the curves [30]. The time–activity curves are then fitted with operational equations derived from 2-compartment tracer kinetic models, which describe the exchange of radiotracer between

tissue compartments and the volume of tracer distribution in each compartment. The operational equations then yields regional MBFs in absolute terms, as denoted in Figure 4.1c on a polar map display. Tracer kinetic models also entail corrections for flow-dependent decline of the radiotracer "retention" fraction at higher flows, physical decay of the radioisotope, partial volume-related underestimations of the true myocardial tissue concentrations by assuming a uniform myocardial wall thickness of 1 cm, and spillover of radioactivity between the left ventricular blood pool and myocardium [43].

[15]O-Water

[15]O-Water is a freely diffusable tracer, the kinetics of accumulation and clearance of which are less complicated than tracers that are partially extractable. Quantitative assessment of regional ^{15}O-water perfusion correlates closely with perfusion as assessed by microspheres [31]. Since ^{15}O-water is both in the vascular space and in the myocardium, visualization of myocardial activity requires correction for activity in the vascular compartment. This is accomplished by acquiring a separate scan after inhalation of ^{15}O-carbon monoxide which labels red blood cells and delineates the vascular space. Subtraction of ^{15}O-carbon monoxide images from the ^{15}O-water images results in visualization of the myocardium [31,44]. Alternatively, a factor analysis may be employed for the separation between blood pool and myocardial tracer uptake and their alterations over time [45], avoiding the necessity for blood pool imaging. To eliminate a second scan with ^{15}O-carbon monoxide, the early phase of ^{15}O-water distribution which reflects first pass of the tracer through the cardiac blood pool may be analyzed separately [46]. Myocardial uptake of ^{15}O-water parallels regional blood flow even at hyperemic range [47–49].

Methodology for Absolute MBF Measurement with ^{15}O-water

Given the shorter half-life of only 2.4 minutes, the assessment of MBF with ^{15}O-water is logistically and technically more challenging than that of ^{13}N-ammonia [42]. After intravenous

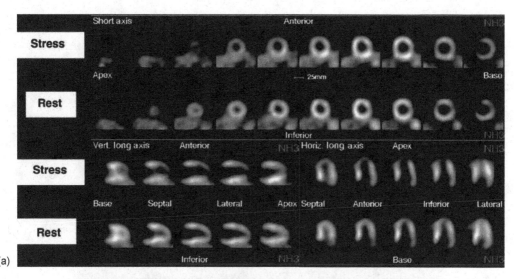

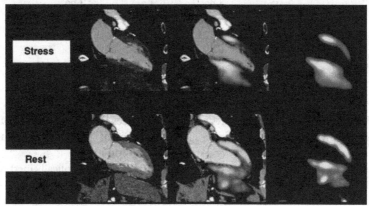

Figure 4.4 (a) Example of a stress and rest myocardial perfusion study with ^{13}N-ammonia PET in a 61-year-old patient with arterial hypertension. The myocardial display demonstrates a regional myocardial perfusion defect antero-septo-apical during hyperemic flow stimulation with dipyridamole that resolves on the resting perfusion images. (b) Corresponding integrated vertical PET/CT images. CT-contrast image with delineation of the left ventricular cavity and myocardial wall *(left panel)*. Integrated PET/CT image allows an accurate co-registration of relatively low spatial resolution of the ^{13}N-ammonia perfusion signal of PET with the high-resolution anatomic signal of the CT-contrast image *(middle panel)*. For direct comparison, ^{13}N-ammonia PET perfusion images alone *(right panel)*. (c) Corresponding polar-map display of regional myocardial blood flow (MBF) quantification in mL/g/min with ^{13}N-ammonia PET during stress with dipyridamole stimulation, at rest, and its difference *(upper panel)* (Munich Heart Program software package, S. Nekolla). Regional MBF values of the left anterior descending artery (LAD), right coronary artery (RCA), and left circumflex artery (LCX) *(middle panel)*. The summarized quantitative data *(lower panel)*, signify a distinct impairment of the MFR not only in the LAD territory with a stress-induced perfusion defect (Figure 4.2a and b) but also in the myocardial territory of the LCX and RCA (MFR<2.5) with apparently normal regional stress perfusion or visually estimated radiotracer-uptake as Figure 4.2a suggests. Subsequent invasive coronary angiography in this patient demonstrated a proximal occlusion of the LAD, and stenoses of 80% diameter in the proximal segments of the LCX and RCA. This example denotes the usefulness of MBF quantification with ^{13}N-ammonia PET and the calculation of the MFR to improve the identification of flow-limiting epicardial lesions in multivessel CAD. (*Continued on next page*)

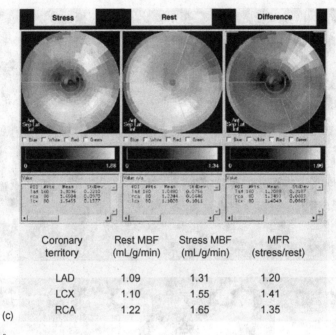

Coronary territory	Rest MBF (mL/g/min)	Stress MBF (mL/g/min)	MFR (stress/rest)
LAD	1.09	1.31	1.20
LCX	1.10	1.55	1.41
RCA	1.22	1.65	1.35

(c)

Figure 4.4 (*Continued*)

application of ^{15}O-water, it rapidly distributes into and clears from the myocardium in proportion to blood flow and its concentration in the blood. Applying a 1-compartment tracer kinetic model, estimates of MBF are then determined from the rate of clearance of ^{15}O-water from the left ventricular myocardium [31,48]. Such estimates of MBF, as measured with ^{15}O-water and PET, have also been reported to closely parallel independent microsphere blood flow measurements in animals [31,49]. The subtraction of the blood pool from the ^{15}O-water images, in concert with the rapid clearance of ^{15}O-water and its short half-life, however, may result in statistically low-count images of the myocardium. Thus, the visual evaluation and semi-quantitative analysis of the relative distribution of MBF of the "static" myocardial ^{15}O-water image have limited diagnostic value for the evaluation of flow-limiting coronary artery lesion. On the other hand, the short physical half-life of ^{15}O-water allows for repeated MBF measurements at short intervals of 10–15 minutes, e.g., rest and vasomotor stress myocardial perfusion studies during the same study session, while the patient is kept in the PET camera.

Differences Between Absolute MBF Measurement with ^{15}O-water and ^{13}N-ammonia

Because of the metabolically inert characteristics of ^{15}O-water, it is theoretically better suited for blood flow measurement than ^{13}N-ammonia. ^{15}O-water does not exhibit a plateau effect at high-flow rates. However, unlike ^{13}N-ammonia, ^{15}O-water persists in the cardiac blood pool, and is present both in the cardiac chambers and the myocardium. The result is a poor contrast image, requiring subtraction of cardiac blood pool activity for accurate semi-quantitative and quantitative assessment of left ventricular myocardial uptake and distribution.

The ^{15}O-water approach to measure MBF differs from that of ^{13}N-ammonia. The properties of ^{13}N-ammonia are such that a quantified average of transmural MBF is obtained [42]. Whereas the ^{15}O-water technique measures flow only in the fraction of the myocardium that is able to rapidly exchange water and not in scar tissue. This difference of ^{15}O-water and ^{13}N-ammonia is worthy of some considerations. Histopathologic studies have shown that myocardial infarctions frequently manifest in a nontransmural or "patchy" pattern. Under such circumstances, viable myocardium exists in the proximity or between scar tissues and ^{13}N-ammonia determines the average transmural MBF, while the ^{15}O-water approach measures only the water exchanging viable fraction of the myocardium [50]. As a consequence, in areas of myocardial infarctions with remaining viable myocardium, the MBF in the hypoperfused infarcted region will be diminished with ^{13}N-ammonia, whereas it may be normal or near normal with ^{15}O-water. Given the latter limitation of ^{15}O-water, some investigators have explored the ability of ^{15}O-water to assess myocardial viability through the modification of the blood flow information [47]. Rather than reliance on the net transmural blood flow, the volume of perfusable and nonperfusable tissue within a myocardial region was measured [31,47]. When this perfusable tissue index method of ^{15}O-water was tested in patients with acute and chronic ischemic heart disease, the determination of myocardial viability was comparable to that obtained using ^{18}F-fluorodeoxyglucose metabolism [47].

[82]Rubidium

[82]Rubidium is a generator-produced, short-lived cation, whose uptake depends on myocardial perfusion [51]. The extraction of [82]Rubidium from the plasma into myocardial cells is flow-dependent, while the washout of [82]Rubidium is dependent on sarcolemmal membrane integrity and the Na^+/K^+ ATPase pump. Uptake and retention of [82]Rubidium are a function of both blood flow and of myocardial cell integrity, respectively. The half-life of [82]Rubidium is only 75 seconds, with peak energy of 3.3 MeV. It is eluted from a commercially available [82]Strontium generator.

Like potassium and thallium, intracellular uptake of rubidium across the sarcolemmal membrane reflects active cation transport. Experimental studies have suggested that myocardial uptake of [82]Rubidium reflects absolute blood flows up to 2–3 mL/min/g tissue. However, net uptake of rubidium plateaus at hyperemic flows with pharmacologic stress [52,53]. There are several studies that suggest that myocardial ischemia or ischemia followed with reperfusion reduces extraction fraction of [82]Rubidium, presumably due to diminished cation transport across the sarcolemmal membrane [52,54,55]. Nonetheless, qualitative as-

sessment of relative [82]Rubidium perfusion defects have correlated well with those obtained from microspheres [56]. Clinically, [82]Rubidium PET has both high sensitivity and specificity for detecting CAD [6–8,17,36,57]. As a result, clinical assessment of myocardial perfusion with [82]Rubidium PET has received US Food and Drug Administration approval.

The ultra-short physical half-life of [82]Rubidium is an advantage for repeat sequential assessments of rest and stress myocardial perfusion studies, at short time intervals (e.g., 10 minutes), while the patient is still in the PET camera. On the other hand, the ultra-short physical half-life of [82]Rubidium necessitates the intravenous injection of high-activity doses ranging between 50–60 mCi in order to properly visualize the myocardium after 1–2 physical half-lives along with the biological half-life for clearance of [82]Rubidium from the blood. More recently, several investigations have proposed tracer kinetic models for quantifying [82]Rubidium MBF in absolute terms [37,38]. The intravenous injection of high-activity doses of [82]Rubidium, however, leads to substantial deadtime related count losses of the PET detectors that may limit the accuracy of the radiotracer input function and the myocardial tissue response needed for the quantification of the MBF through tracer kinetic modeling. Consequently, estimates of hyperemic MBF increases in response to pharmacologic vasodilation have been performed using semi-quantitative analysis by normalizing the myocardial [82]Rubidium activity concentration to the dose of activity injected intravenously [58,59]. Because the semi-quantitative analysis of [82]Rubidium uptake does not take into account flow-related nonlinear increases in myocardial activity, it tends to underestimate the true hyperemic flow increases. Despite this limitation, quantification of MBF with [82]Rubidium PET combined with 1- or 2-compartment tracer kinetic models appears to be feasible as recent investigations suggest [36–38].

Methodology for Absolute MBF Measurement with [82]Rubidium

Quantification of MBF with [82]Rubidium has been more challenging because of its noisy myocardial and blood-pool time–activity curves [36,38]. The kinetic behavior of [82]Rubidium in tissue can be described by a one or two-compartment model, which can be fitted using the arterial input function (obtained from the blood pool concentration of the left ventricular cavity) and myocardial time–activity curves at each segment, or even (with sufficient statistics) at each pixel [35,38,60]. The parameters of the model, which include flow, can be estimated using nonlinear regression or other similar techniques. The large number of free parameters and the high noise levels frequently encountered in [82]Rubidium images mean that simultaneous estimation of all parameters cannot always be performed reliably [61]. The variability of flow estimates can be reduced by fixing certain parameters to physiologically realistic values, but the fact that the extraction fraction of [82]Rubidium is flow dependent remains a challenge for accurate quantification. Semi-quantitative indices of flow such as dividing the mean tissue uptake over a certain period by the integral of the blood concentration may prove more practical for routine use. Many of the error sources nearly cancel out when MFR is calculated and first-order corrections can be applied for the variable extraction fraction of [82]Rubidium [62].

Previous animal validation studies [34,35], using a 2-compartment tracer kinetic model, yielded precise MBF values at rest, while the hyperemic flow was generally underestimated and highly variable. On the other hand, recent clinical investigations, applying [82]Rubidium with a 1-compartment tracer kinetic model reported of more promising results for MBF quantification [37,38]. For example, in 14 healthy volunteers PET determined estimates of MBF with [82]Rubidium as flow tracer, both at rest and during hyperemic flow increases were closely paralleled by flow values obtained with ^{13}N-ammonia ($r = 0.85$) [38]. Further support comes from a comparative study [36] which investigated PET measurements of MBF with [82]Rubidium using a wavelet-based noise reduction protocol [63] and a 2-compartment model and myocardial flows as determined with ^{15}O-water. In 11 healthy volunteers, [82]Rubidium PET measured estimates of MBF at rest and during hyperemia stimulation correlated well with those determined with ^{15}O-water ($r = 0.94$, $p < 0.001$), reinforcing the potential of the flow tracer [82]Rubidium and PET in the quantitative evaluation of MBF [63]. Nevertheless,

while [82]Rubidium PET combined with tracer kinetic models appears to be feasible to quantify MBF, further studies assessing the inter-study and inter-observer variability of [82]Rubidium determined MBF are warranted. Such studies will provide important information on the exact range of measurement-related errors of this approach [64]. This will help to better denote the utility of [82]Rubidium PET measurements in the identification and characterization of the subclinical and clinically manifest CAD process.

Prognostic Value of PET Perfusion Measurements

Similar to myocardial perfusion SPECT studies, the diagnostic and prognostic value of myocardial perfusion PET in patients with suspected or known CAD is emerging in the literature [4–6,65]. Among 685 patients undergoing [82]Rubidium PET myocardial perfusion studies, a normal scan was associated with a 90% cardiac event-free survival for 41 months. In contrast, among patients exhibiting small, moderate or extensive stress perfusion defects, the event-free survival declined to 87, 75 and 75%, respectively [5]. Further support for the incremental prognostic value of PET perfusion imaging comes from a recently conducted clinical study in 367 patients who underwent [82]Rubidium PET perfusion imaging during dipyridamole vasodilation and were followed for a mean of 3 years [6]. In this study, a normal [82]Rubidium PET myocardial perfusion scan was associated with 0.4% annual hard event rate (cardiac death and/or myocardial infarction), while the presence of mild or moderate-to-severe perfusion abnormalities predicted an annual event rate of 2.3 and 7%, respectively [6].

A more recent investigation with a single PET-CT exam in 695 consecutive intermediate-risk patients suggest that the combination of [82]Rubidium PET perfusion imaging and coronary artery calcium scoring with CT may improve the coronary risk stratification [4]. Among patients with a normal PET perfusion scan and no coronary artery calcification, there was an annualized event rate (death and/or myocardial infarction) of 2.6%, while the presence of coronary artery calcium score ≥ 1000 in these patients increased the annualized event rate to 12.3%. The annualized event rate in patients with ischemia on PET, without or with coronary artery calcium score of ≥ 1000 was 8.2 and 22.1%, respectively [4]. Notably, risk-adjusted survival analysis demonstrated a stepwise increase in event rates (death and/or myocardial infarction) with increasing coronary artery calcium scores in patients with and without ischemia on PET myocardial perfusion imaging. These observations suggest that adding CT measurements of coronary artery calcification to PET perfusion imaging may improve coronary risk stratification in patients at an intermediate risk.

Assessment of Coronary Circulatory Function

Measurements of MBF with PET at rest and its responses to physiologically or pharmacologically stimulated coronary flow increases allows the noninvasive identification and characterization of coronary circulatory function in normal and diseased states [9,10,12]. Intracoronary resistance is dependent on the velocity of the coronary flow and inversely on the fourth power of the coronary arterial diameter [66]. Under normal conditions, a flow-mediated vasodilation'of the coronary circulation during higher flows offsets the velocity-related increase in coronary resistance and, as a consequence, the coronary resistance is maintained low. Abnormalities in coronary vasomotor function and/or CAD-related structural alterations of the arterial wall, however, are commonly associated with an impairment of a flow-mediated coronary vasodilation. This leads to a paradoxical increase in coronary resistance during hyperemic flow increases with a proximal-to-distal decline in intracoronary pressure along the epicardial artery [55], which most likely accounts for a longitudinal base-to-apex relative decline in myocardial flow as recent clinical investigations with PET suggest [20,67–69].

The assessment of a longitudinal decrease in myocardial perfusion with PET could provide insight into functional and/or structural abnormalities of CAD in its early stages, before hemodynamically significant lesion develops. This area remains investigational and awaits further validation through comparative studies between PET measurements of regional MBF and invasive angiographic investigations of coronary blood flow and intracoronary pressure gradients.

Total Integrated Vasodilator Capacity

The most commonly applied approach for the evaluation of coronary circulatory function is the pharmacologically induced hyperemic MBF increase [11,12,65]. Vascular smooth muscle relaxing substances such as dipyridamole, adenosine, adenosine triphosphate, or adenosine receptor agonists, lower the resistance to flow at the site of the coronary arteriolar resistance vessels and, thereby, cause maximal or submaximal hyperemic increases in MBF. The hyperemic flow is thought to be an indicator of a predominantly endothelium-independent flow response owing to the relaxation of the vascular smooth muscle cells of the arteriolar vessels during pharmacologic vasodilation. However, shear sensitive components of the coronary endothelium contribute through flow-mediated coronary vasodilation to the overall hyperemic flow during pharmacologic vasodilation. This has been evidenced by the inhibitory effect of intravenous infusion of N^{G}-nitro-L-arginine methyl ester (L-NAME) on the endothelial nitric-oxide-synthase (eNOS), which resulted in a decrease in adenosine-induced MBF by 21–25% as measured with PET [70,71] (Figure 4.5). As pharmacologically induced hyperemic MBF increases reflect smooth muscle cell function of the coronary arteriolar vessels and up to 21–25% flow-mediated and, thus, endothelium-related vasodilatory effects, it is also frequently reported as the "total integrated coronary circulatory function" [11,12].

CPT and Endothelial Vasoreactivity

In contrast to pharmacologically induced hyperemic MBF increases, reflecting the total integrated coronary circulatory function, PET measurements of MBF at rest and its response to sympathetic stimulation with CPT provides more specific information on coronary endothelial function [9,72]. CPT with immersion of a hand into ice water causes a sympathetically mediated increase in heart rate and blood pressure and, thus, an increase in myocardial workload. Increases in myocardial workload and myocardial oxygen demand during CPT lead to a vasodilation of the coronary arteriolar resistance vessels through the presumed release of endogenous adenosine, as the metabolic vasodilator. This decrease in coronary vascular resistance then induces an increase in coronary inflow, which

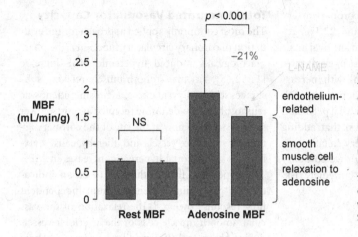

Figure 4.5 Hyperemic MBF increase to adenosine stimulation and its alteration to the intravenous infusion of the nitric oxide (NO) synthase inhibitor *N*G-nitro-L-arginine methyl ester (4 mg L-NAME /body weight i.v.). In the presence of L-NAME the hyperemic MBF response was attenuated by 21% that is likely to reflect the impairment of the flow-mediated and, thus, endothelium-derived and NO-mediated vasodilation by L-NAME. (Adapted from Schindler *et al.* [9].)

in turn leads to a flow-mediated and endothelium-dependent dilation of the upstream coronary artery segments. Consequently, an increase in myocardial workload is normally accompanied by commensurate flow-mediated coronary vasodilation and an increase in MBF as determined by PET. On the other hand, the CPT-induced increase in coronary inflow may not translate into a flow-mediated vasodilation of the upstream vessel segments in the presence of a dysfunctional coronary endothelium. At the same time, the sympathetically mediated vasoconstrictor effects of the vascular smooth muscle cells prevail, and are not offset by normal flow-related and endothelium-dependent coronary vasodilation. The CPT-related MBFs are then attenuated, absent, or even paradoxically decreased, which signifies coronary endothelial dysfunction.

PET Assessment of Coronary Circulatory Function and Clinical Implications

The noninvasive assessment of coronary circulatory function with PET measurements of MBF at rest and its responses to vasomotor stress has contributed to our understanding of CAD pathophysiology, both in the development and in the progression of CAD [9,11,12]. Normal functioning of the vascular endothelium plays a central and integrative role in the regulation and modulation of the vasomotor tone, metabolism of the vascular wall, and hemostasis. Thus, it exerts numerous anti-atherosclerotic and anti-thrombotic effects, predominantly mediated by a coronary

flow-stimulated production and release of nitric oxide (NO). Although endothelial-derived NO reflects the predominant vasoactive mediator, causing a NO-mediated relaxation of the vascular smooth muscle cells with a subsequent vasodilation, others such as prostacyclin and endothelium-derived hyperpolarizing factor (EDHF) contribute to it and may play a pivotal role in the coronary microcirculation [9]. The NO mediated vasodilatory effect, however, offsets possible vasoconstrictor effects of elevated endothelin-1 and angiotensin-II levels, and/or sympathetic activation.

Risk factors for CAD, such as smoking, hypercholesterolemia, hypertension, hyperglycemia, insulin resistance, obesity, menopausal state, or a family history of premature atherosclerotic disease have all been associated with an attenuation or loss of endothelium-dependent vasodilation. While the mechanisms underlying endothelium-dependent vasomotor dysfunction in individuals with risk factors is likely to be multifactorial, increases in vascular production of reactive oxygen species (ROS) derived from the superoxide producing endothelial enzymes, such as NAD(P)H oxidase, xanthine oxidase, and uncoupled NO synthase, have been put forth to account for reductions in the bioavailability of endothelium-derived NO, which is considered as an important cause and common final pathway of abnormal coronary vasodilatory function. Apart from this, increased amounts of ROS in the vascular endothelium and subintimal space not only diminishes the bioavailability of endothelial-derived NO associated with impaired endothelium-mediated vasodilator function, but may also induce the activation of a whole array of inflammatory genes, such as nuclear factor-κB (NF-κB), activator protein-1 (AP-1), or the peroxisome proliferator-activated receptors (PPARs) to further contribute to impaired coronary circulatory function in more advanced stages of CAD. In particular, abnormalities in vascular endothelial function are also associated with the loss of a potent antithrombotic endothelial surface [73]. This increase in thrombogenicity is likely to mediate an increased risk for atherothrombotic events and its sequelae [15]. Abnormalities in vascular endothelial function or commonly so-called *"endothelial activation,"* reflecting an initial injury of the vascular wall associated with inflammation, proliferation or apoptosis, and the expression of vascular cellular adhesion molecules (ICAM), may initiate and accelerate the CAD process. Further, this "endothelial activation" is considered to play a pivotal role in the manifestation of acute coronary syndromes, characterized by coronary plaque vulnerability, and paradoxical vasoconstriction paralleled by endothelial dysfunction, which is likely to contribute to plaque rupture, and increased thrombogenicity due to loss of a potent antithrombotic endothelial surface [73]. Abnormalities in coronary circulatory function may, in part, reflect the vulnerability of plaques, which may explain the independent predictive value of an impairment of coronary circulatory function for future cardiovascular events [13–15].

As recent investigations suggest [4,21,23], there may be a substantial number of patients with subclinical CAD and normal myocardial perfusion SPECT or PET studies. In these patients, the assessment of reductions of MFR, indicative for early functional stages of developing CAD, by the concurrent ability of PET to quantify MBF could emerge as an important tool to identify those individuals at increased risk for cardiovascular events. In patients with normal or mildly diseased epicardial coronary arteries, an inverse relationship between reductions in hyperemic coronary flow increases (owing to intracoronary papaverine stimulation) and MFR was associated with an increase risk of future cardiovascular events [14]. Similarly, attenuation of PET-measured flow responses to sympathetic stimulation with CPT and its MFR in patients with angiographically normal coronary vessels but with coronary risk factors were associated with a higher risk for cardiac events as compared to those with normal flow increases [13]. Notably, the incidence of cardiovascular events increased with the extent of abnormal flow response to CPT as determined with PET (Figure 4.6) or during hyperemic coronary flow owing to

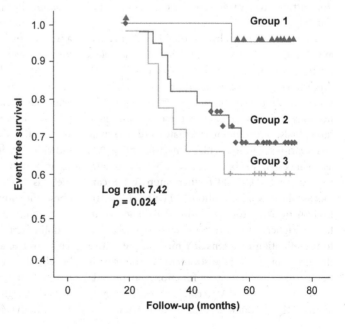

Figure 4.6 Prognostic value of PET-measured, endothelium-related myocardial blood flow responses to sympathetic stimulation with CPT. The Kaplan–Meier analysis demonstrates an association between the incidence of cardiovascular events and the degree of the diminished myocardial blood flow (MBF) response to CPT (group 1: ΔMBF $\geq$40%; group 2: ΔMBF<40% and; group 3: ΔMBF$\leq$0%). (Adapted from Schindler et al. [13].)

intracoronary papaverine application. Such observations may suggest abnormalities in coronary circulatory function as an integrating index of the overall stress burden imposed by various coronary risk factors on the arterial wall. The observations of an impairment of the coronary vasodilator capacity to vasomotor stress as a predictor of cardiovascular events in patients with normal coronary angiograms or without flow-limiting epicardial lesions may, at the first sight, be contradictory to the more favorable outcome of a normal SPECT or PET stress-rest perfusion imaging study [3,5,6,65]. Cardiovascular events predicted by PET-assessment of coronary circulatory dysfunction or invasively during coronary angiography in patients without flow-limiting epicardial lesions normally ensue after 2–3 years, while cardiovascular events predicted by the presence of stress-induced perfusion defects on SPECT or PET normally manifest during shorter time periods. This gives rise to the concept that PET assessment of coronary circulatory dysfunction may signify those asymptomatic individuals at greatest risk of developing CAD and subsequent cardiovascular events rather than identifying the presence of advanced stages of CAD. This could also explain, at least in part, the apparent superiority of functional abnormalities of the coronary circulation over CAD-related structural alterations of the epicardial wall in the prediction of the future cardiovascular clinical outcome [74,75].

A survey conducted by National Health and Examination (NHANES) indicates that about 40–50% asymptomatic individuals with an intermediate risk for cardiovascular events are not considered for preventive medical intervention and/or life style modifications [76]. Conceptually, in these asymptomatic individuals, with an intermediate cardiovascular risk, various cardiovascular imaging modalities assessing directly subclinical stages of CAD or surrogates for CAD, could further improve the cardiovascular risk stratification [9,11,12,27]. Identification of asymptomatic individuals who are in fact at higher cardiac risk could most likely lead to the initiation or intensified medical preventive therapy. Notably, PET assessment of abnormalities in coronary circulatory function may precede and/or accompany CAD related structural alterations of the arterial wall [22,23]. Further, it may be

possible that functional abnormalities of the coronary circulation may in fact reflect the short-term cardiac risk, whereas measures of structural alterations of the arterial wall such as carotid IMT or coronary artery calcium may denote the long-term cardiovascular outcome [74,75]. Whether the application noninvasive cardiovascular imaging modalities for the identification the subclinical atherosclerotic process and, at the same time, monitoring of its response to medical preventive therapy results in an improved clinical outcome remains to be confirmed by large-scale clinical endpoint studies.

Mechanistic Insight of Coronary Circulatory Function and Monitoring Therapy with PET

The noninvasive assessment of coronary circulatory function with PET has provided important mechanistic insight underlying the development and progression of the CAD process. For example, the assessment of coronary circulatory function with PET demonstrated that increased body weight, paralleled by an increase in plasma markers of the insulin-resistance syndrome and chronic inflammation, is independently associated with abnormal coronary circulatory function [21]. This functional abnormality of the coronary circulation in individuals with increasing body weight advanced from a dysfunctional coronary endothelium in overweight, as determined by the MBF response to CPT, to an impairment of the vascular smooth muscle cell relaxation of the coronary arteriolar vessels in obesity as measured with hyperemic flow response to dipyridamole stimulation (Figure 4.7). Similar observations were reported in individuals with increasing severity of insulin resistance and clinically manifest type 2 diabetes mellitus [77]. Notably, it was observed that in obese individuals, increased leptin plasma levels were significantly associated with relatively higher endothelium-related MBF increases to CPT [21]. This positive association might be suggestive of a beneficial effect of leptin on the coronary endothelium to counteract the adverse effects of increases in body weight on coronary vasomotor function. Such findings support the value of the assessment of

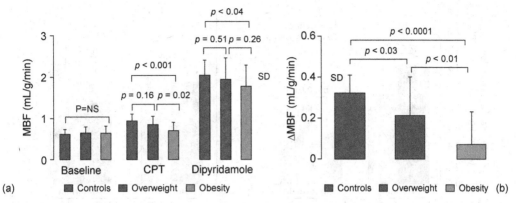

Figure 4.7 Myocardial blood flow (MBF) at rest, during cold pressor testing (CPT), and during stress-stimulation with dipyridamole for the three study groups. (a) The dipyridamole-stimulated MBF was lower in overweight than in controls, but not significantly. In obesity the hyperemic MBFs during dipyridamole stimulation were lowest. (b) Change of endothelium-related MBF during CPT (ΔMBF) for the three study groups. As it can be observed, there is a progressive decrease of the endothelium-related MBF response to CPT from control, to overweight and obesity. (Adapted from [21].)

coronary circulatory function with PET and plasma markers of various coronary risk factors as unique means by which to investigate and to tease out the adverse or even beneficial effects of various factors on coronary circulatory function in complex in vivo conditions [9,11,65]. In healthy individuals without evidence for CAD but with classical coronary risk factors, PET imaging has identified abnormalities in coronary circulatory function as early functional state of the development of CAD. For example, patients with familial hypercholesterolemia and with secondary hypercholesterolemia demonstrated a reduction in hyperemic flow increases during pharmacologic vasodilation [43]. The hyperemic flow increases and MFR were inversely correlated with the severity of abnormal serum lipid levels [78]. There was a marked impairment of hyperemic flows in type 1 and type 2 diabetes mellitus [79,80], which was related to euglycemic control and that also correlated inversely with plasma glucose concentrations averaged over several months.

PET measurements of MBF may be used to monitor the effects of pharmacologic interventions or lifestyle modification on coronary circulatory function in patients with and without manifest CAD [42]. In patients with advanced CAD, the main pillars of medical therapy consist of lipid lowering agents, nitrates, ACE inhibition, and beta-blockers. These treatment options have all been shown to improve mortality and morbidity significantly in the appropriate patient groups. Quantitative PET flow measurements have been used to demonstrate improvement in endothelial dysfunction and myocardial ischemia in patients with advanced CAD after medical treatment with beta-blocker (Figure 4.8), with vitamin C, and a regular exercise program [81–84]. A main advantage of medical therapy is that beyond its beneficial effect on the isolated coronary artery lesion, its systemic effect on all vessels (coronary, carotid, peripheral, etc.) may prevent further progression of atherosclerosis. An example of a patient exhibiting improvement in adenosine-stimulated hyperemia after 1 year of treatment with 3-hydroxy-3-methylglutaryl coenzyme A reductase inhibitor is shown in Figure 4.9 [85].

In chronic smokers placed on acute antioxidant intervention with vitamin C, improvement in hyperemic MBFs during pharmacologic vasodilation or MBF response to CPT was demonstrated [86], indicating that microvascular dysfunction in chronic smokers is largely dependent on the vascular release of reactive oxygen species (ROS). Among patients who underwent 6 weeks of cardiovascular conditioning, near 20% increase in the MFR was shown [81]. In untreated essential hypertension patients, angiotensin II receptor blocker (ARB) improved endothelium-related MBF increases to sympathetic stimulation with CPT [87]. Such improvement in coronary endothelial function was related to ARB-induced elevation of superoxide-dismutase

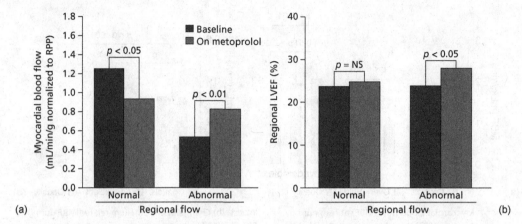

Figure 4.8 Quantitative PET flow measurements can be used to study the effects of six months of medical treatment with metoprolol on absolute myocardial blood flow and function in patients with ischemic cardiomyopathy. (a) There is a favorable redistribution of absolute blood flow from normally perfused myocardium to abnormally perfused myocardium from before to after metoprolol therapy. (b) Increased myocardial blood flow is associated with improvement in regional left ventricular ejection fraction (LVEF) in the abnormally perfused regions of myocardium while myocardial regions with normal baseline perfusion show no change in regional LVEF. The reduction in blood flow in nonischemic regions by beta blockade most probably reflects the reduction in myocardial oxygen demands induced by the reduction in myocardial contractility and work. On the other hand, the decrease in myocardial oxygen demand of the ischemic area by beta blockade may restore vascular autoregulation and allow the ischemic vasculature to regulate its blood flow. By decreasing myocardial oxygen demand (decrease in heart rate) and increasing myocardial oxygen supply (increased subendocardial blood flow in ischemic myocardium), treatment with metoprolol results in an improvement in oxygen balance of the ischemic myocardium. RPP, rate-pressure product, NS, not significant. (Adapted from Bennett *et al.* [84], with permission.)

(SOD). These observations denote specific anti-oxidative effects of ARB inhibition, possibly mediated by inhibition of the endothelial NADPH oxidase activation associated with a decrease in reactive oxygen species (ROS) or increases in antioxidative superoxide dismutase concentrations, responsible for the beneficial effect on coronary endothelial function in these hypertensive patients. Similarly, euglycemic control with glyburide and metformin in type 2 diabetes mellitus resulted in an improvement in CPT-stimulated and endothelium-related MBF increases [88]. This decrease in plasma glucose levels significantly correlated with the improvement in coronary endothelial function ($r = 0.67$, $p < 0.01$), unraveling a direct adverse effect of elevated plasma glucose but not necessarily insulin resistance on diabetes-related coronary vascular disease.

Improvements or even normalization of coronary circulatory dysfunction in patients with subclinical or clinically manifest CAD are likely to reflect a reduction in the coronary risk and improvement in long-term cardiovascular outcome.

In this scenario, improvement of functional abnormalities of the coronary circulation by a variety of interventions, such as angiotensin-converting-enzyme inhibitors, beta-hydroxymethylglutaryl-coenzyme A reductase inhibitors, euglycemic controls in diabetes and physical exercise, has emerged as a primary therapeutic goal in the prevention of the atherosclerotic process [81,88]. Although the latter considerations are intuitively correct, it remains to be shown that an improvement in coronary circulatory dysfunction or its MFR to various forms of vasomotor stress stimulation, for example, by statin or ACE inhibitor therapy, is indeed directly related to the well-known beneficial effects of primary and secondary preventive medical intervention in the prognosis of patients with atherosclerotic heart disease. If the latter holds true, then noninvasive assessment of coronary circulatory function or its vasodilatory capacity with PET could serve as surrogate endpoints for long-term beneficial effects of pharmacologic agents, which remains to be investigated in future large-scale, clinical trials.

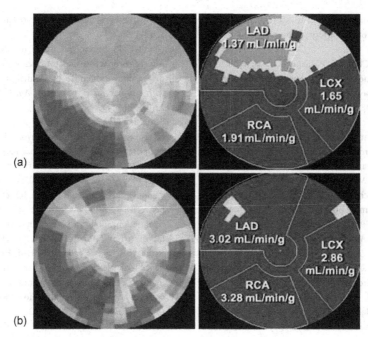

Figure 4.9 An example of a patient exhibiting improvement in adenosine-stimulated hyperemia after 1-year treatment with pravastatin. When compared to baseline quantitative myocardial blood flow reserve values with ^{13}N-ammonia PET (a), follow-up polar maps show significant improvement in myocardial flow reserve in all three vascular territories (b). The extent of the stress-induced defect decreased from 51% of the left anterior descending (LAD) vascular territory to only 3% 1-year post medical therapy. Moreover, there is increase and normalization in myocardial blood flow reserve in the left circumflex artery (LCX) and right coronary artery (RCA) vascular territories, which could only be detected on quantitative measurements of myocardial blood flow but not on the evaluation of the relative radiotracer uptake. (Adapted from Schindler *et al.* [85], with permission.)

Conclusion

The application of PET in concert with short-lived myocardial perfusion tracers has emerged as a reliable noninvasive imaging modality for the detection of CAD. By computing MBF in absolute terms, PET may identify early functional and/or structural abnormalities of the coronary artery circulation before its progression to symptomatic CAD. Likewise, characterization of the vasodilator capacity and endothelial reactivity of the coronary circulation may guide decisions for medical therapy as well as monitor the effects of pharmacologic interventions, risk factor modification, or lifestyle changes, on regional and global MBF. The goal of image-guided personalized medicine may soon be attainable with PET technology.

References

1. Sharir T, Ben-Haim S, Merzon K, *et al.* High-speed myocardial perfusion imaging: initial clinical comparison with conventional dual detector anger camera imaging. *J Am Coll Cardiol Imaging.* 2008;1:156–163.

2. Shaw LJ, Berman DS, Maron DJ, *et al.* Optimal medical therapy with or without percutaneous coronary intervention to reduce ischemic burden: results from the Clinical Outcomes Utilizing Revascularization and Aggressive Drug Evaluation (COURAGE) trial nuclear substudy. *Circulation.* 2008;117(10):1283–1291.

3. Berman DS, Hachamovitch R, Shaw LJ, *et al.* Roles of nuclear cardiology, cardiac computed tomography, and cardiac magnetic resonance: noninvasive risk stratification and a conceptual framework for the selection of noninvasive imaging tests in patients with known or suspected coronary artery disease. *J Nucl Med.* 2006;47(7): 1107–1118.

4. Schenker MP, Dorbala S, Hong EC, *et al.* Interrelation of coronary calcification, myocardial ischemia, and outcomes in patients with intermediate likelihood of coronary artery disease: a combined positron emission tomography/computed tomography study. *Circulation.* 2008;117(13):1693–1700.

5. Marwick TH, Shan K, Patel S, Go RT, Lauer MS. Incremental value of rubidium-82 positron emission

tomography for prognostic assessment of known or suspected coronary artery disease. *Am J Cardiol.* 1997;80(7):865–870.

6. Yoshinaga K, Chow BJ, Williams K, *et al.* What is the prognostic value of myocardial perfusion imaging using rubidium-82 positron emission tomography? *J Am Coll Cardiol.* 2006;48(5):1029–1039.

7. Go RT, Marwick TH, MacIntyre WJ, *et al.* A prospective comparison of rubidium-82 PET and thallium-201 SPECT myocardial perfusion imaging utilizing a single dipyridamole stress in the diagnosis of coronary artery disease. *J Nucl Med.* 1990;31(12):1899–1905.

8. Stewart RE, Schwaiger M, Molina E, *et al.* Comparison of rubidium-82 positron emission tomography and thallium-201 SPECT imaging for detection of coronary artery disease. *Am J Cardiol.* 1991;67(16):1303–1310.

9. Schindler TH, Zhang XL, Vincenti G, Mhiri L, Lerch R, Schelbert HR. Role of PET in the evaluation and understanding of coronary physiology. *J Nucl Cardiol.* 2007;14(4):589–603.

10. Di Carli MF, Hachamovitch R. New technology for noninvasive evaluation of coronary artery disease. *Circulation.* 2007;115(11):1464–1480.

11. Kaufmann PA, Camici PG. Myocardial blood flow measurement by PET: technical aspects and clinical applications. *J Nucl Med.* 2005;46(1):75–88.

12. Camici PG, Crea F. Coronary microvascular dysfunction. *N Engl J Med.* 2007;356(8):830–840.

13. Schindler TH, Nitzsche EU, Schelbert HR, *et al.* Positron emission tomography-measured abnormal responses of myocardial blood flow to sympathetic stimulation are associated with the risk of developing cardiovascular events. *J Am Coll Cardiol.* 2005;45(9):1505–1512.

14. Britten MB, Zeiher AM, Schachinger V. Microvascular dysfunction in angiographically normal or mildly diseased coronary arteries predicts adverse cardiovascular long-term outcome. *Coron Artery Dis.* 2004;15(5):259–264.

15. Lerman A, Zeiher AM. Endothelial function: cardiac events. *Circulation.* 2005;111(3):363–368.

16. Di Carli MF. Advances in positron emission tomography. *J Nucl Cardiol.* 2004;11(6):719–732.

17. Sampson UK, Dorbala S, Limaye A, Kwong R, Di Carli MF. Diagnostic accuracy of rubidium-82 myocardial perfusion imaging with hybrid positron emission tomography/computed tomography in the detection of coronary artery disease. *J Am Coll Cardiol.* 2007;49(10):1052–1058.

18. Huggins GS, Pasternak RC, Alpert NM, Fischman AJ, Gewirtz H. Effects of short-term treatment of hyperlipidemia on coronary vasodilator function and myocardial perfusion in regions having substantial impairment of baseline dilator reverse. *Circulation.* 1998;98(13):1291–1296.

19. Uren NG, Marraccini P, Gistri R, de Silva R, Camici PG. Altered coronary vasodilator reserve and metabolism in myocardium subtended by normal arteries in patients with coronary artery disease. *J Am Coll Cardiol.* 1993;22(3):650–658.

20. Schindler TH, Facta AD, Prior JO, *et al.* PET-measured heterogeneity in longitudinal myocardial blood flow in response to sympathetic and pharmacologic stress as a non-invasive probe of epicardial vasomotor dysfunction. *Eur J Nucl Med Mol Imaging.* 2006;33(10):1140–1149.

21. Schindler TH, Cardenas J, Prior JO, *et al.* Relationship between increasing body weight, insulin resistance, inflammation, adipocytokine leptin, and coronary circulatory function. *J Am Coll Cardiol.* 2006;47(6):1188–1195.

22. Reddy KG, Nair RN, Sheehan HM, Hodgson JM. Evidence that selective endothelial dysfunction may occur in the absence of angiographic or ultrasound atherosclerosis in patients with risk factors for atherosclerosis. *J Am Coll Cardiol.* 1994;23(4):833–843.

23. Schindler TH, Facta AD, Prior JO, *et al.* Structural alterations of the coronary arterial wall are associated with myocardial flow heterogeneity in type 2 diabetes mellitus. *Eur J Nucl Med Mol Imaging.* 2009;36(2):219–229.

24. Yoshinaga K, Katoh C, Noriyasu K, *et al.* Reduction of coronary flow reserve in areas with and without ischemia on stress perfusion imaging in patients with coronary artery disease: a study using oxygen 15-labeled water PET. *J Nucl Cardiol.* 2003;10(3):275–283.

25. Heller LI, Cates C, Popma J, *et al.* Intracoronary Doppler assessment of moderate coronary artery disease: comparison with 201Tl imaging and coronary angiography. FACTS Study Group. *Circulation.* 1997;96(2):484–490.

26. Donohue TJ, Miller DD, Bach RG, *et al.* Correlation of poststenotic hyperemic coronary flow velocity and pressure with abnormal stress myocardial perfusion imaging in coronary artery disease. *Am J Cardiol.* 1996;77(11):948–954.

27. Cecchi F, Olivotto I, Gistri R, Lorenzoni R, Chiriatti G, Camici PG. Coronary microvascular dysfunction and prognosis in hypertrophic cardiomyopathy. *N Engl J Med.* 2003;349(11):1027–1035.

28. Shikama N, Himi T, Yoshida K, *et al.* Prognostic utility of myocardial blood flow assessed by ^{13}N-ammonia positron emission tomography in patients with idiopathic dilated cardiomyopathy. *Am J Cardiol.* 1999;84:434–439.

29. Neglia D, Michelassi C, Trivieri MG, *et al.* Prognostic role of myocardial blood flow impairment in idiopathic left ventricular dysfunction. *Circulation.* 2002;105:186–193.

30. Kuhle WG, Porenta G, Huang SC, *et al.* Quantification of regional myocardial blood flow using ^{13}N-ammonia

and reoriented dynamic positron emission tomographic imaging. *Circulation.* 1992;86(3):1004–1017.

31. Bergmann SR, Fox KA, Rand AL, *et al.* Quantification of regional myocardial blood flow in vivo with $H_2^{15}O$. *Circulation.* 1984;70(4):724–733.

32. Nitzsche EU, Choi Y, Czernin J, Hoh CK, Huang SC, Schelbert HR. Noninvasive quantification of myocardial blood flow in humans. A direct comparison of the [^{13}N]ammonia and the [15O]water techniques. *Circulation.* 1996;93(11):2000–2006.

33. Bol A, Melin JA, Vanoverschelde JL, *et al.* Direct comparison of [^{13}N]ammonia and [15O]water estimates of perfusion with quantification of regional myocardial blood flow by microspheres. *Circulation.* 1993;87(2):512–525.

34. Huang SC, Williams BA, Krivokapich J, Araujo L, Phelps ME, Schelbert HR. Rabbit myocardial 82Rb kinetics and a compartmental model for blood flow estimation. *Am J Physiol.* 1989;256(4 Pt 2):H1156–1164.

35. Herrero P, Markham J, Shelton ME, Weinheimer CJ, Bergmann SR. Noninvasive quantification of regional myocardial perfusion with rubidium-82 and positron emission tomography. Exploration of a mathematical model. *Circulation.* 1990;82(4):1377–1386.

36. Lin JW, Sciacca RR, Chou RL, Laine AF, Bergmann SR. Quantification of myocardial perfusion in human subjects using 82Rb and wavelet-based noise reduction. *J Nucl Med.* 2001;42(2):201–208.

37. El Fakhri G, Sitek A, Guerin B, Kijewski MF, Di Carli MF, Moore SC. Quantitative dynamic cardiac 82Rb PET using generalized factor and compartment analyses. *J Nucl Med.* 2005;46(8):1264–1271.

38. Lortie M, Beanlands RS, Yoshinaga K, Klein R, Dasilva JN, DeKemp RA. Quantification of myocardial blood flow with 82Rb dynamic PET imaging. *Eur J Nucl Med Mol Imaging.* 2007;34(11):1765–1774.

39. Bergmann SR, Hack S, Tewson T, Welch MJ, Sobel BE. The dependence of accumulation of N-13 ammonia by myocardium on metabolic factors and its implications for quantitative assessment of perfusion. *Circulation.* 1980;61:34–43.

40. Krivokapich J, Huang S-C, Phelps ME, MacDonald NS, Shine KI. Dependence of N-13 ammonia myocardial extraction and clearance on flow and metabolism. *Am J Physiol: Heart Circ Physiol.* 1982;242:H536–H542.

41. Kitsiou AN, Bacharach SL, Bartlett ML, *et al.* ^{13}N-Ammonia myocardial blood flow and uptake: Relation to functional outcome of asynergic regions after revascularization. *J Am Coll Cardiol.* 1999;33:678–686.

42. Schelbert HR. Quantifying myocardial perfusion for the assessment of preclinical CAD. In: Di Carli, Lipton. *Cardiac PET and PET/CT Imaging.* New York: Springer, 2007, pp. 166–177.

43. Schelbert HR. Positron emission tomography of the heart: Methodology, findings in the normal and the diseased heart, and clinical applications. In: Phelps M.(ed.) *PET: Molecular Imaging and Its Biological Applications.* New York: Springer-Verlag, 2005, pp. 389–508.

44. Walsh MN, Bergmann SR, Steele RL, *et al.* Delineation of impaired regional myocardial perfusion by positron emission tomography with O-15 water. *Circulation.* 1988;78:612–620.

45. Hermansen F, Ashburner J, Spinks TJ, Kooner JS, Camici PG, Lammertsma AA. Generation of myocardial factor images directly from the dynamic oxygen-15-water scan without use of an oxygen-15-carbon monoxide bloodpool scan. *J Nucl Med.* 1998;39(10):1696–1702.

46. Bacharach SL, Cuocolo A, Bonow RO, *et al.* Arterial blood concentration curves by cardiac PET without arterial sampling or image reconstruction. In: *Computers in Cardiology 1988.* Washington, D.C.: IEEE Computer Society Press, 1989, p. 219.

47. Bergmann SR, Herrero P, Markham J, Weinheimer CJ, Walsh MN. Noninvasive quantitation of myocardial blood flow in human subjects with oxygen-15-labeled water and positron emission tomography. *J Am Coll Cardiol.* 1989;14:639–652.

48. Iida H, Kanno I, Takahashi A, *et al.* Measurement of absolute myocardial blood flow with $H_2^{15}O$ and dynamic positron-emission tomography. Strategy for quantification in relation to the partial-volume effect. *Circulation.* 1988;78(1):104–115.

49. Araujo LI, Lammertsma AA, Rhodes CG, *et al.* Noninvasive quantification of regional myocardial blood flow in coronary artery disease with oxygen-15-labeled carbon dioxide inhalation and positron emission tomography. *Circulation.* 1991;83(3):875–885.

50. Iida H, Tamura Y, Kitamura K, Bloomfield PM, Eberl S, Ono Y. Histochemical correlates of (15)O-water-perfusable tissue fraction in experimental canine studies of old myocardial infarction. *J Nucl Med.* 2000;41(10):1737–1745.

51. Love WD, Burch GE. Influence of the rate of coronary plasma flow on the extraction of rubidium-86 from coronary blood. *Circ Res.* 1959;7:24–30.

52. Selwyn AP, Allan RM, L'Abbate A, *et al.* Relation between regiona myocardial uptake of rubidium-82 and perfusion: Absolute reduction of cation uptake in ischemia. *Am J Cardiol.* 1982;50:112–121.

53. Goldstein RA, Mullani NA, Marani SK, Fisher DJ, Gould KL, O'Brien HA, Jr. Myocardial perfusion with rubidium-82. II, Effects of metabolic and pharmacologic interventions. *J Nucl Med.* 1983;24:907–915.

54. Fukuyama T, Nakamura M, Nakagaki O, Matsuguchi H, Mitsutake A, Kikuchi Y. Reduced reflow and diminished uptake of rubidium-86 after temporary coronary

occlusion. *Am J Physiol: Heart Circ Physiol.* 1978;234: H724–H729.

55. Wilson RA, Shea M, De Landsheere C, *et al.* Rubidium-82 myocardial uptake and extraction after transient ischemia: PET characteristics. *J Comput Assist Tomogr.* 1987;11:60–66.

56. Jeremy RW, Links JM, Becker LC. Progressive failure of coronary flow during reperfusion of myocardial infarction: documentation of the no reflow phenomenon with positron emission tomography. *J Am Coll Cardiol.* 1990;16:695–704.

57. Demer LL, Gould LK, Goldstein RA, *et al.* Assessment of coronary artery disease severity by positron emission tomography. Comparison with quantitative arteriography in 193 patients. *Circulation.* 1989;79:825–835.

58. Chow BJ, Ananthasubramaniam K, dekemp RA, Dalipaj MM, Beanlands RS, Ruddy TD. Comparison of treadmill exercise versus dipyridamole stress with myocardial perfusion imaging using rubidium-82 positron emission tomography. *J Am Coll Cardiol.* 2005;45(8):1227–1234.

59. Parkash R, deKemp RA, Ruddy TD, *et al.* Potential utility of rubidium 82 PET quantification in patients with 3-vessel coronary artery disease. *J Nucl Cardiol.* 2004; 11(4):440–449.

60. Herrero P, Markham J, Shelton ME, Bergman SR. Implementation and evaluation of a two-compartment model for quantification of myocardial perfusion with rebidium-82 and positron emission tomography. *Circ Res.* 1992;70:496–507.

61. Coxson PG, Huesman RH, Borland L. Consequences of using a simplified kinetic model for dynamic PET data. *J Nucl Med.* 1997;38:660–667.

62. Yoshida K, Mullani N, Gould KL. Coronary flow and flow reserve by PET simplified for clinical applications using rubidium-82 or nitrogen-13-ammonia. *J Nucl Med.* 1996;37:1701–1712.

63. Lin JW, Laine AF, Akinboboye O, Bergmann SR. Use of wavelet transforms in analysis of time-activity data from cardiac PET. *J Nucl Med.* 2001;42(2):194–200.

64. Schindler TH, Zhang XL, Prior JO, *et al.* Assessment of intra- and interobserver reproducibility of rest and cold pressor test-stimulated myocardial blood flow with (13)N-ammonia and PET. *Eur J Nucl Med Mol Imaging.* 2007;34(8):1178–1188.

65. Vesely MR, Dilsizian V. Nuclear cardiac stress testing in the era of molecular medicine. *J Nucl Med.* 2008;49(3): 399–413.

66. De Bruyne B, Hersbach F, Pijls NH, *et al.* Abnormal epicardial coronary resistance in patients with diffuse atherosclerosis but "Normal" coronary angiography. *Circulation.* 2001;104(20):2401–2406.

67. Hernandez-Pampaloni M, Keng FY, Kudo T, Sayre JS, Schelbert HR. Abnormal longitudinal, base-to-apex my-ocardial perfusion gradient by quantitative blood flow measurements in patients with coronary risk factors. *Circulation.* 2001;104(5):527–532.

68. Schindler TH, Zhang XL, Vincenti G, *et al.* Diagnostic value of PET-measured heterogeneity in myocardial blood flows during cold pressor testing for the identification of coronary vasomotor dysfunction. *J Nucl Cardiol.* 2007;14(5):688–697.

69. Gould KL, Nakagawa Y, Nakagawa K, *et al.* Frequency and clinical implications of fluid dynamically significant diffuse coronary artery disease manifest as graded, longitudinal, base-to-apex myocardial perfusion abnormalities by noninvasive positron emission tomography. *Circulation.* 2000;101(16):1931–1939.

70. Buus NH, Bottcher M, Hermansen F, Sander M, Nielsen TT, Mulvany MJ. Influence of nitric oxide synthase and adrenergic inhibition on adenosine-induced myocardial hyperemia. *Circulation.* 2001;104(19):2305–2310.

71. Tawakol A, Forgione MA, Stuehlinger M, *et al.* Homocysteine impairs coronary microvascular dilator function in humans. *J Am Coll Cardiol.* 2002;40(6):1051–1058.

72. Schindler TH, Nitzsche EU, Olschewski M, *et al.* PET-measured responses of MBF to cold press or testing correlate with indices of coronary vasomotion on quantitative coronary angiography. *J Nucl Med.* 2004;45(3):419–428.

73. Topol EJ, Yadav JS. Recognition of the importance of embolization in atherosclerotic vascular disease. *Circulation.* 2000;101(5):570–580.

74. Rozanski A, Gransar H, Wong ND, *et al.* Clinical outcomes after both coronary calcium scanning and exercise myocardial perfusion scintigraphy. *J Am Coll Cardiol.* 2007;49(12):1352–1361.

75. Chan SY, Mancini GB, Kuramoto L, Schulzer M, Frohlich J, Ignaszewski A. The prognostic importance of endothelial dysfunction and carotid atheroma burden in patients with coronary artery disease. *J Am Coll Cardiol.* 2003;42(6):1037–1043.

76. Verma S, Buchanan MR, Anderson TJ. Endothelial function testing as a biomarker of vascular disease. *Circulation.* 2003;108(17):2054–2059.

77. Prior JO, Quinones MJ, Hernandez-Pampaloni M, *et al.* Coronary circulatory dysfunction in insulin resistance, impaired glucose tolerance, and type 2 diabetes mellitus. *Circulation.* 2005;111(18):2291–2298.

78. Kaufmann PA, Gnecchi-Ruscone T, Schafers KP, Luscher TF, Camici PG. Low density lipoprotein cholesterol and coronary microvascular dysfunction in hypercholesterolemia. *J Am Coll Cardiol.* 2000;36(1):103–109.

79. Pitkanen OP, Nuutila P, Raitakari OT, *et al.* Coronary flow reserve is reduced in young men with IDDM. *Diabetes.* 1998;47(2):248–254.

80. Di Carli MF, Janisse J, Grunberger G, Ager J. Role of chronic hyperglycemia in the pathogenesis of coronary microvascular dysfunction in diabetes. *J Am Coll Cardiol.* 2003;41(8):1387–1393.

81. Czernin J, Barnard RJ, Sun KT, *et al.* Effect of short-term cardiovascular conditioning and low-fat diet on myocardial blood flow and flow reserve. *Circulation.* 1995; 92(2):197–204.

82. Baller D, Notohamiprodjo G, Gleichmann U, *et al.* Improvement in coronary flow reserve determined by positron emission tomography after six months of cholesterol lowering therapy in patients with early stages of coronary atherosclerosis. *Circulation.* 1999;99:2871–2875.

83. Gould KL, Martucci JP, Goldberg DI, *et al.* Short term cholesterol lowering decreases size and severity of perfusion abnormalities by positron emission tomography after dipyridamole in patients with coronary artery disease. *Circulation.* 1994;89:1530–1538.

84. Bennett SK, Smith MF, Gottlieb SS, *et al.* Effect of metoprolol on absolute myocardial blood flow in patients with heart failure secondary to ischemic or non-ischemic cardiomyopathy. *Am J Cardiol.* 2002;89:1431–1434.

85. Schindler TH, Schelbert HR. PET quantitation of myocardial blood flow. In: Dilsizian V, Narula J (eds). *Atlas of Nuclear Cardiology*, 2nd edition. Current Medicine, Inc., Philadelphia, 2006, pp. 67–95.

86. Schindler TH, Nitzsche EU, Munzel T, *et al.* Coronary vasoregulation in patients with various risk factors in response to cold pressor testing: contrasting myocardial blood flow responses to short- and long-term vitamin C administration. *J Am Coll Cardiol.* 2003;42(5): 814–822.

87. Naya M, Tsukamoto T, Morita K, *et al.* Olmesartan, but not amlodipine, improves endothelium-dependent coronary dilation in hypertensive patients. *J Am Coll Cardiol.* 2007;50(12):1144–1149.

88. Schindler TH, Facta AD, Prior JO, *et al.* Improvement in coronary vascular dysfunction produced with euglycaemic control in patients with type 2 diabetes. *Heart.* 2007;93(3):345–349.

CHAPTER 5

Myocardial Metabolism in Health and Disease

Robert J. Gropler[1], Linda R. Peterson[1] & Vasken Dilsizian[2]
[1] Edward Mallinckrodt Institute of Radiology *and* Washington University School of Medicine, St. Louis, MO, USA
[2] University of Maryland School of Medicine, Baltimore, MD, USA

Introduction

The heart utilizes various metabolic substrates for energy production in the form of adenosine triphosphate (ATP). For a given physiologic environment, the heart consumes the most efficient metabolic fuel as an adaptive response to meet its energy demands. The flexibility of switching from one metabolic substrate to another permits the heart to respond efficiently to various stimuli, depending on the workload, hormonal milieu, regional myocardial perfusion, and substrate availability [1,2]. Metabolic substrate switch can occur as an acute or a chronic adaptation in response to either short or prolonged alterations in the physiological environment.

In acute or short-term increase in workload, the heart immediately mobilizes its metabolic reserve contained in glycogen (transient increase in glycogen oxidation) and meets the needs for additional energy from the oxidation of carbohydrate substrates (glucose and lactate). These rapid changes in metabolism are regulated by a host of enzymes, such as pyruvate dehydrogenase complex and enzyme carnitine palmitoyl transferase 1, which is regulated by the malonyl-CoA concentration [3–7]. In contrast, chronic metabolic adaptations reflect alterations in gene expression regulating various metabolic pathways. These changes are thought to occur primarily at the transcriptional level through the coordinated upregulation of enzymes and proteins involved in key metabolic pathways. For example, in diabetes mellitus, the nuclear receptor peroxisome proliferator-activated receptor alpha (PPARα) activity is increased, leading to an upregulation in genes controlling fatty acid uptake, oxidation, and storage [8,9]. In contrast, in pressure-overload hypertrophy, PPARα activity is decreased, leading to a downregulation of genes controlling fatty acid metabolism and an upregulation of glucose metabolism [10]. These chronic adaptations can induce numerous detrimental effects that extend beyond alterations in energy production and may include enhanced oxygen free radical production, impaired energetics, stimulation of apoptosis, and the induction of left ventricular dysfunction. Important unresolved questions include the extent to which metabolic perturbations in the acute or chronic setting that are adaptive may in fact become maladaptive and cause irreversible myocardial damage? What are the key determinants of these metabolic alterations? How do they impact prognosis? What are their implications for medical therapy?

Perhaps the most dramatic clinical application of metabolic imaging is in hibernation, which represents dysfunctional but viable myocardium that is most likely the result of extensive cellular reprogramming due to repetitive episodes of chronic ischemia. In hibernation, when the oxygen supply to the myocardium is decreased, the heart helps

Cardiac CT, PET and MR, 2nd edition. Edited by Vasken Dilsizian and Gerry Pohost. © 2010 Blackwell Publishing Ltd.

protect itself from an oxygen-lacking fate of infarction by switching its energy source to glycolysis, downregulating mitochondrial oxidative metabolism, and reducing contractile function. The true mechanism for viability remodeling in hibernation is likely to be much more complex. Nonetheless, because glucose transport and phosphorylation is readily tracked by the uptake and retention of – (FDG), hibernating myocardium is readily detected by enhanced glucose uptake in the same regions by external detectors such as positron emission tomography (PET).

Recent clinical studies have also shown the potential utility of metabolic adaptation in the emergency room as well as for detection of coronary artery disease in the form of "ischemic memory" [11,12]. Ischemic memory represents prolonged but reversible metabolic recovery after transient myocardial ischemia, also known as "metabolic stunning" [13–16]. Other disease entities where metabolic imaging by nuclear techniques can play an important role include identification of microvascular disease and subendocardial ischemia in symptomatic women with nonobstructive coronary artery disease, diabetic heart disease, and left ventricular remodeling in hypertrophy and congestive heart failure. Currently, the detection of ischemic but viable myocardium with FDG PET is the only Food and Drug Administration approved indication for the management of patients with ischemic cardiomyopathy.

PET Assessment of Myocardial Metabolism

Most clinical PET scanners are full ring devices that simultaneously measure projections at all angles, whereas conventional single photon emission computed tomography (SPECT) cameras require time to rotate the detector heads about the patient. This is a significant advantage because it enables PET to image rapidly changing physiologic and metabolic processes. PET systems are generally more sensitive than SPECT systems, have better spatial resolution, and provide more accurate attenuation correction. The consequence of these advantages with PET is the possibility for quantification of tracer concentration in absolute units (MBq/mL).

The functional information depicted in PET images depends upon the radiopharmaceutical employed for that particular study. The positron-emitting radionuclides consist of biologically ubiquitous elements, such as oxygen (^{15}O), carbon (^{11}C), and nitrogen (^{13}N), as well as fluorine (^{18}F) substituting for hydrogen, which can be incorporated into a wide variety of substrates or substrate analogs that participate in diverse biochemical pathways without altering the biochemical properties of the substrate of interest. These isotopes have half-lives that are considerably shorter than those used in SPECT and typically have to be produced in close proximity to the scanner using a cyclotron. Sites without a cyclotron are generally limited to ^{18}F-labeled radiotracers, as ^{18}F has a 110-minute half-life and can be shipped from a central production facility to remote imaging sites. An exception to the ^{18}F includes ^{82}Rubidium, which is produced using a generator. By combining the knowledge of the metabolic pathways of interest with kinetic models that faithfully describe the fate of the tracer in tissue, an accurate interpretation of the tracer kinetics can be achieved. The major disadvantages of PET are its complexity in both radiotracer design and image quantification schemes and expense. Metabolic processes that are typically measured with PET include (1) myocardial oxygen consumption (MVO$_2$), (2) carbohydrate metabolism, and (3) fatty acid metabolism (Figure 5.1).

Myocardial Oxygen Consumption

^{15}O-Oxygen

Oxygen is common in all pathways of aerobic myocardial metabolism and is the final step of electron capture. In biological systems, ^{15}O-oxygen PET imaging has been applied to measure myocardial oxygen extraction and MVO$_2$ directly. Due to its short physical half-life of 2 minutes, ^{15}O-oxygen is readily applicable in studies requiring repetitive assessments such as those with an acute pharmacologic intervention. Its major disadvantages are the need for a multiple-tracer study (to account for myocardial blood flow and blood volume) and fairly complex compartmental modeling to obtain the measurements [17–19].

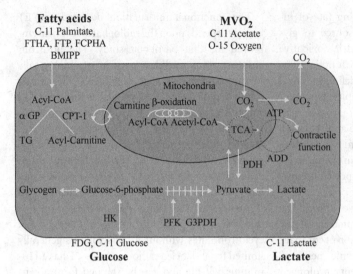

Fatty acids
C-11 Palmitate,
FTHA, FTP, FCPHA
BMIPP

MVO$_2$
C-11 Acetate
O-15 Oxygen

Figure 5.1 Major metabolic pathways and various radiopharmaceuticals to assess myocardial metabolism in a myocyte. FTHA, ^{18}F fluoro-6-thia-heptadecanoic acid; FTP, ^{18}F-fluorothiapalmitate FCPHA, *trans*-9(*RS*)-^{18}F-fluoro-3,4(*RS,RS*) methyleneheptadecanoic acid; BMIPP, ^{123}I-beta-methyl-P-iodophenylpentadecanoic acid; HK, hexokinase; PFK, phosphofructokinase; ADP, adenosine diphosphate; TCA; tricarboxylic acid cycle; PDH, pyruvate dehydrogenase; TG, triglyceride; G3PDH, glyceraldehyde 3-phosphate dehydrogenase; GP, alpha-glycerol phosphate.

[11]C-Acetate

[11]C-acetate PET is the preferred method of measuring MVO$_2$ noninvasively. Acetate is a two-carbon chain free fatty acid that is avidly extracted by the myocardium and is metabolized predominantly by mitochondrial oxidative metabolism. Once in the cytosol, it is rapidly converted to acetyl-CoA and is oxidized through the tricarboxylic acid cycle in the mitochondria to ^{11}C-carbon dioxide and water. Because of the tight coupling of the tricarboxylic acid cycle and oxidative phosphorylation, the myocardial turnover of ^{11}C-acetate reflects overall flux in the tricarboxylic acid cycle and, thus, overall oxidative metabolism or MVO$_2$. Either exponential curve-fitting or compartmental modeling is used to calculate MVO$_2$. The latter is typically preferable in situations of low cardiac output where marked splaying of the input function and spillover of activity from the lungs to the myocardium can decrease the accuracy of the curve-fitting method [20–24].

Carbohydrate Metabolism

[18]F-fluorodeoxyglucose

FDG is a glucose analog that competes with glucose for facilitated transport into the sarcolemma and for hexokinase-mediated phosphorylation. The resultant FDG-6-phosphate is trapped in the cytosol and the myocardial uptake of FDG is thought to reflect overall anaerobic and aerobic myocardial glycolytic flux [25–28]. The myocardial kinetics of FDG has been well characterized, the acquisition scheme is relatively straightforward, and its production has become routine owing in part to the rapid growth of its clinical use in oncology. As such, FDG remains the most widely used tracer for determination of myocardial glucose metabolism. Regional myocardial glucose utilization can be assessed either in relative or in absolute terms (i.e., in nmol/g/min). For quantification, a mathematical correction for the kinetic differences between FDG and glucose, termed "lumped constant," must be used to calculate rates of glucose utilization. The lumped constant thus accounts for differences in the transport and phosphorylation of FDG and glucose and may vary depending upon the prevailing plasma substrate and hormonal conditions [27,29–31]. Once phosphorylated, FDG is trapped in the glycolytic pathway and is not metabolized further. Consequently, the metabolic fate of FDG in tissue (i.e., glycogen formation versus glycolysis) cannot be determined. Moreover, the relatively long physical half-life of [18]F (110 minutes) precludes serial measurements of myocardial glucose utilization.

Carbon-11 Glucose

More recently, quantification of myocardial glucose utilization has been performed with PET using glucose radiolabeled in the 1-carbon position with ^{11}C (^{11}C-glucose). Because ^{11}C-glucose is chemically identical to unlabeled glucose it has the same metabolic fate as glucose, obviating the need for the lumped constant correction. It has been demonstrated that measurements of myocardial glucose utilization based on compartmental modeling of tracer kinetics are more accurate with ^{11}C-glucose than with FDG and can provide estimates of glycogen synthesis, glycolysis, and glucose oxidation [32–34]. Disadvantages of this method include compartmental modeling that is more demanding with ^{11}C-glucose than it is with FDG and the need to correct the arterial input function for the

production of ^{11}CO$_2$ and ^{11}C-lactate, and a fairly complex tracer synthesis process. The shorter physical half-life of ^{11}C (20 minutes) requires an on-site cyclotron.

^{11}C-Lactate

Lactate metabolism in the heart is a key source of energy production, particularly during periods of increased cardiac work. Recently, a multicompartment model was developed for the assessment of myocardial lactate metabolism using PET and L-3-^{11}C-lactate. PET-derived extraction of lactate correlated well with lactate oxidation measured by arterial and coronary sinus sampling over a wide range of conditions (Figure 5.2) [35]. This approach may help delineate the clinical role of lactate metabolism in a variety of pathological conditions such as

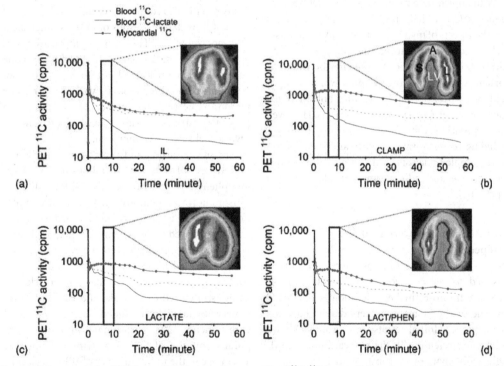

Figure 5.2 Representative PET time–activity curves of L-3-^{11}C-lactate obtained from (a) intralipid (IL); (b)insulin clamp (CLAMP); (c) lactate infusion (LACTATE); or (d) lactate and phenylepherine (LAC/PHEN) studies and corresponding myocardial images obtained 5–10 minutes after tracer injection and depicting primarily early tracer uptake. Images are displayed on horizontal long axis.

Blood ^{11}C, ^{11}C time–activity curves obtained from region of interest (ROI) placed on left atrium; blood ^{11}C-lactate, blood ^{11}C time–activity curves after removing ^{11}CO$_2$, ^{11}C-neutral, and ^{11}C-basic metabolites; myocardial ^{11}C, ^{11}C time–activity curves obtained from ROI placed on lateral wall; A, apical wall; S, septal wall; L, lateral wall; LV, left ventricle. (Adapted from Herrero et al. [35].)

diabetes mellitus and myocardial ischemia. Moreover, when combined with either FDG or ^{11}C-glucose it permits a more comprehensive measurement of myocardial carbohydrate metabolism.

Fatty Acid Metabolism

^{11}C-Palmitate

Under fasting and aerobic conditions, long-chain fatty acids are the preferred fuel in the heart, supplying nearly 70% of the energy for the working heart. As such, early studies in cardiac metabolism focused on the characterization of myocardial kinetics of the long-chain fatty acid, ^{11}C-palmitate with PET. Uptake of ^{11}C-palmitate in the myocardium is dependent on regional perfusion, diffusion across the sarcolemmal membrane, transporter protein, and acceptance in the cytosol by binding to Co-A. With appropriate mathematical modeling techniques, ^{11}C-palmitate permits the assessment of various aspects of myocardial fatty acid metabolism such as uptake, oxidation, and storage [36–39]. Such detailed metabolic analysis may become important when trying to determine which component of myocardial fatty acid metabolism is the main contributor to a pathologic process. However, this approach suffers from several disadvantages including reduced image quality and specificity, a more complex analysis, and the need for an on-site cyclotron and radiopharmaceutical production capability.

Fatty Acid Radiotracers That Are Trapped

Most of the PET tracers in this category have been designed to reflect myocardial β-oxidation. 14-(R,S)-^{18}F-fluoro-6-thiaheptadecanoic acid (FTHA) was one of the first radiotracers developed using this approach. Initial results were promising with uptake and retention in the myocardium accordingly with changes in substrate delivery, blood flow, and workload in animal models [40,41]. Moreover, PET with FTHA was used to evaluate the effects of various diseases such as coronary artery disease and cardiomyopathy on myocardial fatty acid metabolism [42,43]. However, uptake and retention of FTHA has been shown to be insensitive to the inhibition of β-oxidation by hypoxia reducing enthusiasm for this radiotracer to measure

myocardial fatty acid metabolism [44]. To circumvent this problem, 16-^{18}F-fluoro-4-thia-palmitate (FTP) has been developed. This modification retains the metabolic trapping function of the radiotracer, which is proportional to fatty acid oxidation under normal oxygenation and hypoxic conditions [44,45]. Similar to FDG, quantification of myocardial fatty acid metabolism with FTP requires the use of a lumped constant to correct for kinetic differences between the radiotracer and unlabeled palmitate, and the stability of the lumped constant under various conditions is unknown. Nonetheless, FTP is currently undergoing commercialization as it enters early Phase 1 evaluation. Similarly, a new F-18-labeled fatty acid radiotracer, trans-9(RS)-^{18}F-fluoro-3,4(RS,RS) methyleneheptadecanoic acid (FCPHA), has been developed and is undergoing commercialization [46]. This radiotracer is also trapped after undergoing several steps of β-oxidation. Results of initial studies show that uptake of FCPHA into rat myocardium is approximately 1.5% injected dose per gram tissue at 5 minutes with little change over a period of 60 minutes and low blood activity over the same period. However, the impact of alterations in plasma substrates, workload, and blood flow on myocardial kinetics is unknown.

One of the earliest and most promising SPECT radiotracers of fatty acid metabolism was 15-(p-iodophenyl)-pentadecanoic acid (IPPA) [47–49]. This radiotracer demonstrated rapid accumulation in the heart and exhibited clearance kinetics that followed a biexponential function characteristic for ^{11}C-palmitate. Moreover, the clearance rates correlated directly with β-oxidation. Initial studies in humans with coronary atherosclerosis demonstrated reduced uptake and washout in regions subtended by occluded arteries consistent with ischemia [50]. Unfortunately, the poor temporal resolution of SPECT systems did not take advantage of the rapid turnover of IPPA. As a consequence, quantification of myocardial fatty acid metabolism was not possible and image quality was reduced. This led to the development of branched-chain analogs of IPPA, such as ^{123}I-beta-methyl-P-iodophenylpentadecanoic acid (BMIPP) [49–52]. Alkyl branching inhibits β-oxidation shunting radiolabel to the triglyceride pool, thereby increasing radiotracer retention and improving image quality.

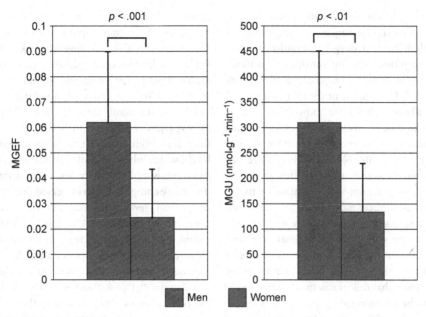

Figure 5.3 Gender-related differences in myocardial glucose extraction fraction (MGEF) and myocardial glucose utilization (MGU). (Adapted from Peterson et al. [55].)

Clinical Applications of Myocardial Metabolism

Gender Differences in Myocardial Substrate Metabolism

Both gender and aging impact the myocardial metabolic phenotype. Results of studies in animal models show that there are gender differences in myocardial substrate metabolism, with female rats exhibiting less myocardial glucose and more fatty acid metabolism [53,54]. Recently, using PET with ^{11}C-glucose and ^{11}C-plamitate, these observations were confirmed in young healthy volunteers [55]. Women exhibited lower levels of glucose metabolism compared with men (Figure 5.3). Although no differences in myocardial fatty acid metabolism were noted, women also exhibited higher MVO_2 compared with men as measured by PET with ^{11}C-acetate. These gender differences in substrate metabolism become more pronounced when transitioning to more pathologic conditions. For example, in addition to the changes in glucose metabolism and MVO_2, obese women exhibited higher fatty acid uptake and oxidation compared with obese men [56]. The differences in myocardial metabolism could not be explained by differences in myocardial blood flow, insulin sensitivity, hemodynamics, myocardial work, or the plasma substrate environment. Differences in hormonal stimulation may play a role in the mechanism of gender-related differences in myocardial substrate metabolism since results of animal studies have shown that estrogen decreases glucose oxidation, gluconeogenesis, and glycogenolysis, and increases fatty acid oxidation in liver and skeletal muscle [57–60]. Myocardial glucose utilization may also be decreased by estrogen because it is known to upregulate nitric oxide synthases, which cause a reduction in GLUT-4 translocation to the cell surface, thereby inhibiting myocardial glucose uptake [61–63]. Indeed, in a small retrospective study, PET-derived measurements of myocardial fatty acid metabolism were higher in postmenopausal women receiving estrogen-based hormonal replacement therapy when compared with either postmenopausal women not receiving hormonal replacement therapy or age-matched men [64].

Altered Myocardial Metabolism with Aging

In various experimental models of aging, the contribution of fatty acid oxidation to overall myocardial substrate metabolism declines with age [65,66].

The cause for the decrease in fatty acid oxidation seems multifactorial, ranging from changes in mitochondrial lipid content, oxygen free radical injury, a decline in carnitine palmitoyltransferase-1 activity, and age-related decline in myocardial PPARα activity [67–69]. Using some of the PET approaches described above, it has been shown that a similar metabolic shift occurs in healthy older humans [70]. However, despite this preference for glucose as an energy substrate, older individuals are not able to increase glucose utilization in response to β-adrenergic stimulation with dobutamine to the same extent as younger individuals. This impaired metabolic response may portend a stress-related energy deprivation state in the aging heart or potentially indicate that the heart is more susceptible to injury during periods of ischemia [71]. Recently, it has been shown that this impairment in metabolic reserve can be ameliorated by endurance exercise training in older subjects [72]. However, it appears that myocardial metabolic response to dobutamine following endurance exercise training is gender-specific, with men demonstrating an increase in myocardial glucose metabolism and a decline in fatty acid use whereas women exhibit an increase in both glucose and fatty acid metabolism. Although requiring further study, these gender and age differences in metabolism may provide a partial explanation for the gender- and age-related outcome differences for various cardiovascular diseases where altered myocardial metabolism plays a role.

Diabetes Mellitus

Cardiovascular disease is the leading cause of morbidity and mortality in patients with diabetes mellitus [73]. The mechanisms responsible for the increased risk are multifactorial and complex with possibilities including an increased prevalence of hyperlipidemia and hypertension, impaired fibrinolysis, abnormal myocardial endothelial function, and reduced sympathetic neuronal function. However, there is extensive evidence to suggest that abnormalities in myocardial substrate metabolism contribute to the cardiovascular abnormalities observed in diabetic patients [74,75].

The metabolic phenotype in diabetes mellitus is an overdependence on fatty acid metabolism and a decrease in glucose use. Multiple mechanisms contribute to this phenotype. These include increased plasma delivery of fatty acids due to peripheral insulin resistance, decreased insulin signaling, and activation of key transcriptional pathways such as the PPAR α/PGC-1 signaling network [74,76,77]. Both insulin-mediated glucose transport and glucose transporter expressions decline in diabetes mellitus. However, rates of myocardial glucose uptake are frequently normal due to the presence of hyperglycemia. The increase in myocardial fatty acid utilization results in increased citrate levels, which inhibit phosphofructokinase. Glucose oxidation is inhibited at the level of pyruvate dehydrogenase complex due to increased mitochondrial acetyl-CoA levels and the phosphorylation of pyruvate dehydrogenase kinase 4 by PPARα activation. Consequently, decrease in the downstream glucose metabolism results in an accumulation of glucose metabolites. Potential detrimental effects associated with this shift in metabolism include impaired mechanical function due to the inability to increase glucose metabolism in response to increase myocardial work, depletion of tricarboxylic acid cycle intermediates due to reduced anapleurosis, electrical instability, a greater sensitivity to myocardial ischemia and myocardial lipid accumulation, or lipotoxicity leading to increased apoptosis.

Small animal imaging has helped clarify the mechanisms responsible for the metabolic alterations that occur in diabetes mellitus. For example, mice with cardiac-restricted overexpression of PPARα demonstrate a metabolic phenotype that is similar to diabetic hearts [78]. Small animal PET studies with ^{11}C-palmitate and FDG in these mice demonstrate an increase in fatty acid uptake and an abnormal suppression of glucose uptake. In contrast, in mice with cardiac-restricted overexpression of PPARβ/σ, small animal PET measurements demonstrated an increase in glucose uptake and a decrease in fatty acid uptake [79]. These observations demonstrate that PPARα and PPARβ/σ drive different metabolic regulatory programs in the heart and that imaging can help characterize genetic manipulations in mouse heart. However, these studies also demonstrate the challenges in imaging the mouse heart due to its small size as only semiquantitative measurements of tracer uptake currently can be performed. However, quantitative measures of myocardial substrate metabolism are now possible with small animal PET in rat heart. For example, rates of myocardial glucose uptake correlate directly and closely with GLUT 4 gene expression in the Zucker-Diabetic-Fat (ZDF) rat, a model of type-2 diabetes mellitus [80]. Moreover, rates of myocardial glucose uptake and fatty acid uptake and oxidation measured with PET in the same disease model demonstrated the importance of increased fatty acid delivery to define the metabolic phenotype in diabetes mellitus [81].

Numerous imaging studies have been performed in humans to assess the impact of diabetes mellitus on myocardial glucose metabolism. These studies have been primarily limited to FDG PET and have generally shown decreased rates of myocardial glucose utilization in patients with either type-1 or type-2 diabetes mellitus compared with nondiabetics [82–84]. Increased myocardial fatty acid uptake measured by arterial–coronary sinus balance studies has been reported in humans with type-1 diabetes mellitus without coronary artery disease [85]. Although the impact of plasma levels of free fatty acids on the level of myocardial fatty acid uptake was not determined, a negative correla-

tion between myocardial glucose uptake and plasma fatty acid levels was observed. Recently, studies using PET and ^{11}C-plamitate and ^{11}C-glucose in patients with type-1 diabetes mellitus have helped verify these findings noninvasively. Patients with diabetes exhibited higher levels of fatty acid uptake and oxidation compared with nondiabetics primarily due to increased plasma fatty acid levels. In contrast, glucose uptake was reduced in these patients primarily due to decreased glucose transport mechanisms [38]. Moreover, the metabolic fate of extracted glucose was shown to be impaired in diabetics with decreased rates of glycolysis and glucose oxidation, which became more pronounced with increases in cardiac work induced by dobutamine (Figure 5.4) [86]. However, the diabetic myocardium was responsive to changes in plasma insulin and fatty acid levels but at a cost. Higher insulin levels were needed to achieve the same level of glucose uptake and glucose oxidation compared with nondiabetics consistent with myocardial

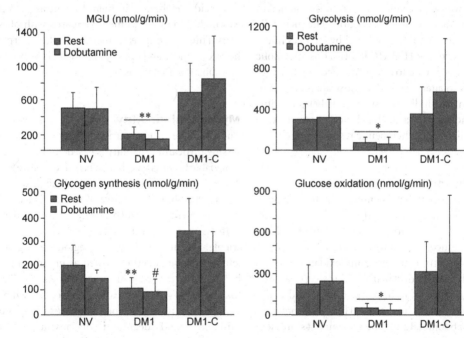

Figure 5.4 Measurements of overall myocardial glucose uptake (MGU), glycolysis, glucose oxidation, and glycogen synthesis for normal volunteers (NV), type-1 diabetic patients studied under baseline metabolic conditions (DM1) and diabetic patients studied during hyperinsulinemic–euglycemic clamp (DM1-C) both at rest (open bars) and during dobutamine (closed bars). (Adapted from Herrero et al. [86].) *P not significant for rest versus dobutamine; $P < .05$ versus NVs (rest and dobutamine) and DM1-C patients (rest and dobutamine). For myocardial glycolysis, $P = .09$ for rest versus dobutamine $P < .05$ versus NVs (rest and dobutamine) and DM1-C patients (rest and dobutamine). **For myocardial glycogen synthesis, $P = .07$ for rest versus dobutamine, $P < .05$ versus NVs (rest) and DM1-C patients (rest); #$P < .05$ versus DM1-C *patients* (rest).

insulin resistance. Similarly, in response to higher fatty acid plasma levels, myocardial fatty acid uptake was increased, however, at a cost of a greater esterification rate [86,87].

The increase in plasma fatty acids are an attractive target to reduce the overdependence of the myocardium on fatty acid metabolism and perhaps improve energetics and function of the left ventricle. For example, the use of the insulin sensitizing agent troglitazone in ZDF rats resulted in decreased plasma fatty acid levels, decreased myocardial lipid accumulation, reduced apoptosis, and improved left ventricular function [88]. In patients with type-2 diabetes mellitus, FDG PET studies performed before and 26 weeks after treatment with rosiglitazone, demonstrated nearly a 40% increase in insulin-stimulated myocardial glucose uptake, implying reduced fatty acid uptake, which was attributed in large part to suppression of plasma fatty acid levels [89]. Of note, similar metabolic changes were not seen with the biguanide, metformin, whose mechanism of action is designed to reduce hepatic glucose production. The metabolic response could not be predicted by changes in the plasma glucose or HgBA1C levels. Thus, metabolic imaging can be used to follow the effects of therapies designed to alter myocardial substrate metabolism in patients with diseases such as diabetes mellitus where more readily available clinical parameters are not predictive of a therapeutic response.

Obesity and Insulin Resistance

It is now apparent that a significant increase in body mass index induces marked increases in myocardial fatty acid metabolism. For example, in either dietary-induced or transgenic models of obesity, myocardial fatty acid uptake and oxidation are significantly increased [88,90]. This increase (at least initially), reflects the increase in fatty acid delivery to the heart due to increased lipolysis from both visceral/abdominal and subcutaneous fat stores secondary to insulin resistance. Similar to diabetes mellitus, the increased delivery of fatty acids likely initiates a cascade of events that lead to increased fatty acid metabolism. Ultimately, fatty acid uptake may exceed oxidation leading to extracted fatty acids entering nonoxidative pathways most likely initially forming triglycerides. The accumulation of

the neutral fats or triglycerides may have detrimental consequences [88].

Imaging obese young women with ^{11}C-acetate and ^{11}C-palmitate, PET has shown that an increase in body mass index is associated with a shift in myocardial substrate metabolism toward greater fatty acid utilization. Moreover, this dependence on myocardial fatty acid metabolism increased with worsening insulin resistance [39]. Of note, little change in myocardial glucose metabolism was observed. Paralleling the preferential use of fatty acids was an increase in MVO_2 and a decrease in energy transduction. These findings suggest that metabolic changes in obesity may play a role in the pathogenesis of cardiac dysfunction. Moreover, the myocardial metabolic response to obesity appears to be gender-dependent [56]. Obese men had a greater impairment in myocardial glucose metabolism per level plasma insulin, suggesting greater myocardial insulin resistance, when compared to obese women. In addition, obesity had less effect on myocardial fatty acid metabolism in men. In contrast, MVO_2 was higher in obese women compared with obese men. Thus, there appears to be a complex interplay between gender and obesity in influencing myocardial substrate metabolism.

Myocardial Viability

The principle of using a metabolic tracer for assessing myocardial viability is based on the concept that viable tissue is metabolically active (Figure 5.5), while scarred or fibrotic tissue is metabolically inactive. The clinical objective of myocardial viability assessment is to prospectively identify patients with coronary artery disease and reversible left ventricular dysfunction in whom regional and global left ventricular function as well as prognosis may be favorably altered with revascularization. FDG may be preserved or increased in hypoperfused but viable myocardium (termed *metabolism/perfusion mismatch*) and decreased or absent in hypoperfused and scarred myocardium (termed *metabolism/perfusion match*). The overall accuracy of FDG mismatch pattern for predicting recovery of function after revascularization is in the range of 80–90% [91]. Furthermore, the extent of the PET "mismatch" pattern correlates with improvement in left ventricle function after revascularization

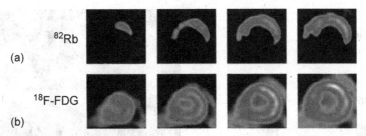

Figure 5.5 PET scan showing perfusion/metabolism mismatch in hibernating myocardium as an example of viable, preserved cardiometabolic reserve. (a) Rubidium-82-labeled PET in short-axis view shows markedly decreased perfusion defects in the apical, inferior, inferolateral, and septal regions of the left ventricle at rest, which extends from distal to basal slices. (b) Images acquired under glucose-loaded conditions, labeled with 18F-fluorodeoxyglucose, show perfusion/metabolism mismatch pattern (the scintigraphic hallmark of hibernation) in all abnormally perfused myocardial regions at rest. An exception is the anteroseptal region, which demonstrates matched perfusion–metabolism pattern (compatible with scarred myocardium). (Adapted from Taegtmeyer and Dilsizian [12].)

(Figure 5.6), as well as with the clinical course, magnitude of improvement in heart failure symptoms (Figure 5.7), and survival after revascularization (Figure 5.8) [91–95]. Patients with heart failure and extensive PET "match" pattern (diminished blood flow and severe reduction in FDG uptake), representing predominant infarction, are unlikely to benefit clinically from revascularization.

The prognostic significance of perfusion/metabolism mismatch pattern has been demonstrated in several nonrandomized, retrospective studies with PET. Patients with perfusion/metabolism mismatch pattern who were treated with revascularization had lower ischemic events and deaths when compared to those treated medically (Figure 5.8). Patients with matched defects (concordant reduction in regional perfusion and metabolism), indicating scarred myocardium displayed no such difference in outcomes between medical and surgical management.

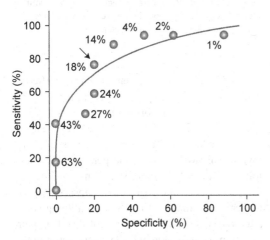

Figure 5.6 Receiver-operating characteristic curve for different anatomic extent of perfusion/metabolism PET mismatch to predict a change (at least one grade) in functional status after revascularization. When the extent of PET mismatch involves 18% or more of the left ventricular mass, the sensitivity for predicting a change in functional status after revascularization is 76% and the specificity is 78% (area under the fitted curve = 0.82). (Adapted from DiCarli et al. [95].)

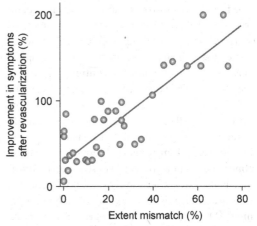

Figure 5.7 The relation between the anatomic extent of perfusion/metabolism PET mismatch pattern (expressed as percentage of the left ventricle) and the change in functional status after revascularization (expressed as percentage of improvement from baseline). The scatterplot shows that the greatest improvement in heart failure symptoms occurs in patients with the largest mismatch defects on quantitative analysis of PET images. (Adapted from DiCarli et al. [95].)

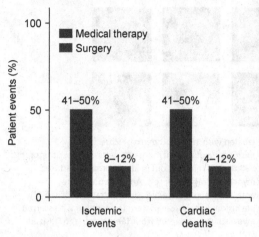

Figure 5.8 The prognostic significance of perfusion/metabolism mismatch pattern in ischemic cardiomyopathy. Patients with perfusion/metabolism mismatch pattern who were treated surgically had lower ischemic event rates and fewer deaths when compared with those treated with medical therapy. In contrast, patients with perfusion/metabolism match pattern displayed no such difference in outcomes between surgical and medical management. (Adapted from Eitzman et al. [92], Di Carli et al. [93], and Lee et al. [94].)

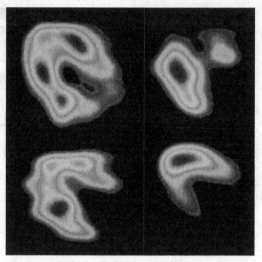

Figure 5.9 Metabolic alterations in postischemic myocardium in a patient with angina. Transaxial rubidium-82 PET images reflecting myocardial blood flow at rest, during exercise, and after exercise are shown along with FDG images after exercise. At rest (top left), the distribution of myocardial blood flow is homogeneous in all myocardial regions. During exercise (top right), there are extensive blood flow abnormalities in the apical and anteroseptal regions that improve on the postexercise images (bottom left) and are comparable to the rubidium-82 rest image (top left). FDG was injected 8 minutes after the termination of exercise. The FDG image recorded 60 minutes after tracer injection (bottom right) shows metabolic alterations in the previously ischemic regions. (Adapted from Camici et al. [98].)

Myocardial Ischemia

Beyond metabolic alterations for differentiating viable from scarred myocardium, with the induction of myocardial ischemia, fatty acid oxidation ceases and anaerobic metabolism supervenes. Glucose becomes the primary substrate for both increased anaerobic glycolysis and for continued oxidative metabolism, albeit diminished [96]. This metabolic switch is a prerequisite for continued energy production and cell survival. When the ischemic insult is reversed, oxygen availability increases and oxidative metabolism resumes. It appears that these abnormalities in myocardial substrate metabolism may persist well after the resolution of ischemia, so-called "ischemic memory" or "metabolic stunning" [11,12]. Demonstration of either accelerated myocardial glucose metabolism or reduced fatty acid metabolism using FDG and BMIPP, respectively, has been used to document this phenomena [13–16].

Nearly two decades ago, it was reported that FDG PET myocardial uptake was increased in patients with unstable angina during pain-free episodes [97] Moreover, in patients with stable angina, increased regional FDG uptake was shown following exercise-induced ischemia in the absence of either perfusion deficits or ECG abnormalities (Figure 5.9) [98]. These earlier observations with PET were recently reproduced with SPECT using BMIPP (Figure 5.10). In patients with acute coronary syndrome, myocardial BMIPP defects may persist 24–36 hours following the resolution of symptoms [99]. Moreover, this "metabolic fingerprint" appears superior to perfusion imaging for either identifying coronary artery disease as the cause of the chest pain or assigning prognosis [99]. This persistence in the metabolic defect is a significant advantage. It increases the flexibility of radiotracer administration for it and allows for delivery of a unit dose after the patient has already been evaluated. This is in contrast to the use of perfusion radiotracers which frequently must be available on-site due to the narrow time window from the resolution of symptoms and normalization of the flow deficit. Based on

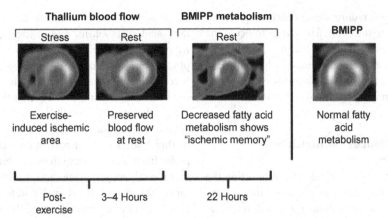

Figure 5.10 Single-photon emission computed tomography showing delayed recovery of regional fatty acid metabolism after transient exercise-induced ischemia, termed ischemic memory. Representative stress (left) and rest reinjection (middle) short-axis thallium tomograms demonstrate a reversible inferior defect consistent with exercise-induced myocardial ischemia. A BMIPP-labeled SPECT image (center) injected and acquired at rest 22 hours after exercise-induced ischemia shows persistent metabolic abnormality in the inferior region despite complete recovery of regional perfusion at rest, as evidenced by thallium reinjection image. The tomogram on the far right shows retention of BMIPP in the heart of a normal adult for comparison. BMIPP, β-methylp-[^{123}I]-iodophenyl-pentadecanoic acid. (Adapted from Taegtmeyer and Dilsizian [12].)

these observations, BMIPP was evaluated in a recent multicenter clinical trial, in which the combination of BMIPP SPECT with initial clinical information resulted in improved sensitivity and negative predictive value for identifying patients with acute coronary syndrome compared to the sensitivity and negative predictive value of the initial clinical diagnosis alone, while maintaining specificity [100].

Metabolic imaging with FDG and BMIPP is also used to detect myocardial ischemia during and/or following transient exercise testing on a treadmill [11]. Results of initial studies where FDG were injected during exercise showed greater sensitivity for detecting moderate-to-severe coronary artery narrowing compared with Tc-99m-labeled perfusion imaging (Figure 5.11) [13]. Despite the promising

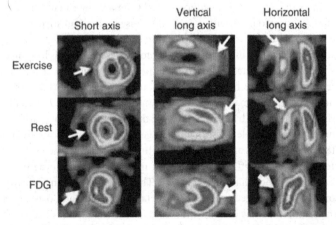

Figure 5.11 Simultaneous myocardial perfusion and metabolism imaging after dual intravenous injection of Tc-99m sestamibi and FDG at peak exercise. Dual isotope simultaneous acquisition was carried out 40–60 minutes after the exercise study was completed. Rest Tc-99m sestamibi imaging was carried out separately. In this patient with angina and no prior myocardial infarction, there is evidence for extensive reversible perfusion defect in the anterior, septal, and apical regions. The coronary angiogram showed 90% stenosis of the left anterior descending and 60% stenosis of the left circumflex coronary arteries. The corresponding FDG image shows intense uptake in the regions with reversible sestamibi defects reflecting the metabolic correlate of exercise-induced myocardial ischemia. (Adapted from He et al. [14].)

results with these radiotracers, numerous questions still remain as to the optimal imaging protocols, the impact of alterations in the plasma substrate environment on diagnostic accuracy, whether added diagnostic and prognostic information is provided over perfusion imaging, and whether this information alters clinical management.

Hypertension/Left Ventricular Hypertrophy

There are several lines of evidence supporting the close relationship between abnormalities in myocardial substrate metabolism and left ventricular hypertrophy. In animal models of pressure-overload left ventricular hypertrophy, reduction in the expression of β-oxidation enzymes, leading to a fall in myocardial fatty acid oxidation and an increase in glucose use has been shown [101,102]. Moreover, interventions in animals that involve inhibition of mitochondrial fatty acid β-oxidation result in cardiac hypertrophy [102]. In humans, variants in genes regulating key aspects of myocardial fatty acid metabolism ranging from PPARα to various key β-oxidative enzymes are associated with left ventricular hypertrophy [103,104].

In a rat model, myocardial FDG uptake with PET increased proportionately with the extent of left ventricular hypertrophy, confirming this shift in substrate preference in vivo [105]. Similar results have been obtained in man. In humans, reduction in myocardial fatty acid oxidation with ^{11}C-palmitate PET was shown to be an independent predictor of left ventricular mass in hypertension [106]. Combining measurements of left ventricular myocardial external work (either by echocardiography or magnetic resonance imaging) with measurements of MVO$_2$ performed by PET with ^{11}C-acetate or ^{15}O-oxygen, it is possible to estimate cardiac efficiency [18,107]. Using this approach, in patients with hypertension-induced left ventricular hypertrophy, the decline in myocardial fatty acid metabolism was shown to be associated with a decline in efficiency, a condition that may increase the potential for developing heart failure.

Another potential application of PET is in phenotyping patients with genetic variants related to myocyte growth. For example, in patients with hypertrophic cardiomyopathy attributable to a known specific variant in the α-tropomyosin gene, it was observed that increased myocardial perfusion, fatty acid metabolism, and efficiency, characterize patients with mild hypertrophy whereas these physiological parameters decrease as hypertrophy becomes more advanced [108]. The results may represent differential penetration of the gene variant or the effect of modifier gene(s), potentially helping in their identification. Although requiring further studies in larger patient populations, these preliminary data suggest that metabolic imaging may identify relevant gene variants without waiting for more end-stage functional manifestations such as left ventricular remodeling and dysfunction.

Dilated, Nonischemic Cardiomyopathy

As with left ventricular hypertrophy, alterations in myocardial substrate metabolism have been implicated in the pathogenesis of contractile dysfunction and heart failure. Animal models of heart failure have shown that during the progression from cardiac hypertrophy to ventricular dysfunction, the expression of genes encoding for enzymes regulating β-oxidation is coordinately decreased, resulting in a shift in myocardial substrate metabolism to primarily glucose use, similar to that seen in the fetal heart [101,109,110]. These metabolic changes are paralleled by re-expression of fetal isoforms of a variety of contractile and calcium regulatory proteins program. The reactivation of the metabolic fetal gene program may have numerous detrimental consequences on myocardial contractile function ranging from energy deprivation to the inability to process fatty acids leading to accumulation of nonoxidized toxic fatty acid derivatives, resulting in lipotoxicity. The importance of this metabolic shift in the pathogenesis of heart failure is underscored by the development of novel therapeutics, which target specific aspects of cellular metabolism, such as the partial fatty acid oxidation antagonists and the insulin sensitizer glucagon-like peptide-1 [111].

The downregulation in myocardial fatty acid metabolism leading to overdependence on glucose use in heart failure has been well documented using both SPECT and PET techniques. For example, SPECT with BMIPP demonstrated reduced myocardial uptake and increased clearance radiotracer in patients with dilated cardiomyopathy compared with controls [112]. Moreover, the magnitude of the perturbations correlated with other measurements of heart failure severity such as left ventricular size and plasma β-natruietic peptide levels. PET using ^{11}C-palmitate and ^{11}C-glucose demonstrated that myocardial fatty acid uptake and oxidation are lower in patients with dilated, nonischemic cardiomyopathy when compared with aged matched control normal subjects. In contrast, myocardial glucose utilization was higher in the cardiomyopathic patients [37]. Similarly, PET has provided mechanistic insights into the myocardial metabolic perturbations associated with heart failure. For example, abrupt lowering of fatty acid delivery with acipimox results in reduced fatty acid uptake, MVO_2, and cardiac work and no change cardiac efficiency in normal volunteers [113]. In contrast, in patients with nonischemic dilated cardiomyopathy, myocardial fatty acid uptake and cardiac work is decreased, with no change in MVO_2 and a decline in efficiency. Although limited by small sample size, these results appear to reinforce the central role of loss of flexibility in myocardial substrate metabolism in the pathogenesis of heart failure with even minor changes in substrate delivery having detrimental consequences on cardiac energy transduction.

Metabolic imaging can also been used to study the mechanisms responsible for the effectiveness of treatment in cardiomyopathy. For example, the efficacy of β-blocker therapy in the treatment of heart failure patients is well established. In patients with ischemic cardiomyopathy, improvement in global left ventricular function during metoprolol therapy may be attributed, in part, to redistribution in absolute myocardial blood flow resulting in increases in regional left ventricular function [114]. However, it appears that other mechanisms of action are key to the improvement in left ventricular function seen in nonischemic cardiomyopathy patients.

Treatment with the selective β-blocker metoprolol results in a reduction in oxidative metabolism and an improvement in cardiac efficiency as measured by PET in patients with heart failure [115]. Cardiac efficiency has been shown to improve following either exercise training or cardiac resynchronization therapy, implicating improved myocardial energy transduction as a potential mechanism [116,117]. Moreover, normalization of the distribution of myocardial glucose metabolism may be partially responsible for the improved energetic following cardiac resynchronization therapy [118].

Partial fatty acid oxidation inhibitors have been proposed for the treatment of heart failure based on the theory that decreasing myocardial fatty acid oxidation should increase the oxidation of glucose leading to a more favorable energetic state and improved left ventricular function. This is because much less oxygen is required to oxidize a glucose compared with fatty acids. In support of this contention is the finding that the administration of trimetizidine to patients with dilated cardiomyopathy results in a significant improvement in left ventricular ejection fraction [119]. However, the improvement in left ventricular function is paralleled by only a mild decrease in myocardial fatty acid oxidation. It appears that with trimetizidine, the improvement in left ventricular function reflects the complex interplay between a mild decrease in myocardial fatty acid oxidation, improved whole-body insulin resistance and synergistic effects with β-blockade. Metabolic imaging can also be used to predict the response to specific therapies in heart failure patients. For example, in patients with dilated cardiomyopathy, it appears that the fraction of myocardial glucose uptake, as measured with FDG PET, predicts the effectiveness of β-blocker therapy [120]. Moreover, in patients with ischemic cardiomyopathy, the extent of viable myocardium as measured with FDG correlated with the hemodynamic response after cardiac resynchronization therapy, suggesting a role for PET in discriminating responders from nonresponders to this therapy [121].

Chronic Kidney Disease

While myocardial infarction and ischemic heart disease account for the significant portion of patients with heart failure and left ventricular remodeling, several sequelae of renal failure which accrue with loss of renal function, can also contribute to left ventricular remodeling, termed uremic cardiomyopathy (Figure 5.12). The United States Renal Data System has reported near-equivalent rates of myocardial infarction and cardiac death in dialysis patients and an approximately 10-fold higher rate of heart failure in the same population [122]. The common occurrence of heart failure in the dialysis population is thought to be related to left

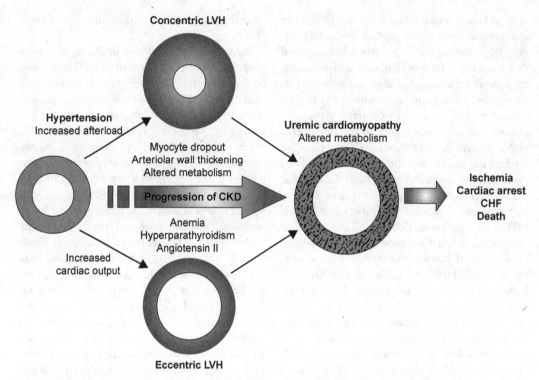

Figure 5.12 Concurrent pathogenic factors contributing to the development of left ventricular remodeling in uremic cardiomyopathy and altered metabolism with declining renal function. (Adapted from Dilsizian and Fink [126].)

ventricular hypertrophy that occurs frequently in patients with chronic kidney disease. Although hypertension is common among patients with kidney disease, several investigators have suggested that elevated blood pressure becomes increasingly volume-dependent with a concomitant increase in arterial stiffening, activation of neurohormones, and endothelial dysfunction as renal function declines. Individuals with chronic kidney disease, therefore, are faced with both pressure- and volume-overload states contributing to the development of left ventricular remodeling and heart failure. The cardiomyopathy typical of chronic kidney disease and the associated uremia is thought to lead to a myocyte/capillary mismatch, with a diminished vascular supply relative to the number and volume of functioning myocytes [123]. The oxygen-poor milieu will lead to diffuse myocardial ischemia with an anticipated decline in aerobic myocardial fatty acid utilization and a shift to anaerobic metabolism, with increased uptake of glucose as the principal energy providing substrate [124,125]. The shift from

a predominance of aerobic (fatty acid) to anaerobic (glucose) metabolism appears to account for a significant portion of the excessive cardiovascular morbidity and mortality observed across all stages of kidney disease [126].

In a prospective study of 130 asymptomatic end-stage renal disease patients undergoing hemodialysis (Figure 5.13), the prevalence of coronary artery disease was assessed by performing dual isotope thallium and BMIPP SPECT at rest followed by coronary angiography [127]. Significant coronary artery luminal narrowing ($\geq 75\%$) was present in 71.5% (93 of 130) of end-stage renal disease patients with additional 5 patients exhibiting coronary vasospasm. When reduced myocardial metabolism with BMIPP (summed score of 6 or more) was used to define an abnormal scan, the sensitivity, specificity, and accuracy for detecting coronary artery disease with rest BMIPP SPECT was 98, 66, and 90%, respectively [127]. In a subsequent publication by the same investigators, the prognostic significance of reduced myocardial metabolism with

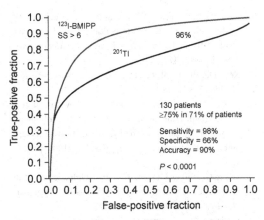

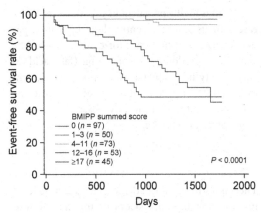

Figure 5.13 Accuracy for BMIPP for detecting CAD in asymptomatic end-stage renal disease patients on hemodialysis. Significant coronary artery luminal narrowing (≥75%) was present in 71.5% (93 of 130) of end-stage renal disease patients with additional 5 patients exhibiting coronary vasospasm. When reduced myocardial metabolism with BMIPP (summed score of 6 or more) was used to define an abnormal scan, the sensitivity, specificity, and accuracy for detecting coronary artery disease with rest BMIPP SPECT was 98, 66, and 90%, respectively [43]. BMIPP, β-methylp-[^{123}I]-iodophenyl-pentadecanoic acid. (Adapted from Nishimura et al. [127].)

Figure 5.14 Relationship between survival rates and severity of BMIPP fatty acid metabolic uptake in patients with end-stage renal disease. Kaplan–Meier survival estimates showed 61% event-free survival at 3 years among patients with summed BMIPP score of 12 or more and 98% in patients with a summed BMIPP score of below 12, with graded relationship between survival and severity of summed BMIPP score. BMIPP, β-methylp-[^{123}I]-iodophenyl-pentadecanoic acid. (Adapted from Nishimura et al. [124].)

BMIPP in conjunction with perfusion abnormalities assessed with thallium in end-stage renal disease patients was examined [124]. Among 318 prospectively enrolled asymptomatic hemodialysis patients without prior myocardial infarction, 50 (16%) died of cardiac events during a mean follow-up period of 3.6 ± 1.0 years. Kaplan–Meier survival estimates showed 61% event-free survival at 3 years among patients with summed BMIPP score of 12 or more and 98% in patients with a summed BMIPP score of below 12, with graded relationship between survival and severity of summed BMIPP score (Figure 5.14). When BMIPP uptake (metabolism) was assessed in relation to regional thallium uptake (perfusion), indicating myocardial ischemia, the sensitivity and specificity of metabolism/perfusion mismatch for predicting cardiac death was 86 and 88%, respectively. Kaplan–Meier survival estimates showed 53% event-free survival at 3 years among patients with BMIPP/thallium mismatch score of 7 or more and 96% in patients with a BMIPP/thallium mismatch score of below 7 (Figure 5.15). These findings support the assertion that altered cardiac metabolism (indicating silent myocardial

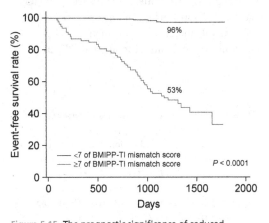

Figure 5.15 The prognostic significance of reduced myocardial metabolism with BMIPP in conjunction with perfusion abnormalities assessed with thallium in patients with end-stage renal disease. BMIPP uptake (metabolism) was assessed in relation to regional thallium uptake (perfusion), indicating myocardial ischemia. The sensitivity and specificity of metabolism/perfusion mismatch for predicting cardiac death was 86 and 88%, respectively. Kaplan–Meier survival estimates showed 53% event-free survival at 3 years among patients with BMIPP/thallium mismatch score of 7 or more and 96% in patients with a BMIPP/thallium mismatch score of below 7. BMIPP, β-methylp-[^{123}I]-iodophenyl-pentadecanoic acid. (Adapted from Nishimura et al. [124].)

ischemia) is highly prevalent in end-stage renal disease patients and can identify the subgroup of patients who are at high-risk for cardiac death. The shift from a predominance of aerobic (fatty acid) to anaerobic (glucose) metabolism appears to account for a significant portion of the excessive cardiovascular morbidity and mortality observed across all stages of kidney disease.

Conclusions

There is a strong clinical demand for accurate non-invasive imaging approaches of myocardial substrate metabolism that provide linkage between the bench and the bedside leading to improved patient management paradigms. The continued growth of metabolic imaging in clinical practice will require the development of new radiotracers in concert with further advances in PET detector design and postdetector electronics. Radiotracers that allow characterization of key metabolic pathways such as uptake, storage, or oxidation that are linked to disease manifestations or provide insights into the pleiotropic aspects of metabolism such as the linkage between substrate metabolism and cell growth, cell survival, and energy transduction will provide additional opportunities for targeted therapy.

References

1. Bing RJ. The metabolism of the heart. *Harvey Lect.* 1955; 50:27–70.
2. Neely JR, Morgan HE. Relationship between carbohydrate and lipid metabolism and the energy balance of heart muscle. *Ann Rev Physiol.* 1974;36:413–459.
3. Goodwin GW, Taegtmeyer H. Regulation of fatty acid oxidation of the heart by MCD and ACC during contractile stimulation. *Am J Physiol.* 1999;277(4, Pt 1): E772–E777.
4. McGarry JD, Brown NF. The mitochondrial carnitine palmitoyltransferase system. From concept to molecular analysis. *Eur J Biochem.* 1997;244(1):1–14.
5. McGarry JD, Mannaerts GP, Foster DW. A possible role for malonyl-CoA in the regulation of hepatic fatty acid oxidation and ketogenesis. *J Clin Invest.* 1977;60(1): 265–270.
6. Sugden MC, Holness MJ. Recent advances in mechanisms regulating glucose oxidation at the level of the pyruvate dehydrogenase complex by PDKs. *Am J Physiol Endocrinol Metab.* 2003;284(5):E855–E862.
7. Young ME, Goodwin GW, Ying J, *et al.* Regulation of cardiac and skeletal muscle malonyl-CoA decarboxylase by fatty acids. *Am J Physiol Endocrinol Metab.* 2001; 280(3):E471–E479.
8. Kelly DP. PPARs of the heart: three is a crowd. *Circ Res.* 2003;92(5):482–484.
9. Finck BN, Han X, Courtois M, *et al.* A critical role for PPARalpha-mediated lipotoxicity in the pathogenesis of diabetic cardiomyopathy: modulation by dietary fat content. *Proc Natl Acad Sci USA.* 2003;100(3):1226–1231.
10. Depre C, Shipley GL, Chen W, *et al.* Unloaded heart in vivo replicates fetal gene expression of cardiac hypertrophy. *Nat Med.* 1998;4(11):1269–1275.
11. Dilsizian V, Bateman TM, Bergmann SR, *et al.* Metabolic imaging with β-methyl-ρ-[^{123}I]-iodophenyl-pentadecanoic acid (BMIPP) identifies ischemic memory following demand ischemia. *Circulation.* 2005; 112(14):2169–2174.
12. Taegtmeyer H, Dilsizian V. Imaging myocardial metabolism and ischemic memory. *Nat Clin Pract Card.* 2008;5:S42–S48.
13. Dilsizian V. Metabolic imaging of the heart: beyond perfusion and anatomy. *J Nucl Cardiol.* 2007;14:S97–S99.
14. He ZX, Shi RF, Wu YJ, *et al.* Direct imaging of exercise-induced myocardial ischemia with fluorine-18-labeled deoxyglucose and Tc-99m-sestamibi in coronary artery disease. *Circulation.* 2003;108(10):1208–1213.
15. Dou KF, Yang MF, Yang YJ, Jain D, He ZX. Myocardial 18F-FDG uptake after exercise-induced myocardial ischemia in patients with coronary artery disease. *J Nucl Med.* 2008;49:1986–1991.
16. Dilsizian V. FDG uptake as a surrogate marker for antecedent ischemia. *J Nucl Med.* 2008;49(12):1909–1911.
17. Iida H, Rhodes CG, Araujo LI, *et al.* Noninvasive quantification of regional myocardial metabolic rate for oxygen by use of $15O_2$ inhalation and positron emission tomography. Theory, error analysis, and application in humans. *Circulation.* 1996;94(4):792–807.
18. Laine H, Katoh C, Luotolahti M, *et al.* Myocardial oxygen consumption is unchanged but efficiency is reduced in patients with essential hypertension and left ventricular hypertrophy. *Circulation.* 1999;100(24):2425–2430.
19. Yamamoto Y, de Silva R, Rhodes CG, *et al.* Noninvasive quantification of regional myocardial metabolic rate of oxygen by $15O_2$ inhalation and positron emission tomography. Experimental validation. *Circulation.* 1996; 94(4):808–816.
20. Armbrecht JJ, Buxton DB, Schelbert HR. Validation of [1-11C]acetate as a tracer for noninvasive assessment

of oxidative metabolism with positron emission tomography in normal, ischemic, postischemic, and hyperemic canine myocardium. *Circulation.* 1990;81(5): 1594–1605.

21. Brown M, Marshall DR, Sobel BE, Bergmann SR. Delineation of myocardial oxygen utilization with carbon-11-labeled acetate. *Circulation.* 1987;76(3):687–696.

22. Brown MA, Myears DW, Bergmann SR. Noninvasive assessment of canine myocardial oxidative metabolism with carbon-11 acetate and positron emission tomography. *J Am Coll Cardiol.* 1988;12(4):1054–1063.

23. Buck A, Wolpers HG, Hutchins GD, et al. Effect of carbon-11-acetate recirculation on estimates of myocardial oxygen consumption by PET. *J Nucl Med.* 1991; 32(10):1950–1957.

24. Sun KT, Yeatman LA, Buxton DB, et al. Simultaneous measurement of myocardial oxygen consumption and blood flow using [1-carbon-11]acetate. *J Nucl Med.* 1998;39(2):272–280.

25. Choi Y, Hawkins RA, Huang SC, et al. Parametric images of myocardial metabolic rate of glucose generated from dynamic cardiac PET and 2-[18F]fluoro-2-deoxy-d-glucose studies. *J Nucl Med.* 1991;32(4):733–738.

26. Gambert S, Vergely C, Filomenko R, et al. Adverse effects of free fatty acid associated with increased oxidative stress in postischemic isolated rat hearts. *Mol Cell Biochem.* 2006;283(1–2):147–152.

27. Iozzo P, Chareonthaitawee P, Di Terlizzi M, Betteridge DJ, Ferrannini E, Camici PG. Regional myocardial blood flow and glucose utilization during fasting and physiological hyperinsulinemia in humans. *Am J Physiol Endocrinol Metab.* 2002;282(5):E1163–E1171.

28. Krivokapich J, Huang SC, Selin CE, Phelps ME. Fluorodeoxyglucose rate constants, lumped constant, and glucose metabolic rate in rabbit heart. *Am J Physiol.* 1987;252(4, Pt 2):H777–H787.

29. Botker HE, Bottcher M, Schmitz O, et al. Glucose uptake and lumped constant variability in normal human hearts determined with [18F]fluorodeoxyglucose. *J Nucl Cardiol.* 1997;4(2, Pt 1):125–132.

30. Hariharan R, Bray M, Ganim R, Doenst T, Goodwin GW, Taegtmeyer H. Fundamental limitations of [18F]2-deoxy-2-fluoro-D-glucose for assessing myocardial glucose uptake. *Circulation.* 1995;91(9):2435–2444.

31. Hashimoto K, Nishimura T, Imahashi KI, Yamaguchi H, Hori M, Kusuoka H. Lumped constant for deoxyglucose is decreased when myocardial glucose uptake is enhanced. *Am J Physiol.* 1999;276(1, Pt 2):H129–H133.

32. Herrero P, Sharp TL, Dence C, Haraden BM, Gropler RJ. Comparison of 1-(11)C-glucose and (18)F-FDG for quantifying myocardial glucose use with PET. *J Nucl Med.* 2002;43(11):1530–1541.

33. Herrero P, Weinheimer CJ, Dence C, Oellerich WF, Gropler RJ. Quantification of myocardial glucose utilization by PET and 1-carbon-11-glucose. *J Nucl Cardiol.* 2002; 9(1):5–14.

34. Herrero P, Kisrieva-Ware Z, Dence CS, et al. PET measurements of myocardial glucose metabolism with 1-11C-glucose and kinetic modeling. *J Nucl Med.* 2007;48(6):955–964.

35. Herrero P, Dence CS, Coggan AR, Kisrieva-Ware Z, Eisenbeis P, Gropler RJ. L-3-11C-lactate as a PET tracer of myocardial lactate metabolism: a feasibility study. *J Nucl Med.* 2007;48(12):2046–2055.

36. Bergmann SR, Weinheimer CJ, Markham J, Herrero P. Quantitation of myocardial fatty acid metabolism using PET. *J Nucl Med.* 1996;37(10):1723–1730.

37. Davila-Roman VG, Vedala G, Herrero P, et al. Altered myocardial fatty acid and glucose metabolism in idiopathic dilated cardiomyopathy. *J Am Coll Cardiol.* 2002; 40(2):271–277.

38. Herrero P, Peterson LR, McGill JB, et al. Increased myocardial fatty acid metabolism in patients with type 1 diabetes mellitus. *J Am Coll Cardiol.* 2006;47(3):598–604.

39. Peterson LR, Herrero P, Schechtman KB, et al. Effect of obesity and insulin resistance on myocardial substrate metabolism and efficiency in young women. *Circulation.* 2004;109(18):2191–2196.

40. DeGrado TR. Synthesis of 14(R,S)-[18F]fluoro-6-thia-heptadecanoic acid (FTHA). *J Label Comp Radiopharm.* 1991;29:989–995.

41. DeGrado TR, Coenen HH, Stocklin G. 14(R,S)-[18F]fluoro-6-thia-heptadecanoic acid (FTHA): evaluation in mouse of a new probe of myocardial utilization of long chain fatty acids. *J Nucl Med.* 1991;32(10): 1888–1896.

42. Schulz G, von Dahl J, Kaiser HJ, et al. Imaging of beta-oxidation by static PET with 14(R,S)-[18F]-fluoro-6-thiaheptadecanoic acid (FTHA) in patients with advanced coronary heart disease: a comparison with 18FDG-PET and 99Tcm-MIBI SPET. *Nucl Med Commun.* 1996;17(12):1057–1064.

43. Taylor M, Wallhaus TR, Degrado TR, et al. An evaluation of myocardial fatty acid and glucose uptake using PET with [18F]fluoro-6-thia-heptadecanoic acid and [18F]FDG in Patients with Congestive Heart Failure. *J Nucl Med.* 2001;42(1):55–62.

44. DeGrado TR, Wang S, Holden JE, Nickles RJ, Taylor M, Stone CK. Synthesis and preliminary evaluation of (18)F-labeled 4-thia palmitate as a PET tracer of myocardial fatty acid oxidation. *Nucl Med Biol.* 2000;27(3): 221–231.

45. DeGrado TR, Kitapci MT, Wang S, Ying J, Lopaschuk GD. Validation of 18F-fluoro-4-thia-palmitate as a PET

probe for myocardial fatty acid oxidation: effects of hypoxia and composition of exogenous fatty acids. *J Nucl Med.* 2006;47(1):173–181.

46. Shoup TM, Elmaleh DR, Bonab AA, Fischman AJ. Evaluation of trans-9-18F-fluoro-3,4-Methyleneheptadecanoic acid as a PET tracer for myocardial fatty acid imaging. *J Nucl Med.* 2005;46(2):297–304.

47. DeGrado TR, Holden JE, Ng CK, Raffel DM, Gatley SJ. Quantitative analysis of myocardial kinetics of 15-p-[iodine-125] iodophenylpentadecanoic acid. *J Nucl Med.* 1989;30(7):1211–1218.

48. Dormehl IC, Hugo N, Rossouw D, White A, Feinendegen LE. Planar myocardial imaging in the baboon model with iodine-123-15-(iodophenyl)pentadecanoic acid (IPPA) and iodine-123-15-(P-iodophenyl)-3-R,S-methylpentadecanoic acid (BMIPP), using time-activity curves for evaluation of metabolism. *Nucl Med Biol.* 1995;22(7):837–847.

49. Eckelman WC, Babich JW. Synthesis and validation of fatty acid analogs radiolabeled by nonisotopic substitution. *J Nucl Cardiol.* 2007;14(Suppl. 3):S100–S109.

50. Reske SN, Sauer W, Machulla HJ, Knust J, Winkler C. Metabolism of 15 (p 123I iodophenyl-)pentadecanoic acid in heart muscle and noncardiac tissues. *Eur J Nucl Med.* 1985;10(5–6):228–234.

51. Ambrose KR, Owen BA, Goodman MM, Knapp FF, Jr. Evaluation of the metabolism in rat hearts of two new radioiodinated 3-methyl-branched fatty acid myocardial imaging agents. *Eur J Nucl Med.* 1987;12(10):486–491.

52. Goodman MM, Kirsch G, Knapp FF, Jr. Synthesis and evaluation of radioiodinated terminal p-iodophenyl-substituted alpha- and beta-methyl-branched fatty acids. *J Med Chem.* 1984;27(3):390–397.

53. Desrois M, Sidell RJ, Gauguier D, Davey CL, Radda GK, Clarke K. Gender differences in hypertrophy, insulin resistance and ischemic injury in the aging type 2 diabetic rat heart. *J Mol Cell Cardiol.* 2004;37(2):547–555.

54. Dyck JR, Lopaschuk GD. Glucose metabolism, H+ production and Na+/H+-exchanger mRNA levels in ischemic hearts from diabetic rats. *Mol Cell Biochem.* 1998; 180(1–2):85–93.

55. Peterson LR, Soto PF, Herrero P, Schechtman KB, Dence C, Gropler RJ. Sex differences in myocardial oxygen and glucose metabolism. *J Nucl Cardiol.* 2007;14(4):573–581.

56. Peterson LR, Soto PM, Herrero P, *et al.* Impact of gender on the myocardial metabolic response to Obesity. *J Am Coll Cardiol Imaging.* 2008;1:424–433.

57. Hatta H, Atomi Y, Shinohara S, Yamamoto Y, Yamada S. The effects of ovarian hormones on glucose and fatty acid oxidation during exercise in female ovariectomized rats. *Horm Metab Res.* 1988;20(10):609–611.

58. Campbell SE, Febbraio MA. Effect of ovarian hormones on mitochondrial enzyme activity in the fat oxidation pathway of skeletal muscle. *Am J Physiol Endocrinol Metab.* 2001;281(4):E803–E808.

59. Matute ML, Kalkhoff RK. Sex steroid influence on hepatic gluconeogenesis and glucogen formation. *Endocrinology.* 1973;92(3):762–768.

60. Kendrick ZV, Ellis GS. Effect of estradiol on tissue glycogen metabolism and lipid availability in exercised male rats. *J Appl Physiol.* 1991;71(5):1694–1699.

61. Lei B, Matsuo K, Labinskyy V, *et al.* Exogenous nitric oxide reduces glucose transporters translocation and lactate production in ischemic myocardium in vivo. *Proc Natl Acad Sci USA.* 2005;102(19):6966–6971.

62. Weiner CP, Lizasoain I, Baylis SA, Knowles RG, Charles IG, Moncada S. Induction of calcium-dependent nitric oxide synthases by sex hormones. *Proc Natl Acad Sci USA.* 1994;91(11):5212–5216.

63. Recchia FA, McConnell PI, Loke KE, Xu X, Ochoa M, Hintze TH. Nitric oxide controls cardiac substrate utilization in the conscious dog. *Cardiovasc Res.* 1999;44(2):325–332.

64. Herrero P, Soto PF, Dence CS, Kisrieva-Ware Z, Delano DA, Peterson LR, *et al.* Impact of hormone replacement on myocardial fatty acid metabolism: potential role of estrogen. *J Nucl Cardiol.* 2005;12(5):574–581.

65. Abu-Erreish GM, Neely JR, Whitmer JT, Whitman V, Sanadi DR. Fatty acid oxidation by isolated perfused working hearts of aged rats. *Am J Physiol.* 1977;232(3):E258–E262.

66. McMillin JB, Taffet GE, Taegtmeyer H, Hudson EK, Tate CA. Mitochondrial metabolism and substrate competition in the aging Fischer rat heart. *Cardiovasc Res.* 1993; 27(12):2222–2228.

67. Iemitsu M, Miyauchi T, Maeda S, *et al.* Aging-induced decrease in the PPAR-alpha level in hearts is improved by exercise training. *Am J Physiol Heart Circ Physiol.* 2002; 283(5):H1750–H1760.

68. Odiet JA, Boerrigter ME, Wei JY. Carnitine palmitoyl transferase-I activity in the aging mouse heart. *Mech Ageing Dev.* 1995;79(2–3):127–136.

69. Paradies G, Ruggiero FM, Gadaleta MN, Quagliariello E. The effect of aging and acetyl-L-carnitine on the activity of the phosphate carrier and on the phospholipid composition in rat heart mitochondria. *Biochim Biophys Acta.* 1992;1103(2):324–326.

70. Kates AM, Herrero P, Dence C, *et al.* Impact of aging on substrate metabolism by the human heart. *J Am Coll Cardiol.* 2003;41:293–299.

71. Soto PF, Herrero P, Kates AM, *et al.* Impact of aging on myocardial metabolic response to dobutamine. *Am J Physiol Heart Circ Physiol.* 2003;285:2158–2164.

72. Soto PF, Herrero P, Schechtman KB, *et al.* Exercise training impacts the myocardial metabolism of older individuals in a gender-specific manner. *Am J Physiol Heart Circ Physiol.* 2008;295(2):H842–H850.

73. Kannel WB, Hjortland M, Castelli WP. Role of diabetes in congestive heart failure: the Framingham study. *Am J Cardiol.* 1974;34:29–34.

74. Stanley WC, Lopaschuck GD, McCormack JG. Regulation of energy substrate metabolism in the diabetic heart. *Cardiovasc Res.* 1997;34(1):25–33.

75. Rodrigues B, Cam MC, McNeill JH. Myocardial substrate metabolism: implications for diabetic cardiomyopathy. *J Mol Cell Cardiol.* 1995;27:169–179.

76. Taegtmeyer H, McNulty P, Young ME. Adaptation and maladaptation of the heart in diabetes: Part I: general concepts. *Circulation.* 2002;105(14):1727–1733.

77. Young ME, McNulty P, Taegtmeyer H. Adaptation and maladaptation of the heart in diabetes: Part II: potential mechanisms. *Circulation.* 2002;105(15):1861–1870.

78. Finck BN, Lehman JJ, Leone TC, *et al.* The cardiac phenotype induced by PPARalpha overexpression mimics that caused by diabetes mellitus. *J Clin Invest.* 2002; 109(1):121–130.

79. Burkart EM, Sambandam N, Han X, *et al.* Nuclear receptors PPARbeta/delta and PPARalpha direct distinct metabolic regulatory programs in the mouse heart. *J Clin Invest.* 2007;117(12):3930–3939.

80. Shoghi KI, Gropler RJ, Sharp T, *et al.* Time course of alterations in myocardial glucose utilization in the Zucker diabetic fatty rat with correlation to gene expression of glucose transporters: a small-animal PET investigation. *J Nucl Med.* 2008;49(8):1320–1327.

81. Welch MJ, Lewis JS, Kim J, *et al.* Assessment of myocardial metabolism in diabetic rats using small-animal PET: a feasibility study. *J Nucl Med.* 2006;47(4):689–697.

82. Monti LD, Landoni C, Setola E, *et al.* Myocardial insulin resistance associated with chronic hypertriglyceridemia and increased FFA levels in Type 2 diabetic patients. *Am J Physiol Heart Circ Physiol.* 2004;287(3):H1225–H1231.

83. Monti LD, Lucignani G, Landoni C, *et al.* Myocardial glucose uptake evaluated by positron emission tomography and fluorodeoxyglucose during hyperglycemic clamp in IDDM patients. Role of free fatty acid and insulin levels. *Diabetes.* 1995;44(5):537–542.

84. vom Dahl J, Herman WH, Hicks RJ, *et al.* Myocardial glucose uptake in patients with insulin-dependent diabetes mellitus assessed quantitatively by dynamic positron emission tomography. *Circulation.* 1993;88(2): 395–404.

85. Avogaro A, Nosadini R, Doria A, *et al.* Myocardial metabolism in insulin-deficient diabetic humans without coronary artery disease. *Am J Physiol.* 1990; 258(4, Pt 1):E606–E618.

86. Herrero P, McGill JB, Lesniak D, *et al.* Pet detection of the impact of dobutamine on myocardial glucose metabolism in women with type 1 diabetes mellitus. *J Nucl Cardiol.* 2008;15(6):598–604.

87. Peterson LR, Herrero P, McGill J, *et al.* Fatty acids and insulin modulate myocardial substrate metabolism in humans with type 1 diabetes. *Diabetes.* 2008;57(1): 32–40.

88. Zhou YT, Grayburn P, Karim A, *et al.* Lipotoxic heart disease in obese rats: implications for human obesity. *Proc Natl Acad Sci USA.* 2000;97(4):1784–1789.

89. Hallsten K, Virtanen KA, Lonnqvist F, *et al.* Enhancement of insulin-stimulated myocardial glucose uptake in patients with Type 2 diabetes treated with rosiglitazone. *Diabet Med.* 2004;21(12):1280–1287.

90. Commerford SR, Pagliassotti MJ, Melby CL, Wei Y, Gayles EC, Hill JO. Fat oxidation, lipolysis, and free fatty acid cycling in obesity-prone and obesity-resistant rats. *Am J Physiol Endocrinol Metab.* 2000;279(4): E875–E885.

91. Tillisch JH, Brunken R, Marshall R, *et al.* Reversibility of cardiac wall-motion abnormalities predicted by positron tomography. *N Engl J Med.* 1986;314:884–888.

92. Eitzman D, Al-Aouar Z, Kanter HL, *et al.* Clinical outcome of patients with advanced coronary artery disease after viability studies with positron emission tomography. *J Am Coll Cardiol.* 1992;20:559–565.

93. Di Carli MF, Davidson M, Little R, *et al.* Value of metabolic imaging with positron emission tomography for evaluating prognosis in patients with coronary artery disease and left ventricular dysfunction. *Am J Cardiol.* 1994;73:527–533.

94. Lee KS, Marwick TH, Cook SA, *et al.* Prognosis of patients with left ventricular dysfunction, with and without viable myocardium after myocardial infarction. Relative efficacy of medical therapy and revascularization. *Circulation.* 1994;90:2687–2694.

95. DiCarli MF, Asgarzadie F, Schelbert HR, *et al.* Quantitative relation between myocardial viability and improvement in heart failure symptoms after revascularization in patients with ischemic cardiomyopathy. *Circulation.* 1995;92:3436–3444.

96. Lopaschuk G. Regulation of carbohydrate metabolism in ischemia and reperfusion. *Am Heart J.* 2000; 139(2, Pt 3):S115–119.

97. Araujo LI, Camici P, Spinks TJ, Jones T, Maseri A. Abnormalities in myocardial metabolism in patients with unstable angina as assessed by positron emission tomography. *Cardiovasc Drugs Ther.* 1988;2(1):41–46.

98. Camici P, Araujo LI, Spinks T, *et al.* Increased uptake of 18F-fluorodeoxyglucose in postischemic myocardium of patients with exercise-induced angina. *Circulation.* 1986;74(1):81–88.

99. Kawai Y, Tsukamoto E, Nozaki Y, Morita K, Sakurai M, Tamaki N. Significance of reduced uptake of iodinated fatty acid analogue for the evaluation of patients with acute chest pain. *J Am Coll Cardiol.* 2001;38(7): 1888–1894.

100. Kontos MC, Dilsizian V, Weiland F, *et al.* Iodofiltic acid I 123 (BMIPP) fatty acid imaging improves initial diagnosis in emergency department patients with suspected acute coronary syndromes: a multicenter trial. *J Am Coll Cardiol* 2010; July 20th issue; in press.

101. Barger PM, Kelly DP. Fatty acid utilization in the hypertrophied and failing heart: molecular regulatory mechanisms. *Am J Med Sci.* 1999;318(1):36–42.

102. Rupp H, Jacob R. Metabolically-modulated growth and phenotype of the rat heart. *Eur Heart J.* 1992; 13(Suppl. D): 56–61.

103. Blair E, Redwood C, Ashrafian H, *et al.* Mutations in the gamma(2) subunit of AMP-activated protein kinase cause familial hypertrophic cardiomyopathy: evidence for the central role of energy compromise in disease pathogenesis. *Hum Mol Genet.* 2001;10(11):1215–1220.

104. Jamshidi Y, Montgomery HE, Hense HW, *et al.* Peroxisome proliferator-activated receptor alpha gene regulates left ventricular growth in response to exercise and hypertension. *Circulation.* 2002;105(8):950–955.

105. Handa N, Magata Y, Mukai T, Nishina T, Konishi J, Komeda M. Quantitative FDG-uptake by positron emission tomography in progressive hypertrophy of rat hearts in vivo. *Ann Nucl Med.* 2007;21(10):569–576.

106. de las Fuentes L, Herrero P, Peterson LR, Kelly DP, Gropler RJ, Davila-Roman VG. Myocardial fatty acid metabolism: independent predictor of left ventricular mass in hypertensive heart disease. *Hypertension.* 2003; 41(1):83–87.

107. de las Fuentes L, Soto PF, Cupps BP, *et al.* Hypertensive left ventricular hypertrophy is associated with abnormal myocardial fatty acid metabolism and myocardial efficiency. *J Nucl Cardiol.* 2006;13(3):369–377.

108. Tuunanen H, Kuusisto J, Toikka J, *et al.* Myocardial perfusion, oxidative metabolism, and free fatty acid uptake in patients with hypertrophic cardiomyopathy attributable to the Asp175Asn mutation in the alpha-tropomyosin gene: a positron emission tomography study. *J Nucl Cardiol.* 2007;14(3):354–365.

109. Buttrick PM, Kaplan M, Leinwand LA, Scheuer J. Alterations in gene expression in the rat heart after chronic pathological and physiological loads. *J Mol Cell Cardiol.* 1994;26(1):61–67.

110. Sack MN, Kelly DP. The energy substrate switch during development of heart failure: gene regulatory mechanisms (Review). *Int J Mol Med.* 1998;1(1):17–24.

111. Taegtmeyer H. Cardiac metabolism as a target for the treatment of heart failure. *Circulation.* 2004;110(8): 894–896.

112. Nakae I, Matsuo S, Koh T, Mitsunami K, Horie M. Iodine-123 BMIPP scintigraphy in the evaluation of patients with heart failure. *Acta Radiol.* 2006;47(8): 810–816.

113. Tuunanen H, Engblom E, Naum A, *et al.* Decreased myocardial free fatty acid uptake in patients with idiopathic dilated cardiomyopathy: evidence of relationship with insulin resistance and left ventricular dysfunction. *J Card Fail.* 2006;12(8):644–652.

114. Bennett SK, Smith MF, Gottlieb SS, *et al.* Effect of Metoprolol on absolute myocardial blood flow in patients with heart failure secondary to ischemic or non-ischemic cardiomyopathy. *Am J Cardiol.* 2002;89: 1431–1434.

115. Beanlands RSB, Nahmias C, Gordon E, *et al.* The effects of b₁-blockade on oxidative metabolism and the metabolic cost of ventricular work in patients with left ventricular dysfunction: a double-blind, placebo-controlled, positron-emission tomography study. *Circulation.* 2000;102:2070–2075.

116. Stolen KQ, Kemppainen J, Ukkonen H, *et al.* Exercise training improves biventricular oxidative metabolism and left ventricular efficiency in patients with dilated cardiomyopathy. *J Am Coll Cardiol.* 2003;41(3): 460–467.

117. Sundell J, Engblom E, Koistinen J, *et al.* The effects of cardiac resynchronization therapy on left ventricular function, myocardial energetics, and metabolic reserve in patients with dilated cardiomyopathy and heart failure. *J Am Coll Cardiol.* 2004;43(6):1027–1033.

118. Nowak B, Sinha AM, Schaefer WM, *et al.* Cardiac resynchronization therapy homogenizes myocardial glucose metabolism and perfusion in dilated cardiomyopathy and left bundle branch block. *J Am Coll Cardiol.* 2003;41(9):1523–1528.

119. Tuunanen H, Engblom E, Naum A, *et al.* Trimetazidine, a metabolic modulator, has cardiac and extracardiac benefits in idiopathic dilated cardiomyopathy. *Circulation.* 2008;118(12):1250–1258.

120. Hasegawa S, Kusuoka H, Maruyama K, Nishimura T, Hori M, Hatazawa J. Myocardial positron emission computed tomographic images obtained with fluorine-18 fluoro-2-deoxyglucose predict the response of idiopathic dilated cardiomyopathy patients to beta-blockers. *J Am Coll Cardiol.* 2004;43(2):224–233.

121. van Campen CM, Visser FC, Van Der Weerdt AP, *et al.* FDG PET as a predictor of response to resynchronisation therapy in patients with ischaemic cardiomyopathy. *Eur J Nucl Med Mol Imaging.* 2007;34(3):309–315.

122. United States Renal Data System. *USRDS 2006 Annual Data Report: Atlas of End-Stage Renal Disease in the US. 2006.* Bethesda, MD: National Institutes of Health, National Institutes of Diabetes and Digestive and Kidney Diseases.

123. Tyralla K, Amann K. (2003) Morphology of the heart and arteries in renal failure. *Kidney Int.* 63:S80–S83.

124. Nishimura M, Tsukamoto K, Hasebe N, Tamaki N, Kikuchi K, Ono T. Prediction of cardiac death in hemodialysis patients by myocardial fatty acid imaging. *J Am Coll Cardiol.* 2008;51(2):139–145.

125. Fink JC, Lodge MA, Smith MF, *et al.* Pre-clinical myocardial metabolic alterations in chronic kidney disease. *Cardiology.* 2010;116:160–167.

126. Dilsizian V, Fink J. Deleterious effect of altered myocardial fatty acid metabolism in kidney disease. *J Am Coll Cardiol.* 2008;51(2):146–148.

127. Nishimura M, Hashimoto T, Kobayashi H, *et al.* Myocardial scintigraphy using a fatty acid analogue detects coronary artery disease in hemodialysis patients. *Kidney Int.* 2004;66:811–819.

CHAPTER 6

PET Innervation and Receptors

Antti Saraste, Hossam Sherif & Markus Schwaiger

Nuklearmedizinische Klinik Technischen Universität München, Munich, Germany

Introduction

The autonomic nervous system plays a role in regulation of cardiac function to meet changing circulatory demands. Its alterations are involved in development and progression of various cardiac diseases, including heart failure, ischemic heart disease and arrhythmic disorders.

Nuclear imaging techniques can provide noninvasive information about global and regional myocardial autonomic nervous function. Conventional nuclear imaging using the catecholamine analog I-123 metaiodobenzylguanidine (MIBG) is widely used for mapping of myocardial presynaptic nerve terminals. Many radiolabeled compounds with distinct functional properties are available to probe the sympathetic nervous system at the pre- and postsynaptic levels by positron emission tomography (PET) imaging. Owing to high spatial and temporal resolutions and routine attenuation correction, PET offers the potential for detailed, quantitative analysis of tracer kinetics.

This chapter provides an overview of PET imaging of myocardial autonomic innervation and receptors. First, a brief overview on structure and physiology of the autonomic nervous system in the heart is given. Then, properties of available radiolabeled neurotransmitters for PET imaging are discussed. Finally, recent PET findings in relevant disease conditions are summarized in the context of their potential clinical implications.

Autonomic Nervous System of the Heart

The autonomic nervous system consists of sympathetic and parasympathetic parts [1,2]. The heart is characterized by dense sympathetic innervation covering both the atria and the ventricles while the parasympathetic system is prevalent mainly in the atria. Sympathetic system mediates cardiac stimulation causing increase in heart rate, atrioventricular conduction, and myocardial contractility while the parasympathetic system mainly exerts negative chronotropic responses.

Sympathetic stimuli are transmitted to the heart via adrenergic fibers traveling along the coronary arteries from the base to the apical regions. They include multiple nerve terminals that are filled with vesicles containing norepinephrine, the major neurotransmitter of the sympathetic nervous system (Figure 6.1). Norepinephrine is synthesized from the amino acid tyrosine within the neuron. First, tyrosine is converted to dopa that is the rate-limiting step in catecholamine biosynthesis. Dopa is converted to dopamine that is transported into storage vesicles by vesicular monoamine transporter. Within the storage vesicles it is converted to norepinephrine. Stimulation of the sympathetic nerves leads to release of norepinephrine from the nerve terminal into synaptic cleft by exocytosis. Apart from the rate of nerve stimulation, norepinephrine release is regulated by several receptors, such as presynaptic α_2-adrenergic receptors providing negative feedback for exocytosis. Most of the released norepinephrine undergoes reuptake into nerve terminals by the uptake-1 mechanism, i.e., presynaptic norepinephrine transporter (NET)

Cardiac CT, PET and MR, 2nd edition. Edited by Vasken Dilsizian and Gerry Pohost. © 2010 Blackwell Publishing Ltd.

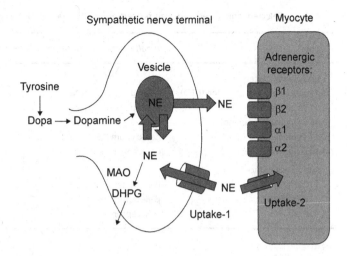

Figure 6.1 Graphical illustration of the sympathetic nerve terminal. For explanation see text. DHPG, dihydroxyphenylglycol; MAO, monoamine oxidase; NE, norepinephrine.

that is a sodium- and chloride-dependent transport protein. The uptake-1 mechanism plays a role in regulating the availability of norepinephrine for the postsynaptic receptors. Structurally related amines, such as epinephrine, guanethidine, and metaraminol are also transported by this system. Norepinephrine can also be removed to some extent into non-neuronal myocardial tissue by uptake-2 system. A small fraction of the released norepinephrine diffuses into vascular space, where it can be measured as norepinephrine spillover in coronary sinus vein blood. In the cytoplasm, norepinephrine is either recycled into the storage vesicles or rapidly degraded to dihydroxyphenylglycol by monoamine oxidase (MAO). Norepinephrine mediates its functions in the heart via three major adrenoceptor types ($\beta 1$, $\beta 2$, and $\alpha 1$) present in the cardiomyocytes. The relative proportions of these vary in diseases.

Acetylcholine is the neurotransmitter of the parasympathetic nervous system. It is synthesized within the parasympathetic nerve terminal from choline and acetyl co-enzyme A by choline acetyltransferase, and subsequently shuttled into storage vesicles. In contrast to amine uptake in sympathetic terminals, the choline uptake system is highly specific to only choline. Upon nerve stimulation, acetylcholine is released into the synaptic cleft, where it interacts with muscarinic receptors. Free acetylcholine is rapidly metabolized by acetylcholine esterase.

Tracers for Presynaptic Cardiac Innervation

A summary of radiotracers available for PET imaging of the myocardial sympathetic innervation is given in Table 6.1 and Figure 6.2. For detailed review see references [3] and [4]. The radiotracers can be divided in true adrenergic neurotransmitters and catecholamine analogs, i.e., so-called "false neurotransmitters." While true neurotransmitters behave identically to endogenous neurotransmitters and follow the entire metabolic catecholamine pathways, analogs are resistant to specific steps of the catecholamine metabolism.

C-11-Hydroxyephedrine

Carbon-11 (C-11) meta-hydroxyephedrine (HED) is the most widely used PET tracer for studying cardiac sympathetic nerve terminals. It is a catecholamine analog synthesized by N-methylation of metaraminol, which reliably yields HED at high specific activity. Studies in experimental models and patients with recent cardiac transplantation demonstrate high affinity to the uptake-1 mechanism, close correlation between HED uptake and NET density, and low nonspecific myocardial uptake [5–7]. Thus, the tracer uptake closely reflects transport by NET. Vesicular storage of HED is lower compared to norepinephrine due to the higher lipophilicity of HED. Moreover, HED is resistant to cytoplasmic metabolism by MAO. When specific inhibitor of uptake-1 (desipramine) is applied

Table 6.1   Selected radiotracers and their properties for PET imaging of the sympathetic innervation.

Tracer	Type/target	Intraneuronal metabolism	Notes
Presynaptic tracers			
C-11 meta-hydroxyephedrine (HED)	Analog	No	High selectivity for uptake-1
C-11 phenylephrine	Analog	Yes	
F-18 6-fluorometaraminol	Analog	No	Experimental
C-11 epinephrine	Catecholamine	Yes	
F-18 6-fluorodopamine	Catecholamine	Yes	
Postsynaptic tracers			
C-11CGP12177	β-Receptor		Nonselective
C-11CGP12388	β-Receptor		Nonselective
C-11GB67	α-Receptor		Experimental

after HED, an accelerated washout of HED can be seen suggesting that its retention is dependent on continuous release and reuptake by the sympathetic neurons [5].

Distribution of HED in healthy normal individuals is regionally homogeneous with high uptake throughout the left ventricular myocardium providing the basis to study specific regional defects of the sympathetic nervous system in diseases (Figure 6.3) [6]. For imaging, 400–700 MBq of C-11 HED is typically injected intravenously as a bolus, followed by a dynamic acquisition lasting 40–60 minutes. For quantification, a "retention index" is commonly calculated by normalizing myocardial radioactivity concentration at a specific time point, typically 40 minutes after injection, to the arterial input derived from the integral of the time–activity curve in the left ventricular arterial blood pool (Figure 6.4). For exact quantification arterial input needs correction for the presence of radiolabeled plasma metabolites. High neuronal affinity of HED makes compartmental modeling of its kinetics difficult because in addition to norepinephrine transporter density, perfusion, and transcapillary transport may significantly influence tracer uptake.

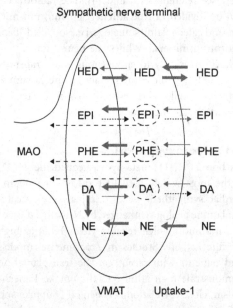

Figure 6.2 Key features of the tracers of presynaptic innervation. Arrow thickness is in proportion to the approximate relative magnitude of rate constants for uptake-1 membrane transporter and vesicular monoamine transporter (VMAT). DA, dopamine; EPI, epinephrine; HED, hydroxyephedrine; MAO, monoamine oxidase; NE, norepinephrine; PHEN, phenylephrine. (Adapted from Raffel and Wieland [3].)

F-18 Fluorodopamine

Dopamine can be labeled with fluorine to produce fluorine-18 (F-18) fluorodopamine that has been used to visualize cardiac sympathetic innervation in several human studies [8]. After tracer injection, sympathetic nerve terminals take up F-18 fluorodopamine mainly via uptake-1 mechanism. Then, fluorodopamine is sequestered into storage vesicles and β-hydroxylated to fluoronorepinephrine that is released in a manner similar to endogenous norepinephrine. Due to the half-life of 110 minutes for F-18, tracer clearance from the heart can be surveyed over a longer period

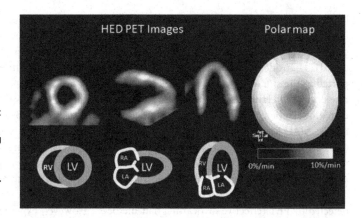

Figure 6.3 Positron emission tomography (PET) study of sympathetic innervation with C-11 meta-hydroxyephedrine (HED) showing normal myocardial uptake in a healthy volunteer. Images of HED uptake and a polar map of HED retention are shown. LA, left atrium; LV, left ventricle; RA, right atrium; RV, right ventricle.

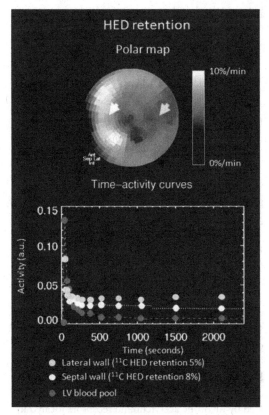

Figure 6.4 Time–activity curves obtained after intravenous injection of C-11 meta-hydroxyephedrine (HED) in a patient with heart failure due to dilated cardiomyopathy. HED retention indexes for two myocardial areas were determined by normalizing myocardial activity at 40 minutes to arterial input function determined from left ventricular blood pool.

than with C-11 labeled tracers. Compared to HED that is highly specific for uptake-1, F-18 fluorodopamine can provide information on both uptake and clearance of norepinephrine. However, its difficult synthesis and complex metabolic fate in the myocardium and plasma have limited its use [9].

C-11 Epinephrine

Epinephrine has a minor role as a physiologic neurotransmitter, but it is released into circulation together with norepinephrine from the adrenal medulla and other chromaffin tissues. Epinephrine can be radiolabeled with C-11 by N-methylation of norepinephrine at high yield and high specific activity. C-11 epinephrine behaves in the myocardium in a manner similar to norepinephrine. It has high affinity for uptake-1 and although it is vulnerable to MAO degradation, efficient vesicular storage in the neurons results in slow clearance of radioactivity from the heart [10]. Compared to C-11 HED that largely reflects uptake-1, C-11 epinephrine imaging reflects also vesicular storage. Its plasma metabolism needs to be taken into account for calculation of quantitative retention indexes. A study comparing healthy subjects with transplant recipients indicated high sensitivity of C-11 epinephrine for neuronal abnormalities [11]. Moreover, its physiologic behavior may be an advantage. However, the number of human studies using C-11 epinephrine for imaging cardiac sympathetic nervous system remains still very limited.

C-11 Phenylephrine

Phenylephrine is a sympathomimetic amine that is commonly used as a nasal decongestant. It can be labeled with C-11 at high specific activity producing the PET tracer C-11 phenylephrine. It is transported by the uptake-1 mechanism at a slower rate than HED. Inside the neuron it is effectively transported to the storage vesicles and diffuses out at a rate slower than HED. The major difference to HED is that C-11 phenylephrine is sensitive to degradation by MAO forming the radiolabeled metabolite C-11 methylamine that diffuses out of the nerve terminals [12]. Human experience with C-11 phenylephrine remains limited, but following its injection of gradual myocardial radioactivity washout can be detected by PET (effective myocardial half-life being about 60 minutes) that probably gives an index of MAO activity [13].

Other Tracers of Sympathetic Innervation

Metaraminol is a catecholamine analog resistant to metabolic degradation by MAO in a similar manner to HED. Metaraminol can be fluorinated to produce F-18 fluorometaraminol for PET imaging of the sympathetic nervous system. However, its application to human studies has been limited by potential risk of vasoactive side-effects. Efforts have also been made to label analogs of the SPECT tracer I-123 MIBG, a guanethidine analog, with positron-emitting isotopes, but they have shown low affinity for uptake-1. Instead of benzylguanidines, phenethylguanidines have been recently investigated as potential compounds for tracer synthesis [14]. They are known to be very potent depletors of cardiac norepinephrine stores due to their avid uptake and retention inside norepinephrine storage vesicles [14].

Tracers of Adrenergic Receptors

Finding of receptor ligands suitable for labeling that would demonstrate high enough specific binding for imaging without toxicity has been challenging. However, two β-adrenoceptor radioligands are currently investigated in clinical studies. C-11CGP12177 is a nonselective, hydrophilic β-receptor antagonist. It has low nonspecific uptake and fast plasma clearance providing good image quality [15]. A method using dual-injection protocol with high and low specific activities of C-11CGP12177 followed by graphical analysis

has been introduced for quantitative assessment of global myocardial density of β-adrenoceptors [16]. However, synthesis of the tracer is laborious and requires C-11 phosgene as a precursor that has prevented broader clinical application. C-11CGP12388 is a more recently introduced nonselective β-adrenoceptor antagonist, which is more easily labeled than CGP12177 [17]. Studies have shown high specific accumulation independent of flow in isolated rat heart [18]. Good image quality and feasibility of quantification of receptor density was demonstrated in humans [19]. However, experience of its use is still limited. Labeled β-adrenoceptor antagonists selective for the β1 adrenoceptor subtype are under development and await application in imaging research [20]. C-11GB67 is an analog of the α1 receptor ligand prazosin that has shown potential for imaging of α1 adrenoceptors [21].

Imaging of the Parasympathetic System

Low density of cholinergic neurons, high specificity of the presynaptic transporter system for acetylcholine and rapid degradation of acetylcholine make imaging of the parasympathetic nervous system difficult [3,4]. Vesamicol, a compound that specifically binds to receptors on parasympathetic neuronal vesicles and inhibits storage of acetylcholine, has been radiolabeled to produce F-18 fluoroethoxybenzovesamicol. However, its specific binding was low and uptake was largely affected by blood flow in isolated perfused heart so that the usefulness of the tracer for clinical cardiac PET imaging was considered to be low. 11-C methylquinuclidinylbenzilat, a specific hydrophilic antagonist of muscarinic receptors, that been used to visualize their density in the heart by PET imaging [22]. In addition to muscarinic receptors, cardiac parasympathetic effects are mediated by nicotinic acetylcholine receptors located in the nerve ganglions intracardially. Recently, it was demonstrated that a specific PET ligand (2-deoxy-2-F-18-fluoro-D-glucose-A85380) showed heart-to-background ratios that indicated feasibility for noninvasive of cardiac nicotinic acetylcholine receptors [23].

PET Imaging of Innervation in Cardiac Diseases

Cardiac Transplantation

Transplanted heart has served as a model to evaluate tracers for imaging as well as study physiologic effects of cardiac sympathetic innervation. The newly transplanted donor heart is initially completely denervated. This is associated with hemodynamic alterations such as increased baseline heart rate, chronotropic incompetence during exercise, and diastolic dysfunction. As a consequence, exercise tolerance is compromised.

PET imaging of HED retention has shown that cardiac allograft becomes reinnervated over time. More than 1 year after transplantation PET measurements showed reappearance of regional HED retention in the basal anterior myocardium [24]. Serial assessment demonstrated progressive increase in the extent and intensity of reinnervation from the basal anterior and septal myocardium toward the apex and lateral wall, consistent with an ingrowth of nerve fibers into the myocardium supplied by the left coronary artery [25]. Figure 6.5 shows examples of transplant reinnervation identified by PET. The pharmacologic integrity of these nerve terminals has been confirmed by studies of neurotransmitter released after injection of precursor tyramine [26]. Notably, reinnervation remained incomplete even 15 years after transplantation, and in some patients the amount of denervation remains very limited [25,27]. Multivariate analysis in 77 transplant recipient revealed several determinants of reinnervation in addition to time after transplantation, including age of the donor and the recipient, duration and complexity of transplant surgery, and extent of allograft rejection [28]. Moreover, the reinnervation process was significantly decreased in diabetic patients when compared to nondiabetics [29].

Comparing denervated and innervated regions of cardiac allograft it has been shown that innervation is associated with improved endothelium-dependent vascular reactivity as measured with cold pressor test [30]. In another study metabolic switch from free fatty acids to prefer glucose was found [31]. The effect of reinnervation on exercise performance has been directly studied in transplant recipients by HED PET and exercise radionuclide angiography. Restoration of sympathetic innervation

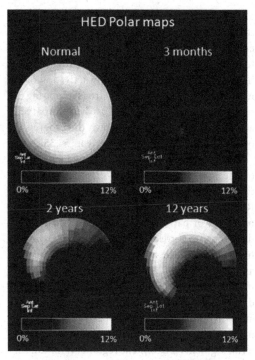

Figure 6.5 Polar maps of myocardial retention of C-11 meta-hydroxyephedrine (HED) in a healthy subject and three cardiac transplant recipients at different times after transplantation showing different degrees of denervation

was associated with improved response of heart rate and global as well as regional contractile function to exercise [32]. These effects were abolished using nonselective β-adrenergic blockade [33]. These results support the functional importance of reinnervation in transplanted hearts and suggest a clinical benefit for the transplant recipient through enhanced exercise capacity [32]. Thus, it seems warranted to develop and test approaches aimed at supporting the process of allograft reinnervation.

Heart Failure

An increased activity of the sympathetic nervous system is a hallmark of heart failure. Plasma levels of noradrenaline are elevated, myocardial noradrenaline stores are depleted, and myocardial β-receptor density reduced reflecting generalized adrenergic activation. Enhanced sympathetic activity increases myocardial contractility, heart rate and via increased preload activates the Frank–Starling mechanism. These responses are capable maintaining ventricular performance and cardiac output for a limited period of time. However, it has been shown that adrenergic activation eventually leads to worsening of myocardial ischemia, cardiotoxicity, deterioration of cardiac function, and progression of heart failure. Drugs counteracting activation of the neurohormonal pathways, i.e., drugs inhibiting the renin–angiotensin system and cardiac sympathetic activity have proven to slow down the progression of heart failure and improve survival [34,35].

Several studies have demonstrated alterations of the presynaptic cardiac sympathetic innervation in the failing heart using HED and PET. Retention of HED was reduced in the failing myocardium of patients with idiopathic dilated cardiomyopathy correlating with clinical markers of heart failure, such as impaired ejection fraction and NYHA class, as well as with elevation of plasma catecholamine levels [36]. In addition reduced global HED uptake, marked regional variation in HED retention has been observed with most pronounced reductions in the apical and inferior segments [36,37]. The regional variation correlated with tissue noradrenaline content and the density of uptake-1 sites in myocardial tissue of explanted failing human hearts [37]. Thus, uptake sites of norepinephrine are decreased in the failing heart due to either loss of neurons or downregulation of uptake-1. An example of HED findings in idiopathic dilated cardiomyopathy is shown in Figure 6.6.

Although mechanisms of presynaptic dysfunction in heart failure remain largely unknown several correlates for reduced HED retention have been found, including blunted vascular sympathetic effector responses responsible for blood pressure maintenance [38], impaired global and regional contractile function as measured by gated blood pool SPECT [39], reduced myocardial efficiency [40], and recently, myocardial insulin resistance [41]. Regional HED uptake was not correlated with ex vivo determined β-adrenergic receptor density but rather with expression of the receptor-inactivating enzyme β-adrenoceptor kinase [42].

In vivo imaging using C-11 CGP12177 PET has demonstrate downregulation of β-receptors in the failing heart as confirmed in tissue biopsies [43] Downregulation was associated with decreased contractile responses to dobutamine, indicating a link between changes in the receptor number and function [43]. On the other hand, upregulation of muscarinic receptor density in patients with idiopathic dilated cardiomyopathy was demonstrated by PET imaging [22]. Using combination of HED and C-11 CGP12177 PET imaging, it was shown that a mismatch between measures of presynaptic norepinephrine uptake-1 mechanism and β-adrenergic receptor density is common in patients with ischemic heart failure, but not in healthy controls [44]. Notably, three out of four patients with

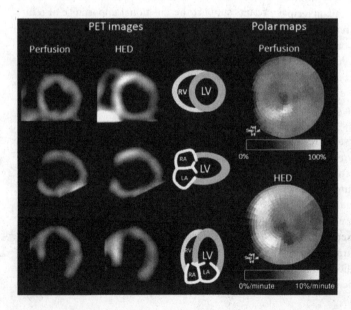

Figure 6.6 Positron emission tomography study of myocardial sympathetic innervation with C-11 meta-hydroxyephedrine (HED) in a patient with symptomatic heart failure due to idiopathic dilated cardiomyopathy. While regional perfusion is very homogeneous, there is a reduction of myocardial HED retention, particularly inferolaterally. In addition to PET images, time–activity curves and retention values 40 minutes after HED injection are shown for blood and two myocardial areas.

adverse events had particularly pronounced mismatch [44].

An association between the extent of presynaptic denervation and adverse clinical outcomes has been reported in heart failure patients using I-123 MIBG and SPECT imaging as well as HED and PET. A recent meta-analysis of 18 studies involving more than 1700 heart failure patients showed that patients with reduced global I-123 MIBG uptake (heart-to-mediastinum ratio) or washout had higher mortality compared with those with normal semi-quantitative MIBG parameters [45]. Consistent with this, reduced global HED retention was an independent predictor of adverse outcome in 46 patients with NYHA class II–III heart failure and an average ejection fraction of 35% [46]. Recently, it was suggested that the extent of mismatch in presynaptic neuronal function assessed with HED and β-receptor density assessed with C-11-CGP12177 PET may be of prognostic value [43]. Serial measurements before and 6 months after start of an exercise training program in heart failure patients revealed improvement in baroreflex sensitivity and heart rate variability, which were associated with an increase of global HED retention, suggesting that physical training induces beneficial changes in cardiovascular autonomic nervous control and a shift toward normalization of the

compensatory autonomic nervous imbalance [47]. Based on these preliminary observations in small numbers of patients larger, prognostic studies seem warranted to determine the value of PET imaging of sympathetic nervous function in prognostic assessment and monitoring the efficacy of therapies in heart failure patients.

Ischemic Heart Disease

Cardiac sympathetic nerve terminals are considered to be sensitive to ischemia. Patient studies demonstrated that early after myocardial infarction the area of reduced HED retention exceeded the perfusion defect—a finding that was especially pronounced in subendocardial infarcts (Figure 6.7) [48]. Moreover, regional reductions in HED retention have been found in the absence of resting perfusion defects in patients with advanced coronary artery disease, but no evidence of myocardial infarction and in a pig model of myocardial hibernation [49,50]. The dependency of myocardial sympathetic innervation on coronary flow reserve was recently analyzed in patients with coronary artery disease. Although C-11 HED retention did not correlate significantly with myocardial resting perfusion a moderate correlation between regional C-11 HED retention and coronary flow reserve was found, particularly in the areas with severely

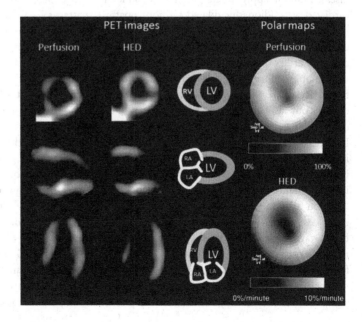

Figure 6.7 Positron emission tomography study of sympathetic innervation with C-11 meta-hydroxyephedrine (HED) after recent acute anterior myocardial infarction. The innervation defect exceeds the anteroapical perfusion defect in septal and apical regions.

impaired reserve. This indicates that sympathetic innervation could be preserved even when there is major impairment in either resting flow or flow reserve [51].

Controversy exists about the occurrence of myocardial reinnervation following regional ischemic damage. In one study no change in HED uptake was observed in the infracted myocardium until 6 months after acute infarction [48]. In another study, a mild increase of initially impaired F-18 fluorodopamine uptake in the infarct area between 2 weeks and 3 months after the event was found [52].

Based on the hypothesis of a higher sensitivity of sympathetic neurons to ischemia compared to cardiomyocytes HED imaging might have potential as a sensitive and early marker of ischemic myocardial damage. Furthermore, more studies are needed on the significance of extensive areas of denervated, but viable myocardium as a potential source of arrhythmias and remodeling as suggested by some SPECT studies with I-123 MIBG [45].

Arrythmias and Sudden Cardiac Death

Sudden cardiac death continues to be a leading cause of death in the Western countries, most often caused by ventricular tachyarrhythmia in the setting of structural heart disease. The single most important underlying etiology is coronary artery disease found in approximately 75–80% of sudden 'cardiac deaths. Idiopathic dilated cardiomyopathy is the second largest cause. Only in about 5–10% of cases, sudden cardiac death occurs in the absence of coronary artery disease or congestive heart failure. Implantable defibrillator has been demonstrated to be an effective treatment modality not only for secondary, but also for primary prevention of sudden cardiac death in selected patient populations. In the MADIT II study, a relative risk reduction in mortality of 31% was achieved by defibrillator implantation in patients with previous myocardial infarction and severe left ventricular dysfunction (ejection fraction $\leq$30%). However, primarily owing to cost implications there is a need to develope better ways of identifying those patients at highest risk for ventricular tachyarrhythmias to be selected for implantation of defibrillator [35].

Experimental and clinical studies have demonstrated a link between sympathetic neuronal function and the presence of arrhythmias [53]. It has been hypothesized that denervated, but viable myocardium can form a substrate for ventricular arrhythmias and thus, imaging of myocardial innervation may contribute to improved selection of patients for ICD implantation. HED and PET have been used to study the relationship between myocardial denervation and ventricular refractoriness as assessed by intraoperative electrophysiologic measurements during placement of an implantable defibrillator in 11 patients with a history of sustained ventricular tachycardia [54]. The refractory period in areas with reduced HED retention was significantly longer than in areas with normal HED retention, documenting effects of innervation as seen with PET imaging on myocardial electrophysiology [54]. Subsequently, involvement of the sympathetic nervous system in specific arrhythmogenic diseases has been evaluated using PET. PET with C-11 HED and C-11CGP12177 for pre- and postsynaptic imaging, respectively demonstrated that in patients with hypertrophic cardiomyopathy [55], arrhythmogenic right ventricular dysplasia [56], and right ventricular outflow tract arrhythmia [57], presynaptic neurotransmitter uptake and postsynaptic receptor density are downregulated. In contrast, in patients with the Brugada syndrome presynaptic neurotransmitter uptake is upregulated while postsynaptic receptor densities were within the normal range [58]. Interestingly, these distinct innervation patterns are associated with a difference in the clinical appearance: while the former cardiomyopathies lead to arrhythmias under stress conditions when sympathetic tone prevails, the Brugada syndrome is associated with potentially lethal arrhythmias occurring at rest when vagal tone predominates. In patients with the familial long QT syndrome, no abnormalities of global ventricular HED retention were identified [59,60]. However, in a study of 11 patients with genotyped long QT syndrome regional reductions in HED retention using a model of 36 small segments for the LV myocardium were still found [60]. It was suggested that sympathetic dysfunction could play a modulatory role also in this disease.

I-123 MIBG imaging with SPECT demonstrated presynaptic innervation defects in patients with idiopathic ventricular fibrillation. During a mean follow-up of 7 years, 18 episodes of lifethreatening ventricular arrhythmias were observed in four patients with abnormal MIBG uptake, as compared to only two episodes in one patient with normal MIBG uptake [61]. Arora *et al.* investigated the relation between MIBG imaging and appropriate defibrillator discharges in 17 patients with a defibrillator implanted due to various reasons. They found a significant difference in the early heart-to-mediastinum ratio between patients with and without appropriate discharges. Moreover, the SPECT images revealed a significantly larger defect score in the patients with appropriate discharges [62]. These results suggest potential for neuronal imaging in improving selection of patients who may be at risk for life-threatening ventricular arrhythmias and may benefit from defibrillator implantation. However, much more data are needed, particularly in patients with ischaemic heart disease and depressed venricular function, to define the incremental value of innervation imaging in the selection of patients for therapy.

Diabetes

Autonomic neuropathy of the heart is a common complication of diabetes having influence on life expectancy and quality of life of the patients. The manifestations include resting tachycardia, exercise intolerance, orthostatic hypotension, and silent myocardial ischemia [63].

Using HED and PET, a pattern of regional myocardial denervation involving the apical, inferior, and lateral walls was found to be associated with cardiac diabetic neuropathy correlating with conventional markers of autonomic dysfunction [64]. In another study regional pattern of HED retention in cardiac diabetic neuropathy was confirmed, but proximal hyperinnervation was also found [65]. Serial assessment of the innervation pattern in diabetic subjects over a period of 3 years demonstrated that innervation defects can regress or progress depending on good or poor glycemic control, respectively [66].

Several studies have contributed to establish a link between diabetic autonomic neuropathy and impairments of myocardial blood flow. Stevens and colleagues found significant reductions of global myocardial blood flow and flow reserve during adenosine-mediated vasodilation in neuropathic diabetic subjects compared to non-neuropathic

diabetic and nondiabetic subjects [67]. Consistent with this it was demonstrated that compared to diabetic patients without microangiopathy, diabetic patients with established microangiopathy showed more severe reduction in HED uptake associated with abnormal response of myocardial perfusion to adenosine and cold pressor test [68]. Di Carli and colleagues reported impaired flow response to adenosine in diabetic patients with and without PET-defined cardiac neuropathy compared to normal controls, while the endothelium-dependent flow response to sympathetic stimulation by cold pressor test was further reduced in diabetic patients with neuropathy than in those without and in normal controls [69].

These studies have provided insights into the pathophysiology of diabetic heart disease, but the relationship between myocardial neuropathy, flow regulation, arrhythmia, and outcome in diabetic subjects remains to be investigated to determine whether imaging of myocardial innervations can provide incremental clinical information over conventional assessment of diabetic neuropathy.

Primary Neurological Disorders

Some primary neurologic disorders causing autonomic neuropathy (dysautonomias) are associated with abnormalities in cardiac sympathetic denervation. They have been classified as idiopathic Parkinson's disease (PD), pure autonomic failure (PAF), and multiple system atrophy (MSA). Studies with PET and F-18 fluorodopamine have demonstrated progressive reduction of catecholamine uptake in the myocardium as well as extracardiac sympathetic system in patients with signs of sympathetic neurocirculatory failure due to idiopathic PD and PAF [70–72].

In contrast, MSA has been associated with increased myocardial uptake of F-18 fluorodopamine when compared with healthy controls [70]. More recently, it was found that cardiac sympathetic denervation was found to occur not only in idiopathic PD but also in other movement disorders, such as MSA and progressive supranuclear palsy. This finding implies that the scintigraphic detection of cardiac sympathetic denervation cannot be used independently to discriminate idiopathic PD from these other movement disorders [72].

Summary and Future Perspectives

In summary, the results of many PET studies evaluating cardiac sympathetic innervation in experimental models and small groups of patients with heart failure or at high risk of ventricular tachyarrhythmia are promising. As with I-123 MIBG, larger, prospective trials seem warranted to define the incremental prognostic value of PET innervation imaging in these disease conditions. For example, it might allow implantation of defibrillators on a more individualized basis to those at the highest risk of arrhythmias.

PET has been established as a tool to monitor integrity of the cardiac neuronal structure in cardiac transplant recipients, diabetics, and patients with neurodegenerative disorders. However, a clear clinical application that would justify the use of this expensive testing modality in these conditions has not emerged so far.

New information about the involvement of autonomic nervous system in pathogenesis of common cardiac disorders, such as atrial fibrillation, together with development of new tracers may provide novel, attractive applications for PET innervation imaging in the future.

References

1. Randall W, Ardell J. Functional anatomy of the cardiac efferent innervation. In: Kulbertus H, Frank G (eds). *Neurocardiology.* New York: Futura Publishing, 1988, pp. 3–24.
2. Bristow MR, Minobe W, Rasmussen R, et al. Beta-adrenergic neuroeffector abnormalities in the failing human heart are produced by local rather than systemic mechanisms. *J Clin Invest.* 1992;89:803–815.
3. Raffel DM, Wieland DM. Assessment of cardiac sympathetic nerve integrity with positron emission tomography. *Nucl Med Biol.* 2001;28:541–559.
4. Langer O, Halldin C. PET and SPECT tracers for mapping of the cardiac nervous system. *Eur J Nucl Med Mol Imaging.* 2002;29:416–434.
5. DeGrado TR, Hutchins GD, Toorongian SA, et al. Myocardial kinetics of carbon-11–meta-hydroxyephedrine: retention mechanisms and effects of norepinephrine. *J Nucl Med.* 1993;34:1287–1293.
6. Schwaiger M, Kalff V, Rosenspire K, et al. Noninvasive evaluation of sympathetic nervous system in human heart by positron emission tomography. *Circulation.* 1990;82:457–464.
7. Raffel DM, Chen W, Sherman PS, et al. Dependence of cardiac 11C-meta-hydroxyephedrine retention on norepinephrine transporter density. *J Nucl Med.* 2006;47:1490–1496.
8. Goldstein DS, Eisenhofer G, Dunn BB, et al. Positron emission tomographic imaging of cardiac sympathetic innervation using 6-[18 F]fluorodopamine: initial findings in humans. *J Am Coll Cardiol.* 1993;22:1961–1971.
9. Goldstein DS, Holmes C. Metabolic fate of the sympathoneural imaging agent 6-[18 F]fluorodopamine in humans. *Clin Exp Hypertens.* 1997;19:155–161.
10. Nguyen NT, DeGrado TR, Chakraborty P, et al. Myocardial kinetics of carbon-11–epinephrine in the isolated working rat heart. *J Nucl Med.* 1997;38:780–785.
11. Munch G, Nguyen NT, Nekolla S, et al. Evaluation of sympathetic nerve terminals with [11C]epinephrine and [11C]hydroxyephedrine and positron emission tomography. *Circulation.* 2000;101:516–523.
12. Raffel DM, Corbett JR, del Rosario RB, et al. Clinical evaluation of carbon-11–phenylephrine: MAO-sensitive marker of cardiac sympathetic neurons. *J Nucl Med.* 1996;37:1923–1931.
13. Raffel DM, Wieland DM. Influence of vesicular storage and monoamine oxidase activity on [11C]phenylephrine kinetics: studies in isolated rat heart. *J Nucl Med.* 1999;40:323–330.
14. Raffel DM, Jung YW, Gildersleeve DL, et al. Radiolabeled phenethylguanidines: novel imaging agents for cardiac sympathetic neurons and adrenergic tumors. *J Med Chem.* 2007;50:2078–2088.
15. Law MP. Demonstration of the suitability of CGP 12177 for in vivo studies of beta-adrenoceptors. *Br J Pharmacol.* 1993;109:1101–1109.
16. Delforge J, Mesangeau D, Dolle F, et al. In vivo quantification and parametric images of the cardiac beta-adrenergic receptor density. *J Nucl Med.* 2002;43:215–226.
17. Elsinga PH, van Waarde A, Jaeggi KA, et al. Synthesis and evaluation of (S)-4-(3-(2′-[11C]isopropylamino)-2-hydroxypropoxy)-2H-benzimidazol-2-one ((S)-[11C]CGP 12388) and (S)-4-(3-((1′-[18F]-fluoroisopropyl)amino)-2-hydroxypropoxy)-2H- benzimidazol-2-one ((S)-[18F]fluoro-CGP 12388) for visualization of beta-adrenoceptors with positron emission tomography. *J Med Chem.* 1997;40:3829–3835.
18. Momose M, Reder S, Raffel DM, et al. Evaluation of cardiac betaadrenoreceptors in the isolated perfused rat heart using (S)-11CCGP12388. *J Nucl Med.* 2004;45:471–477.
19. Doze P, Elsinga PH, van Waarde A, et al. Quantification of betaadrenoceptor density in the human heart with (S)-[11C]CGP 12388 and a tracer kinetic model. *Eur J Nucl Med Mol Imaging.* 2002;29:295–304.

20. Wagner S, Law MP, Riemann B, *et al.* Synthesis of a F-18 labelled high affinity beta1-adrenoceptor PET radioligand based on ICI 89, 406. *J Label Compd Radiopharm.* 2006;49:177–195.

21. Law MP, Osman S, Pike VW, *et al.* Evaluation of [11C]GB67, a novel radioligand for imaging myocardial alpha 1-adrenoceptors with positron emission tomography. *Eur J Nucl Med.* 2000;27:7–17.

22. Le Guludec D, Cohen-Solal A, Delforge J, Delahaye N, Syrota A, Merlet P. Increased myocardial muscarinic receptor density in idiopathic dilated cardiomyopathy: an in vivo PET study. *Circulation.* 1997;96:3416–3422.

23. Bucerius J, Joe AY, Schmaljohann J, *et al.* Feasibility of 2-deoxy-2-[18F]fluoro-D-glucose- A85380-PET for imaging of human cardiac nicotinic acetylcholine receptors in vivo. *Clin Res Cardiol.* 2006;95:105–109.

24. Schwaiger M, Hutchins GD, Kalff V, *et al.* Evidence for regional catecholamine uptake and storage sites in the transplanted human heart by positron emission tomography. *J Clin Invest.* 1991;87:1681–1690.

25. Bengel FM, Ueberfuhr P, Ziegler SI, *et al.* Serial assessment of sympathetic reinnervation after orthotopic heart transplantation. A longitudinal study using PET and C-11 hydroxyephedrine. *Circulation.* 1999;99: 1866–1871.

26. Odaka K, von Scheidt W, Ziegler SI, *et al.* Reappearance of cardiac presynaptic sympathetic nerve terminals in the transplanted heart: correlation between PET using (11)C-hydroxyephedrine and invasively measured norepinephrine release. *J Nucl Med.* 2001;42:1011–1016.

27. Uberfuhr P, Ziegler S, Schwaiblmair M, *et al.* Incomplete sympathetic reinnervation of the orthotopically transplanted human heart: observation up to 13 years after heart transplantation. *Eur J Cardiothorac Surg.* 2000;17:161–168.

28. Bengel FM, Ueberfuhr P, Hesse T, *et al.* Clinical determinants of ventricular sympathetic reinnervation after orthotopic heart transplantation. *Circulation.* 2002;106:831–835.

29. Bengel FM, Ueberfuhr P, Schäfer D, *et al.* Effect of diabetes mellitus on sympathetic neuronal regeneration studied in the model of transplant reinnervation. *J Nucl Med.* 2006;47:1413–1419.

30. Di Carli MF, Tobes MC, Mangner T, *et al.* Effects of cardiac sympathetic innervation on coronary blood flow. *N Engl J Med.* 1997;336:1208–1215.

31. Bengel FM, Ueberfuhr P, Ziegler SI, *et al.* Noninvasive assessment of the effect of cardiac sympathetic innervation on metabolism of the human heart. *Eur J Nucl Med.* 2000;27:1650–1657.

32. Bengel FM, Ueberfuhr P, Schiepel N, *et al.* Effect of sympathetic reinnervation on cardiac performance after heart transplantation. *N Engl J Med.* 2001;345:731–738.

33. Bengel FM, Ueberfuhr P, Karja J, *et al.* Sympathetic reinnervation, exercise performance and effects of β-adrenergic blockade in cardiac transplant recipients. *Eur Heart J.* 2004;25:1726–1733.

34. Bristow MR. The autonomic nervous system in heart failure. *N Engl J Med.* 1984;311:850–851.

35. Swedberg K, Cleland J, Dargie H, *et al.* Guidelines for the diagnosis and treatment of chronic heart failure: executive summary (update 2005): the task force for the diagnosis and treatment of chronic heart failure of the European society of cardiology. *Eur Heart J.* 2005;26:1115–1140.

36. Hartmann F, Ziegler S, Nekolla S, *et al.* Regional patterns of myocardial sympathetic denervation in dilated cardiomyopathy: an analysis using carbon-11 hydroxyephedrine and positron emission tomography. *Heart.* 1999;81:262–270.

37. Ungerer M, Hartmann F, Karoglan M, *et al.* Regional in vivo and in vitro characterization of autonomic innervation in cardiomyopathic human heart. *Circulation.* 1998;97:174–180.

38. Vesalainen RK, Pietilä M, Tahvanainen KU, *et al.* Cardiac positron emission tomography imaging with [11C]hydroxyephedrine, a specific tracer for sympathetic nerve endings, and its functional correlates in congestive heart failure. *Am J Cardiol.* 1999;84:568–574.

39. Bengel FM, Permanetter B, Ungerer M, *et al.* Relationship between altered sympathetic innervation, oxidative metabolism and contractile function in the cardiomyopathic human heart: a noninvasive study using positron emission tomography. *Eur Heart J.* 2001;22: 1594–1600.

40. Bengel FM, Permanetter B, Ungerer M, *et al.* Alterations of the sympathetic nervous system and metabolic performance of the cardiomyopathic heart. *Eur J Nucl Med Mol Imaging.* 2002;29:198–202.

41. Mongillo M, John AS, Leccisotti L, *et al.* Myocardial presynaptic sympathetic function correlates with glucose uptake in the failing human heart. *Eur J Nucl Med Mol Imaging.* 2007;34:1172–1177.

42. Ungerer M, Weig HJ, Kubert S, *et al.* Regional pre- and postsynaptic sympathetic system in the failing human heart—regulation of beta ARK-1. *Eur J Heart Fail.* 2000;2:23–31.

43. Merlet P, Delforge J, Syrota A, *et al.* Positron emission tomography with 11C CGP-12177 to assess beta-adrenergic receptor concentration in idiopathic dilated cardiomyopathy. *Circulation.* 1993;87: 1169–1178.

44. Caldwell JH, Link JM, Levy WC, *et al.* Evidence for pre- to postsynaptic mismatch of the cardiac sympathetic nervous system in ischemic congestive heart failure. *J Nucl Med.* 2008;49:234–241.

45. Verberne HJ, Brewster LM, Somsen GA, van Eck-Smit BL. Prognostic value of myocardial 123I-metaiodobenzylguanidine (MIBG) parameters in patients with heart failure: a systematic review. *Eur Heart J.* 2008;29:1147–1159.

46. Pietilä M, Malminiemi K, Ukkonen H, *et al.* Reduced myocardial carbon-11 hydroxyephedrine retention is associated with poor prognosis in chronic heart failure. *Eur J Nucl Med.* 2001;28:373–376.

47. Pietilä M, Malminiemi K, Vesalainen R, *et al.* Exercise training in chronic heart failure: beneficial effects on cardiac 11C–hydroxyephedrine PET, autonomic nervous control, and ventricular repolarization. *J Nucl Med.* 2002;43:773–779.

48. Allman KC, Wieland DM, Muzik O, *et al.* Carbon-11 hydroxyephedrine with positron emission tomography for serial assessment of cardiac adrenergic neuronal function after acute myocardial infarction in humans. *J Am Coll Cardiol.* 1993;22:368–375.

49. Bulow HP, Stahl F, Lauer B, *et al.* Alterations of myocardial presynaptic sympathetic innervation in patients with multi-vessel coronary artery disease but without history of myocardial infarction. *Nucl Med Commun.* 2003;24:233–239.

50. Luisi AJ, Jr., Suzuki G, deKemp R, *et al.* Regional 11C-Hydroxyephedrine retention in hibernating myocardium: chronic inhomogeneity of sympathetic innervation in the absence of infarction. *J Nucl Med.* 2005;46:1368–1374.

51. Frickel E, Frickel H, Eckert S, *et al.* Myocardial sympathetic innervation in patients with chronic coronary artery disease: is reduction in coronary flow reserve correlated with sympathetic denervation? *Eur J Nucl Med Mol Imaging.* 2007;34:206–211.

52. Fallen EL, Coates G, Nahmias C, *et al.* Recovery rates of regional sympathetic reinnervation and myocardial blood flow after acute myocardial infarction. *Am Heart J.* 1999;137:863–869.

53. Schwartz PJ. The autonomic nervous system and sudden death. *Eur Heart J.* 1998;19:F72–F80.

54. Calkins H, Allman K, Bolling S, *et al.* Correlation between scintigraphic evidence of regional sympathetic neuronal dysfunction and ventricular refractoriness in the human heart. *Circulation.* 1993;88:172–179.

55. Schafers M, Dutka D, Rhodes CG, *et al.* Myocardial presynaptic and postsynaptic autonomic dysfunction in hypertrophic cardiomyopathy. *Circ Res.* 1998;82:57–62.

56. Schafers M, Lerch H, Wichter T, *et al.* Cardiac sympathetic innervation in patients with idiopathic right ventricular outflow tract tachycardia. *J Am Coll Cardiol.* 1998;32:181–186.

57. Wichter T, Schafers M, Rhodes CG, *et al.* Abnormalities of cardiac sympathetic innervation in arrhythmogenic right ventricular cardiomyopathy: quantitative assessment of presynaptic norepinephrine reuptake and postsynaptic beta-adrenergic receptor density with positron emission tomography. *Circulation.* 2000;101:1552–1558.

58. Kies P, Wichter T, Schafers M, *et al.* Abnormal myocardial presynaptic norepinephrine recycling in patients with Brugada syndrome. *Circulation.* 2004;110:3017–3022.

59. Calkins H, Lehmann MH, Allman K, *et al.* Scintigraphic pattern of regional cardiac sympathetic innervation in patients with familial long QT syndrome using positron emission tomography. *Circulation.* 1993;87:1616–1621.

60. Mazzadi AN, Andre-Fouet X, Duisit J, *et al.* Heterogeneous cardiac retention of 11C-hydroxyephedrine in genotyped long QT patients. A potential amplifier role for severity of the disease. *Am J Physiol Heart Circ Physiol.* 2003;285:H1286–H1293.

61. Paul M, Schäfers M, Kies P, *et al.* Impact of sympathetic innervation on recurrent life-threatening arrhythmias in the follow-up of patients with idiopathic ventricular fibrillation. *Eur J Nucl Med Mol Imaging.* 2006;33:866–870.

62. Arora R, Ferrick KJ, Nakata T, *et al.* I-123 MIBG imaging and heart rate variability analysis to predict the need for an implantable cardioverter defibrillator. *J Nucl Cardiol.* 2003;10:121–131.

63. Vinik AI, Maser RE, Mitchell BD, Freeman R. diabetic autonomic neuropathy. *Diabetes Care.* 2003;26:1553–1579.

64. Allman KC, Stevens MJ, Wieland DM, *et al.* Noninvasive assessment of cardiac diabetic neuropathy by carbon-11 hydroxyephedrine and positron emission tomography. *J Am Coll Cardiol.* 1993;22:1425–1432.

65. Stevens MJ, Raffel DM, Allman KC, *et al.* Cardiac sympathetic dysinnervation in diabetes: implications for enhanced cardiovascular risk. *Circulation.* 1998;98:961–968.

66. Stevens MJ, Raffel DM, Allman KC, *et al.* Regression and progression of cardiac sympathetic dysinnervation complicating diabetes: an assessment by C-11 hydroxyephedrine and positron emission tomography. *Metabolism.* 1999;48:92–101.

67. Stevens MJ, Dayanikli F, Raffel DM, *et al.* Scintigraphic assessment of regionalized defects in myocardial sympathetic innervation and blood flow regulation in diabetic patients with autonomic neuropathy. *J Am Coll Cardiol.* 1998;31:1575–1584.

68. Pop-Busui R, Kirkwood I, Schmid H, *et al.* Sympathetic dysfunction in type-1 diabetes association with impaired myocardial blood flow reserve and diastolic dysfunction. *J Am Coll Cardiol.* 2004;44:2368–2374.

69. Di Carli MF, Bianco-Batlles D, Landa ME, *et al.* Effects of autonomic neuropathy on coronary blood flow in patients with diabetes mellitus. *Circulation.* 1999;100:813–819.

70. Goldstein DS, Holmes C, Cannon RO, III, *et al.* Sympathetic cardioneuropathy in dysautonomias. *N Engl J Med.* 1997;336:696–702.

71. Tipre DN, Goldstein DS. Cardiac and extracardiac sympathetic denervation in Parkinson's disease with ortho-static hypotension and in pure autonomic failure. *J Nucl Med.* 2005;46 (11): 1775–1781.

72. Raffel DM, Koeppe RA, Little R, *et al.* PET measurement of cardiac and nigrostriatal denervation in Parkinsonian syndromes. *J Nucl Med.* 2006;47:1769–1777.

CHAPTER 7

MR Angiography: Coronaries and Great Vessels

Patricia Nguyen & Phillip Yang
Stanford University Medical Center, Stanford, CA, USA

Summary

- Magnetic resonance angiography (MRA) of the coronary arteries and great vessels is a promising alternative to invasive angiography.
- The clinical implementation of coronary MRA (C-MRA), however, remains challenging but continued technical advances may enable its more widespread application.
- Most recent developments include high-field imaging, parallel imaging, and whole heart imaging.
- Contrast-enhanced MRA has long been considered the preferred noninvasive imaging modality in great vessel MRA (GV-MRA).
- However, recent reports of nephrogenic systemic sclerosis associated with high-dose gadolinium have prompted research in low dose, contrast-enhanced and unenhanced GV-MRA.
- Although initial results are promising using unenhanced MRA, further evaluation is needed to determine the clinical feasibility of these techniques in GV-MRA.

Introduction

Noninvasive diagnostic imaging of the coronary arteries and great vessels has been one of the most important clinical goals in cardiovascular medicine. The current gold standard for imaging the coronary arteries and great vessels is invasive angiography.

Over 1 million invasive diagnostic coronary angiograms are performed each year to evaluate coronary artery atherosclerosis, with up to 20% of studies showing no evidence of significant disease [1]. The major limitation of this invasive technique is the associated morbidity and mortality ranging from 0.02 to 0.1% [2]. In great vessel MRA (GV-MRCA), the associated morbidity has relegated invasive angiography to a secondary, confirmatory role [3]. Invasive angiography also requires ionizing radiation and provides only projection images of the lumen. Thus, only limited information is available to determine atherosclerotic plaque burden, function, and three-dimensional (3D) anatomical relationships between structures.

Magnetic resonance imaging (MRI) is a promising method for noninvasive imaging of the coronary arteries and great vessels. Submillimeter resolution, exquisite soft tissue contrast, and arbitrary imaging planes are now possible without ionizing radiation [4]. MRI provides flexible imaging capability by combining the chemical sensitivity of nuclear magnetic resonance with high spatial and temporal resolution. The potential of MRI lies in its comprehensive ability to detect physical and chemical processes including flow, motion, morphology, and tissue composition. Its primary advantage is the lack of exposure to ionizing radiation or iodinated contrast media. In addition, MRA can be combined with other techniques to assess cardiac function, structure, blood flow, and viability.

While the potential of MRI has been at least partially realized in GV-MRA, routine clinical implementation of coronary MR angiography (C-MRA)

Cardiac CT, PET and MR, 2nd edition. Edited by Vasken Dilsizian and Gerry Pohost. © 2010 Blackwell Publishing Ltd.

has not been widespread [5]. Challenges still remain including decreasing scan time, improving spatial resolution and increasing the robustness of C-MRA. This chapter addresses the challenges facing both C-MRA and GV-MRA by examining the recent technical advances, resultant clinical implementation, and future development.

Challenges

Optimal spatial and temporal resolution, accurate motion compensation, wide anatomical coverage, and high signal and contrast-to-noise ratios (SNR and CNR) are the inherent challenges in C-MRA [6]. Improvement in one imaging parameter usually occurs at the expense of another. Imaging the coronaries is challenging because the coronaries are small in size (<4 mm) and tortuous, competing MRI signals arise from adjacent tissues, and constant dyssynchrony exist between cardiac and respiratory motions [6]. Other factors that have limited clinical application of both C-MRA and GV-MRA, especially in the acute setting, include restricted patient access, need for transportation to the scanner, longer examination time and the question of adequate cardiac and respiratory monitoring during the scan [7]. New technical developments may facilitate routine application of MRA in the clinical setting.

Technical Advances in Coronary MRA

Hardware Development

Improvements in the gradient strength, receiver coil design, and the magnetic field (strength, homogeneity, and capability) have been critical in coronary MRA (C-MRA). A major advancement has been the development of high performance gradient systems. Higher peak gradient strength and slew rate have enabled imaging with higher temporal and spatial resolution [8]. In spiral C-MRA, for example, earlier gradient systems (amplitude 10 mT/m with a slew rate of 16 mT/m/ms] have yielded a spatial resolution of 1.1–1.3 mm [9], whereas, the newer high-performance gradient system (amplitude 40 mT/m with a slew rate of 150 mT/m/ms] have yielded a resolution in the range of 0.5–0.6 mm [10]. The latest high-performance gradient system

can reach an amplitude of 50 mT/m with a slew rate of 200 mT/m/ms.

Another area of recent innovation is receiver coil design, namely, the development of a 32-channel receiver array and customization of receiver coils for parallel imaging. When parallel MRI techniques were first introduced, the majority of clinical MRI scanners were able to acquire data simultaneously from four to six detector coils. Restrictions on the number of coils in the array have limited the image acceleration and have also led to degradation of image quality. By using time domain multiplexing, an eight-channel receiver was subsequently developed and with further innovations, 16-, 24- and 32-channel receiver coils are now commercially available. Recently, a 128-channel receiver only coil was developed and evaluated at 3 T. Compared to the 24- and 32-channel coils at 3 T, signal-to-noise ratio (SNR) was similar but there was a sevenfold and twofold increase in acceleration for the 24- and 32-channel coil respectively [11]. Current research has also focused on customizing sensitivity profiles of individual detectors and exploring novel geometric arrangements [12].

In addition, imaging at higher fields has improved SNR although the gains are not directly proportional to increases in field strength [13]. High-field imaging, however, presents new technical challenges. The readout duration is limited by larger susceptibility effects, leading to off-resonance blurring [14,15]. Radio-frequency (RF) pulses and echo time (TE) need to be shortened to improve both flow characteristics and T_2 signal loss [16,17]. Slice profile may worsen, leading to partial volume effect. Magnetic field inhomogeneity could also lead to significant difficulties depending on the imagine sequence. Imaging parameters, including timing parameters and flip angles, need to be adjusted [18].

Despite these technical challenges, high-field imaging holds promise. Multiple imaging techniques for C-MRA have been successfully implemented at 3 T [19]. Feasibility was first demonstrated using a 3D-segmented gradient echo (GRE) with respiratory navigator, yielding an in-plane resolution of 0.7–1.0 mm and an average time per scan of 7 minutes [20]. A recent comparison of spiral GRE C-MRA at 1.5 and 3 T showed a significant improvement in overall SNR, CNR, and image quality of the coronary anatomy at 3 T [19] although there was an increase in susceptibility artifacts due to sensitivity of spiral imaging to off-resonance effects. Comparative 1.5 T vs 3 T images are shown in Figure 7.1 [19]. A 3D breath-hold steady-state free precession (SSFP) [21] sequence has also been demonstrated at 3 T. Compared to 1.5 T, however, image quality at 3 T was more variable, with an increase susceptibility artifacts and local brightening as a result of increased field inhomogeneities.

Most recently, parallel imaging techniques have been applied to C-MRA at high fields to capitalize on the higher SNR. One study [22] using a 3D navigator-gated C-MRA at 3 T demonstrated improved spatial resolution and coverage with a decrease in scan. Image quality was preserved although SNR gains were not equal to those gained using nonparallel imaging techniques [Figure 7.2]. Please refer to the section on Advanced Methods for additional details on the evaluation of C-MRA at 3 T.

Software Development

Significant improvement in MRA has also resulted from the development of motion compensation techniques, pulse sequences, k-space acquisition strategies, and methods to enhance CNR. Sequence implementation has been performed in 2D as well as 3D. More recent innovations, including parallel and real-time imaging, have led to further enhancement of MRA. These imaging techniques are discussed in detail in the Advanced Methods section below.

Motion Compensation Techniques

New techniques for motion compensation have been developed to improve image quality and scan efficiency. Accurate cardiac and respiratory gating is critical for coronary MRA. Cardiac gating, as well as patient monitoring, requires precise electrocardiogram (ECG) triggering which can be challenging in the MRI environment. The reliability of ECG gating has been improved by suppressing interference from the RF pulses [23] and gradient switching noise [24], applying advanced algorithms [25] to detect the time of rapid ventricular depolarization (QRS complex) and using a vector cardio-gram reconstructed from multiple ECG channels [26].

The ideal acquisition window needs to minimize cardiac motion while ensuring that enough information is collected so that overall scan time is not too long. Thus, images are generally acquired during the most quiescent time in diastole which is defined by a trigger delay, a delay chosen from the R wave. The trigger delay can be determined by the patient's heart rate [27], from a time resolved prescan [28,29] or adjusted during the acquisition to account for changes in the R-R interval [30]. Some have advocated using a different trigger delay for the right and left coronary arteries [31]. An alternative approach [32] is to collect information during a longer acquisition period and perform cardiac motion correction during the reconstruction.

Respiratory motion compensation has also evolved from simple breath-hold, which is adequate for 2D implementation, to more complex free-breathing and navigator-echo techniques [33]. The most widely used navigator to monitor respiration is the 2D RF excitation pulse which is used to acquire a longitudinal cylinder of tissue through the posterior part of the diaphragm. The diaphragm position is extracted from the navigator using edge detection algorithms. The superior–inferior respiratory motion of the heart is then estimated from the superior inferior position of the diaphragm. The navigator can also be used to detect the anterior and posterior motion of the chest wall. Once the respiratory motion is defined, additional methods, including gating and correction methods, are used to suppress the motion's effect on the images. The gating method acquires images only when the amplitude of detected motion falls within the gating window. Both retrospective and prospective methods have been implemented.

More recently, a novel approach for both cardiac and respiratory gating has been developed. Larson *et al.* [34] introduced a promising new approach called self-gating that may make ECG gating, breath-holding and navigator techniques obsolete. In self-gating, motion synchronization signal is extracted directly from the same MRI signals used for image reconstruction, making ECG gating unnecessary. A study [34] in seven volunteers showed no significant difference in image quality of cine MRI obtained by self-gating and conventional

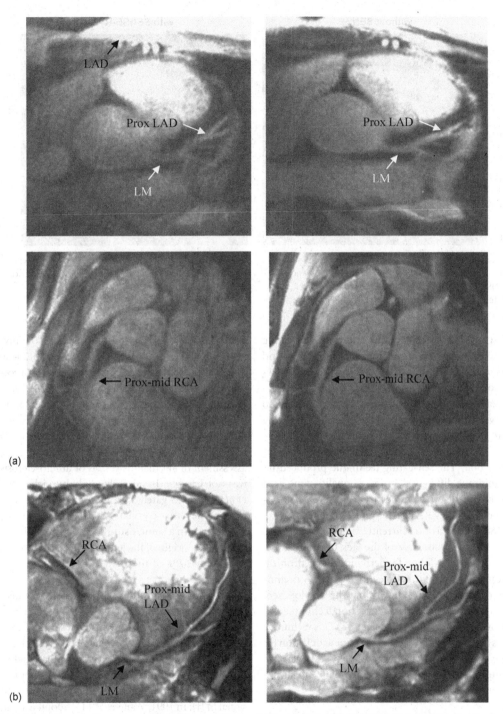

Figure 7.1 (a) Comparative images of the left main (LM) and left anterior descending artery (LAD) at 1.5 T (top, left) and 3 T (top, right) and the right coronary artery (RCA) at 1.5 T(bottom, left) and 3 T (bottom, right) using 2D breath-hold spiral GRE. (b) Comparative images of the LAD using 3D breath-hold SSFP. Higher SNR and anatomic coverage was achieved at 3 T. (Reproduced from Yang *et al.* [19], and Deshpande *et al* [21], Northwestern University, Chicago.)

without SENSE

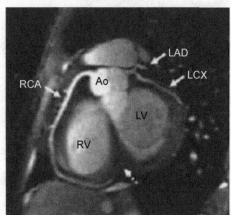

(a)

with SENSE-R=2

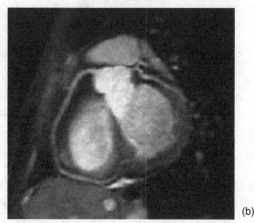

(b)

Figure 7.2 An example of a right coronary artery system obtained in a healthy subject without SENSE (a) and with SENSE (b). The application of SENSE did not affect detection of distal segments of the right coronary artery

(RCA); Ao, aorta; LAD, left anterior descending artery; LCX, left circumflex artery; LV, left ventricle; RV, right ventricle. (Reproduced from Huber *et al*. [22].)

ECG gating techniques. In addition, self-gating can eliminate the need for breath-holding and navigator techniques. Using self-gating, low-resolution images are acquired during the free-breathing acquisition and are then compared to target expiration images. Only raw data-producing images with high correlation to the target images are included in the final high-resolution reconstruction. The self-gating technique produced no significant differences in image quality compared to breath-held techniques [35]; however, demonstration in C-MRA has not yet been published.

Self-gating is not currently used in the clinical setting mainly because of the lack of robust postprocessing algorithms for deriving the synchronization signals from the self-gating signals. A preliminary study [36] has shown that the development of a more complex trigger detection technique improves accuracy of signal detection. This technique has been successfully applied for cine acquisition for the assessment of chamber function and anatomy. Future studies are still needed to evaluate this technique for coronary MRA.

Pulse Sequence Design

Pulse sequence design has evolved from black blood, spine echo (SE) sequences to bright blood sequences such as GRE and (SSFP). The SE sequence generates images in which blood pool appears dark

relative to surrounding soft tissue such as the myocardium [37]. In SE, an initial pulse (TE 20–30 ms) excites the sensitive proton, followed by a second T_2-weighted refocusing pulse (TE 50–90 ms) to produce a coherent signal [38]. Implementation of SE for C-MRA began in the 1980s but was met with limited success. Although SE was occasionally successful at imaging the coronary ostia, reliable assessment of anomalous vessels or atherosclerosis was not feasible. In an early study by Lieberman *et al*. [39], ECG gated SE could only visualize portions of the native coronary arteries in only 30% of 23 subjects. In a similar study, Paulin *et al*. [40] visualized the origin of the left main in all six subjects while only 67% of the right coronary ostia were seen.

Improved visualization with a shorter acquisition can be achieved with fast SE. In fast SE, a long train of echoes is acquired by using a series of 180° RF pulses [41]. A superior black blood effect can be achieved by applying preinversion pulses (additional RF pulses outside the plane used to suppress signal of inflowing blood and to nullify the blood signal [42]). In 1991, Wang *et al*. [43] adopted a fast, breath-hold inversion recovery technique for C-MRA that overcame the respiratory artifacts associated with previous attempts at coronary imaging. Multiple phase encodes per cardiac cycle and incremental flip angle compensated for spin saturation.

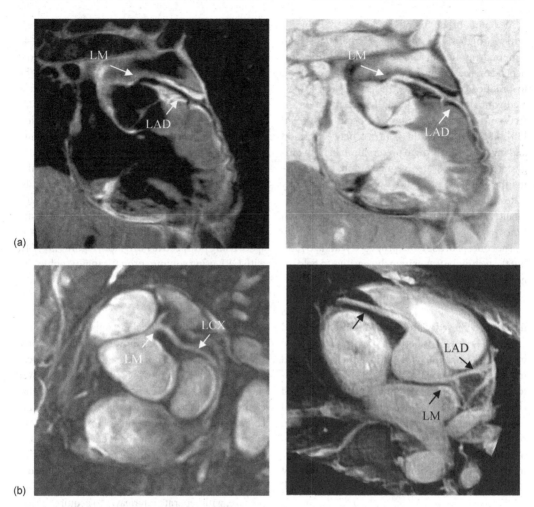

Figure 7.3 Sample images using different pulse sequences: (a) 3D double oblique free-breathing dual inversion fast spin echo, black-blood coronary MRA of a left coronary system in a healthy subject reformatted in the original data set (top, left). The same image data are displayed video inverted (top, right). The figure shows the left main coronary artery (LM) and the left anterior descending artery (LAD). (b) Breath-hold 3D SSFP of the left circumflex artery (LCX) (left). (Reproduced from Stuber *et al.* [45], Deshpande *et al.* [46], and Wielopolski *et al.* [47].)

Successful imaging of the left anterior descending and diagonal branches were achieved. Adding a second prepulse to null the fat signal (dual inversion) has resulted in higher SNR, CNR, and spatial resolution [44]. Ten years later, Stuber *et al.* [45] developed a fast, dual inversion, navigator-gated SE sequence with 400 um in-plane resolution for C-MRA as shown in Figure 7.3.

In contrast to the SE and dual inversion FSE sequences, the GRE sequence produces an increased signal intensity of blood pool (bright blood). The bright blood signal on GRE images results from flow related enhancement obtained by applying RF pulses to saturate a volume of tissue. With a short TR (20–40 ms) and a low flip angle, maximal signal is emitted by inflowing blood [48,49]. The first robust approach to C-MRA utilized GRE, initially described in an isolated heart and an in vivo animal model by Burstein *et al.* [50] and subsequently in humans by Edelman *et al.* [51]. Currently, GRE is the chosen acquisition scheme in the vast majority of reported C-MRA studies [52–57].

A second bright blood technique, SSFP [58], achieves high tissue contrast yet maintains high temporal resolution. Unlike GRE, SSFP does not depend on the inflow of unsaturated spins or blood to produce contrast; thus, the signal loss associated with slow flow, resulting from saturation effects common in GRE, does not occur with SSFP [38]. SSFP enhances the contrast between blood and myocardium through preservation of both longitudinal and transverse magnetizations by refocusing the gradients in all three axes [59]. The steady state achieved by the magnetization provides high-quality images using both T_1 and T_2 relaxation times [60,61].

The concept of SSFP was proposed years ago [58], but the technique was extremely sensitive to field inhomogeneities and, thus, not applicable to cardiac imaging [46]. With recent improvement in gradient capabilities, short TRs on the order of 3–4 ms have been achieved. Combined with improved field capabilities, SSFP has become practical for cardiac imaging. Deshpande *et al.* [46] first demonstrated increase in SNR (55%), CNR (178%) and anatomical coverage using 3D-SSFP [Figure 7.3] and compared it with 3D-GRE in volunteers. Several modifications to the original sequence have been performed to improve image quality including addition of intrinsic/extrinsic contrast [62,63], asymmetric sampling (GRE occurs before the center of the readout period) [21], and parallel imaging [64].

k-space Acquisition

In an effort to improve scan efficiency, k-space acquisition strategies have evolved from rectilinear segmented k-space to more complex echo planar, spiral imaging, and radial imaging [9,65–67].

Over the last decade, rectilinear segmented k-space imaging has dominated C-MRA [43,49]. In rectilinear segmented k-space, multiple phase encoding steps are acquired during the cardiac cycle. Successful visualization of native coronary arteries has been demonstrated in numerous studies using 2D-segmented k-space [52–57,68,69]. However, limited anatomical coverage was shown using this technique.

Echo-planar imaging (EPI) was developed over two decades ago to improve scan efficiency [70]. Instead of acquiring multiple segmented k-space lines per cardiac cycle, EPI acquires the complete data sets to rapidly form a complete image within 30–40 ms; however, flow and susceptibility phase errors can severely degrade image quality [65]. With the introduction of segmented EPI [37], these phase errors are minimized. For fast breath-hold [71,72] or free-breathing 3D C-MRA [73], 2–4 excitation pulses are followed by a short EPI readout train, thus, taking advantage of the EPI speed while keeping the echo and acquisition time short to minimize artifacts related to flow and motion [38]. Feasibility of 3D-segmented EPI was first demonstrated by Wieloposki *et al.* [71]. More recently, successful implementation of 3D EPI with 3D-segmented k-space using prospective navigator [Figure 7.3] [74], with GRE using volume coronary angiography with targeted scans [75], and with inversion recovery with extrinsic contrast enhancement [76] has been shown.

Variations of the original EPI approach may provide great potential in cardiovascular applications. Interleaved or multishot EPI significantly reduces image artifacts by employing several echoes to cover the data space [37]. Other techniques to more efficiently cover data space and reduce flow artifacts include "partial flyback" and "inside-out" EPI [77]. In "partial flyback" EPI, only the even echoes near the center of k-space are used, reducing artifacts arising from flow in the readout direction. In "inside-out" EPI, data collection begins at the center of k-space, with separate interleaves to acquire the top and bottom halves of k-space, reducing artifacts arising from flow in the phase encoding region. A combination of "partial flyback" and "inside out" with partial Fourier EPI demonstrates better flow properties and does not require partial k-space reconstruction [77].

Another k-space acquisition strategy for rapid imaging is the spiral acquisition technique adapted to C-MRA by Meyer *et al.* in 1992 [9]. This non-Cartesian acquisition technique generates images by sampling the data space from the center and spiraling outward, providing several advantages [65]. Image artifacts are reduced because of lower sensitivity to flow by using a short TE [9]. In comparison to EPI, spirals are less sensitive to flow-dependent phase shifts [78]. In addition, spirals achieve higher SNR because fewer excitations per heartbeat are required, allowing application of larger flip angles [9,79]. Data space coverage of EPI and spiral acquisition techniques with comparative images of the right coronary artery using identical GRE pulse sequence are depicted in Figure 7.4. Spirals also provide more efficient k-space coverage, resulting in shorter acquisition time [79]. Thus, blurring from coronary artery motion often seen in segmented k-space strategies is reduced. Improved spatial resolution is obtained through full k-space coverage instead of partial k-space coverage as used in the segmented approach. Meyer *et al.* [9] achieved a spatial resolution of 0.5×0.5 mm^2 with an acquisition time of 37 ms using spiral acquisition compared to a spatial resolution of $1.4–1.9 \times 0.9$ mm^2 with an acquisition time of 78–104 ms using 2D segmented GRE [6]. Several studies have confirmed improved temporal and spatial resolution in C-MRA using the spiral k-space acquisitions [79–82]. In 1997, Hu *et al.* introduced a multislice 2D spiral acquisition sequence which imaged 5–15 slices with 3–5 cm in thickness while maintaining acquisition time of 37 ms per slice during a single breath-hold [10,83]. Sample images using the 2D breath-hold spiral GRE technique with real-time (RT) localization are shown in Figure 7.4. However, spiral imaging has its drawbacks, namely, sensitivity to off-peak resonance, field inhomogeneity and susceptibility artifacts. [79–81].

Another non-Cartesian strategy for k-space sampling is radial imaging which defines the k-space trajectory by a set of radial lines starting from the origin of the coordinate system. Radial k-space sampling has been shown to be less susceptible to motion artifacts [66,67] caused by respiratory and cardiac motion. In addition, the robust undersampling of point spread function [84] enables the aliasing to appear as streaks as opposed to severe ghost images with Cartesian sampling. Thus, radial imaging allows a high degree of undersampling which permits scan time to be reduced to a single breath-hold for targeted volume acquisition and whole heart imaging [85,86]. Short readout times and echo times also enable faster imaging. However, image reconstruction from radial data requires a nonuniform quadratic weighting of data along a radial line, which results in a loss of SNR by a factor of 0.81 compared to Cartesian k-space sampling [87]. In addition, standard implementation does not support anisotropic field of view shapes which are used to match the imaging parameters to the object of interest. Recently, a set of fast simple algorithms was introduced to match the sampling density in the frequency space for the desired field of view shape reducing artifacts and scan times and imaging of elongated regions or thin slabs.

Intrinsic/Extrinsic Contrast Agents

Both intrinsic and extrinsic contrast agents have been used to differentiate blood and surrounding tissue (myocardial fat and myocardium). The intrinsic contrast between coronary blood pool and surrounding tissue can be altered by using the effect of inflowing blood or by application of prepulses [38]. Because most epicardial arteries are surrounded by fat, fat must be suppressed for coronary visualization. Selective fat suppression is performed using a fat saturation prepulse [52,68] or a spectral spatial RF pulse [88]. Because fat has a relatively short T_1 with a resultant signal intensity similar to flowing blood, frequency selective fat saturation prepulses are used to minimize fat signal and, thus, allow coronary visualization [52,68]. Spectral spatial pulse, used in spiral acquisitions, suppresses fat by selectively exciting water [88].

Coronaries are also located close to myocardium. T_1 relaxation times between blood and myocardium are similar [38]. Muscle suppression employing magnetization transfer (MT) [68,89] and T_2 preparation (T_2 prep) improve intrinsic contrast [78,90]. In MT saturation, an off resonance RF pulse is used to saturate bound protons, which in turn, transfer their magnetization to mobile protons in the muscle, thus, reducing the signal strength of muscle. Short MT pulses, however, do not affect flowing blood [89]. Li *et al.* [68] adopted this technique in 3D imaging. Improved MT pulse designs using the Shinnar–Le Roux algorithm, adiabatic pulses and off-resonance spectral spatial pulses are under investigation [91–93]. Another intrinsic contrast mechanism, T_2 prep, induces T_2-weighted imaging using a train of refocusing 180° excitations. Brittain *et al.* [78] developed and demonstrated this contrast mechanism for coronary imaging. Successful implementation by Botnar *et al.* [69] followed, as shown in Figure 7.5. Additional RF pulse

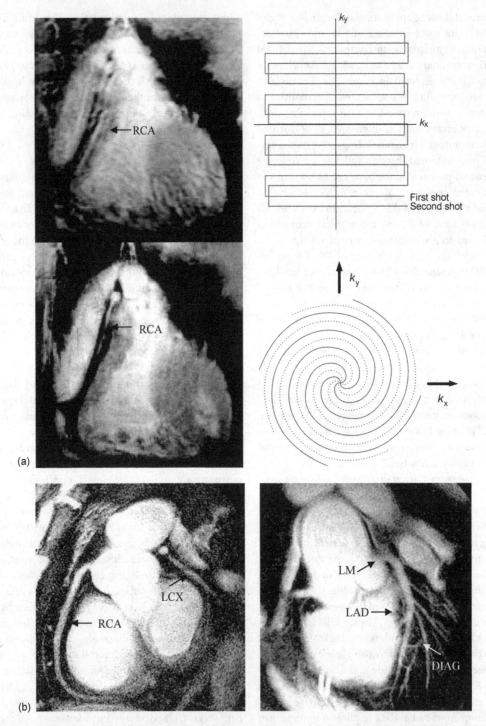

Figure 7.4 (a) Coronary MRA of the right coronary artery (RCA) using echo planar imaging and spiral GRE. (b) Two-dimensional breath-hold spiral GRE images of the RCA and the left circumflex (LCX) (left) and left main (LM), left anterior descending artery (LAD) and diagonals (DIAG) (right). (Reproduced from Meyer *et al.* [10], Stanford University.)

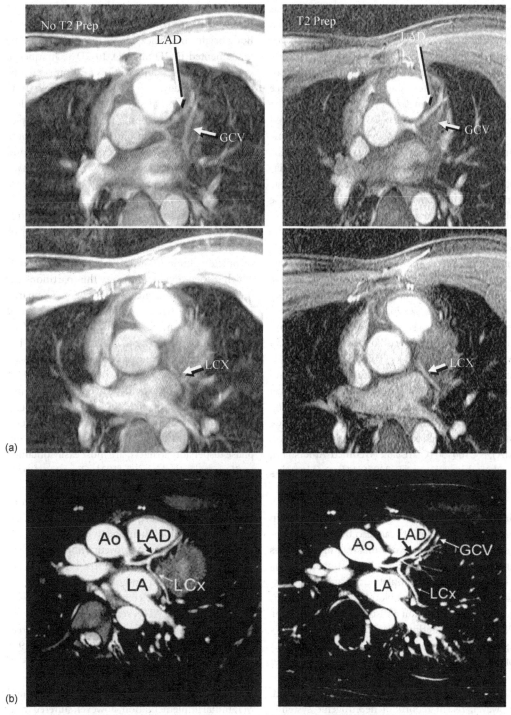

Figure 7.5 (a) Baseline images (left) and T_2 prepulse enhanced images (right) using a three-dimensional, free-breathing GRE sequence. T_2 prepulse suppresses signal from the cardiac muscle as well as skeletal muscle. .(b) T_2 prep enhanced images (right) using a three-dimensional free-breathing GRE and after administration of an intravascular contrast agent, B2256 (left). Ao, aorta; GCV, greater cardiac vein; LA, left atrium; LAD, left anterior descending artery; LCX, left circumflex artery. (Reproduced from Botnar et al. [69] and Paetsch et al. [301]. Cardiology, German Heart Institute, Berlin)

design work to enhance CNR from T_2 prep has been ongoing, including shorter duration, paired adiabatic pulses, and selective excitation [94]. For example, nonuniform magnetization preparation by T_2 prep at 3 T has prompted the development of a new adiabatic refocusing T_2 prep [95] sequence in which the magnetization is tipped into the transverse plane with a hard RF pulse and refocused using a pair of adiabatic fast-passage RF pulses. Improved quantitative and qualitative coronary MRA image measurement was achieved using the adiabatic T_2 prep at 3 T. One shortcoming of intrinsic contrast mechanisms, however, is the compromise of SNR in higher resolution images.

Extrinsic contrast agents may alleviate some of the problems of reduced SNR. The T_1 shortening effects of the agents enhance contrast without significant signal loss. Several studies have demonstrated significantly improved CNR using gadolinium agents [23,76,96]. Most recently, in a preliminary study, a slow infusion of a gadolinium analog contrast agent was successfully applied in whole heart imaging [97]. Gadolinium, however, is an extravascular contrast agent and quickly diffuses into the intracellular space, limiting its clinical utility in C-MRA. Several intravascular pooling agents which have undergone clinical trials include MS-325 (Angiomark; EPIX medical, Cambridge, MA), NC100150 (Clariscan; Nycomed-Amersham, Buckingshire, UK), and B-22956/1 (Bracco Imaging Spa, Milano, Italy). While only phase I and II trial results are available, significant improvement in CNR has been observed [74,98–100] as demonstrated in Figure 7.5. These agents can also be applied to inversion pulse and/or myocardial nulling sequences and may enable fluoroscopic, projectional imaging of the coronaries if complete myocardial suppression is achieved. The first blood pool contrast agent gadofosveset trisodium (Vasovist, Bayer Schering Pharma AG, Berlin, Germany) was recently approved in Europe for contrast-enhanced MRA of the vessels in the abdomen, pelvis, and lower extremity in adults [101]. Application in the coronaries and great vessels has not yet been studied. However, recent reports of nephrogenic systemic sclerosis associated with gadolinium administration have created less enthusiasm for additional research in enhanced MRA using gadolinium based contrast agents.

Two-dimensional and Three-dimensional Imaging

Both bright and black blood techniques may be implemented in 2D and 3D. In 2D techniques, a series of thin, overlapping slices (<2 mm) are obtained sequentially. This technique provides strong blood to background signal in conditions of slow flow. Although 2D techniques are easy to implement, several limitations, including partial volume effects, poor overall SNR, slice misregistration, and long scan times, exist which can result in image blurring and inadequate coverage of the coronary tree [6].

These limitations, particularly slice misregistration, can be resolved by using 3D [68,69,102] or 2D multislice acquisitions [10]. In 3D imaging, a complete volume or single slab is acquired [103] which is then divided into very thin partitions using a second, phase encoding gradient. The partitions are reconstructed with slice thickness equal or less than 1 mm, finer than 2D techniques. The 3D technique is effective for relatively fast flow, because blood can be pulsed several times and loses its signal before it traverses the width of the slab [103], allowing for extended coverage of anatomical structures, improved SNR, isotropic spatial resolution and a variety of postprocessing techniques. Small voxels and short TE, which reduce flow and phase dispersion artifacts, are most easily obtained in 3D imaging techniques [103]. Operator dependence is also diminished [38]. Three-dimensional techniques, however, usually result in reduced contrast and prolonged acquisition, much longer than any patient can hold their breath [38,104].

These hurdles were removed with the application of suppression pulses and free-breathing navigator techniques, in addition, to the recent development of volume coronary angiography with targeted scans (VCATS), resulting in a widespread adoption of 3D-acquisition techniques [38]. Three-dimensional implementation began as early as 1993 when a free-breathing method using averages of multiple acquisitions enabled Li *et al.* [68] to image a 64-mm thick volume using fat saturation and MT. Initial implementation, however, suffered from poor contrast between blood and myocardium. Botnar *et al.* [69] then used T_2 prep to shorten the acquisition window and achieved improved contrast and coronary delineation. Stuber *et al.*

[105] subsequently successfully combined a 3D-segmented *k*-space and EPI acquisition technique with prospective navigator gating to reduce the long acquisition time associated with traditional 3D techniques. Comparable results were obtained by Deshpande *et al.* [46] using 3D VCATS and SSFP (spatial resolution 1.7 mm × 1 mm; acquisition time of 95 ms). In addition to the 3D volume techniques, a different approach utilizing 2D multislice was developed using spiral acquisition by Hu *et al.*. [10].

Advanced Methods

Despite many advances over the past decades, SNR and the speed of data acquisition remain limited. To overcome these limitations, a number of novel strategies have been developed including RT, parallel, time resolved, and whole heart imaging.

Real-time Imaging

RT imaging was developed from a rapid acquisition method using EPI [106]. RT imaging enables continuous image acquisition at high frame rates, providing valuable insights into cardiovascular dynamics and eliminating the need for respiratory and cardiac gating. Data acquisition techniques such as wavelet encoding, sliding reconstruction windows [5], and innovative *k*-space acquisition techniques [9,37] have facilitated rapid data acquisition, thereby, allowing frame rates up to 12 frames per second at 2.0 mm resolution [107]. A clinically robust, reliable RT system has been developed which enables interactive selection of scan planes and provided RT image reconstruction and display for instantaneous image-based feedback [108]. The rapid access of raw data and direct control of reconstruction and display generates interactive images with lag-time of less than 500 ms. RT localization to acquire high-resolution coronary images has been successfully demonstrated [83,109,110].

Another innovative RT approach is the implementation of C-MRA using the adaptive RT architecture [111]. This integrated system dynamically reconfigures pulse sequences on a per-acquisition basis and switches between the coil elements in the phased arrays in RT. The conventional MR scanners consist of sequencers that proceed through each acquisition based on downloaded waveforms and timing commands. Utilizing a modern PC, a sequencer that is capable of running selected parameters of different pulse sequences simultaneously has been designed. Utilizing this system, the operator can switch dynamically between spiral RT localization and high-resolution imaging in 39 ms, which allows adjustment of scan planes to optimize high-resolution image acquisition [Figure 7.6]. In addition to RT localization, high-resolution RT C-MRA has been achieved at 3 T with a spatial resolution of 1.25 mm^2 and a temporal resolution of 190 ms [18].

Parallel Imaging

Another novel approach is parallel imaging, first introduced in 1997 to increase temporal resolution. The two most common parallel imaging methods are simultaneous acquisition of spatial harmonics (SMASH) [112,113] and spatial sensitivity encoding (SENSE) [114]. These techniques accelerate image acquisition by factors of 2–3 by using spatial encoding information from sensitivity maps of multiple coil arrays, thereby, allowing partial *k*-space sampling [38]. The remaining lines of *k*-space are reconstructed using the sensitivity information from individual coil elements. Parallel image encoding can be combined with common MRA approaches [64,115–117]. The gain in imaging speed may be used for larger volume acquisition without longer acquisition time, resulting in greater anatomic coverage [64,116]. Parallel imaging has also been combined with RT to increase frame rate [118].

The potential disadvantages of parallel encoding include extended computation power, requirement for prescanning, reduced SNR, and potential artifacts in reconstruction. The SNR reduction is more critical for coronary imaging given its lower scanning efficiency and need for high resolution, thus, potentially limiting its application for C-MRA. Although feasibility was initially demonstrated at 1.5 T, preliminary results have not been satisfactory despite a reported 50% reduction in acquisition time [117,119]. More encouraging results have been seen at 3 T by Huber *et al.* [22] who demonstrated a twofold decrease in acquisition time while maintaining equivalent SNR and image quality using 3D navigator-gated segmented GRE. The use of intravascular contrast agents has also improved anatomic coverage in parallel imaging although the loss of SNR and CNR is not fully recovered

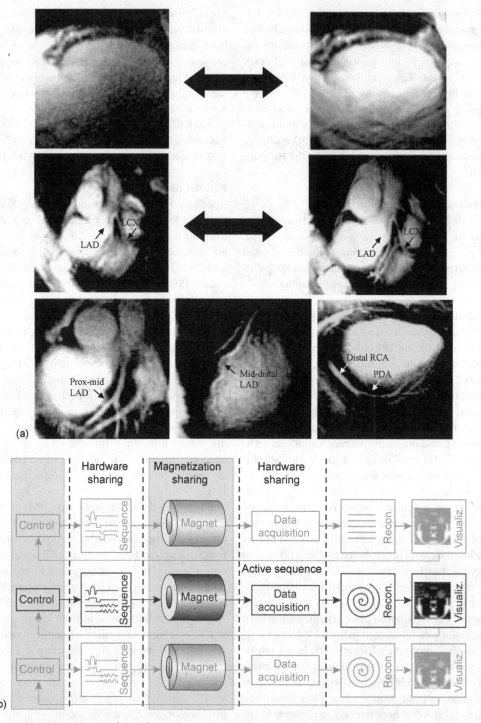

Figure 7.6 (a) Real-time images of the left anterior descending artery (LAD) and left circumflex artery (LCX) demonstrating optimization of scan plane localization during breath-hold (middle row). High-resolution images of the proximal-mid LAD (bottom, left), mid-distal LAD (bottom, middle) and distal right coronary artery (RCA) and posterior descending artery (PDA) (bottom, right). (b) Structure of the adaptive real-time architecture that enables dynamic selection of different pulse sequences and coils.

[120]. Several investigators have recently demonstrated the utility of multielement array coils with a high intrinsic SNR and spatial encoding capability [121,122]. A preliminary study by Nierendorf et al. [116] achieved higher SNR and greater anatomic coverage using a 32-channel array versus 4 and 8 multichannel arrays with the same acquisition time, as shown in Figure 7.7.

Another potential disadvantage for parallel imaging is the need for a separate scan to determine coil sensitivities. Because coronaries move within the heart, separate coil sensitivities scans can lead to misregistration between the coil and cardiac breath-hold positions which results in residual aliasing artifacts and random noise in the reconstructed images [64]. Implementation of auto-calibration methods such as AUTO-SMASH [123] and generalized auto-

calibrating partially parallel acquisition (GRAPPA) [124] can enhance spatial resolution by reducing aliasing artifacts. GRAPPA reconstruction provides improved coronary artery definition with up to 0.7–1.0 mm × 0.7 mm in-plane resolution with acceptable artifact suppression and SNR. The use of segmented k-space coil calibration with variable density sampling enables coverage of almost twice the area of k-space along the phase encoding direction compared to that obtained in a conventional 3D breath-hold acquisition [64]. Self-calibrating parallel imaging has also been performed with non-Cartesian k-space sampling [115].

Time Resolved 3D Imaging (4D Imaging)

Coronary magnetic angiography is usually acquired during mid-diastole of each heartbeat to minimize

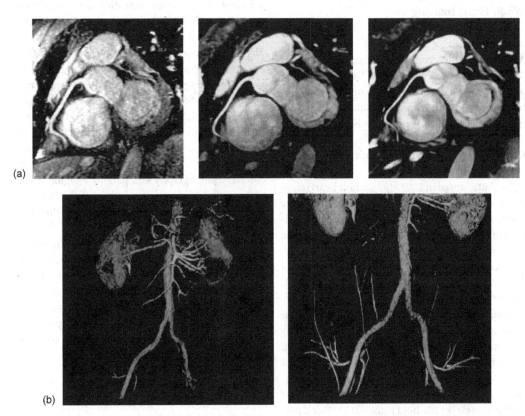

(a)

(b)

Figure 7.7 (a) Comparison of breath held 3D fiesta images of the right coronary artery (RCA) using 4-channel, 8-channel (20% increase in SNR), and 32-channel parallel imaging arrays (40% increase in SNR). With parallel imaging, the distal RCA is better visualized; (b) Contrast-enhanced MRA with parallel imaging of the abdominal aorta in a 22-second breath-hold with spatial resolution of 1.7 mm × 1.7 mm × 2.2 mm and acceleration factor of 12. Result corresponding to arterial phase (left); zoomed view of subsequent acquisition (right). (Reproduced from Niendorf et al. [116] and Zhu et al. [122])

cardiac motion related artifacts. A proper trigger delay must be determined for each patient for optimal acquisition. A time resolved acquisition (i.e., acquiring contiguous cardiac images through the cardiac cycle) has eliminated this complication. Bi et al.. [125] successfully acquired 3D cine coronary artery images at 3 T with high temporal resolution using radial sampling parallel acquisition and interleaved sliding window reconstruction. A recent study [126] also confirmed the feasibility of 4D magnetic resonance contast enhanced coronary angiography with 100 ms temporal resolution at 1.5 T using a whole heart imaging in pigs. CNR was 38% higher compared to conventional inversion recover GRE imaging, Additional clinical studies are needed to evaluate whether 4D imaging can be incorporated into current techniques.

Whole Heart Imaging

One of the major limitations of coronary MRA is the complexity of its application and long scan times. A comparison to computed tomography angiography highlights these limitations. Despite exposure to radiation and use of potentially nephrotoxic contrast agents, CTA is technically simpler, image acquisition is straightforward, and advanced software enables analysis in multiple planes. These features have increased its adoption in clinical settings relative to C-MRA.

First introduced in 2003 [127], whole heart imaging is a promising approach to simplify coronary MRA. Similar to CTA, the upper and lower boundaries of the heart are used to define a single imagine volume that includes the coronary arteries. Separate acquisitions for the coronary arteries are not needed. Not only does it simplify coronary MRA, improved visualization of all the coronary arteries compared with the standard techniques has also been shown. A whole heart imaging scan is typically 4 minutes in duration and utilizes free-breathing, navigator techniques. However, a preliminary study by [116] has successfully demonstrated comprehensive volumetric coverage of the coronary arteries within a single breath-hold using 3D SSFP and parallel imaging with a 32-channel receiver.

The major limitation of whole heart imaging is reduced spatial resolution. Despite the use of SSFP and parallel imaging, spatial resolution remains at 1.1 mm compared to 0.8 mm with standard

techniques. Increasing spatial resolution would require unacceptably long scan times. More recently, a slow infusion (0.3 mL/second) of a newly improved gadolinium agent has been applied to whole heart imaging to improve the depiction of coronary arteries with breath-hold MRA [97]. Ultrashort TR (3 ms) and parallel data acquisition were used to enable whole heat MRA in 5 minutes. Improved SNR and CNR were noted with average scan time of 4.5 minutes.

Comparison studies

Given the complexity of technical developments and the diverse range of innovations, a direct comparison of each technique is not feasible. Therefore, a summary of the various techniques developed for C-MRA is shown in Table 7.1. Unfortunately, little information is available regarding the comparative evaluation of MRA techniques in the same subjects. A recent study [128] comparing six free-breathing, 3D, magnetization prepared sequences found that the optimal sequence was the Cartesian SSFP followed by the spiral GRE (2 shots per heartbeat) and the radial SSFP in terms of visible vessel length and SNR and CNR. Evaluation, however, was performed only in the RCA. A preliminary study in 20 volunteers compared whole heart imaging with targeted volume acquisition using 3 T navigator coronary angiography and parallel imaging. Both techniques had similar navigator efficiencies and similar anatomic coverage but image quality was better with the targeted volume approach. The possible causes for the reduced image quality in whole heart imaging include increased variability of shimming over a larger volume and increased motion artifact which is more common with longer acquisition times. While investigators are appropriately attempting to generate a more unified approach, the most optimal sequence for C-MRA is yet to be determined.

Clinical Implementation of C-MRA

While high-quality images of the coronary arteries have been obtained with various techniques [Table 7.2] [6,19,47,53–57,68,69,74,102,127,129], clinical implementation has not achieved consistent coronary coverage, image quality, and disease detection.

Table 7.1 MRA methods.

Cardiac motion compensation	Breath-hold
	Free-breathing
Pulse sequences	
Black blood	Spin echo
	Double inversion recovery
Bright blood	Gradient recalled echo
	Steady-state free precession
Acquisition Strategies	
k-space acquisition	Rectilinear segmented *k*-space
	Echo planar imaging
	Spiral imaging
	Radial imaging
Contrast-enhanced MRA	Intrinsic contrast
	Extrinsic contrast
2D and 3D acquisitions	2D single slice
	2D multislice
	3D complete volume
	3D single slab
	3D volume targeted
Advanced techniques	Real-time imaging
	Parallel imaging
	Time resolved 3D imaging (4D imaging)
	Whole heart imaging

Currently, the only well defined role for C-MRA is in the diagnosis of coronary anomalies [38].

Anomalous Coronary Arteries

Unlike X-ray angiography, C-MRA provides a 3D spatial relationship to great vessels, allowing evaluation of the origin and course of anomalous coronaries and determining risk and possible surgical intervention [130]. The accuracy of coronary MRA for the identification of coronary anomalies has been shown in several studies. Accurate delineation of the proximal course has been shown with sensitivities of 88–100% and specificity of 100% [Table 7.3] [131–136]. MRI can often provide a definitive diagnosis in patients whose X-ray angiography is inconclusive [131,133].

Coronary Artery Disease

The role of C-MRA in the diagnosis and management of coronary artery disease (CAD) is still undefined. Clinical trials have produced variable results in the evaluation of native CAD [Table 7.4] [6,25,52,74,94,101,102,137–149,150–160] and bypass grafts [23,161–169]. Most clinical trials have utilized either 2D or 3D GRE. In GRE, rapidly moving blood with laminar flow appears bright while areas of stagnant flow or flow turbulence appear dark due to local saturation or dephasing. Amount of signal loss in areas of focal stenosis is thought to be proportionate to the degree of stenosis [170]. However, bright blood coronary MRA methods can sometimes be misleading [38]. Signal loss due to slow flowing blood distal to the lesion can occasionally be mistaken for a stenosis. Moreover, these techniques are insensitive to direction of blood; therefore, a stenosis will not be detected in a total occlusion that has adequate collateral or retrograde filling.

Initial implementation of C-MRA was performed by Manning and Edelman [6] using a 2D-segmented GRE. In a double-blinded study of 39 patients with suspected CAD, sensitivity and specificity were 90 and 92%, respectively. Subsequent trials using 2D-segmented GRE [6,54,170, 171] generated variable results with sensitivity of 53–90% and specificity of 56–92%. With the advent

Table 7.2   Visualization of native coronary arteries.

Reference	n	Technique	Respiratory compensation	RCA (%)	LM (%)	LAD (%)	LCX (%)
Manning and Edelman [6]	25	2D seg GRE	BH	100	96	100	76
Pennell et al. [53]	26	2D seg GRE	BH	95	95	91	76
Duerinckx and Urman [54]	20	2D seg GRE	BH	100	95	86	77
Sakuma et al. [55]	18	2D seg GRE cine	BH	100	100	100	67
Masui et al. [56]	13	2D seg GRE	BH	85	92	100	92
Davis et al. [57]	33*	2D seg GRE	BH	100	100	100	100
Yang et al. [19]	23	2D spiral GRE (1.5 and 3 T)	BH	100	100	100	100
Nguyen et al. [129]	14	2D spiral RT (3 T)	BH	100	100	100	100
Li et al. [68]	14	3D seg GRE	Multi averages	100	100	86	93
Post et al. [102]	20	3D seg GRE	retro nav	100	100	100	100
Botnar et al. [69]	32	3D seg GRE	pro nav	97	100	100	97
Stuber et al. [74]	15	3D seg, contrast GRE EPI	pro nav	100	100	100	100
Wielopolski et al. [47]	32	3D seg EPI	BH	100	100	100	100
Weber et al. [127]	12	3D seg SSFP, whole heart	pro nav	100	100	100	100

*Including 18 heart transplant recipients.

n, number of subjects; RCA, right coronary artery; LM, left main; LAD, left anterior descending artery; LCX, left circumflex; seg GRE, segmented gradient recalled echo; seg EPI, segmented echo planar imaging; RT, real-time; BH, breath-hold; retro nav, retrospective navigator-gated; pro nav, prospective navigator-gated; SSFP, steady-state free precession.

of free-breathing techniques, several centers have adopted 3D-GRE C-MRA [74,94,139–145,147] for ease of patient acceptance and improved SNR. Data from studies using 3D-segmented k-space have been recently published. Kim et al. [27] performed the first multicenter trial using 3D-segmented GRE with EPI in 109 patients with suspected CAD. Overall sensitivity and specificity was 93 and 42%, respectively in the proximal and mid segments with at least diagnostic image quality in 84% of the coronary segments. More recently, spiral acquisition has enabled the detection of distal stenosis

Table 7.3   Anomalous coronary MRA.

Reference	n	Technique	Correctly classified anomalous vessel (%)
McConnell et al. [132]	16	2D seg GRE, BH	14 (93)
Post et al. [135]	19	2D seg GRE, BH	19 (100)*
Vliegen et al. [133]	12	2D seg GRE, BH	11 (92)†
Taylor et al. [134]	16	3D seg GRE, navigator	14 (88)
Bunce et al. [131]	26	3D seg GRE, navigator	26 (100)‡
Gharib et al. [136]	12	3D seg GRE, navigator	9 (100)§

*Including three misclassified by X-ray angiography.
†Including five patients unable to be classified by angiography and one patient reclassified by MRA.
‡Including one patient unable to be classified by angiography and 11 patients whose course could not be defined by X-ray angiography.
§Only nine patients had X-ray angiography to confirm diagnosis; n, number of subjects; seg GRE, segmented GRE; BH, breath-hold.

Table 7.4 Summary of coronary MRA studies for detection of significant coronary artery disease (50% stenosis).

Reference	Technique	n	No. (%) vessels with stenosis	Overall sensitivity % (per vessel)	Overall specificity % (per vessel)
Manning and Edelman [6]	2D seg GRE, BH	39	52 (35)	90 (LM 100, LAD 87, LCX 71, RCA 100)	92 (LM 100, LAD 92, LCX 90, RCA 78)
Duerinckx and Urman [54]	2D seg GRE, BH	20	27 (34)	63 (LM 50, LAD 73, LCX 0, RCA 62)	56 (LM 56, LAD 84, LCX 37, RCA 82)
Post et al. [171]	2D seg GRE, BH	35	35 (28)	n/a (LM 100, LAD 53, LCX 0, RCA 71)	n/a (LM 93, LAD 73, LCX 96, RCA 82)
Pennell et al. [170]	2D seg GRE, BH	39	55 (35)	85 (LM, LAD 88, LCX 75, RCA 75–100)	n/a
Yang et al. [109]	2D spiral GRE, BH	40	31 (76)	76 (LM n/a, LAD 87, LCX 25, RCA 76)	91 (LM 100, LAD 88, LCX 89, RCA 79)
Yang et al. [110]	2D spiral GRE, BH	45	40 (22)	93 (LM 100, LAD 94, LCX 78, RCA 100)	88 (LM 93, LAD 83, LCX 89, RCA 84)
van Geuns et al. [75]	3D GRE, BH	38	39 (34)	68 (LM 77, LAD 77, LCX 50, RCA 64)	97 (LM 97, LAD 97, LCX 100, RCA 94)
Regenfus et al. [172]	3D CE-MRA, BH	50	59 (39)	94 (overall result)	57 (overall result)
Woodard et al. [173]	3D GRE, navigator	10	10 (30)	70–73 (overall result)	n/a
Kessler et al. [174]	3D GRE, navigator	73	87 (33)	65 (overall result)	88 (overall result)
Huber et al. [175]	3D GRE, navigator	20	53 (66)	73–79 (LM 75, LAD 62–71, LCX 67–80, RCA 86–89)	50–54 (LM 25–36, LAD 46–50, LCX 58–63, RCA 67–69)
Sandstede et al. [176]	3D GRE, navigator	30	37 (31)	81 (overall result)	89 (overall result)
Sardanelli et al. [177]	3D GRE, navigator	39	67 (43)	82 (prox segments 90, distal segments 68)	89 (prox segments 90, distal 81)
Post et al. [102]	3D GRE, retro navigator	20	21 (27)	63 (overall result)	89 (overall result)
Muller et al. [178]	3D GRE, retro navigator	35	54 (31)	83 (overall result)	94 (overall result)
Kim et al. [27]	3D, GRE EPI, free-breathing	109	58 (59)	93 (LM 67, LAD 88, LCX 53, RCA 93)	42 (LM 90, LAD 52, LCX 70, RCA 72)
Sommer et al. [179]	3D GRE, RT navigator, 1.5 T + 3 T*	18	17 (16)	82 (overall result)	88 (overall result)
So et al. [180]	3D, SSFP, BH navigator	15	49 (36)	80 (overall result for BH) 75 (overall result for navigator)	100 (overall result for BH) 100 (overall result for navigator)
Sakuma et al. [181]	Whole heart, 3D SSFP, navigator	131	95 (24)	82 (overall result)	90 (overall result)
Maintz et al. [182]	Whole heart, 3D, SSFP, navigator	15	n/a	82 (overall result)	88 (overall result)

*Although SNR and CNR increased for 3 T compared to 1.5 T, image quality and detection of stenosis were comparable.
n, number of subjects; GRE, gradient recalled echo; seg GRE, segmented GRE; EPI, echo planar imaging; SSFP, steady-state free precession; RT, real time; CE-MRA, contrast-enhanced magnetic resonance angiography; BH, breath-hold; retro navigator, retrospective navigator gated.

as well as proximal and mid disease. A prospective clinical trial [109] using 2D multislice spiral GRE of proximal, middle and distal segments in 40 patients generated a sensitivity of 79 and 90%, respectively. Implementation of a new dynamic architecture that allows optimization of scan plane localization in a clinical trial of 45 patients showed improved sensitivity and specificity of 93 and 88%, respectively [110]. Comparative MRI images using 2D-multislice spiral GRE, 3D-VCATS segmented FLASH and 3D-SSFP, along with their corresponding X-ray angiograms, are shown in Figure 7.8. In comparison with native coronaries, saphenous vein and internal mammary grafts are relatively easier to image due to their larger size and relatively stationery position; thus, relative to native coronaries, C-MRA of bypass grafts has a higher sensitivity, specificity and accuracy [38] [Table 7.5] [23,161–169].

Whole heart imaging has also undergone clinical validation. Sakuma *et al.* [181] have evaluated over 130 patients with significant CAD. Using patient specific acquisition periods, the study [181] found per patient sensitivity of 82% and specificity of 90%, with an overall accuracy of 87% which is similar to other single center studies using targeted volume techniques. Whole heart imaging was recently compared with CTA in 20 patients with CAD [182]. Whole heart imaging was inferior to CTA with regard to image quality and the number of interpretable segments, but both had similar diagnostic accuracy when only interpretable segments were included.

Technical Strategies Specific to GV-MRA

Several techniques previously described for C-MRA are also applied in GV-MRA including the traditional SE and GRE and the more advanced RT and parallel imaging techniques. Unlike for C-MRA where the application of SE is limited, conventional T_1-weighted SE has been the mainstay for great vessel imaging because it provides the best anatomic detail of the great vessel wall [7,183]. The advent of fast SE has enabled the implementation of T_2-weighted imaging, which may be useful in tissue characterization of the great vessel wall and blood components [7].

In GV-MRA, additional diagnostic information can be provided by cine GRE [184,185], which displays laminar-moving blood as a bright signal in contrast to stationary tissues [7]. Signal reduction [186,187] and signal voids [188] suggest anomalous flow disturbance and are associated with specific pathology. One major limitation of cine GRE, however, was a relatively lengthy imaging time per slice location compared with ECG-gated SE [137]. The typical imaging time for images with a 256 × 128 matrix with conventional cine GRE is 4–5 minutes (256 heartbeats). Performing cine GRE became more practical with the advent of fast cine GRE with k-space segmentation [49]; imaging time was reduced from 4 to 5 minutes to less than 16 seconds and flow and respiratory artifacts were minimized [138].

Additional techniques to reduce scan time, namely RT and parallel imaging, have been recently applied in GV-MRA. RT application in GV-MRA, however, has been limited. In a recent case series, successful visualization of the aortic arch and extracardiac shunts was demonstrated using RT color flow imaging [139]. More recently, parallel imaging has been applied to GV-MRA to visualize the abdomen [140,141] and thoracic vasculature [142]. In order to offset the acquisition and reconstruction related SNR losses associated with parallel imaging, several investigators have demonstrated the utility of multielement array coils with a high-intrinsic SNR and spatial encoding capability for GV-MRA [121,122]. Zhu *et al.* [122] demonstrated successful MRA of the abdominal aorta with up to 16-fold acceleration using a 32-element array, shown in Figure 7.7. Recent studies have also demonstrated improvement in image quality and acquisition speed with view sharing compared to without view sharing as shown in Figure 7.9 [143].

In addition to the techniques common to both C-MRA and GV-MRA, there are several strategies specific to GV-MRA including multiple overlapping thin slab acquisition (MOTSA), gadolinium-enhanced MRA associated with unique timing techniques, and projectional imaging. Like sequences for C-MRA, GV-MRA techniques can be implemented in 2D or 3D, usually bright blood techniques more commonly referred to as time of flight (TOF). In order to provide better flow enhancement than single slab 3D techniques and less

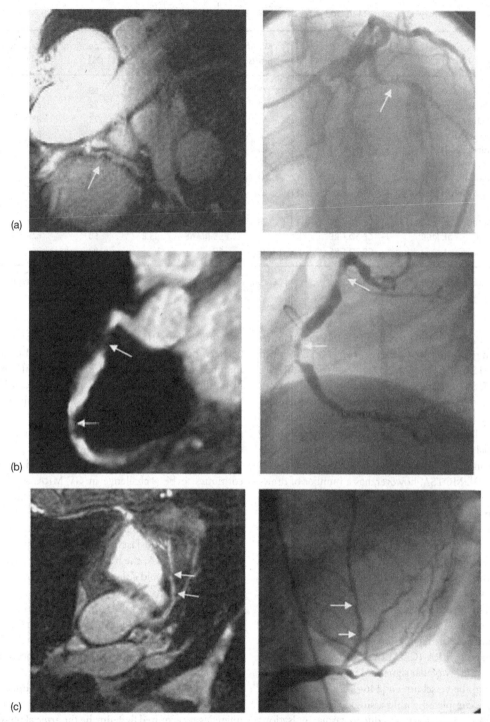

Figure 7.8 (a) 2D multislice breath-hold spiral GRE of a significant stenosis in the proximal left circumflex with corresponding X-ray angiogram. (b) 3D breath-hold (VCATS) segmented GRE of a significant stenosis in the mid right coronary artery with corresponding X-ray angiogram. (c) 3D SSFP of sequential high-grade lesions in the mid left anterior descending artery with corresponding X-ray angiogram. High grade stenosis denoted by arrows. (Reproduced with courtesy of P. Yang, Stanford, CA, Wiepolski *et al.* [71], R. McCarthy, D. Li, NWU, Chicago.)

Table 7.5   Summary of coronary MRA studies for detection of graft patency.

Reference	Technique	n	No. of grafts	Patency (%)	Sensitivity (%)	Specificity (%)	Accuracy (%)
White et al. [161]	2D spin echo	25	72	69	86	59	78
Rubenstein et al. [162]	2D spin echo	20	47	62	90	72	83
Jenkins et al. [142]	2D spin echo	16	41	63	89	73	83
Galjee et al. [164]	2D spin echo	47	98	74	98	85	89
White et al. [165]	2D GRE	28	28	50	93	86	89
Aurigemma et al. [166]	2D GRE	45	45	73	88	100	91
Galjee et al. [164]	2D GRE	47	98	74	98	88	96
Engelmann et al. [167]	2D GRE	40	55	100 (IMA)	100	100	
				66 (SVG)	92	85	89
Wintersperger et al. [168]	CE-3D GRE	27	76	79	95	81	95
Brenner et al. [169]	CE-3D GRE	85	222	95 (IMA)	93.8	50	n/a
Vrachliotis et al. [23]	CE-3D GRE	15	45	67	93	97	95

n, number of subjects; GRE, gradient recalled echo; CE, contrast enhanced; IMA, internal mammary artery; SVG, saphenous vein graft.

dephasing than 2D techniques while maintaining high resolution [144], Parker et al. [145] developed MOTSA, a hybrid of 2D and 3D techniques. In MOTSA, multiple thin 3D slabs are placed orthogonal to the direction of flow and acquired sequentially, as in 2D TOF. Because the slabs are relatively thin, blood can travel through the volume and the signal can be refreshed between RF pulses, resulting in better retention of signal in distal vessels [7,103]. MOTSA, however, has a number of drawbacks. First, to avoid bands of signal loss at the slab edges where the RF profile trails off, consecutive slabs are overlapped, which increases total scan time. Another disadvantage is that patient motion occurring between slab acquisitions is seen as discontinuity of the luminal edge that can be mistaken for stenosis. Moreover, signal intensity variations within the individual slabs due to saturation effects can cause a "venetian blind" artifact [103].

Instead of relying on blood flow, contrast-enhanced MRA (CE-MRA) utilize gadolinium to create intravascular signal and increase blood signal within the vessel lumen [146–148]. Because imaging is completed within a single breath-hold, CE-MRA eliminates artifacts due to cardiac pulsations and respiration and is more sensitive to in-plane flow, enabling more accurate detection of stenosis [149,150]. In CE-MRA, however, correct timing of injection is important to ensure synchronization between the transit of contrast material and scanning because gadolinium quickly diffuses into the intracellular space [151]. Accurate timing can be achieved by [152] estimating transit time, applying a small test bolus, and using an automated detection of contrast bolus passage or MR fluoroscopy to observe contrast bolus passage [153].

Because distinction between arteries and veins continues to be a challenge in GV-MRA, several innovative strategies have been recently developed to differentiate arterial and venous circulation in 3D CE-MRA including novel k-space acquisition techniques and ultra-fast imaging techniques [103]. Ideally in CE-MRA, the maximal arterial contrast enhancement should coincide with the acquisition of the center of k-space, which contains low spatial frequency information and controls image contrast [152,153]. In current sequences, the center of k-space are acquired at the midpoint of the acquisition period [154,155]; thus, timing of contrast injection can be challenging [153]. A new technique consists of applying a centric phased [156] or an elliptical centric encoding [157] where the lower spatial frequencies are acquired first, during the arterial phase of the contrast enhancement. This provides efficient venous signal suppression when the sequence is manually or automatically triggered at the arrival of

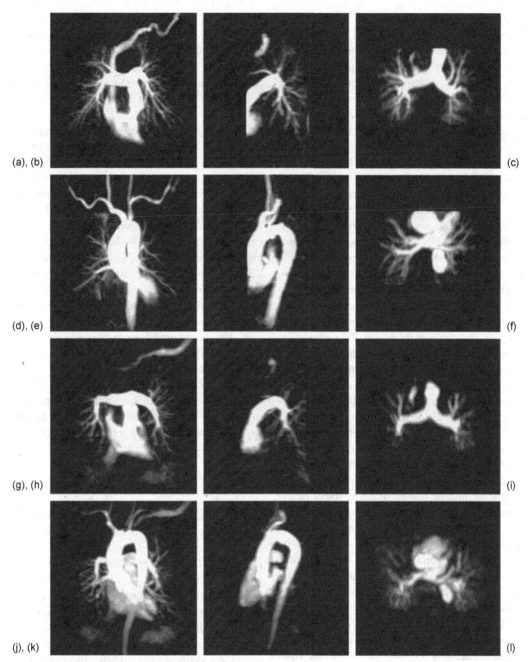

(a), (b)

(c)

(d), (e)

(f)

(g), (h)

(i)

(j), (k)

(l)

Figure 7.9 Maximum intensity projections (MIPs) of time-resolved MRA acquired with parallel imaging with view sharing (a–f) and conventional parallel-MRA protocol. MIPs were reconstructed from data sets with a peak-enhancement of the pulmonary artery (a–c and g–i) and aorta (d–f, j–l). Because of the better spatial resolution, images acquired with the parallel imaging with view sharing show a much sharper delineation of the vascular structures. (Reproduced from Fink *et al.* [142]).

contrast material, lessening motion artifact and venous contamination; however, poor timing of contrast injection time may be more common.

In addition to novel k-space acquisition strategies, ultra-fast imaging techniques including the time resolved imaging of contrast kinetics (TRICKS) [158] have been developed to differentiate arterial and venous circulation. TRICKS [152,159] involves sampling low spatial frequency information more frequently than high spatial information to create a 3D data set with the desired temporal window. This allows depiction of the passage of contrast agent, first through arteries then though the veins, similar to X-ray angiography. With this technique, only the center of k-space is acquired every 2–8 seconds with the periphery interpolated between consecutive time frames. A precise timing strategy is not needed because the image is updated every 2–8 seconds. However, depending on the magnitude of undersampling of the peripheral data, the temporal resolution of the edge information may be compromised, resulting in artifacts at the edges of enhancing vessels [160].

Another interesting approach, commonly referred to as time resolved CE-MRA, involves acquiring multiple 2D or 3D data sets using an ultra-fast sequence with a temporal resolution between 0.3 and 5 seconds [189–191]. By using this method, synchronization between data collection and contrast material injection is not required because the vessels are imaged during different stages of the passage of contrast medium. The main disadvantage of this technique is poorer spatial resolution that is inadequate for the visualization of small arteries like the vertebral arteries [190–192]. Recently, time resolved MRA has been combined with parallel imaging with impressive results as shown in Figure 7.9 [170].

The final technique unique to GV-MRA is projection imaging. Although rarely used in C-MRA, projection imaging is standard for GV-MRA. Postprocessing reconstruction techniques [193], like the maximum intensity projection (MIP) algorithm [104], have enabled display of blood vessels in a projective format similar to X-ray angiography. With the MIP algorithm, the brightest pixels along a user-defined direction are extracted to create a projection image. The quality of the MIP can be greatly improved by reduction of pixel size and suppression of signal from stationery tissues, especially in areas of poor flow contrast (i.e., the edges of blood vessels and small vessels with slow flow) which may be obscured by brighter stationary tissue [194]. Postprocessing can now be performed while the patient is within the magnet and images can be rotated in space [104].

Of note, the current direction of research in GV-MRA is to discover an alternative to CE-MRA requiring high-dose gadolinium administration which has been driven by reports of nephrogenic systemic fibrosis (NSF) due to the administration of high-dose gadolinium in patients with renal disease. A recent study [195] compared low dose, contrast enhanced, time resolved, 3D MRA (TR-MRA) and high-resolution CE-MRA. This study found that TR-MRA produced diagnostic images; however, spatial resolution was inferior to CE-MRA. Perhaps more promising is the successful application of unenhanced free-breathing 3D SSFP. Previous studies [196–198] have found comparable and even better image quality, anatomic coverage and diagnostic accuracy using unenhanced 3D SSFP. The major drawback of this technique is an increase in the number of artifacts. Further evaluation is needed to determine whether unenhanced 3D SSFP can be applied routinely for imaging the great vessels.

Clinical Implementation of GV-MRA

Unlike C-MRA, GV-MRA has a proven clinical role [7]. In comparison to other noninvasive modalities including ultrasound (U/S) and computed tomography (CT), MR provides higher sensitivity and specificity as well as a more comprehensive exam [7,179,199,200]. However, due to limited patient access, need for transportation to the scanner, longer examination time, and question of adequate monitoring while in the scanner, MR has been relegated to a secondary role for acute processes [7].

Thoracic and Abdominal Aorta

Aortic Dissection
Aortic dissection is characterized by laceration of the intima and inner layer of the aorta allowing blood to flow through a false lumen. Early and accurate detection of the dissection and its anatomical

delineation are critical for successful management [201]. The anatomic characteristics of the dissection determine whether medical or surgical management is indicated, and, if surgery is indicated, the type of surgical technique that will provide the highest long-term success [7]. Thus, the imaging modality must be able to clearly delineate the intimal flap and its extension, the entry and re-entry sites, the presence and degree of aortic insufficiency and the flow in the aortic branches [202]. Moreover, defining involvement of the iliac vessels may be important for the placement of stent grafts [203,204].

MRI fulfills these necessary requirements for the noninvasive diagnosis of aortic dissection. The initial MR study for suspected aortic dissection begins with a SE sequence with high-resolution parameters and prepulses to null the blood signal and to obtain a better definition of the aortic wall [7]. The intimal flap appears as a straight line in the axial plane. The true lumen usually appears as a signal void, whereas, the false lumen has higher signal intensity. Sagittal planes are required to determine the extent of dissection in the thoracic, abdominal and aortic arch branches [205]. Gradient recalled sequences [138,187] should be performed to identify aortic insufficiency, entry or re-entry sites, and slow flow but is usually reserved for stable patients. If SE images are negative, 3D contrast MRA [206] should be performed to avoid missing a dissection. With SE, artifacts caused by imperfect ECG gating, respiratory motion, or a slow blood pool can result in intraluminal signal simulating or obscuring the intimal flap [7]. In CE-MRA, the intimal flap and the relationship to great vessels is clearly identified. Entry and re-entry sites appear as segmented interruption of the linear intimal flap as shown in Figure 7.10 [7,199,207]. Compared to other imaging modalities, MR is the most accurate modality for detecting aortic dissection with sensitivity and specificity approaching 100% [179,199,200,208]

All patients undergoing aortic repair should have imaging surveillance. MR is the imaging modality of choice for postoperative surveillance [210–212]. MR measurement parameters are highly reproducible which is critical for surveillance because rupture is often preceded by increases in diameter. Residual dissection can be easily seen on SE, and thrombosis is readily detected GRE [209]. Contrast-enhanced MRA is also valuable in assessing postop-

erative complications including anastomotic leakage and thrombosis, dissection and aneurysm of the re-implanted coronaries [7,213].

Intramural Hematoma

Intramural hematoma refers to dissection without intimal tear. The diagnosis of intramural hematoma depends on the visualization of intramural blood, manifested as a locally thickened aortic wall but can be confused with clot or plaque [214]. In comparison with various imaging modalities, MRI demonstrates the best sensitivity for the detection of intramural hematoma [215] and can determine the age of the hematoma [216] based on the different degradation products of hemoglobin. On T_1-weighted SE images, the intramural hematoma appears as a crescent shaped area of abnormal signal within the aortic wall. Acute hematoma (less than 7 days of symptom onset) show an intermediate signal intensity due to oxyhemoglobin content compared to subacute hematoma that show high signal intensity due to methemoglobin. Intramural hematoma can be difficult to distinguish from thrombus if signal intensity is medium to low [7]. In those cases, T_2-weighted SE can differentiate hemorrhage, which has a high signal, from thrombus, which has a lower signal. Because of poor sensitivity, TOF and CE-MRA must be combined with SE to detect intramural hematoma or extravascular fluid collections [217].

Aortic Ulcers

An aortic ulcer is characterized by rupture of an atheromatous plaque and disruption of the internal elastic lamina. Extension into the media may result in intramural hematoma, dissection or pseudoaneurysm. MR diagnosis of aortic ulcer [218] is based on visualization of a crater-like ulcer in the aortic wall in SE or CE-MRA. Mural thickening with high or intermediate signal may indicate extension into the medium or development of an intramural hematoma [219].

Aortic Aneurysms

An aortic aneurysm is a localized or diffuse dilatation (>1.5 times the expected diameter) involving all layers of the aortic wall. MRI is effective in identifying and characterizing thoracic aneurysms [220]. Spin echo sequences can help evaluate

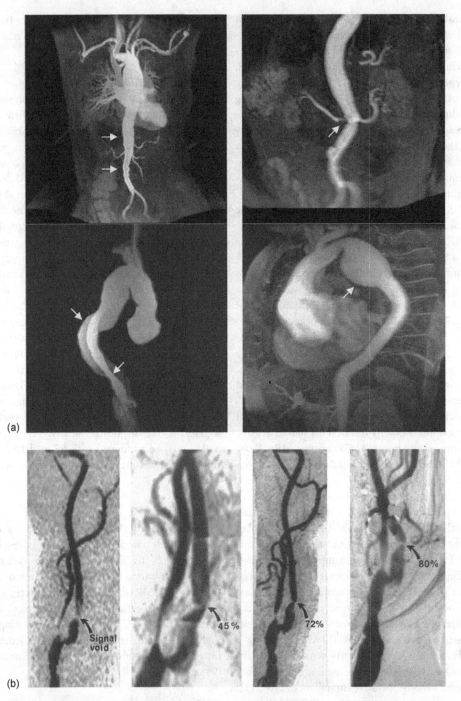

(a)

(b)

Figure 7.10 (a) Three-dimensional contrast-enhanced MRA showing diffuse atherosclerosis of the thoracic and abdominal aorta (top, left), stenosis of the right renal artery (top, right), dissection of the thoracic aorta extending to the abdominal aorta (bottom, left), and aneurysm of the ascending aorta and arch (bottom, right). (b) Classic 2D TOF showing signal void (far, left), followed by MOTSA with 45% measured stenosis, and 3D contrast-enhanced MRA with 72% measured stenosis in a patient with carotid stenosis. The discrepancy was resolved with conventional X-ray angiogram (far, right), confirming 80% stenosis. (Reproduced with courtesy of F. Chan, Stanford University and De Marco *et al.* [209]).

alterations in the wall and periaortic space in the thoracic aorta [184]. Spin echo easily visualizes instability of the aneurysm suggested by periaortic hematoma and areas of high signal intensity within thrombus. Atherosclerotic lesions appear as areas of increased thickness with high signal intensity and irregularity. Accurate measurement of the aneurysm diameter requires fat suppression techniques to differentiate the outer aneurysm wall from periadventitial fat [7]. The addition of 3D CE-MRA [217,221,222] provides precise topographic information about the extent of the aneurysm and its relationship to aortic branches [Figure 7.10], important in the preoperative management of these patients.

Unlike thoracic aneurysms, the role of MRI in the evaluation of abdominal aneurysms is still yet to be defined [103,223]. Monitoring of abdominal aneurysms can be easily performed with CT or U/S, both capable of accurately determining the size of the aneurysm and its relationship to the iliac and renal arteries. Computed tomography [224] and U/S [225], however, are inadequate for preoperative planning which requires more precise anatomic detail regarding the vessels of the lower extremities [226]. Moreover, the success of endovascular stenting procedures requires more exquisite detail including the distance of the aneurysm from the renal arteries, involvement of the iliac arteries, and angle of the aneurysm neck or iliac-femoral axis [227]. In studies using TOF MRA [228–230], often in conjunction with T_1-weighted inversion recovery MRI, accurate classification of aneurysms as suprarenal or infrarenal is sufficient but suffers from inadequate detection of accessory renal arteries, renal artery stenosis, and iliac vascular disease [103].

Results with CE-MRA are more promising for imaging the abdominal aorta [227,231–233]. The use of CE-MRA enables higher resolution and provides high blood signal without the need for fast flow. A study of 27 patients revealed that a combination of CE MRA, SE, and noncontrast 3D TOF detected 7 out of 9 accessory renal arteries, 8 of 9 renal artery stenosis, all celiac stenosis and all iliac aneurysmal and stenotic disease [227]. MRA correlated with surgical findings as well as X-ray angiography for defining the proximal extent of the aneurysm. A subsequent study in patients with

peripheral vascular disease [233] showed that MRA accurately defined the proximal extent of the abdominal aneurysm in 87% of patients. Sensitivities for ileo-femoral occlusive and aneurysmal disease were 83 and 79%, respectively. Sensitivities for renal artery stenosis and accessory renal arteries were 71%. In terms of surgical planning, MRA correctly predicted 87% of the cross-clamp sites, 95% of the proximal anastamotic sites, the need for renal revascularization in 91% of the cases, and the use of a bifurcated aortic prosthesis in 75% of the patients. Contrast-enhanced MRA, in combination with noncontrast techniques, correctly defined the maximum aneurysm diameter, as well as its proximal and distal extent in all 43 subjects. For the detection of aortic branch artery stenosis involving the celiac, mesenteric, renal, or iliac arteries, sensitivity was 94% and specificity 98% [231]. Based on these studies demonstrating accurate anatomical delineation, CE-MRA enables surgical decision between the placement of an aortic tube graft or aorto-bifemoral graft [103]. In addition, CE-MRA can determine candidates for endoluminal repair [234] and may be more sensitive than CT in detecting small endoleaks after surgical or endoluminal repair [235]. Spin echo combined with CE-MRA can also identify inflammatory abdominal aneurysms, which are known to be associated with a higher operative mortality and requires a specialized procedure [7]. Potential limitations include the inability to define the severity of branch vessel stenosis and inadequate visualization of the mesenteric arteries [103]. CE-MRA of the abdominal aorta in a patient with renal artery stenosis is shown in Figure 7.7.

Aortic Rupture

Aortic rupture usually caused by trauma is a lesion that extends from the intima to the adventitia [236]. In the past, TEE and spiral CT had the advantage over MRI in terms of rapid, timely diagnosis especially in patients with severe hemodynamic compromise. Recent developments have shortened MR imaging time making it a viable option in even the most critically ill patients [7]. A recent study in 24 consecutive patients showed that the diagnostic accuracy of MRI was 100% compared to 84% using angiography (two false negatives) and 69% using CT (2 false negatives and 2 false positives) [237]. The advantage of MR lies in its ability to visualize hemorrhagic components of a lesion. On SE images in the sagittal plane, MRI can distinguish between a tear limited to the anterior or posterior wall and a lesion encompassing the entire aortic circumference, which is more likely to rupture. Other signs of instability easily identified by MRI are the presence of periadventitial hematoma and of pleural and mediastinal hemorrhagic effusion. MR can also evaluate trauma outside the heart including lung contusion and edema, pleural effusion, and rib fractures [238].

Aortitis

MRI is the procedure of choice in the diagnosis of inflammatory lesions of the aorta [239]. X-ray angiography can only visualize late changes including aneurysms, and vascular stenosis and should be avoided due to a high risk for pseudoaneurysm at the puncture site [240]. Computed tomography cannot detect subtle changes during the early phase of aortitis. Using contrast-enhanced T_1-weighted and T_2-weighted SE imaging, active inflammation has been demonstrated as mural thickening of the aortic wall which enhances with gadolinium. In chronic stages characterized by fibrosis, lower signal intensity is observed and there is no contrast enhancement [241]. MRA is also useful in diagnosing stenosis and aneurysms and for serial evaluation.

Congenital Disease

Aortic Arch Anomalies and Aortic Coarctation

Several congenital diseases can be diagnosed using MRI including aortic arch anomalies, coarctation and pseudo-coarctation [242]. Spin echo and CE-MRA can detect abnormal vessels, origin, relationship to other structures, and any compression of structures in the mediastinum [243,244]. Because of its ability to provide 3D information, MRI is more effective than X-ray angiography in the preoperative assessment of patients with congenital arch anomalies.

One of the most common congenital diseases of the aorta is coarctation, which is caused by the formation of a fibrous ridge that protrudes into the aorta and forms a stenosis [245]. The stenosis can be a focal segment (aortic coarctation), diffuse (hypoplastic aortic isthmus or complete (aortic arch interruption). It is best viewed on sagittal SE images. The severity of the coarctation can be estimated by the length of signal void on cine MRI [7]. Flow mapping can quantify the flow pattern and the volume of collateral flow down the descending aorta [246]. Three-dimensional MRA can also display the extent of the coarctation and its severity [247]. Postoperative complications including re-stenosis, aortic dissection, aneurysm and pseudoaneurysms can be readily detected by MR [248,249]. Compared to ultrasound, which is the standard for postoperative assessment, MR can provide additional detail including improved visualization of the arch and proximal portion of the descending aorta and is not limited by acoustic windows [7].

Carotid and Vertebral Arteries

Carotid and Vertebral Artery Stenosis

Several MRI techniques are used for imaging the carotid and vertebral arteries including 2D-TOF [250], 3D-TOF [251], and CEMRA [148,189,209]. 2D-TOF provides a strong vascular signal, even when the arterial velocity is low. Two-dimensional TOF should be used to differentiate near and complete internal carotid artery occlusion. Three-dimensional TOF provides superior, submillimeter resolution, however, at the expense of flow sensitivity. The weak vascular signal of 3D-TOF in slow-flow states can be improved with MOTSA [145]. Three-dimensional TOF acquisition may demonstrate some features of the plaque directly. The area covered by TOF sequences remains limited and complete visualization of both the anterior and posterior circulation from the aortic arch to the skull base is not possible [153]. In addition, scan time is long, leading to frequent image degradation by motion artifacts. Signal loss is also observed in areas of tight stenosis because of turbulent flow.

Contrast-enhanced MRA is a quick and robust technique that is not impaired by slow flow but requires appropriate timing of contrast [103]. In head and neck imaging, the blood–brain barrier prevents the extraction of gadolinium from the intracerebral circulation. This can lead to a rapid enhancement of veins that can hinder visualization of the carotid and vertebral arteries, especially in case of large or duplicated jugular veins. A preliminary study by Slosman *et al.* [252] in 50 patients with atherosclerotic carotid disease using a long scan time of

Table 7.6   Summary of TOF MRA studies of the carotid arteries.

Reference	TOF	Comparison	n	Stenosis threshold	Sensitivity (%)	Specificity (%)
Anderson et al. [255]	2D/3D	XRA/DUS	50	70	92	95
Mittle et al. [262]	2D	XRA/DUS	38	70	92	75
Young et al. [263]	2D/3D	XRA/DUS	70	70	86	93
Vanninen et al. [265]	3D	XRA	55	70	93	88
Kent et al. [261]	3D	XRA/DUS	81	70	98	85
Nicholas et al. [260]	2D/3D	XRA/DUS	40	70	92	98
Patel et al. [259]	2D/3D	XRA/DUS	88	70	94	85
Levi et al. [256]	2D/3D	XRA	45	70	95	77
Liberopoulous et al. [258]	3D	XRA/DUS/surgery	52	60	100	80
Link et al. [183]	3D	XRA	40	70	90	92
Nederkoorn et al. [268]	3D	XRA	51	70	86	73
Serfaty et al. [269]	3D	XRA/DUS	33	70	88	94

TOF, time of flight; n, number of subjects; XRA, X-ray angiography; DUS, duplex ultrasound.

150 seconds showed an inability to assess 29 carotid arteries because of venous overlap. Better results were obtained with shorter acquisition time. Levy et al. [253], who assessed the bolus timing of a single dose of gadolinium with a 29-second scan time, achieved complete isolation of the arterial phase in about half of patients. Most recent studies [153] show that appropriate timing of gadolinium infusion with selective reconstruction of carotid arteries allowed elimination of overlapping vessels in most cases. A feasibility study [254] of this technique to image supra-aortic vessels in 98 patients showed the carotid bifurcation could be assessed in 95% of cases, whereas the entire lengths of vertebral arteries were visualized in 82%.

Results from recent prospective studies comparing 2D TOF, 3D TOF, and X-ray angiography for the evaluation of carotid stenosis are shown in Table 7.6 [255–265]. The median sensitivity for a high-grade lesion was 93%, whereas, median specificity was 88% with 2D and 3D TOF. An overestimation of stenosis severity, however, can occur in an area of turbulent flow where there is a signal void or signal loss [266]. The tendency to overestimate stenosis is greatly reduced if interpretation is performed from source or reformatted images rather than projection images [255,267]. Overestimation is also reduced by 3D acquisitions, because of the additional gradient generation and the use of submillimeter voxels, which results in less phase dispersion. In addition, overestimation is reduced if a quantitative measure is used rather than a qualitative visual estimate [103].

In comparison to TOF, CE-MRA minimizes the problems with overestimation because of the T_1-shortening of gadolinium in areas of turbulent or residual flow. Sardenilli et al. [270] demonstrated that CE-MRA overestimated the degree of stenosis in 2 out of 30 cases, whereas 3D-TOF overestimated the degree of stenosis in 9 cases. All severe stenoses were correctly detected with 100% sensitivity and specificity using CE MRA. Compared to 3D-TOF, CE-MRA demonstrated better ulcer detection and better depiction of the length of stenosis and slow flow beyond a critical lesion [7,103]. However, in cases of high-grade stenosis, a signal loss and reduced diameter were observed throughout the distal portion of the internal carotid artery despite absence of complete occlusion [271]. Moreover, the SNR of CE-MRA was found to be inferior to noncontrast techniques if peak arterial enhancement was missed because of incorrect timing of acquisition. The combination of CE-MRA combined with noncontrast techniques, however, has resulted in exceptionally high rates of accuracy in comparison with X-ray angiography [103]. Sample images of a patient with carotid stenosis using 2D TOF, 3D MOTSA, CE-MRA, and X-ray angiography are shown in Figure 7.10. Results from prospective studies comparing CE-MRA and X-ray

Table 7.7   Summary of contrast-enhanced MRA studies of the carotid arteries.

Reference	CE-MRA	Comparison	n	Stenosis threshold	Sensitivity (%)	Specificity (%)
Huston et al. [170]	3D	XRA	50	70	93.3	85.1
Alvarez-Linera et al. [272]	3D	XRA/CT	40	70	97.1	95.2
Borisch et al. [273]	3D	XRA/DUS	39	70	94.9	79.1
Serfaty et al. [269]	3D	XRA/DUS	33	70	94	85
Randoux et al. [274]	3D	XRA/CT	22	70	93	100
Remonda et al. [275]	3D	XRA	120	70	96	95
Nederkoorn et al. [268]	3D	XRA	51	70	90	77
Butz et al. [276]	2D/3D	XRA	50	70	95.64	90.39
Lenhart et al. [277]	3D	XRA	43	70	98	86

CE-MRA, contrast-enhanced MR angiography; n, number of subjects; XRA, X-ray angiography; CT, computed tomography; DUS, duplex ultrasound.

angiography for the evaluation of carotid stenosis are shown in Table 7.7 [157,272–277].

These previous studies used X-ray angiography as the gold standard which may be problematic [103]. A comparison of X-ray angiography, MRA, and ultrasound [278] with surgical specimens found that both ultrasound and MRA correlated better with the endarterectomy specimen than X-ray angiography. The discrepancy may occur because X-ray angiography may not appreciate the smallest diameter in an elliptical or complex lesion [103]. Rotational angiography, a technique that obtains images in many orientations following a single catheter injection commonly used in coronary angiography, demonstrated that catheter angiography may underestimate the severity of lesions by not viewing it from the most stenotic region [279]. Thus, MRA may not be overestimating lesions but catheter angiography is in fact underestimating lesions [7,103].

Current recommendations for the evaluation of carotid artery stenosis include initial screening with ultrasound followed by confirmation with MRA in cases of >70% stenosis. X-ray angiography is currently recommended if there is discrepancy between ultrasound and MRA findings, possible hairline patency, or atypical lesions, which can only be understood by an invasive study. MRA is especially advisable when results of ultrasound are technically limited including the presence of a shadowing plaque, deep course of the internal carotid artery, discordant gray scale and Doppler measurements, and evidence of tandem lesions [103,280].

For the posterior circulation, the detection of significant vertebral stenosis of greater than 50% in diameter remains difficult on the CE-MRA because of the small diameter of vertebral arteries and frequent anatomic variants [271,281]. Preliminary studies show that sensitivity and specificity appear lower than the anterior circulation [281]. Randoux et al. [282] reported sensitivity and specificity for vertebral ostial stenosis was 100 and 85%, respectively, while the positive predictive value was only 58%. This is largely due to overestimation caused by partial volume effect.

Carotid and Vertebral Dissection

Various techniques have been employed for the detection of dissection. On T_1 and T_2-weighted images [281,283], a dissection is suggested by an eccentric signal void surrounded by a crescent-shaped hyperintensity [284]. Stenosis or complete vascular occlusion may be present but these findings lack specificity for dissection. TOF techniques [285,286] have the advantage of better demonstration of the intramural hematoma than phase-contrast techniques. Two-dimensional TOF can image a long segment of artery in a short time but suffers from signal loss in regions of turbulent flow that can simulate stenosis. Three-dimensional TOF MRA [287] may reveal an "increased" external diameter of the artery due to superimposed intramural hematoma containing methemoglobin. This finding is more useful for the diagnosis of carotid artery dissection, but it is of limited use in vertebral dissection owing to the small diameter and marked variation in caliber of the vertebrals [283]. Studies have shown that sensitivity and specificity of MRI and 3D-TOF for carotid dissection is 92 and 99%, respectively [283,284,287,288]. However, the sensitivity and specificity of MRI and 3D-TOF MRA for the detection of vertebrobasilar dissection has been reported as low as 20 and 60%, respectively [283]. MRI may also be insufficient to detect pseudoaneurysm, mild stenosis, and fibromuscular dysplasia, which can predispose to dissection. The application of additional sequences may aid in the diagnosis of dissection. Contrast-enhanced MRA can help differentiate residual flow from intramural hematoma with greatly improved resolution. The addition of SE T_1-weighted transverse images may also aid in identifying the false lumen [289].

Studies have reported successful serial monitoring of patients with carotid dissection using MRI [286,290]. Features showing evidence of healing included stenosis and mural hematoma/intimal flap. Persistent luminal irregularities were associated with persistent dissection and late cerebrovascular events [286]. Moreover, several studies [286,291] have reported encouraging results of combined CE-MRA/MRI for the follow up of vertebral artery dissection. In one study [291], contrast enhancement was seen in 71% of vertebrobasilar dissecting aneurysms up to 8 weeks after the initial injury when T_1 SE signal of intramural hematoma has disappeared. Enhancement was still present in more than 50% of cases 24 weeks post injury.

Pulmonary Vessels

Pulmonary MRA has been slow in its clinical implementation. Initial approaches used 2D or 3D-TOF with promising results; however, techniques were not reliable for widespread clinical use. Recently, CE-MRA has been applied to the pulmonary arteries [292], with the entire pulmonary tree covered in one breath-hold. A report of 30 patients showed sensitivities ranging from 75 to 100% plus specificities from 95 to 100% for the detection of pulmonary embolism among three readers with spatial resolution of 1.25 mm × 2.5 mm × 3.0 mm. In a prospective study by Oudkerk *et al.* [293], sensitivity of MRA for isolated subsegmental, segmental, and central or lobar pulmonary embolism was 40, 84, and 100%, respectively ($p < 0.01$). Selected visualization of pulmonary arteries and veins has

also been demonstrated with high spatial resolution (1.9 mm × 1.4 mm × 2 mm) [294]. Recently, it has been shown that 3D CE-MRA can identify pulmonary and systemic venous anomalies as well as catheterization in 61 patients [295].

Future Direction

The most significant question in MRA today is how to improve this imaging modality to meet the high standard of routine, robust and safe implementation for the diagnosis of a wide spectrum of vascular diseases in addition to safe acquisition in all patient subsets. Clearly, impressive technological progress has been made in the past decades.

To ensure a future for C-MRA in the clinical evaluation of patients with suspected CAD, acquisition methods need to be simplified and spatial resolution improved. Further development is needed in whole heart imaging [127,296,297] with the goal of acquiring the entire coronary tree with high spatial resolution within one breath-hold, akin to acquisition using CT angiography. Improvement in parallel imaging, the application of intravascular contrast agents, time resolved imaging, and real-time imaging may help realize this goal.

For GV-MRA, in the short term, research will likely focus on the development of low-dose contrast-enhanced or unenhanced MRA to address the recent controversy over the administration of gadolinium to ensure safety of image acquisition in all patients. Recent studies [196–198] have suggested that unenhanced MRA may even provide improve diagnostic accuracy compared to contrast-enhanced techniques.

The ultimate goal of MRA will be imaging the entire vasculature. Recently, the global coherent free precession sequence [298] has been developed which enables dynamic images of vascular morphology and flow, similar to X-ray angiography. Global coherent free precession (GCFP) [299] enables dynamic images of both vascular morphology and blood flow similar to X-ray angiography. In the GCFP state, excited protons continue to yield signal regardless of where they travel, even in the absence of additional RF excitation. RF excitations can be applied every few milliseconds, creating a continuous outward flow of excited protons. Thus, spatially selective RF pulses produce a continuous stream of coherently excited blood whose spins freely precess

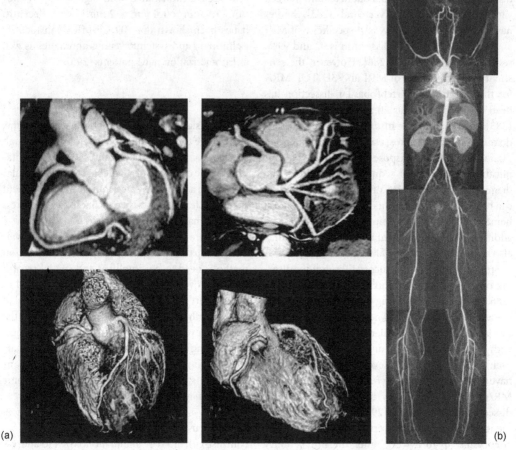

(a)   (b)

Figure 7.11 (a) Right coronary artery and left circumflex (LCX) (right) and left anterior descending artery (LAD) (right) of a volunteer as imaged using a targeted sequence (top row) and reformatted using the whole heart sequence (bottom row). Note longer segments of the LAD and LCX are visualized using the whole heart sequence. (Reproduced with kind permission from Springer Science+Business Media from Sakuma, Mie University, Japan and Bernd, *Eur Radiol* 2004; 14: M26–M27.) (b) Whole body MRA images using contrast enhancement and parallel imaging techniques. (Reproduced from Tombach, Whole-body CE-MRA with Gadovist, *Eur Radiol* 2004; Suppl 5: M26–27.)

as the blood flows through regions of space unaffected by the ongoing excitation.

Similarly, recent advances have enabled the implementation of whole body MRA. Contrast agent dose limitations had initially restricted 3D MRA to the display of arteries contained in a single 40- to 48-cm field of view [7]. Before bolus-chase MR imaging, extended coverage could be achieved with separate injections in one examination. Two contiguous areas were studied with separate doses of gadolinium-based contrast agent [300]. Implementation of bolus-chase techniques extended coverage to two or three territories with a single administration of contrast agent. Several studies have demonstrated the feasibility of whole body MRA as demonstrated in Figure 7.11 [286–288,290].

Conclusion

A great deal of progress has been achieved in the MR angiography over the past two decades. Currently, GV-MRA is considered the noninvasive gold standard for imaging the great vessels. C-MRA remains a research tool but further research aimed at simplifying acquisition and improving spatial resolution may enable its application in clinical setting. The exquisite tissue contrast of MRI without exposure to ionizing radiation allows this imaging modality to be a promising tool for the evaluation of the human vascular system.

References

1. Johnson L, Lozner E, Johnson S, *et al.* Coronary arteriography 1984–1987: a report of the Registry of the Society for Cardiac Angiography and Interventions. I. Results and complications. *Cathet Cardiovasc Diagn.* 1989;17: 5–10.

2. Lozner E, Johnson L, Johnson S, *et al.* Coronary arteriography 1984–1987: a report of the Registry of the Society for Cardiac Angiography and Interventions II. An analysis of 218 deaths related to coronary arteriography. *Cathet Cardiovasc Diagn.* 1989;17:11–14.

3. Kunz KM, Skillman JJ, Whittenmore AD, *et al.* Carotid endardarectomy in asymptomatic patients—is contrast angiography necessary? A morbidity analysis. *J Vasc Surg.* 1995;22:706–714.

4. Cranney G, Lotan C, Pohost G. *Cardiovascular Applications of Magnetic Resonance Imaging.* Boston, Massachusetts: Little, Brown and Company, 1991.

5. Blackwell G, Pohost G. The evolving role of MRI in the assessment of coronary artery disease. *Am J Cardiol.* 1995;75:74D–78D.

6. Manning W, Li W, Edelman R. A preliminary report comparing magnetic resonance coronary angiography with conventional angiography. *N Engl J Med.* 1993; 328:828–832.

7. Higgins C, De Roos A. *Cardiovascular MRI and MRA.* Philadelphia: Lippincott Williams and Wilkins, 2003.

8. Schmitt F, Arz W. An ultra-high performance gradient system for cardio and neuro MR imaging. Proceedings of the ISMRM, 7th Annual Meeting, Toronto, Canada, 1999, p. 470.

9. Meyer C, Hu B, Nishimura D, Macovski A. Fast spiral coronary artery imaging. *Magn Reson Med.* 1992;28: 202–213.

10. Meyer C, Hu B, Kerr A, *et al.* High-resolution multislice spiral coronary angiography with real-time interactive localization. Proceedings of the ISMRM, 5th Annual Meeting, Vancouver, Canada, 1997, p. 439.

11. Schmitt M, Potthast A, Sosnovik DE, *et al.* A 128-channel receive-only cardiac coil for highly accelerated cardiac MRI at 3 Tesla. *Magn Reson Med.* 2008;59(6): 1431–1439.

12. Niendorf T, Sodickson DK. Highly accelerated cardiovascular MR imaging using many channel technology: concepts and clinical applications. *Eur Radiol.* 2008; 18(1):87–102.

13. Rinck PA. *Magnetic Resonance in Medicine,* 3rd edition. London: Blackwell Scientic Publications, 1993.

14. Noll D, Pauly J, Meyer C, Nishimura D, Macovski A. De-blurring for non-2D Fourier transform magnetic resonanance imaging. *Magn Reson Med.* 1992;25:319–333.

15. Man L, Pauly J, Macovski A. Improved automatic off-resonance correction without a field map in spiral imaging. *Magn Reson Med.* 1997 (37):906–913.

16. Noeske R, Siefert F, Rhein KH, Rinneberg H. Human cardiac imaging at 3T using phased array coils. *Magn Reson Med.* 2000;44:978–982.

17. Singerman RW, Denison TJ, Wen H, Balaban RS. Simulation of B1 field distribution and intrinsic signal-to-noise in cardiac MRI as a function of static magnetic field. *J Magn Reson.* 1997;125:72–83.

18. Nayak K, Cunningham C, Santos J, Pauly J. Real-time cardiac MR at 3 Tesla. *Magn Reson Med.* 2004;51: 655–660.

19. Yang PC, Nguyen PK, Shimakawa A, Brittain J, Hu BS, McConnell MV. Spiral MR coronary angiography at 1.5T and 3T – clinical comparison. *J Cardiovasc Magn Reson.* 2004;6(4):877–884.

20. Stuber M, Botnar R, Larmerichs R, *et al.* A preliminary report on in-vivo coronary MRA at 3T in humans. Proceedings of the ISMRM, 10th Annual Meeting, Glasgow, Scotland, 2002, p. 116.

21. Deshpande VS, Shea SM, Chung YC, McCarthy RM, Finn JP, Li D. Breath-hold three-dimensional true-FISP imaging of coronary arteries using asymmetric sampling. *J Magn Reson Imaging.* 2002;15(4):473–478.

22. Huber ME, Kozerke S, Pruessmann KP, Smink J, Boesiger P. Sensitivity-encoded coronary MRA at 3T. *Magn Reson Med.* 2004;52(2):221–227.

23. Vrachliotis TG, Bis KG, Aliabadi D, Shetty AN, Safian R, Simonetti O. Contrast-enhanced breath-hold MR angiography for evaluating patency of coronary artery bypass grafts. *Am J Roentenol.* 1997;168(4):1073–1080.

24. Polson MJ, Barker AT, Gardiner S. The effect of rapid rise-time magnetic fields on the ECG of the rat. *Clin Phys Physiol Meas.* 1982;3(3):231–234.

25. Fischer SE, Wickline SA, Lorenz CH. Novel real-time R-wave detection algorithm based on the vectorcardiogram for accurate gated magnetic resonance acquisitions. *Magn Reson Med.* 1999;42(2):361–370.

26. Steenbeck J, Pruessmann K. Technical developments in cardiac MRI: 2000 update. *Rays.* 2001;26:15–34.

27. Kim R, Danias P, Stuber M, *et al.* Coronary magnetic resonance angiography for the detection of coronary stenoses. *N Engl J Med.* 2001;345:1863–1869.

28. Jahnke C, Paetsch I, Nehrke K, *et al.* A new approach for rapid assessment of the cardiac rest period for coronary MRA. *J Cardiovasc Magn Reson.* 2005;7(2):395–399.

29. Ustun A, Desai M, Abd-Elmoniem KZ, Schar M, Stuber M. Automated identification of minimal myocardial motion for improved image quality on MR angiography at 3 T. *AJR Am J Roentgenol.* 2007;188(3):W283–W290.

30. Leiner T, Katsimaglis G, Yeh EN, *et al.* Correction for heart rate variability improves coronary magnetic resonance angiography. *J Magn Reson Imaging.* 2005;22(4):577–582.

31. Manke D, Bornert P, Nehrke K, Nagel E, Dossel O. Accelerated coronary MRA by simultaneous acquisition of multiple 3D stacks. *J Magn Reson Imaging.* 2001;14(4):478–483.

32. Stehning C, Bornert P, Nehrke K, Dossel O. Free breathing 3D balanced FFE coronary magnetic resonance angiography with prolonged cardiac acquisition windows and intra-RR motion correction. *Magn Reson Med.* 2005;53(3):719–723.

33. Stehning C, Boernert P, Nehrke K. Advances in coronary MRA from vessel wall to whole heart imaging. *Magn Reson Med Sci.* 2007;6(3):157–170.

34. Larson AC, White RD, Laub G, McVeigh ER, Li D, Simonetti OP. Self-gated cardiac cine MRI. *Magn Reson Med.* 2004;51(1):93–102.

35. Larson AC, Kellman P, Arai A, *et al.* Preliminary investigation of respiratory self-gating for free-breathing segmented cine MRI. *Magn Reson Med.* 2005;53(1):1.

36. Nijm GV, Sahakian AV, Swiryn S, Larson AC. Comparison of signal peak detection algorithms for self-gated cardiac cine MRI. *Comput Cardiol.* 2007;34:407–410.

37. McKinnon G. Ultrafast interleaved gradient-echoplanar imaging on a standard scanner. *Magn Reson Med.* 1993; 30:609–616.

38. Manning W, Pennel D. *Cardiovascular Magnetic Resonance,* 1st edition. Philadelphia: Churchill Livingston, 2002.

39. Lieberman L, Botti R, Nelson A. Magnetic Resonance of the heart. *Radiol Clin North Am.* 1984;22:847–858.

40. Paulin S, von Schulthess G, Fossel E. Magnetic resonance of the heart. *Am J Roentenol.* 1987;148:665–670.

41. Hennig J, Nauerth A, Friedburg H. RARE imaging: a fast imaging method for clinical MR. *Magn Reson Med.* 1986;3(6):823–833.

42. Simonetti OP, Finn JP, White RD, Laub G, Henry DA. "Black blood" T 2-weighted inversion recovery MRA imaging of the heart. *Radiology.* 1996;1996(199):49–57.

43. Wang S, Hu B, Macovski A, Nishimura D. Coronary angiography using fast selective inversion recovery. *Magn Reson Med.* 1991;18:417–423.

44. Edelman RR, Chien D, Kim D. Fast selective black blood MR imaging. *Radiology.* 1991;181:655–660.

45. Stuber M, Botnar RM, Spuentrup E, Kissinger KV, Manning WJ. Three-dimensional high-resolution fast spin-echo coronary magnetic resonance angiography. *Magn Reson Med.* 2001;45:206–211.

46. Deshpande VS, Shea SM, Laub G, Simonetti OP, Finn JP, Li D. 3D magnetization-prepared true-FISP: a new technique for imaging coronary arteries. *Magn Reson Med.* 2001;46(3):494–502.

47. Wielopolski PA, van Geuns RJ, de Feyter PJ, Oudkerk M. Breath-hold coronary MR angiography with volume-targeted imaging. *Radiology.* 1998;209(1):209–219.

48. Haase A, Frahm J, Matthaei D, *et al.* FLASH imaging: rapid NMR imaging using low flip-angle pulses. *J Magn Reson.* 1986;67:258–266.

49. Atkinson D, Edelman R. Cineangiography of the heart in a single breath hold with a segmented turbo-FLASH sequence. *Radiology.* 1991;178:357–360.

50. Burstein D. MR Imaging of coronary artery flow in isolated and in vivo hearts. *J Magn Reson Imaging.* 1991; 1.

51. Edelman R, Manning W, Burstein D, Paulin S. Coronary arteries: breath-hold MR angiography. *Radiology.* 1991; 641–643.

52. Manning WJ, Li W, Boyle NG, Edelman RR. Fat-suppressed breath-hold magnetic resonance coronary angiography. *Circulation.* 1993;87(1):94–104.

53. Pennell DJ, Keegan J, Firmin DN, Gatehouse PD, Underwood SR, Longmore DB. Magnetic resonance imaging of coronary arteries: technique and preliminary results. *Br Heart J.* 1993;70(4):315–326.

54. Duerinckx AJ, Urman MK. Two-dimensional coronary MR angiography: analysis of initial clinical results. *Radiology.* 1994;193(3):731–738.

55. Sakuma H, Caputo GR, Steffens JC, *et al.* Breath-hold MR cine angiography of coronary arteries in healthy volunteers: value of multiangle oblique imaging planes. *Am J Roentgenol.* 1994;163(3):533–537.

56. Masui T, Isoda H, Mochizuki T, *et al.* MR angiography of the coronary arteries. *Radiat Med.* 1995;13(1):47–50.

57. Davis SF, Kannam JP, Wielopolski P, Edelman RR, Anderson TJ, Manning WJ. Magnetic resonance coronary angiography in heart transplant recipients. *J Heart Lung Transplant.* 1996;15(6):580–586.

58. Oppell A, Graumann R, Berfuss H, *et al.* FISP – a new fast MRI sequence. *Electromedica.* 1986;54:15–18.

59. Sekihara K. Steady-state magnetization in rapid NMR imaging using small flip angles and short reptition intervals. *IEEE Trans Med Imaging.* 1987;6:157–164.

60. Heid O. True FISP cardiac fluoroscopy. ISMRM, 4th Annual Meeting; 1997. Berkely, CA: International Society of Magnetic Resonance in Medicine, 1997, p. 320.

61. Deimling M, Heid O. True FISP imaging with inherent fat cancellation. ISMRM 7th Annual Meeting; 2000.

Berkely, CA: International Society of Magnetic Resonance in Medicine, 2000, p. 1500.

62. Shea SM, Deshpande VS, Chung YC, Li D. Three-dimensional true-FISP imaging of the coronary arteries: improved contrast with T2-preparation. *J Magn Reson Imaging.* 2002;15(5):597–602.

63. Li D, Carr J, Shea S, *et al.* Coronary arteries: magnetization-prepared contrast-enhanced three-dimensional volume-targeted breath-hold MR angiography. *Radiology.* 2001;219:270–277.

64. Park J, McCarthy R, Debia L. Feasibility and performance of breath-hold 3D TRUE-FISP Coronary MRA using self calibrating parallel acquisition. *Magn Reson Med.* 2004;52:7–13.

65. Nishimura D, Irarrazabal P, Meyer C. A velocity k-space analysis of flow effects in echo-planar and spiral imaging. *Magn Reson Med.* 1995; 549–556.

66. Spuentrup E, Katoh M, Buecker A, *et al.* Free-breathing 3D steady-state free precession coronary MR angiography with radial k-space sampling: comparison with cartesian k-space sampling and cartesian gradient-echo coronary MR angiography–pilot study. *Radiology.* 2004; 231(2):581–586.

67. Spuentrup E, Katoh M, Stuber M, *et al.* Coronary MR imaging using free-breathing 3D steady-state free precession with radial k-space sampling. *Rofo.* 2003; 175(10):1330–1334.

68. Li D, Pascal C, Haacke E, Adler L. Coronary arteries: three dimensional MR imaging with fat saturation and magnetization transfer contrast. *Radiology.* 1993;187: 401–406.

69. Botnar R, Stuber M, Danias P, Kissinger K, Manning W. Improved coronary artery definition with T2-weighted, free-breathing, three-dimensional coronary MRA. *Circulation.* 1999;99:3139–3148.

70. Mansfield P. Multi-planar image formation using NMR spin echos. *J Phys C: Solid State Phys.* 1977 (Solid State Physics):L55–58.

71. Wielopolski PA, Manning WJ, Edelman RR. Single breath-hold volumetric imaging of the heart using magnetization-prepared 3-dimensional segmented echo planar imaging. *J Magn Reson Imaging.* 1995;5(4): 403–409.

72. Slavin GS, Riederer SJ, Ehman RL. Two-dimensional multishot echo-planar coronary MR angiography. *Magn Reson Med.* 1998;40:883–889.

73. Botnar R, Stuber M, Danias P, Kissinger K, Manning W. A fast 3D approach for coronary MRA. *J Magn Reson Imaging.* 1999;10:821–825.

74. Stuber M, Botnar RM, Danias PG, *et al.* Contrast agent-enhanced, free-breathing, three-dimensional coronary magnetic resonance angiography. *J Magn Reson Imaging.* 1999;10:790–709.

75. van Geuns R, Wielopolski P, de Bruin H, *et al.* MR coronary angiography with breath-hold targeted volumes: preliminary clinical results. *Radiology.* 2000;217: 270–277.

76. Deshapande V, Wielopolski P, Shea S, Carr J, Zheng J, Li D. Coronary artery imaging using contrast enhanced 3D segmented EPI. *J Magn Reson Imaging.* 2001;13(5): 676–681.

77. Luk Pat GT, Meyer CH, Pauly JM, Nishimura DG. Reducing flow artifacts in echo-planar imaging. *Magn Reson Med.* 1997;37(3):436–447.

78. Brittain J, Hu B, Wright G, Meyer C, Macovski A, Nishimura D. Coronary angiography with magnetization prepared T2 contrast. *Magn Reson Med.* 1995;33: 689–696.

79. Bornert P, Stuber M, Botnar R, *et al.* Direct comparison of 3D spiral vs. cartesian gradient-echo coronary magnetic resonance angiography. *Magn Reson Med.* 2001;46:789–794.

80. Taylor A, Keegan J, Jhooti P, Gatehouse P, Firmin D, Pennell D. A comparison between segmented k-space FLASH and interleaved spiral MR coronary angiography sequences. *J Magn Reson Imaging.* 2000;11:394–400.

81. Keegan J, Gatehouse P, Taylor A, Yang G, Jhooti P, Firmin D. Coronary artery imaging in 0.5-tesla scanner: implemention of real-time, navigator echo-controlled segmented k-space FLASH and interleaved spiral sequences. *Magn Reson Med.* 1999;41:392–399.

82. Maintz D, Botnar R, Heindel W, Manning W, Stuber M. Coronary magnetic resonance angiography: an objective quantitative comparison between four different MR techniques. Proceedings of the ISMRM, 10th Annual Meeting, Glasgow, Scotland, 2002, p. 108.

83. Hu B, Meyer C, Macovski A, Nishimura D. Multi-slice spiral magnetic resonance coronary angiography. Proceedings of the ISMRM, 4th Annual Meeting, Denver, Colorado, 1996, p. 176.

84. Peters DC, Korosec FR, Grist TM, *et al.* Undersampled projection reconstruction applied to MR angiography. *Magn Reson Med.* 2000;43(1):91–101.

85. Barger AV, Block WF, Toropov Y, Grist TM, Mistretta CA. Time-resolved contrast-enhanced imaging with isotropic resolution and broad coverage using an undersampled 3D projectin trajectory. *Magn Reson Med.* 2002;2002(48):297–305.

86. Stehning C, Bornert P, Nehrke K, Eggers H, Dossel O. Fast isotropic volumetric coronary MR angiography using free-breathing 3D radial balanced FFE acquisition. *Magn Reson Med.* 2004;52:197–203.

87. Lauzon ML, Rutt BK. Effects of polar sampling in k-space. *Magn Reson Med.* 1996;36(6):940–949.

88. Meyer C, Pauly J, Macovski A, Nishimura D. Simultaneous spatial and spectral selective excitation. *Magn Reson Med.* 1990;35:521–531.

89. Balaban RS, Ceckler TL. Magnetization transfer contrast in magnetic resonance imaging. *Magn Reson Q.* 1992;8:116–137.

90. Hu B, Conolly S, Wright G, Nishimura D, Macovski A. Pulsed saturation transfer contrast. *Magn Reson Med.* 1992;33:689–696.

91. Pauly J, Le Roux P, Nishimura D, Macovski A. Parameter relations for Shinnar-Le Roux RF pulse design algorithm. *IEEE Trans Med Imaging.* 1991;10:53–65.

92. Henkelman R, Stanisz F, Graham S. Magnetization transfer in MRI: a review. *NMR Biomed.* 2001;14:57–64.

93. Cunningham CH, Wright GA, Wood ML. High-order multiband encoding in the heart. *Magn Reson Med.* 2002; 48(4):689–698.

94. Parrish T, Hu X. A new T2 preparation technique for ultrafast gradient-echo sequence. *Magn Reson Med.* 1994; 32:652–657.

95. Nezafat R, Stuber M, Ouwerkerk R, Gharib AM, Desai MY, Pettigrew RI. B1-insensitive T2 preparation for improved coronary magnetic resonance angiography at 3 T. *Magn Reson Med.* 2006;55(4):858–864.

96. Lorenz C, Johansson L. Contrast-enhanced coronary MRA. *J Magn Reson Imaging.* 1999;10:703–708.

97. Bi X, Carr JC, Li D. Whole-heart coronary magnetic resonance angiography at 3 Tesla in 5 minutes with slow infusion of Gd-BOPTA, a high-relaxivity clinical contrast agent. *Magn Reson Med.* 2007;58(1):1–7.

98. Taylor AM, Panting JR, Keegan J, et al. Safety and preliminary findings with the intravascular contrast agent NC100150 injection for MR coronary angiography. *J Magn Reson Imaging.* 1999;9:220–227.

99. Cavagna F, La Noce A, Maggioni F, et al. MR coronary angiography with the new intravascular contrast agent B-22956/1: first human experience. Proceedings of the ISMRM, 10th Annual Meeting, Glasgow, Scotland, 2002, p. 114.

100. Paetsch I, Huber M, Bornstedt A, et al. Improved 3D free breathing coronary MRA using gadocoletic acid (B-22956) for intravascular contrast enhancement. *J Magn Reson Imaging.* 2004;20:2888–2293.

101. Fink C, Goyen M, Lotz J. Magnetic resonance angiography with blood-pool contrast agents: future applications. *Eur Radiol.* 2007;17(Suppl. 2):B38–B44.

102. Post JC, van Rosum AC, Bronzwear JG, et al. Three-dimensional respiratory-gated MR angiography of coronary arteries: comparison with conventional coronary angiography. *Am J Roentgenol.* 1996;166:1399–1404.

103. Yucel Anderson C, Edelman R, Grist T, et al. Magnetic resonance angiography: update on applications for extracranial arteries. *Circulation.* 1999;100:2284–2301.

104. Wang Y, Grist TM, Korosec FR, et al. Respiratory blur in 3D coronary MR imaging. *Magn Reson Med.* 1995; 33(4):541–548.

105. Stuber M, Botnar RM, Danias PG, et al. Double-oblique free-breathing high resolution three-dimensional coronary magnetic resonance angiography. *J Am Coll Cardiol.* 1999;34(2):524–531.

106. Mansfield P. Real-time echo-planar imaging by NMR. *Br Med Bull.* 1984;40:187–190.

107. Nayak K, Yang P, Pauly J, Hu B, Nishimura D. Real-time interactive MRA. *Magn Reson Med.* 2001;46:430–435.

108. Kerr A, Pauly J, Hu B, et al. Real-time interactive MRI on a conventional scanner. *Magn Reson Med.* 1997;38: 355–367.

109. Yang P, Meyer C, Kerr A, et al. Spiral magnetic resonance coronary angiography with real-time localization. *J Am Coll Cardiol.* 2003;41:1134–1141.

110. Yang PC, Santos JM, Nguyen PK, et al. Dynamic real-time architecture in magnetic resonance coronary angiography–a prospective clinical trial. *J Cardiovasc Magn Reson.* 2004;6(4):885–894.

111. Santos J, Wright G, Yang P, Pauly J. Adaptive architecture of real-time imaging systems. Proceedings of the ISMRM, 10th Annual Meeting, Glasgow, Scotland, 2002, p. 468.

112. Sodickson D, Griswold M, Jakob P. SMASH imaging. *Magn Reson Imaging Clin N Am.* 1999;7:237–254.

113. Sodickson W, Manning D. Simultaneous acquisition of spatial harmonics (SMASH): fast imaging with radiofrequency array coils. *Magn Reson Med.* 1999;38:591–603.

114. Pruessmann KP, Weiger M, Scheidegger MB, Boesiger P. SENSE: sensitivity encoding for fast MRI. *Magn Reson Med.* 1999;42:952–962.

115. Yeh E, Botnar R, Leiner T, McKenzie C, Sodickson D. Adaptation of coronary imaging pulse sequences for self-calibrated non-Cartesian parallel imaging. Proceedings of the ISMRM, 11th Annual Scientific Meeting, Toronto, Canada, 2003, p. 1882.

116. Niendorf T, Sodickson D, Hardy CJ, et al. Towards whole heart coverage in a single breath-hold coronary artery imaging using a true 32 channel phased array MR system. Proceedings of the International Society of Magnetic Resonance Medicine, 11th Annual Scientific Meeting, Kyoto, Japan, 2004, p. 703.

117. Sodickson D, Stuber M, Botnar R, et al. Accelerated coronary MR angiography in volunteers and patients using double oblique 3D acquisitions combined with SMASH. *J Cardiovasc Magn Reson.* 1999;1:260–265.

118. Wieger M, Pruessmann K, Boesiger P. Cardiac real time imaging using SENSE sensitivity encoding scheme. *Magn Reson Med.* 2000;43:177–184.

119. Muthupillai R, Smink J, Hong S, *et al.* Flamm1, 4SENSE or k-MAG to accelerate free breathing navigator-guided coronary MR angiography. *AJR* 2006;186:1669–1675.

120. Waltering K, Nassentein K, Massing S, Schlosser T, Hunold P, Barkhausen J. Coronary magnetic resonance angiography using parallel acquisition techniques and intravascular contrast media. *SCMR,* Eighth Annual Proceedings, Orlando, 2005, p. 211.

121. Weiger M, Pruessmann KP, Leussler C, Roschmann P, Boesiger P. Specific coil design for SENSE: a six-element cardiac array. *Magn Reson Med.* 2001;45:495–504.

122. Zhu Y, Hardy CJ, Sodickson DK, *et al.* Highly parallel volumetric imaging with a 32-element RF coil array. *Magn Reson Med.* 2004;52(4):869–877.

123. Heidemann RM, Griswold MA, Haase A, Jakob PM. VD-AUTO-SMASH imaging. *Magn Reson Med.* 2001; 45:1066–1074.

124. Griswold MA, Jakob PM, Heidemann RM, *et al.* Generalized autocalibrating partial parallel acquisitions (GRAPPA). *Magn Reson Med.* 2002;47:1202–1210.

125. Bi X, Park J, Larson AC, Zhang Q, Simonetti O, Li D. Contrast-enhanced 4D radial coronary artery imaging at 3.0T within a single breath-hold. *Magn Reson Med.* 2005;54(2):470–475.

126. Warmuth C, Schnorr J, Kaufels N, *et al.* Whole-heart coronary magnetic resonance angiography: contrast-enhanced high-resolution, time-resolved 3D imaging. *Invest Radiol.* 2007;42(8):550–557.

127. Weber O, Alastair J, Higgins. Whole-heart steady-state free precession coronary artery magnetic resonance angiography. *Magn Reson Med.* 2003;50:1223–1228.

128. Weber O, Pujadas S, Martin A, Higgins C. Free-breathing, three-dimensional coronary artery magnetic resonance angiography: comparison of sequences. *J Magn Reson Imaging.* 2004;20:395–402.

129. Nguyen PK, Nayak KS, Cunningham CH, *et al.* Real time coronary MR angiography at 3T. ISMRM, The 12th Scientific Meeting and Exhibition, Kyoto, Japan, 2004; Kyoto, Japan. 2004.

130. Kragel A, Roberts WC. Anomalous origin of either the right or left main coronary artery from the aorta with subsequent coursing between aorta and pulmonary trunk: analysis of 32 necropsy cases. *Am J Cardiol.* 1988; 62:771–777.

131. Bunce NH, Lorenz CH, Keegan J, *et al.* Coronary artery anomalies: assessment with free-breathing three-dimensional coronary MR angiography. *Radiology.* 2003;227(1):201–208.

132. McConnell MV, Ganz P, Selwyn AP, Li W, Edelman RR, Manning WJ. Identification of anomalous coronary arteries and their anatomic course by magnetic resonance coronary angiography. *Circulation.* 1995;92(11): 3158–3162.

133. Vliegen HW, Doornbos J, de Roos A, *et al.* Value of fast gradient echo magnetic resonance angiography as an adjunct to coronary angiography in detecting and confirming the course of clinically significant coronary artery anomalies. *Am J Cardiol.* 1997;79:773–776.

134. Taylor AM, Thorne SA, Rubens MB, *et al.* Coronary artery imaging in grown up congenital heart disease: complementary role of magnetic resonance and X-ray coronary angiography. *Circulation.* 2000;101(14): 1670–1678.

135. Post JC, van Rossum AC, Bronzwaer JG, *et al.* Magnetic resonance angiography of anomalous coronary arteries. A new gold standard for delineating the proximal course? *Circulation.* 1995;92(11):3163–3171.

136. Gharib A, Ho VB, Rosing D, *et al.* Coronary artery anomalies and variants: technical feasibility of assessment with coronary MR angiography at 3T. *Radiology.* 2008;247:220–227.

137. Sechtem U, Pflugfelder PW, White RD, *et al.* Cine MR imaging: potential for the evaluation of cardiovascular function. *AJR.* 1987;148:239–246.

138. Sakuma H, Bourne M, O'Sullivan M, *et al.* Evaluation of thoracic aortic dissection using breath-holding cine MRI. *J Comput Assist Tomogr.* 1996;20(1):45–50.

139. De La Pena E, Nguyen PK, Nayak KS, *et al.* Real time color-flow MRI in adults with congenital heart disease. *J Cardiovasc Magn Reson.* 2006;8(6):809–815.

140. Weiger M, Pruessmann K, Kassner A, *et al.* Contrast-enhanced 3D MRA using sense. *J Magn Reson Imaging.* 2000;12:671–677.

141. Sodickson D, McKenzie C, Li W, Wolff S, Manning W, Edelman R. Contrast-enhanced 3D MR angiography with simultaneous acquisition of spatial harmonics: a pilot study1. *Radiology.* 2000;217:284–289.

142. Fink C, Ley S, Kroeker R, Requardt M, Kauczor H, Bock M. Time-resolved contrast-enhanced three dimensional magnetic resonance angiography of the chest: combination of parallel imaging with view sharing (TREAT). *Invest Radiol.* 2005;40(1):40–48.

143. Wu Y, Goodrich K, Buswell H, Katzman G, Parker D. HIgh-resolution time-resolved contrast enhanced 3D MRA by combining SENSE with keyhole and SLAM strategies. *Magn Reson Imaging.* 2004;22(9):1161–1168.

144. Davis WL, Blatter DD, Harnsberger HR, *et al.* Intracranial MR angiography: comparison of single-volume three-dimensional time-of-flight and multiple overlapping thin slab acquisition techniques. *Am J Roentenol.* 1994;163:915–920.

145. Parker DL, Yuan C, Blatter DD. MR acquisition by multiple thin slab 3D acquisition. *Magn Reson Med.* 1991; 17:434–451.

146. Prince MR, Yucel EK, Kaufman JA, Harrison DC, Geller SC. Dynamic gadolinium-enhanced three dimensional

abdominal MR angiography. *J Magn Reson Imaging.* 1993;3:877–881.

147. Prince MR. Gadolinium-enhanced MR aortography. *Radiology.* 1994;191:155–164.

148. Cloft H, Murphy K, Prince M, Brunberg J. 3D Gadolinium-enhanced MR angiography of the carotid arteries. *Magn Reson Imaging.* 1996;14(6):593–600.

149. Riederer SJ. Current technical development of magnetic resonance imaging. *IEEE Eng Med Biol Mag.* 2000; 19(5):34–41.

150. Willig DS, Turski PA, Frayne R, *et al.* Contrast enhanced 3D MR DSA of the carotid artery bifurcation: preliminary study of comparison with unenhanced 2D and 3D time-of-flight MR angiography. *Radiology.* 1998;208: 447–451.

151. Saloner D. Determinants of image appearance in contrast-enhanced magnetic resonance angiography. *Invest Radiol.* 1998;33:488–495.

152. Carroll TJ, Grist TM. Technical developments in MR angiography. *Radiology.* 2002;40:921–951.

153. Leclerc X, Pruvo J-P. Recent advances in magnetic resonance angiography of carotid and vertebral vessels. *Curr Opin Neurol.* 2000;13:75–82.

154. Maki JH, Prince MR, Londy FJ, Chenevert TL. The effects of time varying signal intravascular signal intensity and K space acquisition order on three dimensional angiography image quality. *J Magn Reson Imaging.* 1996; 6(4):642–651.

155. Mezrich R. A perspective on K-space. *Radiology.* 1995; 195(2):297–315.

156. Steffens JC, Link J, Gressner J, *et al.* Contrast enhanced K-space centered, breath hold MR angiography of the renal arteries and abdominal aorta. *J Magn Reson Imaging.* 1997;7(4):617–622.

157. Huston J III, Fain SB, Riederer SJ, William AH, Bernstein MA, Busse RF. Carotid arteries: maximizing arterial to venous contrast in fluoroscically triggered contrast enhanced MR angiography with elliptic centric view ordering. *Radiology.* 1999;211:265–273.

158. Korosec FR, Frayne R, Grist TM, Mistretta CA. Time-resolved contrast enhanced 3D MR angiography. *Magn Reson Med.* 1996;36:345–351.

159. Mistretta CA, Grist TM, Korosec FR, *et al.* 3D time-resolved contrast-enhanced MR DSA: advantages and trade offs. *Magn Reson Med.* 1998;40:571–581.

160. Naganawa S, Koshikawa T, Fukatsu H, *et al.* Contrast-enhanced MR angiography of the carotid artery using 3D time-resolved imaging of contrast kinetics: comparison with real-time fluoroscopic triggered 3D-elliptical centric view ordering. *Radiat Med.* 2001;19(4):185–192.

161. White RD, Caputo GR, Mark AS, Modin GW, Higgins CB. Coronary artery bypass graft patency: noninvasive evaluation with MR imaging. *Radiology.* 1987;164(3): 681–686.

162. Rubenstein RI, Askenase AD, Thickman D, Feldman MS, Agarwal JB, Helfant RH. Magnetic resonance imaging to evaluate patency of aortocoronary bypass grafts. *Circulation.* 1987;76(4):786–791.

163. Jenkins JPR, Love HG, Foster CJ, *et al.* Detection of coronary artery bypass graft patency as assessed by magnetic resonance imaging. *Br J Radiol.* 1988;61(721):2–4.

164. Galjee MA, van Rossum AC, Doesburg T, van Eenige MJ, Visser CA. Value of magnetic resonance imaging in assessing patency and function of coronary artery bypass grafts. An angiographically controlled study. *Circulation.* 1996;93(4):660–666.

165. White RD, Pflugfelder PW, Lipton MJ, Higgins CB. Coronary artery bypass grafts: evaluation of patency with cine MR imaging. *Am J Roentgenol.* 1988;150(6): 1271–1274.

166. Aurigemma GP, Reichek N, Axel L, Schiebler M, Harris C, Kressel HY. Noninvasive determination of coronary artery bypass graft patency by cine magnetic resonance imaging. *Circulation.* 1989;80(6):1595–1602.

167. Engelmann MG, Knez A, von Smekal A, *et al.* Noninvasive coronary bypass graft imaging after multivessel revascularisation. *Int J Cardiol.* 2000;76(1):65–74.

168. Wintersperger BJ, Engelmann MG, von Smekal A, *et al.* Patency of coronary bypass grafts: assessment with breath-hold contrast-enhanced MR angiography – value of a non-electrocardiographically triggered technique. *Radiology.* 1998;208(2):345–351.

169. Brenner P, Wintersperger B, von Smekal A, *et al.* Detection of coronary artery bypass graft patency by contrast enhanced magnetic resonance angiography. *Eur J Cardiothorac Surg.* 1999;15(4):389–393.

170. Pennell D, Bogren H, Keegan J, Firmin K, Underwood S. Assessment of coronary artery stenosis by magnetic resonance imaging. *Heart.* 1996;75:127–133.

171. Post JC, van Rossum AC, Hofman MB, de Cock CC, Valk J, Visser CA. Clinical utility of two-dimensional magnetic resonance angiography in detecting coronary artery disease. *Eur Heart J.* 1997;18:426–433.

172. Regenfus M, Ropers D, Achenbach S, Kessler W, Laub DG, Moshage W. Noninvasive detection of coronary artery stenosis using contrast enhanced three dimensional breath-hold magnetic resonance coronary angiography. *J Am Coll Cardiol.* 2000;36:44–50.

173. Woodard PK, Li D, Haacke EM, *et al.* Detection of coronary stenoses on source and projection images using three-dimensional MR angiography with retrospective respiratory gating: preliminary experience. *Am J Roentenol.* 1998;170(4):883–888.

174. Kessler W, Achenbach S, Moshage W, *et al.* Usefulness of respiratory gated magnetic resonance coronary

angiography in assessing narrowings $\geq$ or $=$ 50% in diameter in native coronary arteries and in aorto-coronary bypass conduits. *Am J Cardiol.* 1997;80:989–993.

175. Huber M, Nikolaou K, Gonschior P, Knez A, Stehling M, Reiser M. Navigator echo-based respiratory gating for three-dimensional MR coronary angiography: results from healthy volunteers and patients with coronary artery stenosis. *Am J Roentenol.* 1999;173:95–101.

176. Sandstede JJ, Pabst T, Beer M, Geis N, Kenn W, Neubauer S, et al. Three dimensional MR coronary angiography suing the navigator technique compared with conventional coronary angiography. *Am J Roentenol.* 1999;172:135–139.

177. Sardanelli F, Molinari G, Zandrino F, Balbi M. Three-dimensional, navigator-echo MR coronary angiography in detecting stenosis of the major epicardial vessels, with conventional coronary angiography as the standard of reference. *Radiology.* 2000;214:808–814.

178. Muller MF, Fleisch M, Kroeker R, et al. Proximal coronary artery stenosis: three-dimensional MRI with fat saturation and navigator echo. *J Magn Reson Imaging.* 1997;7:644.

179. Sommer T, Fehski W, Holzknecht, et al. Aortic dissection: a comparative study of diagnosis with spiral CT, multiplanar transesophageal echocardiography and MR imaging. *Radiology.* 1996;199:347–352.

180. So NM, Lam W, Li D, Chan AK, Sanderson JE, Metreweli C. Magnetic resonance coronary angiography with 3D TrueFISP: breath-hold versus respiratory gated imaging. *Br J Radiol.* 2005;78(926):116–121.

181. Sakuma H, Ichikawa Y, Chino S, Hirano T, Makino K, Takeda K. Detection of coronary artery stenosis with whole-heart coronary magnetic resonance angiography. *J Am Coll Cardiol.* 2006;48(10):1946–1950.

182. Maintz D, Ozgun M, Hoffmeier A, et al. Whole-heart coronary magnetic resonance angiography: value for the detection of coronary artery stenoses in comparison to multislice computed tomography angiography. *Acta Radiol.* 2007;48(9):967–973.

183. Link KM, Lesko NM. The role of MR imaging in the evaluation of the thoracic aorta. *Am J Roentenol.* 1992;158:115–1125.

184. Hartnell GG, Finn JP, Zenni M, et al. MR imaging of the thoracic aorta: comparison of spin-echo, angiographic, and breath-hold techniques. *Radiology.* 1994;191(3):697–704.

185. Solomon SL, Brown JJ, Glazer H, Mirowitz SA, Lee JKT. Thoracic aortic dissection: pitfalls and artifacts in MR imaging. *Radiology.* 1990;177:223–228.

186. Seelos KC, Funari M, Higgins CB. Detection of aortic arch thrombus using MR imaging. *J Comput Assist Tomogr.* 1991;15:224–247.

187. Sonnabend SB, Colletti PM, Pentecost M. Demonstration of aortic lesions via cine magnetic resonance imaging. *Magn Reson Imag.* 1990;8:613–618.

188. Dumoulin CL, Hart HR. Magnetic resonance angiography. *Radiology.* 1986;161:717–720.

189. Enochs WS, Ackerman RH, Kaufman JA, Candia M. Gadolinium-enhanced MR angiography of the carotid arteries. *J Neuroimaging.* 1988;8:185–190.

190. Levy RA, Maki JH. Three dimensional contrast enhanced MR angiography of the extracranial carotid arteries: two techniques. *Am J Neuroradiol.* 1998;1998:688–690.

191. Ramonda L, Heid O, Schroth G. Carotid artery stenosis, occlusion, and pseudo-occlusion; first pass, gadolinium-enhanced, three-dimensional MR angiography; preliminary study. *Radiology.* 1998;209:95–102.

192. Wang Y, Donald LJ, Breen JF, et al. Dynamic MR digital subtraction angiography using contrast enhanced, fast data acquisition, and complex subtraction. *Magn Reson Med.* 1996;36:551–556.

193. Laub G. Displays for MR angiography. *Magn Reson Med.* 1990;14:222–229.

194. Anderson CM, Saloner D, Tsurada JS, Shapeero LG, Lee R. Artifacts in maximum-intensity-projection display of MR angiograms. *Am J Roentenol.* 1990;154:623–629.

195. Krishnam MS, Tomasian A, Lohan DG, Tran L, Finn JP, Ruehm SG. Low-dose, time-resolved, contrast-enhanced 3D MR angiography in cardiac and vascular diseases: correlation to high spatial resolution 3D contrast-enhanced MRA. *Clin Radiol.* 2008;63(7):744–755.

196. Krishnam MS, Tomasian A, Deshpande V, et al. Non-contrast 3D steady-state free-precession magnetic resonance angiography of the whole chest using nonselective radiofrequency excitation over a large field of view: comparison with single-phase 3D contrast-enhanced magnetic resonance angiography. *Invest Radiol.* 2008;43(6):411–420.

197. Gebker R, Gomaa O, Schnackenburg B, Rebakowski J, Fleck E, Nagel E. Comparison of different MRI techniques for the assessment of thoracic aortic pathology: 3D contrast enhanced MR angiography, turbo spin echo and balanced steady state free precession. *Int J Cardiovasc Imaging.* 2007;23(6):747–756.

198. Koktzoglou I, Kirpalani A, Carroll TJ, Li D, Carr JC. Dark-blood MRI of the thoracic aorta with 3D diffusion-prepared steady-state free precession: initial clinical evaluation. *AJR Am J Roentgenol.* 2007;189(4):966–972.

199. Bogaert J, Meyns B, Rademakers FE, et al. Follow-up of aortic dissection: contribution of MR angiography for the evaluation of the abndominal aorta and its branches. *Eur Radiol.* 1997;7:695–702.

200. Nienaber CA, Von Kodolitsch Y, Nikolas V. The diagnosis of thoracic aortic dissection by non invasive imaging procedures. *N Engl J Med*. 1993;328:1–9.

201. Coady MA, Rizzo JA, Goldstein LJ, *et al*. Natural history, pathogenesis and etiology of thoracic aneurysms and dissection. *Cardiol Clin*. 1999;17:615–633.

202. Cigarroa JE, Isselbacher EM, De Sanctis RW, *et al*. Diagnostic imaging in the evaluation of suspected aortic dissection. Old standards and new directions. *N Engl J Med*. 1993;328:35–43.

203. Nienaber CA, von Kodolitsch Y, Nikolas V. Non-surgical reconstruction of thoracic aortic dissection by stent-graft placement. *N Eng J Med*. 1999;140:1338–1345.

204. Dake MD, Kato N, Mitchell RS. Endovascular stent-graft placement for the treatment of acute aortic dissection. *N Eng J Med*. 1999;140:1546–1552.

205. Kersting-Somerhoff BA, Higgins CB, White RD, Sommerhoff CP, Lipton MJ. Aortic dissection: sensitivity and specificity of MR imaging. *Radiology*. 1988;166(3):651–655.

206. Fernandez GC, Tardaguila FM, Duran D, Trinidad C, Rodriguez M, Hortas M. Dynamic 3-dimensional contrast-enhanced magnetic resonance angiography in acute aortic dissection. *Curr Probl Diagn Radiol*. 2002;31(4):134–145.

207. Kunz RP, Oberholzer K, Kuroczynski W, *et al*. Assessment of chronic aortic dissection: contribution of different ECG-gated breath-hold MRI techniques. *Am J Roentgenol*. 2004;182(5):1319–1326.

208. Fisher U, Vossherich R, Kopka L. Dissection of the thoracic aorta: pre- and postoperative findings of turbo-FLASH MR images in the plane of the aortic arch. *Am J Roentenol*. 1994;163:1069–1072.

209. De Marco JK, Huston J, Bernstein M. Evaluation of classic 2D time-of-flight MR angiography in the depiction of severe carotid stenosis. *Am J Roentenol*. 2004;183:787–793.

210. Moore NR, Parry AJ, Trottman-Dickenson B, *et al*. Fate of the native aorta after repair of acute Type A dissection: a magnetic resonance imaging study. *Heart*. 1996;75:62–66.

211. Mesana TG, Caus T, Gaubert J, *et al*. Late complications after prosthetic replacement of the ascending aorta: what did we learn from routine magnetic resonance imaging follow-up? *Eur J Cardiothorac Surg*. 2000;18:313–320.

212. Gaubert J, Moulin G, Mesana T, *et al*. Type A dissection of the thoracic aorta. Use of MR imaging for long-term follow-up. *Radiology*. 1995;1996:363–369.

213. Cesare ED, Giordano AV, Cerone G, De Remigis F, Deusanio G, Masciocchi C. Comparative evaluation of TEE, conventional MRI and contrast-enhanced 3D breath-hold MRA in the post-operative follow-up of dissecting aneurysms. *Int J Card Imaging*. 2000;16(3):135–147.

214. Nienaber CA, von Kodolitsch Y, Petersen B. Intramural hemorrhage of the thoracic aorta: diagnostic and therapeutic implications. *Circulation*. 1995;92:1465–1472.

215. Moore A, Oh J, Bruckman D, *et al*. Transesophageal echocardiography in the diagnosis and management of aortic dissection. An analysis of data from the International Registry of Aortic Dissection (IRAD). *J Am Coll Cardio*. 1999;1999(33–2 (A)):470A.

216. Murray JG, Manisali M, Flamm SD. Intramural hematom of the thoracic aorta: MR imaging findings and their prognostic implications. *Radiology*. 1997;204:349–355.

217. Krinsky G, Rofsky N, De Corato DR, *et al*. Thoracic aorta: comparison of gadolinium-enhanced three dimensional angiography with conventional MR imaging. *Radiology*. 1997;202:183–193.

218. Yucel EK, Steinberg FL, Egglin TK, Geller SC, Waltman AC, Athanasoulis CA. Penetrating aortic ulcers: diagnosis with MR imaging. *Radiology*. 1990;177(3):779–781.

219. Hayeshi H, Matsuoka Y, Sakamoto I, *et al*. Penetrating atherosclerotic ulcer of the aorta: imaging features and disease concept. *Radiographics*. 2000;20:995–1005.

220. Hartnell GG. Imaging of aortic aneurysms and dissection: CT and MRI. *J Thorac Imaging*. 2001;16(1):35–46.

221. Neimatallah MA, Ho VB, Dong Q, *et al*. Gadolinium-enhanced 3D magnetic resonance angiography of the thoracic vessels. *Magn Reson Imaging*. 1999;10:758–770.

222. Prince MR, Narasimham DL, Jacoby WT, *et al*. Three dimensional gadolinium-enhanced MR angiography of the thoracic aorta. *Am J Roentenol*. 1996;166:1387–1397.

223. Nasim A, Thompson MM, Sayers RD, *et al*. Role of magnetic resonance angiography for assessment of abdominal aortic aneurysm before endoluminal repair. *Br J Surg*. 1998;85(5):641–644.

224. Papanicolaou N, Wittenberg J, Ferrucci JT Jr, *et al*. Preoperative evaluation of abdominal aortic aneurysms by computed tomography. *AJR Am J Roentgenol*. 1986;146(4):711–715.

225. Pavone P, Di Cesare E, Di Renzi P, *et al*. Abdominal aortic aneurysm evaluation: comparison of US, CT, MRI, and angiography. *Magn Reson Imaging*. 1990;8(3):199–204.

226. Gomes MN, Choyke PL. Pre-operative evaluation of abdominal aortic aneurysms: ultrasound or computed tomography? *J Cardiovasc Surg (Torino)*. 1987;28(2):159–166.

227. Kaufman JA, Geller SC, Petersen MJ, Cambria RP, Prince MR, Waltman AC. MR imaging (including MR angiography) of abdominal aortic aneurysms: comparison with conventional angiography. *Am J Roentenol*. 1994;163:203–210.

228. Kaufman JA, Yucel EK, Waltman AC, *et al*. MR angiography in the preoperative evaluation of abdominal aortic

aneurysms: a preliminary study. *J Vasc Interv Radiol.* 1994;5:489–496.

229. Durham JR, Hackworth CA, Tober JC, *et al.* Magnetic resonance angiography in the preoperative evaluation of abdominal aortic aneurysms. *AM J Surg.* 1993;166: 173–177.

230. Ecklund K, Hartnell GG, Hughes LA, Stokes KR, Finn JP. MR angiography as the sole method of evaluating abdominal aortic aneurysms: correlation with conventional techniques and surgery. *Radiology.* 1994; 192: 345–350.

231. Prince MR, Narasimham DL, Stanley JC, *et al.* Gadolinium-enhanced magnetic resonance angiography of abdominal aortic aneurysms. *J Vascu Surg.* 1995; 21:656–669.

232. Liassy JP, Soyer P, Tebboune D, Tiah D, Hvas U, Menu Y. Abdominal aortic aneurysms: assessment with gadolinium-enhanced time of flight coronal MR angiography (MRA). *Eur J Radiol.* 1995;20:1–8.

233. Petersen MJ, Cambria RP, Kaufman JA, *et al.* Magnetic resonance angiography in the preoperative evaluation of abdominal aortic aneurysms. *J Vasc Surg.* 1995;21: 891–898.

234. Lookstein RA, Goldman J, Pukin L, Marin ML. Time-resolved magnetic resonance angiography as a noninvasive method to characterize endoleaks: initial results compared with conventional angiography. *J Vasc Surg.* 2004;39(1):27–33.

235. Insko E, Kulzer L, Fairman R, Carpenter J, Stavropoulous W. MR imaging for the detection of endoleaks in recipients of abdominal aortic stent-grafts with low magnetic susceptibility. *Acad Radiol.* 2003;10: 509–513.

236. Pate JW, Fabian TC, Walker W. Traumatic rupture of the aortic isthmus: an emergency? *World J Surg.* 1995; 19:119–126.

237. Fattori R, Celletti F, Bertraccini P, *et al.* Delayed surgery of traumatic aortic rupture: role of magnetic resonance imaging. *Circulation.* 1996;94:2865–2870.

238. Fattori R, Celletti F, Descovich B, *et al.* Evolution of post traumatic aneurysm in the subacute phase: magnetic resonance imaging follow-up as a support of the surgical timing. *Eur J Cardiothorac Surg.* 1998;13:582–587.

239. Yamada I, Nakagawa T, Himeno Y, Kobayashi Y, Numano F, Shibuya H. Takayasu arteritis: diagnosis with breath-hold contrast-enhanced three-dimensional MR angiography. *J Magn Reson Imaging.* 2000;11(5):481–487.

240. Kissin EY, Merkel PA. Diagnostic imaging in Takayasu arteritis. *Curr Opin Rheumatol.* 2004;16(1):31–37.

241. Choe YH, Kim DK, Koh EM, *et al.* Takayasu arteritits: diagnosis with MR imaging and MR angiography in acute and chronic stages. *J Magn Reson Imaging.* 1999; 10:751–757.

242. Thiene G, Frescura C. Etiology and pathology of aortic arch malformations. In: Nienaber CA, Fattori R (eds). *Diagnosis and Treatment of Aortic Diseases.* New York: Kluwer Academic Publishers, 1999.

243. Kersting-Somerhoff BA, Sechtem V, Fisher MR, Higgins CB. MR imaging of congenital anomalies of the aortic arch. *Am J Roentenol.* 1987;149:9.

244. Carpenter JP, Holland GA, Golden MA, *et al.* Magnetic resonance angiography of the aortic arch. *J Vasc Surg.* 1997;25:145–151.

245. Fixler DE. Coarctation of the aorta. *Cardiol Clin.* 1988; 6(4):561–571.

246. Julsrud PR, Breen JF, Felmlee JP, *et al.* Coarctation of the aorta: collateral flow assessment with phase-contrast MR angiography. *Am J Roentenol.* 1997;169:1735–1742.

247. Godart F, Labrot G, Devos P, McFadden E, Rey C, Beregi JP. Coarctation of the aorta: comparison of aortic dimensions between conventional MR imaging, 3D MR angiography, and conventional angiography. *Eur Radiol.* 2002;12(8):2034–2039.

248. Paddon AJ, Nicholson AA, Ettles DF, *et al.* Long-term follow up of percutaneous balloon angioplasty in adult aortic coarctation. *Cardiovasc Interv Radiol.* 2000;23: 364–367.

249. Bogart J, Kuzo R, Dymor K, *et al.* Follow-up of patients with previous treatment for coarctation of the thoracic aorta: comparison between contrast-enhanced MR angiography and fast spin echo. *Eur Radiol.* 2000; 10:1047–1054.

250. Keller PJ, Drayer BP, Fram EK, Dumoulin Cl, Souza SP. MR angiography with two dimensional acquisition and three dimensional display. *Radiology.* 1989;173: 527–532.

251. Masaryk TJ, Modic MT, Ruggieri PM, *et al.* Three dimensional (volume) gradient echo imaging of the carotid bifurcation: preliminary clinical experience. *Radiology.* 1989;171:801–806.

252. Slosman F, Stolpen AH, Lexa FJ, *et al.* Extracranial atheroslerotic carotid artery disease: evaluation of non-breath-hold three dimensional gadolinium-enhanced MR angiography. *Am J Roentenol.* 1998;170:489–495.

253. Levy RA, Prince MR. Arterial-phase three-dimensional contrast-enhanced MR angiography of the carotid arteries. *Am J Roentenol.* 1996;167:211–215.

254. Leclerc X, Gauvrit JY, Nicol L, Martinat P, Pruvo JP. Gadolinium-enhanced fast three dimensional angiography of the neck: technical aspect. *Invest Radiol.* 1999; 34:204–210.

255. Anderson CM, Lee RE, Levin DL, de la Torre Alonso S, Saloner D. Measurement of internal carotid stenosis

from source MR angiograms. *Radiology.* 1994;193:219–226.

256. Levi CR, Mitchell A, Fitt G, Donnan GA. The accuracy of magnetic resonance angiography in the assessment of extracranial carotid occlusive disease: a comparison with digital subtraction angiography using NASCET criteria for stenosis measurement. *Cerebrovasc Dis.* 1996; 6:231–236.

257. Korogi Y, Takahashi M, Mabuchi N, *et al.* Intracranial vascular stenosis and occlusion: diagnostic accuracy of three-dimensional, Fourier transform, time-of-flight MR angiography. *Radiology.* 1994;193:187–193.

258. Liberopoulous K, Kaponis A, Kokkins K, *et al.* Comparative study of magnetic resonance angiography, digital subtraction angiography, duplex ultrasound examination with surgical and histological findings of atheroslerotic carotid bifurcation disease. *Int Angiol.* 1996;15:131–137.

259. Patel MR, Kuntz KM, Klufas RA, *et al.* Preoperative assessment of carotid bifurcation: can magnetic resonance angiography and duplex ultrasonography replace contrast angiography? *Stroke.* 1995;26:1753–1758.

260. Nicholas GG, Osborne MA, Jaffe JW, Reed JF III. Carotid stenosis: preoperative noninvasive evaluation in a community hospital. *J Vasc Surg.* 1995;22:9–16.

261. Kent KC, Kuntz KM, Patel MR, *et al.* Perioperative imaging strategies for carotid endarterectomy: an analysis of morbidity and cost effectiveness. *JAMA.* 1995;274: 888–893.

262. Mittle RL Jr, Broderick M, Carpenter JP, *et al.* Blinder-reader comparison of magnetic resonance angiography and duplex ultrasonography for carotid artery bifurcation stenosis. *Stroke.* 1994;25:4–10.

263. Young GR, Humphrey PR, Shaw MD, Nixon TE, Smith ET. Comparison of magnetic resonance angiography, duplex ultrasound and digital subtraction angiography in the assessment of extracranial internal carotid artery stenosis. *J Neurol Neurosurg Psychiatry.* 1994;57: 1466–1478.

264. Young GR, Sandercock PA, Slattery J, Humphrey PR, Smith ET, Brock L. Observer variation in the interpretation of intra-arterial angiograms and the risk of inappropriate decisions about carotid endarterectomy. *J Neurol Neurosurg Psychiatry.* 1996;60:152–157.

265. Vanninen R, Manninen H, Soimakallio S. Imaging of carotid artery stenosis: clinical efficacy and cost effectiveness. *Am J Neuroradiol.* 1995;16:1875–1883.

266. Urchuk SN, Plewes DB. Mechanisms of flow-induced signal loss in MR angiography. *J Magn Reson Imaging.* 1992;2:453–462.

267. De Marco JK, Nesbit GM, Wesbey GE, Richardson D. Prospective evaluation of extracranial carotid stenosis: MR angiography with maximum-intensity projections and multiplanar reformation compared with conventional angiography. *Am J Roentenol.* 1994;163: 1205–1212.

268. Nederkoorn PJ, Elgersma OE, Van Der Graaf Y, Eikelboom BC, Kappelle LJ, Mali WP. Carotid artery stenosis: accuracy of contrast-enhanced MR angiography for diagnosis. *Radiology.* 2003;228(3):677–682.

269. Serfaty JM, Chirossel P, Chevallier JM, Ecochard R, Froment JC, Douek PC. Accuracy of three-dimensional gadolinium-enhanced MR angiography in the assessment of extracranial carotid artery disease. *Am J Roentenol.* 2001;175(2):455–463.

270. Sardanelli F, Zandrino F, Parodi RC, De Caro G. MR angiography of internal carotid arteries: breath-hold gd-enhanced 3D fast imaging with steady-state free precession versus unenhanced 2D and 3D time of flight techniques. *J Comput Assist Tomogr.* 1999;23:208–215.

271. Leclerc Martinat P, Goldefroy O, Lucas C, Giboreau F, Soto Ares G. Contrast-enhanced three dimensional with steady state (FISP) MR angiography of supraaortic vessels: preliminary study. *Am J Neuroradiol.* 1998;19: 1405–1413.

272. Alvarez-Linera J, Benito-Leon J, Escribano J, Campollo J, Gesto R. Prospective evaluation of carotid artery stenosis: elliptic centric contrast-enhanced MR angiography and spiral CT angiography compared with digital subtraction angiography. *Am J Neuroradiol.* 2003;24(5): 1012–1019.

273. Borisch I, Horn M, Butz B, *et al.* Preoperative evaluation of carotid artery stenosis: comparison of contrast-enhanced MR angiography and duplex sonography with digital subtraction angiography. 2003;24(6): 1117–1122.

274. Randoux B, Marro B, Koskas F, *et al.* Carotid artery stenosis: prospective comparison of CT, three-dimensional gadolinium-enhanced MR, and conventional angiography. *Radiology.* 2001;220(1):179–185.

275. Remonda L, Senn P, Barth A, Arnold M, Lovblad KO, Schroth G. Contrast-enhanced 3D MR angiography of the carotid artery: comparison with conventional digital subtraction angiography. *Am J Neuroradiol.* 2002;23(2): 213–219.

276. Butz B, Dorenbeck U, Borisch I, *et al.* High-resolution contrast-enhanced magnetic resonance angiography of the carotid arteries using fluoroscopic monitoring of contrast arrival: diagnostic accuracy and interobserver variability. *Acta Radiol.* 2004;45(2):164–170.

277. Lenhart M, Framme N, Volk M, *et al.* Time-resolved contrast-enhanced magnetic resonance angiography of the carotid arteries: diagnostic accuracy and interobserver variability compared with selective catheter angiography. *Invest Radiol.* 2002;37(10):535–541.

278. Pan XM, Saloner D, Reilly LM, *et al.* Assessment of carotid artery stenosis by ultrasonography, conventional angiography, and magnetic resonance angiography: correlation with ex vivo measurement of plaque stenosis. *J Vasc Surg.* 1995;21:82–88.

279. Elgersma OE, Wust AFJ, Buijs PC, *et al.* Multidirectional depiction of internal carotid artery stenosis: three dimensional time-of-flight MR angiography versus rotational and conventional digital subtraction angiography. *Radiology.* 2000;216:511–516.

280. Culebras A, Kase CS, Masdeu JC, *et al.* Practice guidelines for the use of imaging in transient ischemic attacks and acute stroke. A report of the Stroke Council, American Heart Association. *Stroke.* 1997;7:1480–1497.

281. Tay K, U-King Im J, Trivedi R, *et al.* Imaging the vertebral artery. *Eur Radiol.* 2005;15:1329–1343.

282. Randoux B, Marro B, Koskas F, *et al.* Proximal great vessels of the aortic arch: comparison of three dimensional gadolinium-enhanced MR angiography and digital subtraction angiography. *Radiology.* 2003;229:697–702.

283. Levy C, Laissy JP, Raveau V, *et al.* Carotid and vertebral artery dissections: three-dimensional time-of-flight MR angiography and MR imaging versus conventional angiography. *Radiology.* 1994;190:97–103.

284. Goldberg HI, Grossman RI, Gomori JM, Ashbury AK, Bilaniuk LT, Zimmerman RA. Cervical internal carotid dissection hemorrhage: diagnosing using MR. *Radiology.* 1986;158:157–161.

285. Oelerich M, Stogbauer F, Kurlemann G, Schul C, Schuierer G. Craniocervical artery dissection: MR imaging and MR angiographic findings. *Eur Radiol.* 1999; 9(7):1385–1391.

286. Kasner S, Hankins L, Bratina P, Morgenstern L. Magnetic resonance angiography demonstrates vascular healing of carotid and vertebral artery dissections. *Stroke.* 1997;28:1993–1997.

287. Stringaris K, Liberopoulos K, Giaka E, *et al.* Three-dimensional time-of-flight MR angiography and MR imaging versus conventional angiography in carotid artery dissections. *Int Angiol.* 1996;15(1):20–25.

288. Klufas RA, Hsu L, Barnes PD, Patel MR, Schwartz RB. Dissection of the carotid and vertebral arteries: imaging with MR angiography. *Am J Roentenol.* 1995;164: 673–677.

289. Provenzale JM. Dissection of the internal carotid and vertebral arteries: imaging features. *Am J Roentenol.* 1995;165:1099–1104.

290. Jacobs A, Lanfermann H, Szelies B, Schroder R, Neveling M. MRI- and MRA-guided therapy of carotid and vertebral artery dissections. *Cerebrovas Dis.* 1996; 6(Suppl. 2):80.

291. Nagahiro S, Hamada J, Sakamoto Y, Ushio Y. Follow-up evalluation of dissecting aneurysms of the vertebrobasilar circulation by using gadolinium-enhanced magnetic resonance imaging. *J Neurosurg.* 1997;87:385–390.

292. Meaney JF, Weg JG, Chenevert TL, Stafford-Johnson D, Hamilton BH, Prince MR. Diagnosis of pulmonary embolism with magnetic resonance angi. *N Engl J Med.* 1997;336(20):1422–1427.

293. Oudkerk M, van Beek EJ, Wielopolski P, *et al.* Comparison of contrast-enhanced magnetic resonance angiography and conventional pulmonary angiography for the diagnosis of pulmonary embolism: a prospective study. *Lancet.* 2002;359(9318):1643–1647.

294. Schoenberg SO, Bock M, Floemer F, *et al.* High-resolution pulmonary arterio- and venography using multiple-bolus multiphase 3D-Gd-mRA. *J Magn Reson Imaging.* 1999;3:339–346.

295. Greil G, Powell A, Gildein H, Geva T. Gadolinium-enhanced three-dimensional magnetic resonance angiography of pulmonary and systemic vein anomalies. *J Am Coll Cardiol.* 2002;39:335–341.

296. Santos J, Cunningham C, Hargreaves B, *et al.* Whole-Heart Multislice Imaging using Variable-Density Spirals. 8th SCMR. *J Cardiovasc Magn Reson.* 2005; 7(1):188–189.

297. Maintz D, Ozgun M, Hofmeier A, *et al.* Initial results of free breathing balanced fast field echo whole heart MR angiography. Proceedings of the ISMRM, 11th Annual Scientific Meeting, Kyoto, Japan, 2004, p. 706.

298. Rehwald W, Klem I, Wagner A, Chen EL, Kim R, Judd R. GCFP—a new non-invasive non-contrast cine angiography technique using selective excitation and global coherent free precession. ISMRM, 11th Annual Proceedings, Toronto, Canada, 2004.

299. Klem I, Rehwald W, Heitner J, *et al.* Noninvasive assessment of blood flow based on magnetic resonance global coherent free precession. *Circulation.* 2005;111: 1033–1039.

300. Earls JP, Patel NH, Smith PA, DeSana S, Meissner MH. Gadolinium-enhanced three dimensional MR angiography of the aorta and peripheral arteries: evaluation of a multistation examination using two gadopentetate dimeglumine infusions. *Am J Roentgenol.* 1998;171: 599–604.

301. Paetsch I, Jahnke C, Barkhausen J, *et al.* Detection of coronary stenoses with contrast enhanced, three-dimensional free breathing coronary MR angiography using the gadolinium-based intravascular contrast agent gadocoletic acid (B-22956). *J Cardiovasc Magn Reson.* 2006;8(3):509–516.

CHAPTER 8

Cardiovascular Magnetic Resonance: Evaluation of Myocardial Function, Perfusion, and Viability

Padmini Varadarajan[1], Ramdas G. Pai[1], Krishna S. Nayak[2], Hee-Won Kim[2] & Gerald M. Pohost[1,2]

[1]Loma Linda University Medical Center, Loma Linda, CA, USA
[2]University of Southern California, Los Angeles, CA, USA

Introduction

The present chapter is based on the latest magnetic resonance (MR) approaches to assess cardiac morphology, ventricular function, and myocardial perfusion and viability. In this monograph, we use the most recent term for applications of MR to the cardiovascular system, cardiovascular magnetic resonance (CMR). Chapter 2 describes the physical principals of CMR. As with all MR applications, CMR is based on the work of Felix Bloch [1] at Stanford and Edward Purcell [2] at Harvard, who were the first to report the phenomenon of nuclear magnetic resonance (NMR). Subsequently, remarkable advances have been made in the clinical application of NMR to assess morphology and function (imaging in vivo) and chemical composition (spectroscopy both in isolated organs and in vivo). Nuclear magnetic resonance was adapted in the late 1970s for the clinical evaluation of the cardiovascular system. Imaging was made possible through the introduction of magnetic field gradients as suggested by Paul Lauterbur, PhD [3] and by Peter Mansfield, PhD [4]. Richard

Ernst, PhD used the mathematical operation of Fourier transformation to generate spectra from the information generated after radio-frequency (RF) excitation, in a domain called "*k*-space" [5]. Because of the importance of these discoveries, Purcell, Bloch, Ernst, Lauterbur and Mansfield have all received Nobel prizes, far more than have been awarded for any other medical imaging modality. Another important and early contributor to the field of MRI was Raymond Damadian [6]. He speculated that magnetic resonance signals could characterize tissue as benign or malignant. The history of CMR is described in the manuscript by Pohost [7].

It is now possible to generate images of the heart and blood vessels, with high resolution and in real time. The evolution of CMR has been made possible by the advances in computer technology, advances in the performance of linear magnetic field gradients, and higher field and magnetically homogeneous superconducting magnets [8,9]. With its high spatial resolution and contrast, CMR has become widely regarded as the "gold standard" for the assessment of the morphology and function of the heart, and for the viability of the myocardium. Furthermore, decades of experience have shown it to be safe for biologic tissues, without the use of ionizing radiation such as that produced by X-rays or radionuclides (such as technetium-99 m or thallium-201). Additionally, when used with gadolinium chelate-based paramagnetic contrast agents, there is no nephrotoxicity and allergic reactions are uncommon compared with iodinated X-ray contrast agents. In the presence of end-stage renal disease and/or severe renal dysfunction, the use of gadolinium is generally contraindicated. The major advantage of CMR is that it is able to provide the most comprehensive evaluation of the cardiovascular system. CMR can generate high-resolution images of morphology and function; it can assess myocardial perfusion; it can define myocardial necrosis and scar; it can assess the coronary and peripheral arteries; and it can evaluate myocardial metabolism, (e.g., that of the high energy phosphates, such as phosphocreatine as well as ATP and other intramyocardial phosphates).

If CMR can do so much, why has it not become more widely applied. First, CMR is the most complex of the imaging modalities, requiring two different forms of energy, magnetic and RF. Second, there is a functional complexity inherent to this technique. This stems from the ability to generate considerable information about the heart. Finally, the magnetic and RF fields of CMR can be contraindicated if patients have certain implanted devices, such as a defibrillator.

Brief Review of CMR Principles and Methods

Cardiovascular magnetic resonance (see Chapter 2 for a more comprehensive review on its principles and methods) is the newest of the noninvasive cardiovascular imaging modalities and has become the modality of choice for the optimal evaluation of ventricular volumes and function. It is preferred to catheter-based left ventriculography, which is invasive, requires radio-opaque iodinated contrast medium, and is two-dimensional (2D), although biplane ventriculography improves the volume of ventricle interrogated. CMR of cardiac function requires an elaborate array of equipment including RF coils; instrumentation that allows the generation of RF pulses of varying durations and strengths; a homogeneous magnetic field; hardware to allow selection of tomographic slices in any plane orientation; phase encoding and readout gradients;

Table 8.1   Approximate values of T_1 and T_2 relaxation times at 1.5 T.

Tissue	T_1 (milliseconds)	T_2 (milliseconds)
Myocardium	880	75
Skeletal muscle	1000	30
Blood	1200	360
Fat	260	110

and the software and hardware needed to monitor cardiac and respiratory motion. Understanding the physics of CMR can be challenging. Briefly, CMR images result from a mathematical operation, Fourier transformation, on the signal released in a uniform magnetic field by the sensitive nuclei contained within the organ(s) to be imaged after pulsing with the appropriate RF (the Larmor frequency) for a given magnetic field. For most magnetic resonance imaging, the sensitive nucleus is the proton, i.e., the hydrogen nucleus. The uniform magnetic field generally has a strength of 1.5–3.0 Tesla. A Tesla is the unit of magnetic field equivalent to $\sim 2 \times 10^4$ fold greater than the earth's magnetic field. A second (substantially weaker) unit of magnetic field is the Gauss. The earth's magnetic field is ~ 0.5 Gauss. A Tesla is equivalent to 10,000 Gauss.

First, a RF pulse is used to excite the sensitive nuclei. Then, "relaxation" of the nuclei occurs in two planes and is determined by the longitudinal (T_1) and the transverse (T_2) relaxation times. Intensity of tissue on a CMR image depends on the concentration or density of hydrogen nuclei (or other sensitive nuclei), and the relaxation times, which depend on the strength of the interaction between these nuclei and the surrounding molecular environment [10–12]. Table 8.1 provides the proton relaxation times, T_1 and T_2, for different tissues in the most commonly used magnetic field strength of 1.5 T [13]. The 3 T magnet is now becoming increasingly more popular due to the frequently higher quality of its resultant images.

CMR for Evaluation of Morphology and Function

Pulse sequences consisting of a series of RF pulses and changes in magnetic field gradients are used to generate CMR images include simpler spin-echo and gradient-echo sequences and more complex sequences such as steady state free precession (SSFP), echo-planar imaging (EPI), velocity encoded (VEC) imaging, and RF tagging. Spin echo sequences were among the first pulse sequences to be used to generate cardiovascular images. These sequences consist of a single 90° pulse (i.e., the net magnetization vector **B** within the tissue to be imaged was rotated 90° and this was subsequently followed by a 180° pulse (inverting the net magnetization or **B** vector). In spin-echo images the ventricular blood pool is darker than the myocardium and has become known as "black blood images." Spin-echo images can be acquired more rapidly using an approach known as fast spin-echo imaging which uses multiple echoes generated by a train of 180° pulses known as refocusing pulses that improve the signal-to-noise ratio. Spin-echo sequences are frequently used to assess morphology and myocardial viability using delayed contrast enhancement.

A gradient-echo pulse sequence uses a second gradient with opposite polarity that increases the CMR signal as it leads to the restitution of spin phase coherence. The gradient-echo pulse sequence has been used to assess ventricular function and wall motion, as well as flow patterns in valvular disease, shunts, and great vessels. This pulse sequence depicts the blood pool with a high signal, resulting in "bright blood images." The infusion of paramagnetic contrast agents most commonly a gadolinium-based chelate can further increase the signal-to-noise ratio and highlight differences between various tissues or in pathology within a given tissue (e.g., normal myocardium, reperfused viable myocardium or infarcted or scarred myocardium). In addition, these agents can highlight differences between edematous and nonedematous tissue as well as other differences in the molecular environment within the tissue that affect T_1 and T_2 or the relaxivity of the excited protons (e.g., an increase in both T_1 and T_2 is observed in the presence of myocardial edema) [14]. Chelated gadolinium (e.g., gadolinium DTPA) distributes into the interstitium of edematous tissue. Such chelates however, due to their molecular size do not enter the intracellular space of viable cells [15]. Thus, a contrast agent related increase in signal intensity on delayed imaging provides evidence of infarcted myocardium or myocardial scar [16–20]. Such gadolinium chelate-based contrast agent accumulates in the extracellular volumes in approximately 8–10 minutes after the first-pass of an intravenous injected contrast agent [21].

The pulse sequences described above can be applied in association with a pulse sequence designed to suppress or to null the underlying myocardial signal intensity. The pulse sequence that affects image contrast by nulling the myocardium is known as inversion recovery (IR). Another pulse sequence can lead to suppression of the signal generated by fat or lipid to remove the confounding effects of the bright lipid signal that can obscure the "enhancement" of contrast agent accumulation in necrotic or scarred myocardium.

The use of the SSFP pulse sequence in cine CMR imaging results in a substantial improvement in the image quality compared with those obtained with conventional fast gradient-echo sequences [21,22]. SSFP utilizes high-speed gradients to achieve extremely short repetition times of 3–5 ms. The steady state is achieved and maintained between the transverse and longitudinal magnetization while the magnetic field is exposed to a train of RF pulses that are of equal space uand magnitude. With SSFP, acquisition is less dependent on the inflow of fresh spins (i.e., blood) than with a fast gradient-echo pulse sequence, and signal intensity is related mainly to the inherent properties of the blood and tissue (i.e., the ratio of T_2 to T_1). Thus, the use of SSFP-based pulse sequences has found widespread application in cardiac imaging because of the excellent contrast it can generate between blood and myocardium in addition to its excellent signal-to-noise characteristics. A problem with SSFP is that it behaves well at the most commonly employed field strength of 1.5 T or lower. However, at 3 T artifacts can be problematic. Nevertheless, there are strategies to circumvent the artifact problem with SSFP at 3 T. To combine the virtues of SSFP and of 3 T would provide the best CMRI possible.

EPI, first developed by Mansfield, is among the fastest MR imaging techniques. In EPI, an elongated image acquisition is performed during rapid switching of gradients. This technique can be used to evaluate ventricular function and myocardial perfusion with high temporal resolution.

Phase contrast, phase shift or VEC imaging are used for flow quantification using a pulse sequence specifically designed to produce a phase angle within a pixel where signal is proportional to velocity along one axis. Once pixel-by-pixel velocity is known, flow in a vessel or through a valve can be determined (i.e., multiplying the pixel area by the pixel velocity). Summation of the pixels within the region of interest determines the flow volume. This technique can accurately assess flow and has a wide dynamic range, allowing encoding of a wide range of velocities from several millimeters per second to at least 10 m/second [23,24]. This allows measurement of, for example, cardiac outputs, shunts, and pressure gradients across stenotic valves.

Since the late 1980s, it has been possible to visualize intrinsic myocardial contractile patterns using RF tagging. These patterns are produced by a combination of restricted presaturation localized RF pulses and conventional RF "spoiled" gradient-echo (SPGR) readout gradients [25]. The changes in shape and size of the cardiac chambers throughout the cardiac cycle reflect the function of the atria and ventricles in three dimensions. Parameters such as ventricular eccentricity can be easily determined. The increasing availability of fast-automated post-processing software provides a means for rapid generation of more information about function than is available with any other methodology. RF tag lines have provided CMR images of the heart, which are useful for assessing the detailed contractile function of the myocardium [26]. This includes measurement of left ventricular (LV) circumferential fiber shortening, wall thickening as an indicator of the radial strain, and changes in systolic torsion in patients at baseline and after medical or surgical treatment [27–31]. Figure 8.1 shows a HARmonic Phase image (HARP) analysis of short axis tagged CMR images.

Although successfully used in clinical studies, conventional SPGR tagging has intrinsic disadvantages resulting from the fading of the tag lines during the cardiac cycle (related to repeated RF excitation and T_1 relaxation). Using higher field magnets such as 3 T allows the tag lines to persist for practically the entire cardiac cycle because of T_1 elongation at such higher fields. Current pulse sequences combine partial modulation of magnetization (SPAMM) tagging preparation with fully balanced SSFP acquisition [32,33]. Table 8.2 provides an overview of the terminology for these pulse sequences from the three major manufacturers of CMR instruments and software.

Technical Aspect

Ultimately, images are conventionally acquired to generate a horizontal long-axis (4 chamber), a vertical long-axis (2 chamber), and short-axis planes. Multiple short-axis planes are used to generate ventricular volumes and ejection fraction. Such images are reconstructed as follows: imaging planes are aligned with the coronal (axial) plane and acquired during a breath-hold. Next, the transverse (axial) plane is acquired during a breath-hold. Then, a line is drawn between the LV apex and the middle of the mitral annulus to define the vertical long-axis view. The horizontal long-axis view is then obtained using a comparable cutting line, followed by multiple short-axis planes. Finally, the LV outflow tract view. One must insure that the LV is not shortened and a true long-axis view is obtained. This is accomplished by redoing the long-axis view and prescribing them again from short-axis images of the apex and the mitral valve plane. Images from planes within the principal axes of the body are particularly useful in the evaluation of the anterior right ventricular (RV) wall, but are also useful in the assessment of pericardial thickening or effusion, paracardiac masses, and the aorta.

The optimal management of cardiovascular disease depends on the assessment of LV and RV function. It is widely held that CMR offers the reference standard for the noninvasive assessment of ventricular function and mass [34–40]. It is accurate and reproducible in both normal [41–43] and deformed or asymmetrically contracting ventricles. Such asymmetrical contraction can be caused by a broad spectrum of conditions including myocardial ischemia [44,45], hypertrophy and dilatation [46–49], pulmonary hypertension [50], or after surgical repair [51]. Simpson's rule is the most commonly used approach to measure volume and thereby function. Short-axis cine MR images using gradient-echo pulse sequences are obtained; spanning the whole LV and the volume in each slice is measured and summed over the ventricle. The volumes obtained by this method are independent of geometric assumptions and are dimensionally

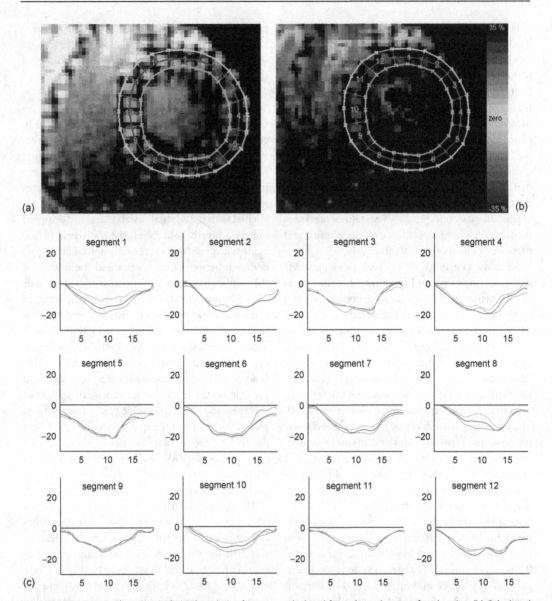

Figure 8.1 HARmonic Phase image (HARP) analysis of short-axis tagged CMR images. (a) A circular grid that contains a variable number of chords of equal size is defined by the user to represent the region of measurement within the left ventricular wall, where the green line represents the subendocardial layer, the red line the mid-wall portion and the blue line the subepicardium. Points on the grid are then automatically tracked through all the image sections in the data set, and strain values are calculated from the trajectory of each point. (b) Calculated strain values are displayed as a color-coded map superimposed on the tagged images. (c) Strain plots showing circumferential shortening in every segment and in all three layers. The x-axis represents the number of imaged phases of the cardiac cycle, and the y-axis is the percentage of change in circumferential shortening. (Reproduced from Castillo et al., Radiographics 2003;23:5127–5140, with permission.)

Table 8.2 Pulse sequence nomenclature for each of the major MR platform manufacturers.

	General electric	Philips	Siemens	Toshiba
Generic				
Spin echo (black blood)				
Standard	SE	SE	SE	SE
Fast breath-hold	FSETSE	TSE		
Ultrafast (single heartbeat)	SSFS E	Single shot TSE	HASTE	HASTE
Gradient echo (bright blood)				
Standard nonbreath-hold	GRASS, GRE	FFE	GRE	FE
Fast breath-hold segmented *k*-space	Fast GRE	TFE	Turbo FLASH	
Steady state free precession (breath-hold segmented *k*-space, high SNR/CNR, real time)	FIESTA	Balanced FFP	True FISP	
Angiographic option				
Velocity encoding imaging	Phase contrast	Phase contrast	Phase contrast	Phase contrast
Suppression techniques				
Inversion recovery	STIR, fseSTIR, fastFLAIR	STIR, tseSTIR, tseFLAIR	STIR, tseSTIR, tseFLAIR	STIR, tseSTIR, tseFLAIR
Fat suppression	fatSAT	SPIR	fatSAT	fatSAT

accurate whether or not the papillary and trabecular volumes are subtracted [52]. Left ventricular volumes also can be determined by the simplified equation of Simpson, i.e., $V = L/2$ (AMV + 2/3 APM), in which the area of the ventricle (V) is measured on two short-axis views (the initial section is obtained just below the mitral valve, (AMV) the second at the level of the papillary muscles, (APM) and the length of the cavities (L) is measured on a four-chamber view. Subtraction of the end-systolic from the end-diastolic volume gives the stroke volume. Multiplying the stroke volume by the heart rate yields the cardiac output, which demonstrates a close correlation with thermodilution catheter methods [53–56]. RV function is also an important determinant of prognosis in coronary artery disease (CAD) [57], in congenital heart disease and in pulmonary hypertension [50]. The Simpson's rule approach can be readily applied to the determination of the volume of the RV since there is no standard geometric model to fit this chamber [58].

Furthermore, right and LV volume measurement using Simpson's equation allows the calculation of the regurgitant fraction, i.e., the ratio of the re-

gurgitant volume (difference in stroke volume between the ventricle with the regurgitant valve and the normal ventricle) and the stroke volume of the regurgitant ventricle, and this calculation correlates with the severity of valvular disease: regurgitation of 15–20%, 20–40%, and greater than 40% represents mild, moderate, and severe regurgitation respectively [59]. Moreover, gradient-echo sequences that depict normally circulating blood as a bright signal depict regurgitant or stenotic valvular high-velocity flow patterns as a signal loss or void [60,61]. Although the area and maximum duration of the signal void vary greatly related to the scanning variables and the "echo time" (TE) in particular [62] these sequences provide specificity, sensitivity and diagnostic accuracy greater than 93, 89, and 92% respectively for severity of aortic and mitral regurgitation [24]. There is also significant correlation with Doppler echocardiography and catheter determined pressure gradients in aortic and mitral stenosis [63–65].

The stroke volumes of the RVs and LVs can also be calculated using VEC CMR imaging to measure flow in the ascending aorta and pulmonary artery in planes either perpendicular to (through-plane velocity measurement) or parallel to (in-plane velocity measurement) the direction of flow [66,67]. This pulse sequence is specifically designed so that the phase angle in each pixel of the selected region-of-interest in each of the 16 time frames constituting the cardiac cycle is proportional to the velocity. The product of the cross-sectional area and the average per pixel velocity within a given region-of-interest yields the instantaneous flow volume and an esti-mated flow volume per heartbeat when integrated [64,68]. The severity of shunt size can be reliably expressed as the ratio of pulmonic-to-systemic flow ratio [69,70]. Thus, the best way to quantify the volume of isolated (mitral, aortic, tricuspid, or pulmonic) regurgitation or stenosis, isolated aortic regurgitation, or isolated is to combine ventricular volume measurements obtained from the LV and RV stroke volumes [71–74]. Of course, this strategy cannot work if there are regurgitant lesions in other valves or an intracardiac shunt.

Global and Regional Systolic Ventricular Function

Cardiovascular magnetic resonance imaging provides precise evaluation of ventricular volumes but also allows assessment of valvular function, and myocardial necrosis and fibrosis. Cardiovascular magnetic resonance imaging has great potential for diagnosis and assessment of risk which are related to its substantial contrast, its large field of view and its ability to image using the intrinsic planes of the heart as opposed to only the axial planes. In order to optimally evaluate ventricular volumes and other relevant parameters, scan planes must be well defined, standardized via cine gradient-echo sequences with measurements of forward flow into the aorta obtained via VEC CMR imaging. This approach optimizes intra and inter-observer agreement (±4.8 and ±7.7%) and has the advantages of being independent of the effects of tricuspid and pulmonary regurgitation, allowing correction for the presence of aortic regurgitation [75–77]. Similarly, pressure gradients across a stenotic valve estimated by VEC MRI vs Doppler echocardiography are closely related for aortic [78–80], mitral [81,82] and pulmonaic stenosis when measured either in the main, the right, or in the left pulmonary arteries [83].

Furthermore, regional ventricular function can be assessed both qualitatively, as with echocardiography [84], and quantitatively. CMR images, especially those acquired in the short axis, have been shown to effectively determine LV regional wall motion [30,85,86]. Outstanding delineation of the endocardial and epicardial borders of the myocardium allows the assessment not only of wall motion but also of wall thinning and thickening, and wall thickness. Wall thickening has been shown to be more sensitive for the detection of abnormal myocardium than the analysis of wall motion [87]. Regional wall thickness can be derived using acquisitions from manually or automatically defined endocardial and epicardial borders in each short-axis image which rely on an approximately circular shape of the LV. As opposed to the center point approach, the centerline method [88,89] relies on a path between the endo- and epicardial contours. Equally spaced perpendicular chords are constructed starting at a clearly visible anatomical reference and spanning the whole circumference of the short-axis ventricular slice. The length of such a chord represents the local wall thickness, and the ratio between the end-systolic and end-diastolic chord length equals the local end-systolic wall thickening. Subsequently, the size, extent, and severity of a wall thickening abnormality can be quantified [88] (Figure 8.2). The use of CMR tag lines and grids in multiple short and long-axis slices provides a means for measurement of three-dimensional (3D) myocardial strain [90,91] at different points within the cardiac cycle reflecting regional ventricular performance. Thus, the CMR with RF tagging provides a means to evaluate normal systolic clockwise rotation at the base and counter clockwise rotation at the apex. Such rotational motion can be demonstrated to be significantly reduced with chronic heart failure and improves with effective treatment [92]. In hypertrophic cardiomyopathy (HCM), the regional dysfunction combines a reduction of both the rotational pattern, mainly in the posterior ventricular wall, and the septal radial strain [26]. In ischemic heart disease, LV circumferential shortening has a strong correlation with the ejection fraction by CMR ventriculography [66] and has proved to be very accurate for the quantitation of the recovery of the segmental LV function after coronary revascularization [29,93].

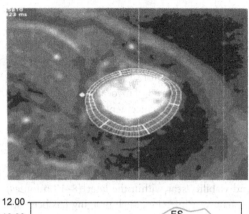

(a)

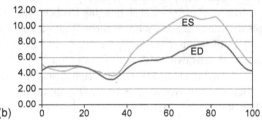

(b)

Figure 8.2 (a) Application of the centerline method for the calculation of regional wall thickness in an end-systolic short-axis MR image. The centerline chords, which are constructed at evenly spaced intervals perpendicular to the centerline, are numbered in a clockwise fashion starting at the white dot. (b) The graph depicts the lengths of the centerline chords. The lack of wall thickening in the region defined by chords 2–35 corresponds to the region of myocardial infarction. ES, end-systolic; ED, end-diastolic. (Reproduced from Van der Geest and Reiber [88], with permission.)

Diastolic Ventricular Function

Not only is CMR effective for the evaluation of systolic LV performance but it is also effective for the assessment of diastolic LV function, including the ability to evaluate ventricular relaxation [94]. Gradient-echo imaging provides a means to generate reproducible measurements of ventricular volumes throughout the cardiac cycle. From the contours describing the endocardial and epicardial borders of the myocardium, ventricular volumes, and mass can be calculated. Additionally, peak (ventricular) filling rate (PFR) and the time to PFR can be determined using the maximal change during the rapid filling phase [94–96]. Prolongation of the time-to-peak during the early filling phase and the time-to-peak wall thickening/thinning rate indicate impaired relaxation. It also correlates with decreased perfusion in HCM [97]. The ratio between early-to-late filling (i.e., the peak early rate divided by the peak late rate) and early filling percentage (i.e., the volume increase from the end of systole to the diastolic midpoint divided by the stroke volume multiplied by 100) can be demonstrated before changes in the classical mitral Doppler pattern in patients with LV hypertrophy occur [98]. Since flow measurements are obtained at high temporal resolution over the complete cardiac cycle, VEC is especially useful for the evaluation of LV

and RV diastolic function parameters. Peak velocity and volume flow of the early (E) and atrial filling waves (A) through both mitral and tricuspid valves [99–101] have been measured using velocity encoding in a reproducible and accurate manner regardless of jet orientation [102]. These measurements show close agreement with Doppler-derived indices in normal [102], hypertrophic [103] and ischemic myocardium [104]. Left ventricular deformation during diastole can be determined by cardiac tagging. Such assessment of the time for ventricular "untwisting" [105] was reported to be prolonged in myocardial infarction (MI) [106] and to be normalized after reperfusion [107]. More recently, the time to peak "untwisting" was found to be an accurate parameter for identifying patients with CAD when evaluated during low dose dobutamine administration [108].

Specific CMR Findings in Cardiomyopathic Heart Disease

Cardiomyopathy of Ischemic Heart Disease

Evaluation of the patient with ischemic heart disease is made possible by the wealth of information provided by CMR, and specifically by its ability to assess ventricular function, myocardial perfusion and ventricular scar. Such imaging data provides a means of assessing cardiovascular risk. Protocols lasting less than 1 hour can combine multiphase cine gradient-echo imaging for function, first pass of paramagnetic contrast agent at rest and during stress with assessment of myocardial perfusion, and delayed contrast enhancement for detection of myocardial scar [109,110]. Perfusion/scar assessment, like the approach using thallium-201, is performed after a single dose of CMR contrast agent, perfusion within the early phase postcontrast injection and viability/scar within the later (8–15 minutes) postcontrast injection. Such imaging has been applied in the emergency room to allow diagnosis and risk stratification in patients presenting with chest pain with sensitivity and specificity of 85% for diagnosis of MI [111,112]. CMR imaging provides a means for determining the total volume rather than only the presence of MI (as indicated, for example, by the presence of the Q waves by electrocardiography) [113,114]. The superior spatial resolution of CMR imaging allows detection of the extent of transmural involvement of MI [115] and adds temporal information to conventional imaging analysis because of its ability to differentiate between acute (<2 weeks old) and chronic (>4 weeks old) MI. Whereas both acute and chronic MI exhibit delayed enhancement [116,117], T_2 weighted CMR imaging allows sensitive detection of infarct associated myocardial edema and the extent of the acute damaged tissue [118]. In combination with delayed enhancement CMR imaging of acute and chronic MI can be differentiated with a specificity of 96% [119]. The reproducibility of CMR imaging has significant cost and time implications in cardiovascular research, as illustrated by the small sample size required to show the efficiency of beta-blockers [120] and angiotensin-converting enzyme inhibitors in reducing LV volumes and improving function by decreasing infarct segment extent, expansion and mass-to-volume ratio [121,122]. Furthermore, using VEC techniques CMR imaging can evaluate the physiologic significance of a native or stented coronary artery stenosis by measuring coronary artery blood flow before and after pharmacologically induced hyperemia [123–126]. The signal–intensity–time curves using first-pass contrast enhanced imaging have been reported to detect significant coronary artery stenosis

(75%) with sensitivity, specificity, and accuracy of 90, 83, and 87% respectively [127,128], and to improve after revascularization procedures [86,129].

Ischemic heart disease is the leading cause of both myocardial diastolic and systolic dysfunction. The underlying cause, i.e., CAD frequently can be detected using cardiovascular magnetic resonance angiography of the coronary arteries [130–145]. This topic has been the focus of several 2D and 3D technical advances in the past few years, which have improved the ability of CMR for assessing CAD severity and extent. Furthermore the role of CMR for characterizing plaque is promising, but still under investigation [146–149]. Approximately, 72% of patients have been accurately diagnosed as having CAD and 87% as having left main or three-vessel coronary disease [150]. For saphenous vein coronary artery bypass grafts that are typically of larger diameter and more fixed in position than native coronary arteries, the sensitivity and specificity for detection of occlusion or of stenosis of 70% or greater were 83 and 99% (for occlusion), and 73 and 83% (for stenosis) [151]. The current method of choice for coronary artery imaging uses fat-saturated ECG-triggered SSFP imaging with or without gadolinium contrast agent administration or respiratory gating. Coronary imaging with CMR requires further refinement to improve its ability to provide consistent visualization of more than the proximal and mid-portions of the major coronary artery branches with a resolution higher than 1.5 mm^3. Several approaches have improved the visualization of the normal and diseased coronary arteries. One approach uses a spin-echo or dark blood approach with a dual-inversion magnetization preparation scheme to suppress the signal of the blood that moves into the imaging plane between the preparation pulses and data acquisition [152–154]. Others include accelerated imaging speed with a receiver coil array and parallel data acquisition [155,156]; development of blood pool contrast agents with greater T_1 shortening effect than the conventional extracellular agents [157,158]; 3 Tesla platform, and [159,160] radial [161,162] and spiral sampling of the k-space with their expected superior signal-to-noise ratio (SNR), contrast-to-noise ratio (CNR), and image quality [163,164]. CMR coronary angiography is not yet adequate for routine diagnosis of CAD, since its spatial resolution is inferior to that of catheter coronary angiography, but its application is regarded as good for identification of the origin and the initial course of anomalous coronary arteries, which frequently present with angina pectoris and may be difficult to delineate by conventional coronary angiography [165–167].

In ischemic cardiomyopathy, mapping the scar distribution and burden in relation to coronary artery anatomy has major implications in treatment planning. Nonscarred muscle or transmural scar distribution of <50% signifies viability [129,168]. Revascularizing ischemic, but viable myocardium would result in improvement of LV function and may facilitate reverse LV remodeling [169]. Using this strategy in patients with ischemic cardiomyopathy may reduce morbidity, mortality and avoidance of unnecessary referral to heart transplantation. In addition to viability, LV endsystolic volume is a powerful determinant of reverse remodeling—larger the LV size, less is the likelihood of functional recovery [170].

In patients with the cardiomyopathy associated with ischemic heart disease, scar burden and scar morphology are predictive of mortality and arrhythmias [171]. The greater the scar burden, the greater the mortality. The appearance of scar seems to be related to arrhythmic risk as well. A heterogeneous scar (delayed contrast enhancement) would indicate islands of scar interspersed with the viable myocardium and has greater arrhythmic potential. Assessment of scar location and extent is helpful in planning for ablation of ventricular arrhythmias, incremental to that provided by electrophysiological mapping [172].

Myocardial scar location and extent predicts response to cardiac resynchronization therapy [173]. Responses are poorer in those with >15% scar burden and those with scarred septum on myocardial delayed enhancement with Gadolinium.

The goals of CMR examination in patients with ischemic cardiomyopathy include assessment of LV function, quantification of myocardial ischemia in relation to coronary anatomy and extent of myocardial scar, and transmural and regional distribution. In addition, CMR is helpful for assessing the anatomy of ischemic mitral regurgitation and excluding significant aortic stenosis that can coexist with ischemic cardiomyopathy (Table 8.3).

Table 8.3   CMR technique and findings in the cardiomyopathy of ischemic heart disease.

Suggested Imaging technique:
- ECG triggered SSFP imaging for assessment of LV and RV morphology and morphology, and valvular morphology and function
- Rest and stress perfusion
- Myocardial delayed enhancement for scar distribution and burden
- VEC of mitral and aortic valves for MR and AS quantitation

Possible Findings:
- Regional wall motion abnormalities
- LV wall thinning – <5.5 mm may indicate infarct, but MDE is better
- LV dilatation, increased volumes, low EF, increased sphericity
- Resting or stress myocardial perfusion deficits
- Myocardial scarring, subendocardial or transmural
- LV thrombus
- RV dysfunction—inferior in inferior MI, global in pulmonary hypertension
- Left atrial enlargement due to MR or high LA pressure; predisposes to atrial fibrillation
- Mitral regurgitation—generally due to tenting of the leaflets, and surrounding the medial commissure (A3 and P3 segments) in inferior MI; tends to involve both leaflets in LV dilitation; is related to the ability to repair the valve.
- Aortic stenosis—can be associated with the presence of CAD

Myocarditis

Delayed contrast enhancement (DCE) is by no means specific for MI. It can detect necrotic or scarred myocardium in a number of other conditions including myocarditis and cardiomyopathies. Since these conditions can affect myocardial function and the extent of DCE can also predict prognosis. Acute myocarditis is a life-threatening inflammatory myocardial disease process [174–176]. It may progress to an autoimmune phase, then to progressive cardiac dilatation and may ultimately lead to dilated cardiomyopathy. Gadolinium DCE provides a marker of inflammation associated with myocardial necrosis. Myocardial inflammatory involvement can spreads from focal to disseminated within the first 2 weeks after the onset of symptoms [177]. The extent of DCE correlates with LV dysfunction in the early stages of myocarditis and to clinical presentation later. The presence of heart failure symptoms after 3 months seems to be accompanied by sustained elevation of global myocardial DCE after administration of gadolinium diethyltriaminetetraacetic acid (Gd-DTPA) [178]. This technique is more sensitive than the single photon radionuclide technique using gallium-67, to visualize inflammation or radiolabeled antimyosin antibody to visualize myocardial necrosis [179,180]. The standard for diagnostic approach for myocarditis is endomyocardial biopsy which also allows demonstration of progression or regression of disease when performed serially [166,174,181].

T_2 weighted imaging also is useful for the diagnosis of myocarditis. The myocardial edema that is a feature of myocarditis is diffuse compared to acute MI which is segmental. The myocardial T_2 weighted signal intensity is compared to that of skeletal muscle. Reduced myocardial signal intensity is found in association with an increase in myocardial mass suggesting myocardial edema [182]. It has been shown that about 50% of the patients presenting with chest pain, increased cardiac markers, and normal coronary arteries have DCE consistent with myocarditis [183]. Table 8.4 summarizes the useful imaging sequences and probable findings that may be encountered in myocarditis.

Table 8.4   CMR techniques and findings in myocarditis.

Suggested Technique:
- ECG gated SSFP for evaluation of LV and RV function
- Delayed enhancement for detection of myocardial necrosis and scar
- T_2 weighted imaging for detection of myocardial edema (edema leads to an increase in T_2 and the relaxation parameter T_2 can be visualized by imaging using the appropriate pulse sequence)

Possible Findings:
- Regional and global LV and RV dysfunction
- Pericardial effusion
- Myocardial delayed enhancement in noncoronary distribution
- Myocardial edema
- Functional mitral regurgitation

Left Ventricular Noncompaction Cardiomyopathy

Left ventricular noncompaction (LVNC) cardiomyopathy is a unique unclassified congenital disorder of endomyocardial morphogenesis with a pattern of inheritance suggesting genetic heterogeneity [157–167,174]. This cardiomyopathy is associated with congestive heart failure, thromboembolism, and malignant ventricular arrhythmias [174,176] in both the pediatric and the adult age ranges [177]. The morphological features of LVNC is inconsistently identified by 2D echocardiography which depicts prominent trabeculations and deep intertrabecular recesses in hypertrophied and hypokinetic segments most commonly affecting apical and mid-ventricular segments of the inferior and lateral walls in more than over 80% of patients [175], with or without concomitant RV involvement [178–180]. Indeed, a high prevalence of anomalous images (47%) as false tendons (75%), trabeculations (23%), or thrombi (2%) of the LV were reported by Tamborini *et al.* [181] for patients with or without pathologic hearts, suggesting the need to update the imaging tools for this misdiagnosed disease [184]. Imaging using CMR is considered the diagnostic modality of choice for patients in whom LVNC is suspected. Cine CMR image using an SSFP pulse sequence shows the numerous trabeculations and intertrabecular recesses in communication with the LV cavity (Figure 8.3) and hypokinesis of the noncompacted ventricular wall during the cardiac cycle [185]. It also allows estimation of LV mass both with and without the incorporation of trabeculations from a stack of contiguous short-axis images. When expressed as a percentage of total mass, trabecular mass of greater than 20% of the total mass suggested the diagnosis of LVNC [186]. Analysis of CMR first-pass perfusion imaging suggests reduced trabecular perfusion without demonstration of either LV thrombus on the early inversion-recovery images or myocardial fibrosis on the later images demonstrating delayed enhancement [186,187].

Dilated Cardiomyopathy

Dilated cardiomyopathy may be primary and associated with alcoholism or secondary to viral infections or ischemic heart disease. There are also

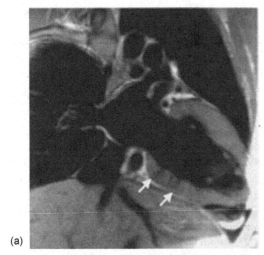
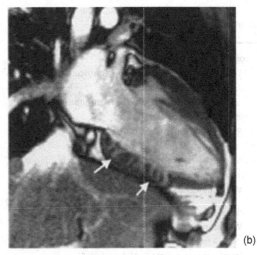

(a)   (b)

Figure 8.3 Vertical long axis of the left ventricle in diastole using SSFP sequence showing multiple inferior wall intertrabecular recesses in communication with the left ventricular cavity (arrows). (Adapted from McCrohon *et al.* [189].)

familial dilated cardiomyopathies. Ischemic cardiomyopathy will be discussed separately.

In dilated cardiomyopathy, there is global, relatively diffuse hypokinesis of the LV and frequently the RV, though in ischemic cardiomyopathy wall motion may be segmental. The atria may be dilated secondary to both direct cardiomyopathic involvement as well as increased atrial pressures. Dilated LV and RV may tether mitral or tricuspid leaflets causing functional MR or TR. In functional regurgitation, the leaflets are intrinsically normal, but prevented from closing because of apically/laterally directed pull by the chordae due to the dilated ventricles. Mitral and pulmonary vein flows may show patterns of elevated LA pressure and the IVC may be dilated if RA pressure is high. Delayed contrast enhancement may be observed due to LV scarring which may be patchy, mid myocardial or subendocardial in ischemic cardiomyopathy in the presence of previous MI. Significant subendocardial scar is indicative of an ischemic etiology. Performance of DCE imaging may be helpful before implantable cardiac defibrillator (ICD) implant, in view of the possibility that many of these patients live long enough to have intractable ventricular arrhythmia which may need electrophysiological ablative therapy. Scar distribution and morphology can be helpful in planning VT ablation along with electroanatomic mapping during ablation. The pres-

ence and amount of myocardial scar is predictive of adverse cardiovascular events [188]. Cardiomyopathy also can be caused by non-compaction of the left ventricle [189]. Table 8.5 summarizes suggested imaging techniques and possible abnormalities.

Hypertrophic Cardiomyopathy

HCM is an autosomal-dominant disorder characterized by LV hypertrophy, myofibrillar disarray, and a high prevalence of sudden death [190–194]. The most frequent cause of death is ventricular arrhythmia [194,195]. Although no single test can reliably predict outcome in HCM, CMR provides excellent morphological definition and noninvasive tissue characterization contributing to risk stratification. Most often the thickness of the interventricular septum as can be assessed in the four-chamber or short-axis view is at least 15 mm in end-diastole [196–198]. Serial CMR studies provide a means to identify concerning changes [199] such as alterations in the three-dimensional distribution [200,201] of myocardial mass. Myocardial mass is normal in about 20% of the patients and hypertrophy is not a prerequisite for the diagnosis of HCM. However, increased mass is a sensitive predictor of adverse outcome [202]. RF tagging provides a means for CMR to demonstrate [28,203] abnormally enhanced LV torsion. The use of CMR determined abnormalities in myocardial perfusion [204]

Table 8.5 CMR techniques and findings in dilated cardiomyopathy.

Suggested imaging technique:
● ECG triggered SSFP imaging for ventricular and valvular function and anatomy
● GRE for better visualization of regurgitant jets—four chamber and LV long axis views
● Rest and stress perfusion if coronary angiogram has not been done
● Myocardial delayed enhancement for scar burden and distribution
● VEC of mitral and aortic valves

Findings:
● Wall motion abnormalities
● LV wall thinning
● LV dilatation, increased volumes, low EF
● Resting or stress myocardial perfusion deficits
● Myocardial scarring: patchy, midmyocardial or subendocardial
● LV thrombus
● RV dysfunction
● Left atrial enlargement
● Mitral regurgitation (functional)
● Features of raised LA or RA pressure

Table 8.6 CMR techniques and findings in hypertrophic cardiomyopathy.

Suggested CMR approaches in HCM:
● ECG triggered SSFP imaging allows optimal assessment of ventricular and valvular function and morphology Myocardial perfusion imaging at rest and with stress provides a means to evaluate ischemic burden
● Delayed myocardial enhancement imaging allows detection of the presence, extent and distribution of myocardial scar
● VEC of mitral valve for MR and LVOT for gradient–

Possible findings:
● LV hypertrophy, often asymmetric (severity correlates with sudden death risk)
● Myocardial fibrosis (extent and heterogeneity correlates with risk of ventricular arrhythmias)
● Systolic anterior motion (SAM) of the anterior mitral leaflet
● Mitral regurgitation related to systolic anterior motion of the anterior leaflet of the mitral valve or SAM; mitral regurgitation is occasionally related to another mechanism
● Dynamic LV outflow tract obstruction
● RV hypertrophy
● Myofibrillar disarray by diffusion-tensor imaging
● Increased mitral leaflet length
● Left atrial enlargement
● Myocardial perfusion defects
● Reduced myocardial velocities and strain despite normal EF

and myocardial transmural wall motion and, the presence of delayed contrast enhancement [205,206], provide a means to detect changes that may predict problematic clinical course in HCM patients. It has been postulated that an important anatomic component of the arrhythmogenic substrate in HCM is the presence of areas of plexiform fibrosis [193] shown to occur in hypertrophied regions, predominantly in the junction of the septum and the RV free wall in a patchy manner [205]. The extent of septal hypertrophy and scarring in young patients with HCM has been identified by CMR in patients experiencing ventricular tachycardia and sudden death [206,207]. This underscores the important role of CMR imaging for risk assessment in patients with HCM. The abnormal systolic anterior motion of the anterior mitral valve leaflet and the resultant eccentric mitral regurgitation are easily detected. As noted above, the extent of myocardial scarring that can be assessed by using CMR imaging of delayed contrast enhancement is associated with a risk of ventricular arrhythmias [208]. Approximately 2% of patients with HCM have apical

aneurysms that are often missed by echocardiography [209]. Such aneurysms are associated with a high risk of death [209]. Both morphology and scar in these aneurysms is optimally assessed by CMR. A summary of suggested imaging techniques for the evaulation of patients with HCM and possible findings are listed in Table 8.6.

Arrhythmogenic RV Dysplasia
Assessment of the morphology and function of the RV is difficult [42] and CMR imaging provides an optimal approach for its evaluation. Isolated involvement of the RV is observed in arrhythmogenic RV dysplasia (ARVD), an autosomal dominant familial cardiomyopathy [210,211] that can lead to sudden death in young patients due to ventricular arrhythmias [212–216]. Unfortunately, CMR as an isolated approach for the diagnosis of ARVD is not

Table 8.7   Diagnostic criteria for ARVD.

There is no pathognomonic feature of ARVD. The diagnosis of ARVD is based on a combination of several major and minor criteria. To make a diagnosis of ARVD either 2 major criteria, 1 major and 2 minor criteria, *or* 4 minor criteria is required [215].

Major criteria

(1) Right ventricular dysfunction:

Severe RV dilatation and reduction of RVEF with little or no impairment of LV function

Localized RV aneurysms

Severe segmental dilatation of the RV

(2) Tissue characterization

Fibrofatty replacement of myocardium on endomyocardial biopsy

(3) Conduction abnormalities

Epsilon waves in $V_1 - V_3$.

Localized prolongation (>110 ms) of QRS in $V_1 - V_3$

(4) Family history

Familial disease confirmed on autopsy or surgery

Minor Criteria

(1) Right ventricular dysfunction

Mild global RV dilatation and/or reduced ejection fraction with normal LV.

Mild segmental dilatation of the RV

(2) Regional RV hypokinesis

(3) Tissue characterization: none

(4) Electrophysiological abnormalities

Inverted T waves in V_2 and V_3 in an individual over 12 years old, in the absence of a RBBB Arrhythmias

Late potentials on signal averaged EKG.

Ventricular tachycardia with LBBB

Frequent PVCs (>1000 PVCs/24 hours)

(5) Family history

Family history of sudden cardiac death before age 35

Family history of ARVD (even if not confirmed at autopsy or surgery)

Table 8.8   CMR techniques and findings in ARVD.

Suggested CMR technique:

• ECG gated "black blood" imaging for morphology, preferably using a double inversion recovery, fast spin-echo pulse sequence

• SSFP imaging to evaluate RV volume, EF, regional function: axial slices preferable

• Delayed enhancement contrast imaging to depict fibrosis in the RV free wall

CMR Imaging Findings in ARVD:

• RV hypokinesis, dyskinesis, aneurysm, especially in triangle of dysplasia consisting of subtricuspid area, apex and RVOT

• Enlargement of RVOT area, larger than aortic root or bulging during systole

• Low RVEF (≤35%)

• Fat in RV myocardium (may need smaller FOV with anterior coil elements only to prevent wrap around artifact)

• Late gadolinium enhancement of the RV free wall

• Blurring of the line of demarcation between epicardial fat and RV myocardium

• Areas of RV wall thinning (<2 mm) and wall thickening (>8 mm)

• Giant Y-shaped trabeculae and hypertrophy of the RV moderator band

as helpful as originally hoped. Diagnosis depends on a combination of clinical and imaging criteria as outlined in Tables 8.7 and 8.8 [215]. Nevertheless, using appropriate pulse sequences, CMR can be of substantial value for the diagnosis of ARVD. A unique aspect of ARVD that can be detected by CMR is the fibro-fatty infiltration in the RV free wall growing from epicardium to endocardium that appears as territory with high signal intensity on T_1 weighted scanning [212–216]. As an isolated find-

ing, intramyocardial fat is neither specific nor relevant to the assessment of ARVD and may be a source of false positive diagnosis [217]. However, when other morphologic features associated with this disease are added to the presence of intramyocardial lipid by CMR the diagnosis becomes more certain. These additional findings include dilatation of the RV and its outflow tract [218,219], and variable size ventricular aneurysmal change detected by inversion-recovery segmented fast-spin-echo imaging [220]. Global and regional systolic function is generally best assessed by a SSFP pulse sequence. Several studies have addressed the presence of RV diastolic dysfunction as an early marker of ARVD, even when systolic function is preserved [221,222], and this might be considered by some as an additional criterion for diagnosis of ARVD [223].

Constrictive Pericarditis

The clinical and hemodynamic features of restrictive cardiomyopathy can overlap with those of

Table 8.9 CMR technique and findings in constrictive pericarditis (CP).

CMR methods:

1) Spin echo imaging for measurement of pericardial thickness

2) ECG gated SSFP with axial images as well as using cardiac axes

3) Real time imaging available on many new generation CMR imaging devices, to assess interventricular motion (paradoxical in CP)

MRI findings:

● Pericardial thickness >4 mm
● Pericardial tethering to underlying cardiac chamber walls
● Biatrial enlargement
● Ventricular septal bounce in diastole
● Dilated IVC suggesting high RA pressure
● Demonstration of marked septal shift during respiration on real-time imaging (interventricular dependence)

Table 8.10 CMR findings in cardiac amyloidosis.

● Morphologic LV hypertrophy (with low QRS voltage and./or Q waves on ECG)
● Low myocardial signal intensity
● Patchy scarring by late gadolinium enhancement
● Biatrial enlargement
● RV wall thickness
● Thickened interatrial septum
● Valve leaflet thickening
● Dilated inferior vena cava (related to elevated RA pressure)
● Dilated pulmonary veins (related to elevated LA pressure)

constrictive pericarditis. Differentiation between the two can be provided by CMR imaging. Although Talreja *et al.* reported normal pericardial thickness in 18% (5 of 26) of patients with constrictive pericarditis [224], the CMR measurement of pericardial thickness improves the diagnosis of constrictive pericarditis. When spin-echo CMR imaging showed a pericardial thickness that exceeded 4 mm, the sensitivity, specificity and accuracy for of constrictive pericarditis were 88, 100, and 93% respectively [225]. Early posterior motion of the interventricular septum during inspiration is another finding that assists with diagnosis of constrictive pericarditis, indicating interventricular dependence. This abnormal septal motion can be detected using spin-echo imaging or even more effectively using real time CMR imaging. Other features include evidence of high ventricular filling pressures and biatrial dilatation (Table 8.9).

Infiltrative Myocardial Diseases

Certain infiltrative diseases of the myocardium can cause typical changes in myocardial signal intensity. For example, in amyloid involvement of the myocardium, restrictive physiology is associated with increased right and left atrial volumes, right atrial

wall thickness and RV free wall thickness and reduced wall motion and ejection fraction. An increase in myocardial mass with reduced voltage or infarct patterns on the electrocardiogram is highly suggestive of an infiltrative process such as cardiac amyloid. These measurements differentiate amyloid cardiomyopathy from hypertrophic cardiomyopathy. Furthermore, CMR imaging can differentiate amyloid involvement of the myocardium in patients with hypertrophic cardiomyopathy from that in a group of healthy volunteers. Myocardial signal intensity in cardiac amyloidosis is significantly lower both at an echo delay (TE) of 20 ms and a TE of 60 ms [226]. Patchy delayed enhancement is also seen in patients with cardiac amyloid (Table 8.10).

Sarcoidosis

Cardiac involvement in patients with sarcoidosis can precede, occur concurrently, or follow involvement in other organs. It has no specific clinical signs. Two-dimensional echocardiography can miss structural or functional changes due to granuloma formation and fibrosis [197]. Thallium-201 (^{201}Tl) myocardial imaging findings have no prognostic value when positive [227] and when absent, do not exclude the presence of cardiac involvement if normal [228]. Furthermore, the sensitivity of myocardial biopsy can be as low as 20% [229]. The ability of CMR imaging to diagnose sarcoid heart disease has been demonstrated in several case reports [230–233]. CMR imaging findings were recently shown to correlate with clinical findings

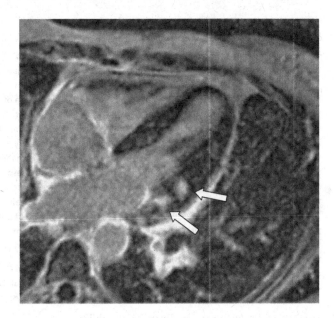

Figure 8.4 Delayed enhancement CMR images in a four-chamber view showing patchy infiltration of the left ventricular lateral wall (multiple foci with increased intensity, depicted by white arrows) due to sarcoid involvement.

and immunosuppressive treatment responses at follow-up [234]. The patchy sarcoid infiltrate progresses through three successive histologic stages: granulomatous, exudative, and fibrotic. All are visible on CMR images as zones of increased intramyocardial signal intensity that are more pronounced on T_2 weighted images (Figure 8.4) most likely related at least in part to the edema associated with inflammation and enhanced after gadolinium injection [235]. Early aggressive treatment of sarcoidosis diagnosed with CMR imaging can avoid the serious consequences of myocardial involvement. The most serious consequence of myocardial sarcoid involvement is sudden death due to conduction system involvement or ventricular arrhythmias. Unfortunately, in patients with older pacemakers or automated implantable cardioverter-defibrillators CMR imaging is generally contraindicated [236]. In these patients the radionuclide perfusion imaging allows estimation of the extent of myocardial damage. Sarcoidosis can also involve the RV and resultant severe RV dysfunction can be present which may mimic ARVD. The CMR findings for sarcoidosis are summarized in Table 8.11.

Congenital Heart Diseases

CMR is of immense value in patients with complex and simple congenital heart disease. It complements echocardiography and catheter lab angiography for

Table 8.11   CMR technique and findings in sarcoidosis.

Suggested technique:

(1) ECG gated SSFP sequence to assess LV and RV function

(2) T_2 weighted imaging for myocardial characterization including detection of the presence of edema reflecting active inflammatory process and potentially the presence of other agents associated with inflammation such as free radicals

● Delayed gadolinium enhancement for detection of myocardial scarring

MRI findings:

● Regional or global LV dysfunction

● RV dysfunction that may mimic ARVD

● In early myocardial sarcoid T_2 increases which may help with diagnosis but also with response to intense therapy

● Patchy myocardial scarring on late gadolinium enhancement

the diagnostic value for the assessment of patients with possible congenital heart disease. In the planning of CMR in evaluation for congenital heart disease (CHD), it is important to bring up the clinical questions and formulate a customized imaging protocol to answer these questions. These may vary from patient to patient. In general, the unique capabilities of CMR that are useful include the ability to

Table 8.12 General CMR approach to patients with congenital heart diseases.

- Obtain and review the 2D echocardiogram
- Formulate the goals of the CMR examination
- Acquire an axial stack of ECG gated thick SSFP slices from hepatic IVC to aortic arch
- Additional targeted cine SSFP images with thin slices focusing on structures of interest
- If there are metal artifacts, use static TSE with blood suppression to assess morphology
- 3D dynamic MRA to evaluate entire course of blood transit from vena cavae to aorta.
- Late contrast enhancement to search for scar particularly if ventricular arrhythmias are present
- VEC for pulmonary and aortic flow and any areas of flow disturbance both for volumetric assessment and obtain gradients

Table 8.13 CMR in patients with repair of TOF.

Suggested CMR approach:
(1) ECG gated SSFP for LV and RV function, especially RV volumes in patients with pulmonic regurgitation, evaluation of RVOT morphology, and detection of RVOT aneurysms
(2) Dynamic 3D MRA for assessment of the RVOT, pulmonary artery and branches, and ascending aorta
(3) Late gadolinium enhancement for myocardial scarring, especially in the area of the RVOT and VSD patch area, moderator band, inferior RV insertion, LV apex, and LV free walls
(4) VEC of pulmonary valve flow to look at velocity profile, amount of regurgitation and evaluation of stenoses at any level

Possible MRI findings:
- Residual RVOT obstruction
- Aneurysm in the region of the RVOT
- Peripheral pulmonary artery stenosis, stent in PA branch
- Presence and degree of pulmonic regurgitation
- Increased RV volume and reduced EF from severe pulmonic regurgitation.
- Residual RV hypertrophy
- Residual VSD
- Ascending aortic dilatation
- Aortic regurgitation
- Tricuspid regurgitation due to RV dilatation from RV volume overload
- Scar in RVOT area and VSD patch area, moderator band, inferior RV insertion, LV apex, and LV free wall

assess LV and RV volumes and function, the ability to assess detailed morphology, the ability to define connections between different chambers, vessels and conduits and their patency, and the ability to assess myocardial scarring. A general approach to patients with congenital heart diseases is summarized in Table 8.12. Some of the specific problems frequently encountered in adult patients are discussed briefly.

Tetralogy of Fallot

Cardiovascular magnetic resonance imaging is commonly performed as a means to diagnose Tetrology of Fallot in children and in young adults especially following surgical correction (Table 8.13). The fundamental defect is underdevelopment of the subpulmonary infundibulum resulting in RV outflow tract stenosis or atresia, large nonrestrictive VSD, larger over-riding aorta and RV hypertrophy. The aorta receives blood from both ventricles resulting in pulmonary oligemia and cyanosis. Surgical repair involves resection of infundibular stenosis or pulmonary valvotomy or an RV to PA conduit depending on the anatomy to direct venous blood into the lungs and closure of the VSD with a patch to direct LV blood flow into the aorta. The ascending aorta may be dilated and the aortic valve may be secondarily regurgitant. There may also be peripheral pulmonary artery stenosis or an ASD. The major sequelae after

repair include VT from scar in the RVOT and severe pulmonary regurgitation causing RV enlargement and dysfunction which may also result in atrial arrhythmias.

The clinical questions postrepair include assessment of any residual lesions, degree of pulmonary regurgitation, size and function of the RV as the possible consequences of RV volume overload, and myocardial scarring as a source of ventricular tachycardia. In patients with severe pulmonary regurgitation but with no symptoms, reliable serial follow-up of RV volume and EF are critical, to detect the presence and severity of RV volume overload as an indication for pulmonary valve surgery. CMR is the most reproducible way for assessing RV volume and function [237] without the risk or ionizing radiation as with CT scanning in this pediatric and adolescent patient population. There is no clear threshold at which to perform pulmonary valve replacement, but a RVEDV index of <160 cc/m2 and RVESV index of <82 cc/m^2 are likely indications [238]. Larger volumes and lower EF are associated with reduced exercise tolerance and irreversibility of postoperative RV dysfunction [239]. DCE imaging of postrepair patients uniformly shows scarring in the RVOT and septal patch areas [240]. Other areas where DCE are of interest include the insertion of the moderator band, inferior RV insertion point, LV apex at vent site and rarely the LV free walls as a reflection of previous MI. This DCE indicates scarring and is more common in older individuals, and is associated with worse symptoms, RV dysfunction and ventricular arrhythmias [240].

Transposition of Great Arteries (TGA)

In TGA, the great arteries (aorta and pulmonary artery) come from the wrong ventricles such that the venous blood from RV is ejected into the aorta and LV ejects into pulmonary artery such that the infant is profoundly cyanotic. To sustain life, there should be a connection between the two closed circuits at some level through an ASD, VSD or a PDA or an iatrogenically created ASD by septostomy. Surgical correction is done early in life and hence in adulthood only postsurgical patients are seen.

Though many anatomic variants of TGA do exist, the most common variety has viscero-atrial situs solitus (i.e., liver, right atrium and trilobed bronchus on the right side), atrioventricular concordance (RA connected to RV and LA connected to LV), d-loop (RV on right side) and ventriculo-arterial discordance (aorta connected to RV and PA to LV).

There are two basic types of surgical corrections: venous switch and arterial switch. Venous switch is the older operation where vena caval blood is directed into the mitral valve and hence to LV and PA into the lungs either with a pericardial patch (Mustard procedure) or native atrial tissue (Senning procedure) and pulmonary venous blood is directed into tricuspid valve, and hence into RV and aorta for systemic circulation. Hence, RV will be pumping into the systemic circulation which may lead to RV dysfunction and functional tricuspid regurgitation. The other problems may be baffle leaks, pulmonary venous inflow stenosis, obstruction of the vena caval inflow, sinus node dysfunction and atrial and ventricular arrhythmias. Arterial switch involves normalizing the arterial connections so that the ventricles pump into the correct great arteries. In patients with VSD and pulmonary stenosis or atresia, the Rastelli procedure is performed, which involves VSD patch closure with direction of LV flow into aorta and a valve conduit from RV to pulmonary artery.

The goals of the examination in those with atrial switch include assessment of systemic and pulmonary vemous inflows, any baffle leaks or obstructions, assessment of the function of the systemic ventricle, regurgitation of systemic atrioventricular valve, any myocardial scarring and any outflow obstructions. Pulmonary venous inflow obstruction can cause pulmonary hypertension and significant baffle leaks can cause cyanosis. Time resolved contrast enhanced MRA with 3D reconstruction are excellent for evaluation of intrathoracic great veins and arteries, their sequential anatomy and detection of any shunts [241]. MRI is excellent for assessment of systemic RV and subpulmonic LV functions [242,243]. Same group of investigators have also shown that the RV shortening becomes more circumferential that longitudinal and that the subpulmonic LV strain is intermediate between that of a normal LV and RV (Table 8.14).

Coarctation of the Aorta

Coarctation of the aorta commonly manifests as a discrete stenosis just distal to the subclavian artery, though a longer hypoplastic segment may be found. This results in a gradient and flow acceleration across the narrowing and development of collaterals across the narrowing involving the intercostal arteries which result in rib notching. Most popular surgical therapy is coarctation resection with end to end anastomosis and patch enhancement of the arch if necessary. Angioplasty or stenting is more popular with recurrent coarctation. MRI is uniquely suited for a comprehensive assessment of coarctation in terms of anatomy, gradient, functional significance and collaterals.

The goals of the examination broadly are to show the anatomy of the lesion, evaluate the gradient and assess amount of collateral flow. When flows are evaluated by phase contrast imaging in patients with coarctation, the aortic flow at the level of the

Table 8.14   CMR in patients with repair of TGA (venous or atrial switch).

Suggested technique:
(5) ECG gated SSFP for LV and RV function
(6) Dynamic 3D MRA for assessment of all connections, baffle leaks and aortopulmonary collaterals
(7) Delayed contrast enhancement for myocardial scarring, especially in the RV
(8) Assessment of ventricular outflow tracts for obstruction and tricuspid valve for regurgitation

Possible MRI findings:
● Increased RV volume and reduced EF from supporting systemic circulation
● RV scarring
● Tricuspid regurgitation (systemic AV valve)
● Obstruction to caval inflow
● Obstruction to pulmonary venous inflow causing pulmonary hypertension
● Baffle leak which can cause arterial desaturation
● Aortopulmonary collaterals on MR angiogram
● Small, thin walled LV with SAM causing dynamic subpulmonic (i.e., LVOT) obstruction

Table 8.15   CMR in patients with coarctation of the aorta.

Suggested technique:
(9) ECG gated SSFP for LV function and mass, aortic valve morphology and aorta
(10) 3D MRA with MIP for visualization of the area of coarctation, obtain measurements and assess collaterals
(11) GRE sequence to visualize flow jets in the aorta and aortic valve
(12) TSE with blood signal suppression for high resolution, high contrast images of the area of coarctation. This sequence is less affected by presence of a stent as well.
(13) VEC to measure flow above the coarctation and at the level of the diaphragm to evaluate amount of collateral flow
(14) Maximum flow velocity, peak gradient, mean gradient and diastolic flow signal at the coarctation site.
(15) Flow velocity profile in the descending aorta to look for reduced pulsation and continuous flow.

Possible MRI findings:
● Narrowing or hypoplasia distal to left subclavian artery
● Increased flow velocity across the narrowing
● Diastolic flow with slow deceleration across the narrowing
● Continuous, nonpulsatile flow in descending aorta
● Intercostal collaterals
● Greater flow at the level of the diaphragm below the coarctation compared to just above the coarctation due to collateral flow
● Associated lesions: bicuspid aortic valve, aortic stenosis, aortic regurgitation, LV hypertrophy, ASD, VSD, subvalvular aortic stenosis

diaphragm is substatntially higher compared to just proximal to coarctation in comparison to normals where it is 11% lower [244]. Compared to echocardiography, it provides better anatomy and visualization of the arch and assessment of collateral flow. Well developed collateral flow can reduce the gradient despite severe coarctation [245]. In a study of 31 patients, the degree of narrowing on 3D MR angiography and slow deceleration coarct flow were independent predictors of coarct severity [246]. Suggested imaging routine and expected findings are summarized in Table 8.15.

Single Ventricle Physiology

This encompasses a wide variety of conditions in which all blood is pumped via a single functioning ventricle. The caval blood flows passively (without an intervening ventricle) into the pulmonary arteries through a Fontan type of connection placed surgically. The functioning ventricle could be of an LV or an RV type. The Fontan connection could be atrio-pulmonary (between RA appendage and the left pulmonary aretery), superior cavopulmonary

(SVC to RPA) or a lateral tunnel between IVC and PA. The goals of the examination are to evaluate conduit patency, rule out thrombi (pulmonary emboli will impede passive pulmonary flow), to assess ventricular function, and to assess other associated abnormalities.

Suggested techniques for visualization of anatomy, flows and possible complications are listed in Table 8.16. Time resolved 3D MR angiography is excellent for demonstration of Fontan connections, to rule out leaks, thrombi and any stenoses [247]. Uneven distribution of flow to the lungs is a problem in these patients and generally evaluated by radionuclide pulmonary scanning.

Table 8.16   CMR in patients with single ventricle physiology.

Suggested technique:

(1) ECG gated SSFP for ventricular function, visualization of vena cavae and connections, visualization of PA

(2) Dynamic 3D MRA for assessment of all connections, rule out compression of pulmonary veins, Fontan baffle fenestrations

(3) Delayed contrast enhancement for myocardial scarring

(4) VEC MRI for Fontan pathway, valves and amount of flow in each lung

Possible MRI findings:

● LV or RV morphology of the single ventricle with or without dysfunction

● Scarring of the single ventricle

● Obstruction to Fontan pathway or fenestrations

● Thrombus in Fontan pathway or PA

● Preferential flow into one of the lungs

● Obstruction to pulmonary venous inflow by the Fontan pathway

● Aortopulmonary collaterals

● Regurgitation of atrioventricular valve

● Dilated vena cavae (high pressure) due to increasing pulmonary vascular resistance or left heart failure

However, phase contrast MRI of the flow in the pulmonary artery branches is more accurate for such assessment [248]. MRI has also been used to evaluate flow during stress and nonlinear power loss [249].

Valvular Heart Disease

Echocardiography has evolved as the current gold standard for the assessment of valvular anatomy and function. But many patients have difficult acoustic windows and CMR serves as an alternate imaging modality for the assessment of valves. In addition, valves need to be assessed in patients undergoing CMR for other reasons to complete the cardiac assessment. As volumetric measurements of LV and RV are most accurate on CMR compared to other imaging tools, CMR is best suited for surveillance on ventricular volume and EF in patients with asymptomatic regurgitant lesions.

Basic questions in patients with valvular disease are (1) severity of the lesion; (2) its hemodynamic impact; (3) mechanism of valve dysfunction; (4) impact on ventricular function; and (5) morphology to evaluate reparability in lesions such as MR, TR, and to some extent AR. The following tables summarize in specific terms on some of the common conditions.

Mitral Regurgitation

Mitral regurgitant (MR) jet can be seen in Fiesta and gradient-echo imaging, though with better contrast with GRE. Jet size, origin and extent can be evaluated. Volumetric assessment can be made with one of the two methods in those with isolated MR: as difference in LV and RV stroke volume from Fiesta images or the difference in the forward flows between the mitral and aortic valves by phase velocity imaging (Table 8.17). Regurgitant fraction by the first method correlates well with echocardiographic estimates; a regurgitant fraction >48% correlates with severe MR [250]. The mitral anatomy can be accurately determined by multiple, parallel long-axis cuts through the mitral valve perpendicular to the commissures [251]. Segmental mitral valve anatomy assessed with this technique is very accurate compared to transesophageal echocardiography (TEE) or surgical inspection. CMR is the gold standard for the assessment for LV volumes and would be the technique of choice to monitor LV volumes in patients with asymptomatic chronic severe MR. In patients with ischemic mitral regurgitation, CMR is helpful not only in assessing myocardial ischemia and viability, but also LV geometry and functional anatomy of the mitral apparatus and is extremely helpful in planning surgical therapy [252].

Aortic Regurgitation

As with mitral regurgitation, with MRI one can visualize the AR jet and do volumetric quantitation (Table 8.18). Recently, it has been shown that one can planimeter the regurgitant orifice as well and this correlates well with AR severity by contrast angiography [253]. Assessment of LV volume is important for timing of surgery and follow-up. Both black blood imaging and MR angiography

Table 8.17 CMR in mitral regurgitation.

Suggested technique:

(1) ECG gated SSFP for LV and RV function, left atrial size and mitral anatomy. In isolated MR, difference in LV and RV stroke volume from chamber tracings is regurgitant volume

(2) GRE or SSFP for jet size, location and direction

(3) VEC MRI of mitral and ascending aortic for determination of MR regurgitant volume in those with no AR

(4) Mitral flow and pulmonary vein flow profiles for MR quantitation and hemodynamics

(5) TR velocity for PA pressure measurement

Possible MRI findings:

● MR quantitation: severe if jet reaches the posterior LA wall, there is systolic flow reversal in pulmonary vein or regurgitant fraction >50%

● MR hemodynamics: high LA pressure if mitral E/A ratio >2 or PA pressure is elevated from TR velocity assessment. RV may be hypokinetic in pulmonary hypertension

● MR mechanism: assess for prolapsing or flail mitral leaflets, leaflet tenting which occurs secondary to LV dilation of regional dyssynchrony, mitral annular dilation or mitral leaflet vegetations or perforations

● MV repairability: important assessments are leaflet structure, extent of prolapse, degree of tenting and if both leaflets are tented and mitral annular diameter

● Effect of LV function and LA size: LV EF and LVESV are important for monitoring asymptomatic patients. LA size correlates with atrial fibrillation risk and long term outcomes.

Table 8.18 CMR in aortic regurgitation.

Suggested technique:

(1) ECG gated SSFP for LV and RV function, left atrial size and aortic valve anatomy

(2) GRE or SSFP for jet size, location and direction

(3) VEC MRI of mitral and aortic valves for determination of AR regurgitant volume in those with no MR

(4) VEC of descending thoracic aorta or distal arch to evaluate diastolic flow reversal

Possible MRI findings:

● AR quantitation: severe if jet occupies >50% of LVOT area, or holodiastolic flow reversal in the descending aorta or regurgitant fraction >50%

● Hemodynamics of AR: high LA pressure if mitral E/A ratio >2 or PA pressure is elevated from TR velocity assessment. RV may be hypokinetic in pulmonary hypertension. Pressure half time of AR signal <250 ms generally indicates severe AR.

● Mechanism of AR: assess for bicuspid aortic valve, aortic root dilation and leaflet vegetations or perforations. AR jet is away from the conjoint cusp. Measure aortic annulus, sinus, sinotubular junction and the tubular portion.

● Effect of LV function: LV EF and LVESV are important for monitoring asymptomatic patients.

are excellent for visualization of the ascending aorta for incidental pathology and also evaluate AR mechanism and decide if ascending aortic surgery is needed.

Valvular Aortic Stenosis

Aortic stenosis is the commonest cause of valve replacement in the United States and its prevalence is likely to rise with increasing life expectancy. The gold standard for assessment of its severity and hemodynamics has been echocardiography. However in many patients echocardiographic images are suboptimal and an alternate noninvasive assessment tool is desirable. CMR offers an alternative technique and is accurate for the assessment of aortic valve area by phase velocity mapping [254]

(Table 8.19). Continuity equation is used as in echocardiography. The stroke volume is obtained either by LV tracing or by through plane flow in the LV outflow tract or the ascending aorta as the flow at the valve is less reliable due to turbulence. Stroke volume divided by the time-velocity integral of the transvalvular flow yields the aortic valve area [254]. This also correlates well with planimetered aortic valve area [255]. One other interesting observation from CMR studies is that the LV outflow tract is elliptical rather than circular as assumed in computations using Doppler echocardiography [256].

Conclusions (morphology and function)

Cardiovascular magnetic resonance provides complete and reliable morphologic and functional information about the cardiac chambers. It is harmless to myocardium and other biologic tissue using the magnetic field strengths of 3 Tesla or less. It is a superb high-resolution diagnostic tool that can be

Table 8.19 CMR in aortic stenosis.

Suggested technique:

(1) ECG gated SSFP for LV and RV function, left atrial size and aortic valve anatomy/area

(2) VEC MRI aortic valves for determination of AS jet velocity

(3) Stroke volume from LV tracing and through plane flows at LVOT level or above the aortic valve.

Possible MRI findings:

● Restricted opening of aortic valve; aortic valve area may be planimetered.

● Hemodynamics in AS: from VEC MRI, obtain peak velocity for peak and mean gradients, aortic valve area by dividing stroke volume by peak time velocity integral of the signal at aortic valve level

● Effect on LV function: LV EF, LVESV and mass are important for monitoring asymptomatic patients.

---

used to assess risk. It can reliably measure ejection fraction, ventricular volumes, cardiac outputs, myocardial mass, myocardial wall thickening and even differences in wall motion between the subendo and subepicardium using RF tagging. With the use of nonmagnetic implantable devices and the increasing safety of CMR used with electrical devices such as pacemakers and ICDs and the increase in magnetic field strength, CMR is becoming more involved as an integral diagnostic technique and is becoming the gold standard for imaging of ventricular function.

Cardiovascular Magnetic Resonance Myocardial Perfusion Imaging

Decisions regarding revascularization in CAD are based not only on the anatomic severity of arterial stenoses, but also on their physiological significance [257]. The extent and severity of perfusion abnormalities are directly related to outcomes [258,259]. Radionuclide methods, especially single photon emission computed tomography (SPECT) has been the most widely employed test to evaluate regional myocardial perfusion. Radionuclide methods, though widely employed, have their limitations, including limited resolution and, more

importantly, the confounding effect of attenuation artifacts [260,261]. In addition, SPECT exposes patients to ionizing radiation. In recent times, methods to assess myocardial perfusion and coronary artery blood flow using cardiovascular magnetic resonance imaging have been developed. CMR imaging has high resolution and has no ionizing radiation. While CMR perfusion methods involve the use of paramagnetic contrast agents, they are more suitable for serial studies to evaluate the progression or regression of CAD than radionuclide approaches.

In CAD, myocardial perfusion is frequently normal at rest but, as with radionuclide approaches, abnormal perfusion patterns are induced by physical exercise (treadmill stress testing) or pharmacological vasodilator agents (adenosine or related agents). While physical stress induces perfusion abnormalities in parallel with other evidence of myocardial ischemia (angina pectoris, ST segment depression and wall motion abnormalities), vasodilators generally induce perfusion abnormalities without concomitant myocardial ischemia unless stenoses are severe enough to induce a steal phenomenon. In a study by Gould *et al.*, it was shown that coronary artery stenoses with a greater than 50% reduction in diameter limit hyperemic flow during vasodilation, leading to perfusion deficit [262]. Accordingly, coronary lesions which are angiographically determined to be greater than 50% are considered significant, and are typically treated by percutaneous coronary intervention or bypass graft surgery when clinical circumstances are appropriate. Data from studies such as the coronary artery surgical study or CASS have shown that vessels with significant stenosis are associated with MI [263,264]. Iskandrian *et al.* have shown that the extent and severity of myocardial perfusion defects were strong predictors of future cardiac events [258]. Perfusion imaging with SPECT, positron emission tomography (PET) and CMR imaging are all used for evaluating both myocardial perfusion and viability. In contrast to the radionuclide approaches, CMR uses a method known as delayed contrast enhancement to assess myocardial viability and rather than labeling viable myocardium the technique labels MI and scar [265]. Briefly, CMR perfusion/viability imaging works as follows. After administration of the paramagnetic contrast agent, generally a gadolinium chelate, (e.g., Gd-DTPA) intravenously administered using a nonmagnetic power injector, high speed CMR imaging allows assessment of perfusion during the first pass of the contrast agent through the myocardium. After approximately ten minutes, repeat imaging shows contrast agent localization in myocardial infarct or scar territory.

In conjunction with CMR myocardial perfusion imaging it is possible to compare resting and vasodilated imaging studies to determine coronary flow reserve (CFR): hyperemic flow divided by resting flow. CFR is impaired in patients with cardiac risk factors but anatomically normal coronary arteries (less than 50% diameter stenosis) [266]. PET has been used to estimate CFR. Studies using PET have demonstrated that hyperemic flow data correlated strongly with both the severity of stenosis by coronary angiography and CFR [267–269].

CMR Perfusion Imaging Using First Pass of Contrast Agent

Myocardial perfusion is observed by rapid imaging after the peripheral injection of an extracellular contrast agent (typically Gd-DTPA), which have a T_1-lowering effect. The contrast agent passes from the blood pool via the coronary circulation into the myocardium substantially reducing the T_1 (spin-lattice relaxation time) from 1500 ms for blood and 1100 for myocardium at 3 Tesla [270] to as little as 50 ms depending on the local concentration of the Gd-DTPA. The reduction in tissue T_1 depends on the baseline T_1 of the blood or tissue, the concentration of Gd-DTPA and the tissue parameters relating to water exchange. During the first pass of contrast agent, CMR pulse sequences are used that produce strong T_1 contrast (making short T_1s in the tissue with the contrast agent bright and the longer T_1s of tissue with less contrast agent dark). Accordingly, during the wash-in of paramagnetic contrast agent, the myocardium gets brighter, and during wash-out, the myocardium gets darker (Figure 8.5).

Qualitative assessment of hypoperfused areas using CMR is accomplished by visually estimating the wash-in rates of extracellular contrast agent into the myocardium supplied by normal or insignificantly stenotic coronary arteries compared with coronary arteries with significant stenoses [102,271–273]. Signal intensity time curves can be used to calculate parameters such as peak signal intensity [274,275]; signal change over time (slope) [120,271,276–280], arrival time; time to peak signal; mean transit time [276,281], and area under the signal intensity time curve [282]. Signal intensity is a simple function of T_1 (and the pulse sequence), and T_1 is a simple

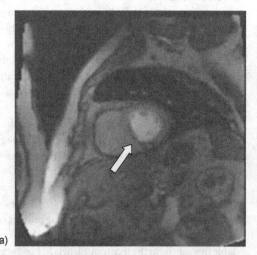
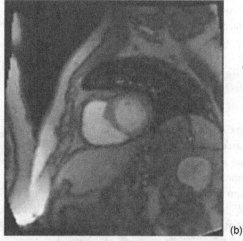

(a)   (b)

Figure 8.5 (a) Subendocardial perfusion defect: short-axis tomographic view during the myocardial phase of the first-pass of gadolinium chelate. The white arrow points to a subendocardial inferior septal perfusion defect. Note the dark rim artifact surrounding the blood pool of right ventricle. (b). First-pass gadolinium study showing no defect. Note the dark rim artifact is still present although less conspicuous.

function of contrast agent concentration, baseline T_1 and water exchange rate. In animal models a close correlation has been shown between microsphere measurements and upslope of the intensity time curve [282]; the upslope is used as a semiquantitative measure of perfusion. The upslope method uses the initial portion of the signal intensity time curve, which lasts up to 20 seconds. In view of the need for a 20-second acquisition time the sensitivity of the measurement can be affected due to motion, since the breath-holding required for high quality imaging is not readily accomplished by all patients. Myocardial upslope data are divided by the upslope data of the signal in the LV blood pool to obtain a measure of input [120,273,277–281].

This method of correction is not optimal as the value may change based on hemodynamic status in patients, as in vasodilator states. In a recent study, upslope of signal intensity during hyperemia divided by the upslope in the LV blood pool was calculated in 32 sectors per heart (eight sectors per slice) and was compared to a normal database of upslope values [271]. This method allowed color coding of the "wash-in" of contrast agent, producing a parametric map and allowing the identification of hypoperfused areas.

Perfusion imaging during the "first pass" is particularly demanding, since whole heart coverage is necessary. One must be able to resolve the first 20 seconds of "wash-in" with high temporal resolution in order to determine rates of perfusion. Current methods typically image three or four short-axis slices, which is sufficient for identifying under perfusion resulting from large-vessel CAD, but may not be sufficient for estimating the volume of affected myocardium.

During CMR perfusion imaging, artifacts are also observed. These artifacts must be eliminated or corrected in order to reliably assess regional myocardial perfusion. Otherwise, regions that have reduced signal intensity due to artifact might be confused with regions that have reduced signal intensity due to reduced myocardial perfusion, as is the case with attenuation artifacts with radionuclide imaging. Artifacts can occur because of the sensitivity of the receiver coil (the coil which detects the signal from the body after a transmitted pulse). Signal intensity decreases with increasing coil distance. This means that the signal intensity

during the "first pass" of contrast agent can be reduced in posterior myocardium compared with anterior myocardium. Cardiovascular magnetic resonance imaging can correct for this reduced signal with increasing coil distance by computing the relative change in signal. Dividing the absolute signal change by the baseline precontrast signal intensities can be used to determine the relative value. In addition, the perfusion data should be corrected for motion artifacts either due to diaphragmatic drift or breathing prior to generating a signal intensity time curve [283–285]. Another artifact, termed "dark rim," refers to abnormally low signal in subendocardial myocardium, which can appear in healthy subjects. It is believed to be related to truncation in k-space [286], and therefore can be resolved by improving spatial resolution. In addition, it is most significant when the contrast agent concentration in the LV reaches its peak, and therefore is readthrough by evaluating later stages of myocardial intensity time curves.

Techniques Used in Clinical Studies

IR has been the most widely used pulse sequence to evaluate perfusion in animals. By appropriate setting of the time between the inversion and the read pulse, signal can be markedly reduced or nulled. Contrast agent then produces the greatest impact on myocardium during its first pass. In human studies, several methods, including IR [120,123,272,276,278,280,287–289]; saturation recovery [271,277,281,290,291]; notched saturation recovery [292], and T_2^* preparation, have been employed [42,43]. Most of these initial studies only examined feasibility of CMR perfusion imaging. They were performed in healthy human volunteers [291,293–297] or in patients with knowledge of their angiographically determined coronary anatomy and disease [123,292,296]. Perfusion was evaluated in the 1990s, using a multislice approach, but the sensitivity and specificity were low. This was in part because of hardware limitations and in part because of artifacts. Al-Saadi and colleagues [120] tried to evaluate perfusion with data acquisition limited to a single slice, using contrast injected into the right atrium. Recent improvements in hardware with fast echo-planar readout and the use of saturation recovery sequences have made it possible to evaluate perfusion in multiple slices [271,281] during a single-injection first-pass experiment. Today, the most widely used protocol (which is supported by the major manufacturers) is based on multislice saturation recovery followed by fast gradient-echo acquisitions. Image acquisition time is on the order of 150–200 ms, allowing imaging of three slices per R-R interval. Typically, six parallel short-axis slices are acquired with a temporal resolution of two R-R intervals. A typical nonselective saturation pulse is used before each slice acquisition, resulting in very short saturation recovery times.

CMR Myocardial Perfusion Imaging: The Future

Scanner hardware, receiver coils, and pulse sequences are constantly improving. Speed and improvement in signal-to-noise ratio (SNR) can be expected with the adoption of parallel imaging [143,297] and SSFP techniques [282]. The availability and prevalence of commercial 3T systems with high-speed gradients are advantageous in evaluating perfusion [298]; these systems also improve SNR and provide longer myocardial T_1s for ease of and improvement in quality of perfusion imaging. It is also now possible to evaluate the entire LV myocardium (without gaps) [299,300], which may provide new prognostic information, and the ability to study spatial patterns of perfusion deficit. Of great interest is the potential of CMR to assess myocardial perfusion without using contrast agents, using T_2 mapping [301], and arterial spin labeling [302,303]. Robust myocardial perfusion using arterial spin labeling. This approach uses the RF to tag the inflowing blood and then to observe that blood as it traverses the myocardium. While there is much to be done to perfect this approach, if done it would provide the ability for myocardial perfusion imaging without ionizing radiation and without paramagnetic contrast agents, i.e., essentially risk free.

Myocardial Viability Using Cardiovascular Magnetic Resonance Imaging

Heart failure is a common consequence of many diseases that affect the myocardium. The leading cause of heart failure in the Western world is CAD [304]. Knowledge of structure, metabolism and function is crucial to understanding the myocardial response to injury such as ischemia. Detection of viable myocardium in patients with LV dysfunction in the setting of CAD is important in deciding between medical and surgical management. Revascularization of dysfunctional yet viable myocardium can improve ventricular function and long-term survival [305–307].

Noncontractile but viable myocardium may result from acute, subacute or chronic reduction in myocardial perfusion and is frequently described as stunning or hibernation. In the 1970s, patients with regional wall motion abnormalities recovered contractile function after coronary artery bypass graft surgery (CABG) [308,309]. Inotropic stimulation, for example involving ventricular contraction after a ventricular premature beat, demonstrated improved wall motion in viable territories. Such postextrasystolic improvement in wall motion was used to identify viable myocardium and thus patients whose abnormal wall motion would benefit from CABG [310,311]. The term "hibernating myocardium" was used to refer to patients with reduced myocardial contractile function at rest in the presence of severe coronary artery stenoses, presumably associated with reduced blood supply [312,313]. Hibernation is a chronic condition of resting LV dysfunction due to reduced coronary blood flow. It can be partially or completely reversed by revascularization. Chronically reduced perfusion is thought to down regulate metabolism, decreasing energy demand and limiting necrosis. Myocardial stunning is characterized by prolonged mechanical dysfunction after coronary reflow and resumption of perfusion without evidence of permanent tissue damage [314,315]. Stunning seems to be related to alterations in contractile proteins in response to ischemic insult [316–318]. Myocardial stunning can occur in conjunction with various conditions, such as unstable angina or exercise-induced ischemia, as well as in other situations, such as following cardiac surgery or early successful reperfusion of acute MI.

Myocardial viability has great influence on patient outcome in terms of mortality and morbidity. Several studies have shown that in the setting of acute LV dysfunction, prognosis is worse in the presence of myocardial necrosis compared to reversible myocardial dysfunction [319,320]. The extent of

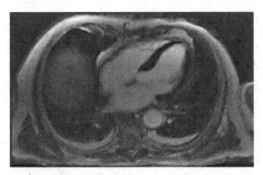

Figure 8.6 No delayed enhancement in a patient with angina but without previous MI. The patient received gadolinium contrast agent 10–15 minutes prior to acquisition of the imaging study in this four-chamber long-axis image.

viable (or nonviable) myocardium dictates the need for and type of further patient management. The detection of stunned myocardium following reperfusion therapy [319,321] and the demonstration of viability in a dysfunctional area may determine the need for early revascularization.

The prognosis in a patient with chronic LV dysfunction may be improved by revascularization, provided there is sufficient viable myocardium to permit recovery of contractile function. Revascularization in the presence of nonviable myocardium may be detrimental to patient outcomes and may be associated with an increase in mortality [322, 323]. The extent of myocardial viability, in addition to its presence, is also useful in selecting patients who are likely to benefit from therapy (Figure 8.6).

Noninvasive Methods to Assess Viability

Techniques currently available to assess myocardial viability include PET using ^{18}F-fluorodeoxyglucose (FDG); SPECT with either ^{201}Tl or technetium-99 m (^{99m}Tc); and low dose dobutamine echocardiography (DobE). Each of these imaging approaches defines myocardial viability in different ways: FDG-PET images the distribution of myocardial glucose metabolic activity or evidence of anaerobic glycolysis, ^{201}Tl-SPECT images sarcolemmal cell membrane integrity, ^{99m}Tc-SPECT images mitochondrial membrane integrity, and dobutamine echocardiography assesses the presence of myocardial contractile reserve. Dobutamine echocardiography, PET, and SPECT have similar predictive ac-

curacy, however, dobutamine CMR is significantly better for detecting myocardial ischemia compared with DE, because of the improved ability of CMR to visualize the LV in 3D.

PET, SPECT, and DobE (or dobutamine CMR) assess different markers of viability. Using dobutamine stimulation, the presence of contractile reserve in hibernating myocardium is demonstrated in the presence of viable myocardium [34].

All of these tests have inherent limitations. Dobutamine echocardiography is limited by adequacy of the acoustic window or suboptimal images in 15% of patients [324]. Additionally, DobE is operator-dependent, endocardial definition in the posterolateral segment is poor, the apical segments may be foreshortened, and the approach is presently inherently two-dimensional. An additional problem is the long period of training necessary to acquire the skills for optimum image display and interpretation [325]. The accuracy of SPECT studies is confounded by attenuation artifacts and poor spatial resolution. PET is limited by the expense of radionuclide tracer production (using either an on-site cyclotron to produce ^{13}N-ammonia and FDG or a generator to produce Rubidium-82 (^{82}Rb)). ^{13}N-ammonia or ^{82}Rb are used to image myocardial perfusion while FDG is used to image anaerobic myocardial glucose utilization. The ^{13}N-ammonia or ^{82}Rb are used to image perfusion and the ^{18}F is used to image anaerobic metabolism. When perfusion is reduced or absent the involved territory may be viable or nonviable. When FDG is present in a region of perfusion deficit, metabolic activity and thus viability has been defined. Like SPECT, PET procedures are also limited by low spatial resolution compared to CMR, with SPECT substantially worse than PET. This section concentrates on the imaging techniques of CMR that allow assessment of myocardial viability. CMR provides several approaches to defining viability, including dobutamine stimulation of asynergic ventricular wall segments, delayed enhancement by paramagnetic contrast agent, and abnormal myocardial high energy phosphate metabolism.

Viability Assessment Using Cine CMR to Determine Regional Function

As noted previously, cine CMR imaging allows high resolution visualization of myocardial wall motion, wall thickness, and wall thickening. Scarred myocardium is associated with loss of myocardial mass, leading to wall thinning. Previous studies have shown that the total thickness of scarred myocardium is usually ≤5 mm [326]. This assumption of thinned and akinetic myocardium representing scar has been studied by comparing CMR with PET and SPECT [327,328]. Observation of morphology and function of the LV at rest cannot detect viability, per se. The presence of even a small amount of wall thickening with low dose dobutamine in an area of asynergy suggests myocardial contractile function and hence some degree of viable myocardium.

Dobutamine CMR to Assess Viability

The question of viability arises in myocardium with regional or global contractile dysfunction. When such dysfunction is associated with heart failure, successful treatment depends on whether or not the dysfunction is associated with ischemic but viable or nonviable myocardium (or scar). Viable myocardium demonstrates improvement in contractile function with infusion of low dose dobutamine. This method of assessing residual function is the same as that used in dobutamine echocardiography. A low dose infusion of dobutamine (5–10 µg/kg/min) is used and two or three sets of cine images are acquired, one before and the other during infusion at each level of dobutamine. The sets of cine images are examined side by side to detect changes in regional wall thickening. Improvement of contractile function compared to resting images indicates viable myocardium. If there is wall motion improvement at the lowest dobutamine dose, testing can be stopped, since viability has been demonstrated.

Newer approaches use fast gradient-echo and high speed SSFP such as fast low angle shot (FLASH), fast imaging with steady-state precession (FISP), balanced fast field echo (FFE), and fast imaging employing steady-state excitation (FIESTA). These newer approaches have greater temporal resolution, permitting the acquisition of cine loops of the beating heart. These sequences make it possible to acquire studies during multiple breath-holds, resulting in high quality short- and long-axis views of the myocardium, both at rest and with the infusion of dobutamine. Image sequences require a breath-hold of about 20 seconds. Images are displayed in cine mode, pairing short-axis cuts in comparable locations. Resolution is high and still frames from end-systole and end-diastole can be displayed with well defined epicardial and endocardial borders. These images allow precise quantification of myocardial volumes, mass, and thickness, as well as assessment of regional wall motion and wall thickening in the cine mode.

Dendale and colleagues [329] were the first to report the use of low dose dobutamine CMR in assessing viability. They studied 25 patients early after acute MI with low dose dobutamine CMR and echocardiography, and quantitative assessment of wall motion was performed using both modalities. Concordance between these two modalities for identifying viable from nonviable segments was 81%. The "gold standard" was recovery of function after revascularization. The positive and negative predictive values for dobutamine CMR ranged from 89 to 100% and 73 to 94%, respectively [330,331], significantly better than dobutamine echocardiography.

Baer *et al.* [332] compared dobutamine CMR, dobutamine TEE, and FDG uptake on PET imaging to detect viable myocardium. The sensitivity and specificity for dobutamine TEE compared to dobutamine CMR were 77 and 94% vs 81 and 100% respectively.

The use of dobutamine CMR was suboptimal until recently because of the lack of availability of fast imaging sequences. Another disadvantage of dobutamine CMR (and echocardiographic studies) is the risk involved in administering dobutamine. The infusion of a positive inotropic agent in a patient with CAD can elicit an ischemic or arrhythmic event. The physical distance between physician and patient while in the scanner precludes optimum patient–physician interaction. In addition, the ECG waveform cannot be utilized to assess ST segment changes due to its alteration by the magnetic field. Considering this problem, i.e., the difficulty in using ST segment depression as a means of detecting ischemia, a number of groups have reported using low dose dobutamine CMR for successfully assessing viability. A few other groups have also reported the use of higher doses of dobutamine to detect ischemia [324,333].

Potential disadvantages of dobutamine CMR also include underestimation of the extent of viable myocardium and inability to estimate the transmural extent of myocardial ischemia. Several manuscripts in the literature regarding dobutamine echocardiography have shown that compared to ^{201}Tl-SPECT, the use of contractile reserve to assess viability will result in higher specificity but lower sensitivity [334–336]. This reduced sensitivity may be due to the development of ischemia at even low levels of inotropic stimulation or the nature of hibernating myocardium, which may cause myofibrillar dropout. In these two situations, myocardium will not be able to respond to inotropic stimulation [337].

Delayed Contrast Enhancement and Viability

Relaxation agents such as gadolinium chelates are large molecules that rapidly diffuse from the intravascular space into the interstitial space and tend to remain in the extracellular compartment. The presence of these contrast agents decreases both the longitudinal (T_1) and the transverse (T_2) relaxation times of the protons (of water and fat). At clinical doses of these agents the effect on T_1 relaxation time is greater, resulting in increased signal intensities on T_1-weighted images. As a direct effect, the CMR pulse sequences used to elucidate contrast are designed to generate image patterns with intensities that are strongly T_1-weighted.

ECG-gated spin-echo images were used earlier to assess viability, in which one k-space line was acquired for each cardiac cycle. Since the duration of cardiac cycle (800 ms) was comparable to myocardial T_1 relaxation time, T_1 weighted images were obtained. Using these approaches MI was first detected in animal and human studies [338,339], and Dendale *et al.* [331] and Yokota *et al.* [340] visualized nontransmural infarction.

Improvement in CMR Techniques

In recent years there have been a number of technical improvements in CMR, one of the most important being the use of k-space segmentation. This has enabled the acquisition of multiple k-space lines of data during each cardiac cycle [341], leading to a reduction in imaging times, even to the point of acquiring images in a single breath-hold. This has translated into improved breath-hold tolerance by

patients, improved image quality, and wider application of CMR in clinical practice.

Advances in imaging pulse sequences to allow increased T_1 weighting have been crucial for imaging myocardial viability. The preparation of magnetization prior to image acquisition by the use of an IR pulse sequence significantly increases the degree of T_1-weighting. When compared to other pulse sequences, a segmented IR sequence resulted in improved visualization of viable myocardium [342]. A much higher contrast between necrotic or scarred myocardium and normal myocardium was achieved with this sequence, with the inversion time set to substantially reduce (or null) the signal from myocardium prior to administration of contrast agent. This sequence has shown a difference in the intensities between normal and enhanced myocardium on the order of 1000% in animals [342], translating to a 10-fold increase in the degree of image contrast compared with older, previously used spin-echo sequences.

Images are acquired in end-diastole to reduce cardiac motion. A nonselective 180° pulse is used to prepare the magnetization of the heart to increase T_1 weighting. The inversion time (TI) is defined as the time between this 180° pulse and the center of acquisition of the segmented k-space lines. This time is chosen so that the magnetization of normal and non-contrast-enhanced myocardium is near its zero-crossing, ensuring that normal myocardium will appear as dark as possible (Figure 8.7).

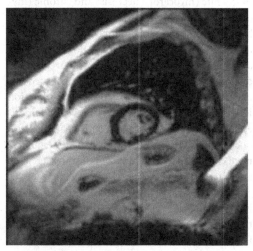

Figure 8.7 Dark myocardium produced by an "inversion recovery" pulse sequence.

Contrast enhanced CMR with spin-echo pulse sequences was able to detect the transmural and overall extent of acute MI in patients with medium to larger infarcts. The transmural extent of smaller infarcts was not measurable because of the low resolution of spin-echo sequences [339,343–345]. Dendale and colleagues [331] used spin-echo techniques to assess viability and differentiate between transmural and subendocardial infarcts. Nontransmural involvement was visualized, but in 15 (27%) of the 56 infarcted segments no visible enhancement was seen. Similarly, Yokota *et al.* [340] did not visualize enhancement in six (13%) of the 44 patients with documented infarctions. The infarcts that were missed were generally small with normal wall motion at rest [331] and had lower peak creatine levels [340]. This inability to detect smaller infarcts is due to the limitations of the spin-echo sequence with image acquisition over several minutes during free breathing. Other factors that decrease the ability to detect smaller infarcts include partial volume effects due to motion averaging over the respiratory cycle, image artifacts caused by respiratory motion, and lower T_1 weighting that limits repetition time. With the advent of newer IR sequences, smaller subendocardial infarcts can be easily visualized [265,346].

Acute and Chronic MI and Delayed Contrast Enhancement

Both acute (myocardial necrosis) and chronic (myocardial scar) infarction show delayed contrast enhancement in laboratory animal and patient studies. Kim and colleagues scanned dogs between 1 and 3 days following reperfused or nonreperfused coronary artery occlusion, and demonstrated enhancement in histologically confirmed infarction [265]. Similar enhancement was shown by Simonetti *et al.* in a study of 18 consecutive patients after documented MI. In each of these patients, enhancement correlated with the appropriate infarct related artery territory [342].

Kim *et al.* have shown that both acute and chronic infarcts enhance even given the difference between the tissue characteristics of acute and chronic infarcts [267]. In their study, dogs were scanned 8 weeks after MI. Using high resolution *ex vivo* imaging, the regions of enhancement observed in chronic infarcts appeared to occur in the same regions as those defined by histology.

Wu and colleagues [346] used segmented IR pulse sequences to systematically evaluate if chronic infarcts enhanced. Patients were enrolled at the time of acute infarction and underwent CMR several months later. At the same time, healthy volunteers and patients with nonischemic cardiomyopathy were also studied. The researchers found a wide variety of enhanced areas, ranging from full transmural enhanced areas to small subendocardial areas of delayed contrast enhancement. In all instances these areas of enhancement correlated with the IRA. Delayed enhancement was not seen in the healthy volunteers or in patients with nonischemic dilated cardiomyopathy, resulting in a specificity of 100%. The sensitivity for detection of old infarcts was 91% in 3-month-old and 100% in 14-month-old infarcts.

Myocardial Viability in Patients with Heart Failure

Chronic heart failure is huge economic burden and accounts at least 5 million patients in the United States. CAD is the etiological factor in 70% of the cases [304]. Though coronary revascularization is one of the main therapeutic options, only one third of the dysfunctional segments improve in function, and only about 40% show an improvement in ejection fraction [347]. Due to the high mortality and morbidity of the revascularization procedures, careful selection of patients is warranted. Myocardial viability using various imaging techniques has been reported by various investigators [314,348–351]. As a general rule viability was detected in about 50% of the dysfunctional segments making it a necessity to search for viability in patients with chronic cardiomyopathy.

The term myocardial hibernation was introduced to describe a condition of chronic sustained abnormal contraction due to chronic underperfusion in patients with CAD and revascularization causes an improvement in LV function [313]. Myocardial stunning has been defined as reversible myocardial contractile dysfunction in the presence of normal blood flow [314]. Various imaging studies assessing viability have used different end points. Bax *et al.*, in a recent analysis of pooled data from 105 studies (3003 patients, nuclear imaging and dobutamine stress) 7941 segments out of a total of 15,045 dysfunctional segments showed an improvement in function. Of these 84% were considered to be viable [352]. Left ventricular ejection fraction has been demonstrated to be a powerful prognostic indicator and hence from a clinical perspective an improvement in global EF may be more important than improvement in regional function. Few studies have assessed improvement in EF with relation to viability [353]. Current evidence suggests that 20–30% of the LV needs to be viable to show an improvement in EF. Other studies have shown an improvement in symptoms and exercise capacity in patients revascularized with viable myocardium [354,355].

Left ventricular volumes are powerful prognostic parameters. Mule *et al.* have shown that patients with ischemia or viability in excess of 20% demonstrated reverse remodeling after revascularization with significant reduction in LV end-systolic and end-diastolic volumes. Patients with predominant scar tissue exhibited ongoing adverse remodeling with increase in volumes [356]. Another important endpoint in these patients is long-term prognosis. Rohatgi *et al.* have demonstrated that revascularization in patients with substantial viable myocardium reduces the number of hospitalizations for congestive heart failure [357]. Allman *et al.* performed a meta analysis of 24 prognostic studies (3088 patients), using various viability techniques and showed an annual death rate of 3.2% in patients revascularized with viable myocardium vs 16% in those treated medically [322]. All these studies were retrospective and the results from the prospective, randomized STICH trial are much awaited.

Viability with MRI in chronic heart failure: MRI can assess resting LV dysfunction; end diastolic wall thickness can be used to assess viability, contractile reserve with low dose dobutamine and probably is the gold standard for visualizing scar tissue.

Viability criteria: Various studies have used an LV end-diastolic dimension of less than 5.5 mm as a marker of scar tissue. Baer *et al.* [328] compared end diastolic wall thickness on MRI with glucose use on ^{18}F-FDG PET and showed that regions with wall thickness <5.5 mm had reduced glucose use compared to preserved glucose use with wall thickness ≥5.5 mm.

Prediction of outcomes: Using wall thickness criteria Kaandorp *et al.*, with data from three pooled studies showed wall thickness to predict functional recovery has a sensitivity of 95% and specificity of 41% [358]. Baer *et al.* showed a systolic wall thickening of greater than 2 mm during dobutamine infusion predicts functional recovery [328]. Similarly Bove *et al.* showed that in areas with limited scar tissue, a normal response to dobutamine helps to determine likely functional recovery [359]. The mean sensitivity is about 73% (50–89%) and specificity 83% (70–95%) with dobutamine MRI [358]. Studies with contrast enhanced MRI depicting transmural scar showed low likelihood of functional recovery. The amount of hyperenhancement is a very good indicator of functional recovery, improvement in function decreases as the amount of transmural scar increases [168,360]. Selvanayagam *et al.* have demonstrated that late-enhancement by CMR to be powerful predictor of viability [169]. Cardiovascular magnetic resonance imaging is also an important tool in evaluating resting myocardial blood flow, scarring, and functional recovery [361,362].

Mechanism of Delayed Contrast Enhancement

The mechanism of late enhancement is not fully understood. The fluid volume of normal myocardial tissue is predominantly intracellular. The volume of distribution of the extracellular contrast agents (e.g., gadolinium chelate) in normal myocardium is quite low, suggesting that viable myocardial cells exclude contrast agents. In MI, the myocyte membranes rupture, allowing the passage of the contrast agent into the intracellular space and giving rise to a higher level of contrast agent. Cell death is thought to be closely related to loss of sarcolemmal membrane integrity, and this correlates with delayed enhancement [363,365]. This also explains the relationship between the spatial distribution of delayed CMR enhancement and histologically observed necrosis [265]. Extracellular contrast agents such as Gd-DTPA are excluded from the myocyte's intracellular space by an intact sarcolemmal membrane [14,365]. Viable myocardium has an intact sarcolemmal membrane which excludes the chelate and helps explain the lack of delayed contrast enhancement.

Chronic infarction or scar, on the other hand, is characterized by dense collagen. The interstitial space between the collagenous scar tissue may be greater than the interstitial space between the densely packed living myocardial cells. Rehwald and associates [124] have shown a greater volume of distribution of contrast agent in a scar compared to viable myocardium.

In the setting of reversible ischemic injury, myocardium is viable and the cell membrane is intact. Thus, delayed enhancement of contrast agent is not seen. This is because the sarcolemmal membrane is intact and the contrast agent is excluded from the intracellular space [363]. Here the volume of distribution of the contrast agent in the reversible ischemic areas will be similar to that of normal myocardium, resulting in no enhancement of these areas [364,365].

Technical Considerations

Partial volume effects can occur whenever the spatial resolution is low. Even with adequate spatial resolution, partial volume effects can occur when the imaging time is long due to either respiratory or patient motion.

Areas of hypo-enhancement or deficits in the distribution of the contrast agent are often observed in the central areas of myocardial infarcts surrounded by areas of delayed enhancement. The area of hypo-enhancement has been related to the phenomenon of no-reflow (microvascular obstruction) [366,367]. This no-reflow territory, characterized by markedly reduced perfusion, is thought to be due to damage or destruction at the microvascular level, impeding the presence of blood flow and the penetration of the MR contrast agent. Since flow in these areas is low but not absolutely zero, they initially appear dark, but slowly enhance as contrast agent accumulates. Accordingly, these hypo-enhanced or darker areas should be included in the quantification of infarct size (Figure 8.8).

Clinical Applications

CMR assessment of wall motion, perfusion and contrast enhancement allows accurate high-resolution evaluation of normal, ischemic viable, and ischemic nonviable myocardium. When wall

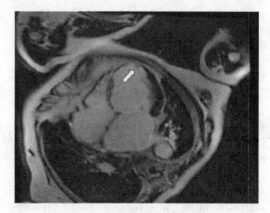

Figure 8.8 Example of a patient with hypertrophic cardiomyopathy who demonstrates a nonischemic etiology for delayed enhancement (DE). Four-chamber long-axis view depicting DE in the apical interventricular septum (arrow).

motion and thickening are normal, perfusion is normal and there is no delayed contrast enhancement, normal myocardium has been defined. When wall motion and thickening are normal, perfusion is abnormal and there is no delayed contrast enhancement, early myocardial ischemia is present. When wall motion and thickening are reduced, perfusion is abnormal and there is no contrast enhancement, a higher level of myocardial ischemia has been defined. When wall motion is akinetic and thickening is absent, perfusion is abnormal and there is no delayed enhancement, myocardium is most likely viable and ischemia severe. Finally, when wall motion is akinetic or dyskinetic, wall thickening is absent or wall thinning is present, when perfusion is absent, and when there is delayed contrast enhancement, myocardium is nonviable. The relationship between ventricular function (wall motion and wall thickening), perfusion pattern (subendocardial and transmural), and contrast enhancement pattern is complex. Ventricular function, perfusion, and contrast enhancement all reflect different physiological processes and therefore, combinations of the three are useful for evaluation of the level of myocardial ischemic process. In the clinical setting of acute MI CMR can fully characterize the ischemic process. DCE determines the presence and extent of the infarct, perfusion imaging determines the presence and extent of the ischemic plus infarcted territory, and the cine study determines the function of the involved myocardial segment). In the case of myocardial stunning after reperfusion wall motion is reduced (stunned), perfusion is normal or can show nontransmural or transmural deficits, and enhancement pattern is generally absent or subendocardial. The combined observation of these three imaging characteristics defines the resulting reperfusion. Likewise, the combined assessment of function, perfusion and enhancement can be applied in the chronic setting to distinguish between scarred, hibernating, and normal myocardium.

In an animal study by Hillenbrand and associates [368], the relationship between the transmural extent of contrast enhancement and myocardial salvage after reperfusion treatment for acute MI was examined. In this study the transmural extent of delayed contrast enhancement on post MI day 3 predicted improvement in contractile function.

Viability assessment weeks or longer after acute MI is also essential to determine the optimal therapeutic strategy. The involved myocardium could be scar or it could have reduced wall motion but still be viable, such as is the case in hibernation. Myocardial dysfunction associated with viable myocardium is usually reversible, but the treatment also depends on the extent of the dysfunction. A very small region of viability and a substantial amount of scar may not be worth an interventional PCI or bypass graft procedure. The total extent of involvement is evaluated by assessment of ventricular function, while the extent of scar (irreversible by revascularization) is identifiable by the extent of delayed contrast enhancement. In a study conducted by Kim *et al.* [129], cine and contrast CMR were performed in 50 consecutive patients before they underwent revascularization by percutaneous intervention (PCI) or coronary artery bypass grafting (CABG) and Cine CMR was repeated at 11 weeks after revascularization to assess changes in regional wall motion. The likelihood of improvement was related to the extent of transmural enhancement in this study. Seventy-eight per cent with no enhancement improved after revascularization whereas only one out of 58 segments with greater than 75% delayed enhancement showed improvement. The relationship between delayed enhancement and contractile dysfunction was the same for severe hypokinesis, akinesis, or dyskinesis at baseline. It was also shown that the greater the extent of dysfunctional but viable myocardium the greater the improvement in wall motion ($p < 0.001$) and ejection fraction ($p < 0.001$) after revascularization.

Contrast CMR has advantages over other imaging modalities used to assess viability. Detection of the transmural extent of delayed enhancement or DE is helpful in predicting functional improvement. Kim *et al.* showed that the mean extent of DE was $10 \pm 7\%$ in patients who improved versus $41 \pm 14\%$ in patients with no improvement ($p < 0.001$). Previous studies have shown that significant viability can exist without functional improvement. This underscores the importance of combining the high-resolution assessment of myocardial function, perfusion pattern, and delayed contrast enhancement by CMR in the assessment of viability.

Future Applications of Contrast Enhanced CMR

Contrast enhanced CMR now allows routine detection of the transmural extent of infarcted or scarred myocardium and even the presence of less extensive subendocardial defects. Cine CMR and contrast CMR allow evaluation of the intricate relationship between infarction and contractile function. The application of the method of delayed enhancement to the assessment of viability in patients with suspected CAD will provide an understanding of the incidence of myocardial damage even when wall motion appears normal. Of course, the dynamic importance of such an observation may not be of much clinical importance, but the presence of such findings may have a bearing on outcomes in CAD.

Delayed CMR Contrast Enhancement and Normal Wall Motion

Traditionally it has been assumed that MI is associated with contractile dysfunction. It has been shown by Lieberman and colleagues [369] that contractile dysfunction when used alone results in overestimation of the infarct size. Though the infarct may be small, the extent of the contractile dysfunction itself may be large [370–372]. Recently, Wu *et al.* [346] have shown that the area of contractile dysfunction may be smaller than the infarct itself. In their study of patients with chronic infarction, 25% of segments with subendocardial infarction had normal wall motion. The relationship between transmural infarct and wall thickening is mainly based on studies conducted in patients with acute MI. Mahrholdt and colleagues [373] studied patients with chronic enzyme-positive MI and single vessel CAD. They showed that in a setting of reperfused chronic MI, contractile dysfunction occurs when thickness of the transmural infarction approaches 50% of normal. Hence, contractile function alone cannot be used to rule out chronic MI. These studies suggest that the relationship of contractile function and infarct size are complex. They also show that infarct size can be overestimated in the acute setting and underestimated in the chronic setting. Magnetic resonance imaging techniques cannot evaluate the presence and size of infarction based only on contractile dysfunction. Chronic subendocardial infarcts with normal wall motion may be missed by imaging techniques in the absence of biochemical evidence of infarction or wall thinning.

Performance of CMR when Infarcts are Missed by SPECT

SPECT has lower resolution compared to CMR. An IR CMR pulse sequence provides a voxel size of 1.4 mm × 1.9 mm × 6.0 mm (0.016 cm^3). SPECT has a resolution of approximately 10 mm × 10 mm × 10 mm (1 cm^3) [374,375]. The resolution is almost 50 fold greater for CMR compared with SPECT. Wagner *et al.* [108] conducted a study of 91 patients to determine whether CMR is capable of detecting infarcts that are missed by SPECT. Both CMR and SPECT were analyzed and scored for the presence, location, and extent of infarcts. At the same time, they also conducted delayed contrast enhanced CMR in 12 animals with MI and three without MI. The presence of MI was determined by histochemical staining.

Both CMR and SPECT detected nearly all transmural infarctions. CMR was able to detect subendocardial infarcts in 100 of 109 segments (92%), compared to SPECT which identified infarcts in only 31 (28%) segments. Both SPECT and CMR had high specificity for the detection of infarction: 97% vs 98% respectively. In the nine patients, all transmural infarcts identified by CMR were also detected by SPECT. But of the 181 segments with subendocardial infarction (less than 50% of the transmural thickness of the LV wall), 85 were not detected by SPECT. This means that while six (13%) of the

patients whose subendocardial infarction was visible by CMR, their infarctions were undetected by SPECT.

In conclusion, it can be said that while both CMR and SPECT detect infarction equally, CMR is superior for detecting subendocardial infarcts.

CMR Delayed Enhancement in the Absence of a History of MI

Myocardial infarcts occur without patient or physician knowledge in 30–40% of cases. This estimate is based on the detection of new Q waves by ECG, and does not include some subendocardial infarcts which may not be detectable by routine ECG [376–378].

DCE that has been performed for routine evaluation has been positive in patients without ECG or historical evidence of MI. Kim and associates [379] studied 100 patients who were referred for coronary angiography, with no prior history of MI or revascularization. They detected delayed contrast enhancement in 57% with Q waves on ECG present in only 14%. CMR detection of infarction is fourfold higher than that of routine 12 lead ECG. The prognostic significance of such silent, clinically unrecognized, delayed enhancement needs further investigation.

Myocardial CMR Spectroscopy: Introduction

Another unique aspect of CMR is its ability to evaluate metabolism using its capacity to detect sensitive nuclei that comprise important molecular species within the myocardium. These nuclei include proton (H), carbon-13, fluorine-19, sodium-23, and phosphorus-31. To date, only ^{31}P and ^{1}H MR studies are clinically applicable. Phosphorus-31 spectroscopy has been primarily performed because of the importance of the process of high-energy phosphate (HEP) in the myocardium. Myocardial contractile function is related to metabolism of molecular species containing phosphorus (^{31}P) including adenosine triphosphate (ATP), adenosine diphosphate (ADP), adenosine monophosphate (AMP) and phosphocreatine (PCr). Acquisition of ^{31}P signal from the myocardium using various types of transmitter and surface coil receivers over the chest wall allows direct quantification of ATP, PCr, and inorganic phosphates (Pi). Localized spectroscopy that generates NMR signals from a defined region of interest within the myocardium provides a means, of assessing global myocardial concentrations of the phosphates. The ability to quantify these metabolites is improved at higher magnetic field strengths, where better spectral resolution and sensitivities are obtained. Myocardial Pi peak is usually obscured by a strong 2,3-diphosphoglycerate (2,3-DPG) signal from the blood at 1.5 Tesla, which is the most widely available CMR system. The Pi peak can be resolved at 3.0 Tesla or higher field, and this peak can be used for assessment of intracellular pH (pH) which can be determined as a function of relative frequency of Pi resonance, or chemical shift. When pH decreases, with acidosis due to myocardial ischemia, the Pi peak shifts to the right or downfield. The converse is true with an increase in pH.

Myocardial [31]P Spectroscopy and Ischemic Insult

When the myocardium becomes ischemic, as for example during stress, the PCr and PCr/ATP ratio decrease and Pi peak moves downfield consistent with a decrease in pH. The stress modality is commonly used is handgrip and no contrast agent is used. Intracellular metabolic markers such as PCr and ATP provide a direct means of assessing ischemia and infarction. PCr is a labile molecule that is the first to decrease and does so rapidly when blood supply decreases and/or when work increases, leading to a reduction in PCr/ATP ratio. As the ischemic insult progresses ATP begins to decrease. By the time of cell death, ATP has decreased substantially and there is little if any PCr. Concomitantly, during the early phase of myocardial ischemia, there is a shift in Pi downfield consistent with acidosis. Accordingly, while PCr/ATP provides an excellent definition for myocardial ischemia, it is a less effective means for determination of loss of viability, since the level of ATP that portends cell death is not well defined.

Clinical Applications of [31]P Myocardial Spectroscopy

The cardiac ^{31}P MR spectroscopy has been applied in evaluating clinical severity of heart failure [380,381], assessment of cardiac rejection [382], cardiac hypertrophy [383], and CAD. The most important study describing the use of PCr/ATP with handgrip stress to define myocardial ischemia was that of Weiss et al. [384]. Two groups of patients were compared: those with no significant CAD and those with significant CAD. In patients with significant CAD, the PCr/ATP decreased during exercise ($p < 0.001$). Such direct evaluation of intracellular myocardial metabolism should probably be the "gold standard" to define ischemia clinically.

Another important study that applied ^{31}P spectroscopy is that of Neubauer et al. [380,381], which used PCr/ATP to prognosticate in patients with heart failure due to dilated cardiomyopathy. In this study, patients with normal PCr/ATP ratio (>1.6) had significantly reduced mortality than those with low PCr/ATP ratio (<1.6) at reevaluation after two and half years ($p = 0.016$). A third interesting study [325] using ^{31}P myocardial spectroscopy evaluated women as part of Women's Ischemia Syndrome Evaluation (WISE) supported by the United States National Heart Lung and Blood Institute (NHLBI). Selected women with chest pain, who were referred for coronary angiography but without significant CAD, also underwent ^{31}P myocardial spectroscopy. The study included two control groups, one group of healthy, but age-matched volunteers, and one with significant left anterior descending CAD. The volunteer control group was used to define the abnormal change with handgrip stress in PCr/ATP or mean minus-2SD as the threshold for abnormality. Twenty per cent of the 35 women in the WISE group had abnormal changes in PCr/ATP (below 2SD less than the mean value) with a significant change. Thirty five per cent of the 20 patients with ≥70% stenosis of the LAD had a significant change. These data suggest that a moderate percentage of WISE patients with chest pain but without evidence of angiographically demonstrable significant CAD had an abnormal fall in PCr/ATP, suggesting myocardial ischemia. The change was more dramatic in patients with significant LAD disease. It is likely that the WISE patients had microvascular disease which led to myocardial ischemia in 20%, with a modest level of myocardial stress associated with microvascular disease. In a follow-up study by Johnson et al. [385,386], the WISE patients with the greater fall in PCr/ATP had more frequent hospital admissions and more coronary angiograms, but no increase in morbidity and mortality.

Among other applications, it is reported that the altered expression of dystrophin leads to a reduced

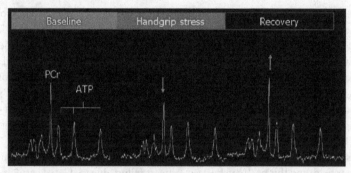

Figure 8.9 ^{31}P MR spectra of positive response to handgrip stress at 3T magnet. Rest (left), stress (middle), and recovery (right). During stress the phosphocreatine level was significantly lowered.

PCr/ATP ratio in the myocardium of the patients with muscular dystrophy [387]. The metabolic change in PCr/ATP during stress ^{31}P spectroscopy correlates with the retinopathy as an indicator of the microvascular dysfunction in type-1 diabetes mellitus patients (Figure 8.9). On the other hand, application of proton MR spectroscopy has also been applied to evaluation of lipid contents in the heart [387,388].

Conclusions

Myocardial viability can be routinely assessed by CMR either by evaluation of the response of abnormal wall motion using cine CMR to low dose dobutamine or by the use of delayed contrast enhancement. Low dose dobutamine cine CMR provides information in a manner similar to that of low dose dobutamine echocardiography but with greater sensitivity and specificity. The definition of viability in this instance is the documentation of improved contractile function with low dose dobutamine providing indirect evidence of myocardial contractile reserve. Delayed contrast enhanced myocardial segments provides evidence of acute and/or chronic MI, and has correlated well with histochemical staining in laboratory animal studies. The absence of delayed contrast enhancement detected by CMR is indicative of viable myocardium. In both the acute and chronic settings, regions of myocardium with contractile dysfunction, but without evidence of delayed enhancement are likely to recover function with revascularization. In routine practice, delayed contrast enhanced CMR is preferable to low dose dobutamine CMR

as the former is safer and gives direct evidence of viability.

Contrast enhanced CMR is able to detect infarcts or scar in regions of normal wall motion, subendocardial infarcts not detected by SPECT, and infarcts that are not clinically recognized. The prognostic significance of such delayed enhancement requires further investigation.

Finally, another unique aspect of CMR, the ability to assess metabolism using ^{31}P spectroscopy, provides a specific way to assess myocardial ischemia, but is less useful to define viability.

References

1. Bloch F. Nuclear induction. *Phys Rev (Physics)*. 1946;70:460–473.
2. Purcell E, Torrey H, Pound R. Resonance adsorption by nuclear magnetic moments in a solid. *Phys Rev (Physics)*. 1946;69:37–38.
3. Lauterbur P. Image formation by induced local interactions: examples employing nuclear magnetic resonance. *Nature*. 1973;242:190–191.
4. Mansfield P. Multiplanar image formation using NMR spin echoes. *J Phys*. 1977;10:L55–L58.
5. Kumar A, Welti D, Ernst RR. NMR Fourier zeugmatography. *J Magn Reson*. 1975;18:69–83.
6. Damadian RV. Tumor detection by nuclear magnetic resonance. *Science*. 1971;171:1151–1153.
7. Pohost GM. Historical perspective: the history of cardiovascular magnetic resonance. *JACC: CV Imaging*. 2008 1:672–678.
8. Goldman MR, Pohost GM, Ingwall JS, *et al*. Nuclear magnetic resonance imaging: potential cardiac applications. *Am J Cardiol*. 1980;46:1278–1283.
9. Blackwell G, Doyle M, Cranney G. Cardiovascular MRI techniques. In: Blackwell GG, Cranney GB, Pohost GM

(eds). *MRI: Cardiovascular System.* New York: Gower Medical Publishing, 1992.

10. McRobbie DW, Moore EA, Graves MJ, *et al. MRI from Picture to Proton.* Cambridge: Cambridge University Press, 2003.

11. Elster AD, Burdette JH. *Questions and Answers in MRI.* London: Mosby, 2001.

12. Bottomley PA, Foster TH, Argersinger RE, *et al.* A review of normal tissue hydrogen NMR relaxation times and mechanisms from 1–100 mHz: dependence on tissue type, NMR frequency, temperature, species, excision and age. *Med Phys.* 1984;11:425–448.

13. Donahue KM, Weisskoff RM, Burnstein D. Water diffusion and exchange as they influence contrast enhancement. *J Magn Reson Imaging.* 1997;7:102–110.

14. Weinmann HJ, Brasch RC, Press WR, *et al.* Characteristics of gadolinium-DTPA complex: a potential NMR contrast agent. *Am J Roentgenol.* 1984;142:619–624.

15. Saeed M, Wagner S, Wendland MF, *et al.* Occlusive and reperfused myocardial infarcts: differentiation with Mn-DPDP enhanced MR imaging. *Radiology.* 1989;172:59–64.

16. Saeed M, Wendland MF, Takehara Y, *et al.* Reversible and irreversible injury in the reperfused myocardium: differentiation with contrast material-enhanced MR imaging. *Radiology.* 1990;175:633–637.

17. Saeed M, Wendland MF, Takehara Y, *et al.* Reperfusion and irreversible myocardial injury: identification with a non-ionic MR imaging contrast medium. *Radiology.* 1992;182:675–683.

18. Saeed M, Wendland MF, Masui T, *et al.* Reperfused myocardial infarctions on T1- and susceptibility-enhanced MRI: evidence for loss of compartmentalization of contrast media. *Magn Res Med.* 1994;31:31–39.

19. Geschwind JF, Wendland MF, Saeed M, *et al.* Identification of myocardial cell death in reperfused myocardial injury using dual mechanisms of contrast enhanced magnetic resonance imaging. *Acad Radiol.* 1994;1:319–325.

20. Adzamli IK, Jolesz FA, Bleier AR, *et al.* The effect of gadolinium DTPA on tissue water compartments in slow- and fast-twitch rabbit muscles. *Magn Reson Med.* 1989;11:172–181.

21. Barkhausen J, Ruehm SG, Goyen M, *et al.* MR evaluation of ventricular function: true fast imaging with steady-state precession versus fast low-angle shot cine MR imaging-feasibility study. *Radiology.* 2001;219:264–269.

22. Plein S, Bloomer TN, Ridgway JP, *et al.* Steady-state free precession magnetic resonance imaging of the heart: comparison with segmented k-space gradient-echo imaging. *J Magn Reson Imaging.* 2001;14:230–236.

23. Pettigrew RI, Oshinski JN, Chatzimavroudis G, *et al.* MRI techniques for cardiovascular imaging. *J Magn Reson Imaging.* 1999;10:590–601.

24. Szolar DH, Sakuma H, Higgins CB. Cardiovascular applications of magnetic resonance flow and velocity measurements. *J Magn Reson Imaging.* 1996;1:78–89.

25. Zerhouni EA, Parish DM, Rogers WJ, *et al.* Human heart tagging with MR imaging—a method for noninvasive assessment of myocardial motion. *Radiology.* 1988;169:59–63.

26. Garot J, Bluemke DA, Osman NF, *et al.* Fast determination of regional myocardial strain fields from tagged cardiac MR images using harmonic phase (HARP) MRI. *Circulation.* 2000;101:981–988.

27. Maier SE, Fischer SE, McKinnon GC, *et al.* Evaluation of left ventricular segmental wall motion in hypertrophic cardiomyopathy with myocardial tagging. *Circulation.* 1992;86:1919–1928.

28. Bogaert J, Maes A, van de Werf F, *et al.* Functional recovery of subepicardial myocardial tissue in transmural myocardial infarction after successful perfusion: an important contribution to the improvement of regional and global left ventricular function. *Circulation.* 1999;99:36–43.

29. Maniar HS, Cupps BP, Potter DD, *et al.* Ventricular function after coronary artery bypass grafting: evaluation by magnetic resonance imaging and myocardial strain analysis. *J Thorac Cardiovasc Surg.* 2004;128:76–82.

30. Fuchs E, Muller MF, Oswald H, *et al.* Cardiac rotation and relaxation in patients with chronic heart failure. *Eur J Heart Fail.* 2004;6:715–722.

31. Dubach P, Myers J, Bonetti P, *et al.* Effects of bisoprolol fumarate on left ventricle size, function, and exercise capacity in patients with heart failure: analysis with magnetic resonance myocardial tagging. *Am Heart J.* 2002;143:676–683.

32. Scheffler K, Heid O, Henning J. Magnetization preparation during the steady state: fat saturated 3D TrueFISP. *Magn Reson Med.* 2001;45:1075–1080.

33. Markl M, Reeder SB, Chan FP, *et al.* Steady state free precession MR imaging improved myocardial tag persistence and signal-to-noise ratio for analysis of myocardial motion. *Radiology.* 2004;230:852–861.

34. Semelka RC, Tomei E, Wagner S, *et al.* Normal left ventricular dimensions and function: interstudy reproducibility of measurements with cine MR imaging. *Radiology.* 1990;174:763–768.

35. Germain P, Roul G, Kastler B, *et al.* Interstudy variability in left ventricular mass measurement. Comparison between M-mode echography and MRI. *Eur Heart J.* 1992;13:1011–1019.

36. Lorenz CH, Walker ES, Morgan VL, *et al.* Normal human right and left ventricular mass, systolic function and gender differences by cine-magnetic resonance imaging. *J Cardiovasc Magn Reson.* 1999;1:7–21.

37. Longmore DB, Klipstein RH, Underwood SR, *et al.* Dimensional accuracy of magnetic resonance in studies of the heart. *Lancet.* 1985;1:1360–1362.

38. Shapiro EP, Rogers WJ, Beyar R, *et al.* Determination of left ventricular mass by MRI in hearts deformed by acute infarction. *Circulation.* 1989;79:706–711.

39. Semelka RC, Tomei E, Wagner S, *et al.* Interstudy reproducibility of dimensional and functional measurements between cine-magnetic resonance studies in the morphologically abnormal left ventricle. *Am Heart J.* 1990;119:1367–1373.

40. Chuang ML, Hibberd MG, Salton CJ, *et al.* Importance of imaging method over imaging modality in non-invasive determination of left ventricular volumes and ejection fraction: assessment by two- and three-dimensional echocardiography and magnetic resonance imaging. *J Am Coll Cardiol.* 2000;35:447–487.

41. Doherty NE, 3rd, Fujita N, Caputo GR, *et al.* Measurement of right ventricular mass in normal and dilated cardiomyopathic ventricles using cine-magnetic resonance imaging. *Am J Cardiol.* 1992;69:1223–1228.

42. Grothues F, Moon JC, Bellenger NG, *et al.* Interstudy reproducibility of right ventricular volumes, function, and mass with cardiovascular magnetic resonance. *Am Heart J.* 2004;147:218–223.

43. Katz J, Whang J, Boxt LM, *et al.* Estimation of right ventricular mass in normal subjects and in patients with primary pulmonary hypertension by nuclear magnetic resonance imaging. *J Am Coll Cardiol.* 1993;21:1475–1481.

44. Lorenz CH, Walker ES, Graham TP, Jr, *et al.* Right ventricular performance and mass by use of cine MRI late after atrial repair of transposition of the great arteries. *Circulation.* 1995;92 (Suppl. II): II233–II239.

45. Sievers B, Kirchberg S, Bakan A, *et al.* Impact of papillary muscles in ventricular volume and ejection fraction assessment by cardiovascular magnetic resonance. *J Cardiovasc Magn Reson.* 2004;6:9–16.

46. Utz JA, Herfkens RJ, Heinsimer JA, *et al.* Cine MR determination of left ventricular ejection fraction. *Am J Roentgenol.* 1987;148:839–843.

47. Culham JA, Vince DJ. Cardiac output by MR imaging: an experimental study comparing right ventricle and left ventricle with thermodilution. *Can Assoc Radiol J.* 1988;39:247–249.

48. Hunter GJ, Hamberg LM, Weisskoff RM, *et al.* Measurement of stroke volume and cardiac output within a single breath-hold with echoplanar MR imaging. *J Magn Reson Imaging.* 1994;4:51–58.

49. Hundley WG, Li HF, Hillis LD, *et al.* Quantitation of cardiac output with velocity encoded, phasedifference magnetic resonance imaging: validation with invasive measurements. *Am J Cardiol.* 1995;75:1250–1255.

50. Zehender M, Kasper W, Kauder E, *et al.* Right ventricular infarction as an independent predictor of prognosis after acute inferior myocardial infarction. *N Engl J Med.* 1993;328:981–988.

51. Rominger MB, Bachmann GF, Pabst W, *et al.* Right ventricular volumes and ejection fraction with fast cine MR imaging in breath-hold technique: applicability, normal values from 52 volunteers, and evaluation of 325 adult cardiac patients. *J Magn Reson Imaging.* 1999;10:908–918.

52. Alfakih K, Plein S, Thiele H, Jones T, Ridgway JP, Sivananthan MU. Normal human left and right ventricular dimensions for MRI as assessed by turbo gradient echo and steady-state free precession imaging sequences. *J Magn Reson Imaging.* 2003;17(3):323–329.

53. Didier D, Ratib O, Friedli B, *et al.* Cine gradient-echo MR imaging in the evaluation of cardiovascular disease. *Radiographics.* 1993;13:561–573.

54. Kondo C, Caputo GR, Semelka R, *et al.* Right and left ventricular stroke volume measurements with velocity encoded cine NMR imaging: *in vitro* and *in vivo* evaluation. *Am J Roentgenol.* 1991;157:9–16.

55. Larose E, Ganz P, Reynolds HG, *et al.* Right ventricular dysfunction assessed by cardiovascular magnetic resonance imaging predicts poor prognosis late after myocardial infarction. *J Am Coll Cardiol.* 2007;49(8):855–862. Epub 2007 Feb 9.

56. Helbing WA, Rebergen SA, Maliepaard C, *et al.* Quantification of right ventricular function with magnetic resonance imaging in children with normal hearts and with congenital heart disease. *Am Heart J.* 1995;130(4): 828–837.

57. Beygui F, Furber A, Delépine S, *et al.* Routine breath-hold gradient echo MRI-derived right ventricular mass, volumes and function: accuracy, reproducibility and coherence study. *Int J Cardiovasc Imaging.* 2004;20 (6): 509–516.

58. Higgins CB, Wagner S, Kondo C, *et al.* Evaluation of valvular heart disease with cine gradient echo magnetic resonance imaging. *Circulation.* 1991;84 (Suppl. 3): I198–I207.

59. De Roos A, Reichek N, Axel L, *et al.* Cine MR imaging in aortic stenosis. *J Comput Assist Tomogr.* 1989;13:421–425.

60. Suzuki J, Caputo GR, Kondo C, *et al.* Cine MR imaging of valvular heart disease: display and imaging parameters affect the size of the signal void caused by valvular regurgitation. *Am J Roentgenol.* 1990;155:723–727.

61. Mohiaddin RH, Pennell DJ. MR blood flow measurement: clinical application in the heart and circulation. *Cardiol Clin.* 1998;16:161–187.

62. Mitchell L, Jenkins JP, Watson Y, *et al.* Diagnosis and assessment of mitral and aortic disease by cine flow magnetic resonance imaging. *Magn Reson Med.* 1989;12:181–197.

63. Cosolo GC, Zampa V, Rega L, *et al.* Evaluation of mitral stenosis by cine-magnetic resonance imaging. *Am Heart J.* 1992;123:1252–1260.

64. Rebergen SA, Niezen RA, Helbing WA, *et al.* Cine gradient echo MR imaging and MR velocity mapping in the evaluation of congenital heart disease. *Radiographics.* 1996;16:467–481.

65. Kayser HV, Stoel BC, Van Der Wall EE, *et al.* MR velocity mapping of tricuspid flow: correction for through-plane motion. *J Magn Reson Imaging.* 1997;7:669–673.

66. Wang ZJ, Reddy GP, Gotway MB, *et al.* Cardiovascular shunts: MR imaging evaluation. *Radiographics.* 2003;23 (Spec No): S181–S194.

67. Hundley WG, Li HF, Lange RA, *et al.* Assessment of left-to-right intracardiac shunting by velocity encoded, phase-difference magnetic resonance imaging. *Circulation.* 1995;91:2955–2960.

68. Hundley WG, Li HF, Willard JE, *et al.* Magnetic resonance imaging assessment of the severity of mitral regurgitation: comparison with invasive techniques. *Circulation.* 1995;92:1151–1158.

69. Fujita N, Chaouilleres AF, Hartiala MM, *et al.* Quantification of mitral regurgitation by velocity encoded cine nuclear magnetic resonance imaging. *J Am Coll Cardiol.* 1994;23:951–958.

70. Kon MW, Myerson SG, Moat NE, *et al.* Quantification of regurgitant fraction in mitral regurgitation by cardiovascular magnetic resonance: comparison of techniques. *J Heart Valve Dis.* 2004;13:600–607.

71. Eichenberger AC, Jenni R, von Schulthess GK. Aortic valve pressure gradients in patients with aortic valve stenosis: quantification with velocity encoded cine MR imaging. *Am J Roentgenol.* 1993;160:971–977.

72. Caruthers SD, Lin SJ, Brown P, *et al.* Practical value of cardiac magnetic resonance imaging for clinical quantification of aortic valve stenosis: comparison with echocardiography. *Circulation.* 2003;108:2236–2243.

73. Heidenreich PA, Steffens J, Fujita N, *et al.* Evaluation of mitral stenosis with velocity encoded cine-magnetic resonance imaging. *Am J Cardiol.* 1995;75:365–369.

74. Lin SJ, Brown PA, Watkins MP, *et al.* Quantification of stenotic mitral valve area with magnetic resonance imaging and comparison with Doppler ultrasound. *J Am Coll Cardiol.* 2004;44:133–137.

75. Sridharan S, Derrick G, Deanfield J, Taylor AM. Assessment of differential branch pulmonary blood flow: a comparative study of phase contrast magnetic resonance imaging and radionuclide lung perfusion imaging. *Heart.* 2006;92 (7): 963–968.

76. Bellenger NG, Burgess M, Ray SG, *et al.* Comparison of left ventricular ejection fraction and volumes in heart failure by two-dimensional echocardiography, radionuclide ventriculography and cardiovascular magnetic resonance: are they interchangeable? *Eur Heart J.* 2000;21:1387–1396.

77. Holman ER, Buller VGM, de Roos A, *et al.* Detection and quantification of dysfunctional myocardium by magnetic resonance imaging: a new three-dimensional method for quantitative wall thickening analysis. *Circulation.* 1997;95:924–931.

78. Van Rugge FP, Van Der Wall EE, Spanjersberg SJ, *et al.* Magnetic resonance imaging during dobutamine stress for detection of coronary artery disease: quantitative wall motion analysis using a modification of the centerline method. *Circulation.* 1994;90:127–138.

79. Haag UJ, Maier SE, Jakob M, *et al.* Left ventricular wall thickness measurements by magnetic resonance: a validation study. *Int J Card Imaging.* 1991;7:31–41.

80. Baer FM, Smolarz K, Theissen P, *et al.* Regional ^{99m}Tc-methoxyisobutyl-isonitrile uptake at rest in patients with myocardial infarcts: comparison with morphological and functional parameters obtained from gradient-echo magnetic resonance imaging. *Eur Heart J.* 1994;15:97–107.

81. Azhari H, Sideman S, Weiss JL, *et al.* Three-dimensional mapping of acute ischemic regions using MRI: wall thickening versus motion analysis. *Am J Physiol.* 1990;259:H1492–H1503.

82. Sheehan FH, Bolson EL, Dodge HT, *et al.* Advantages and applications of the centerline method for characterizing regional ventricular function. *Circulation.* 1986;74:293–305.

83. Von Land CD, Rao SR, Reiber JHC. Development of an improved centerline wall motion model. *Comput Cardiol.* 1990;17:687–690.

84. Bellenger MG, Burgess M, Ray SG, *et al.* Comparison of left ventricular ejection fraction and volumes in heart failure by two-dimensional echocardiography, radionuclide ventriculography and cardiovascular magnetic resonance: are they interchangeable? *Eur Heart J* 2000;21:1387–1396.

85. McVeigh ER, Zerhouni EA. Non-invasive measurement of transmural gradients in myocardial strain with MR imaging. *Radiology.* 1991;180:677–683.

86. Gerber BL, Garot J, Bluemke DA, *et al.* Accuracy of contrast enhanced resonance magnetic imaging in predicting improvement of regional myocardial function in patients after acute myocardial infarction. *Circulation.* 2002;106:1083–1089.

87. Paelinck BP, Lamb HJ, Bax JJ, et al. Assessment of diastolic function by cardiovascular magnetic resonance. Am Heart J. 2002;144:198–205.

88. Van Der Geest RJ, Reiber JH. Quantification in cardiac MRI. J Magn Reson Imaging. 1999;10:602–608.

89. Suzuki JI, Caputo GR, Masui T, et al. Assessment of right ventricular diastolic and systolic function in patients with dilated cardiomyopathy using cinemagnetic resonance imaging. Am Heart J. 1991;122:1035–1040.

90. Fujita N, Hartiala J, O'Sullivan M, et al. Assessment of left ventricular diastolic function in dilated cardiomyopathy with cine-magnetic resonance imaging: effect of an angiotensin converting enzyme inhibitor, benazepril. Am Heart J. 1993;125:171–178.

91. Yamanari H, Kakishita M, Fujimoto Y, et al. Regional myocardial perfusion abnormalities and regional myocardial early diastolic dysfunction in patients with hypertrophic cardiomyopathy. Heart Vessels. 1997;12:192–198.

92. Kudelka AM, Turner DA, Liebson PR, et al. Comparison of cine-magnetic resonance imaging and Doppler echocardiography for evaluation of left ventricular diastolic function. Am J Cardiol. 1997;80:384–386.

93. Mohiaddin RH, Gatehouse PD, Henien M, et al. Cine MR Fourier velocimetry of blood through cardiac valves: comparison with Doppler echocardiography. J Magn Reson Imaging. 1997;7:657–663.

94. Hartiala JJ, Mostbeck GH, Foster E, et al. Velocity encoded cine MRI in the evaluation of left ventricular diastolic function. Measurement of mitral valve and pulmonary vein flow velocities and flow volume across the mitral valve. Am Heart J. 1993;125:1054–1066.

95. Fyrenius A, Wigstrom L, BoDCEr AF, et al. Pitfalls in Doppler evaluation of diastolic function: insights from three-dimensional magnetic resonance imaging. J Am Soc Echocardiogr. 1999;12:817–826.

96. Hartiala JJ, Foster E, Fujita N, et al. Evaluation of left atrial contribution to left ventricular filling in aortic stenosis by velocity encoded cine MRI. Am Heart J. 1994;127:593–600.

97. Karwatowski SP, Brecker SJD, Yang GZ, et al. Mitral valve flow measured with cine MR velocity mapping in patients with ischemic heart disease: comparison with Doppler echocardiography. J Magn Reson Imaging. 1995;5:89–92.

98. Buchalter MB, Weiss JL, Rogers WJ, et al. Noninvasive quantification of left ventricular rotational deformation in normal humans using magnetic resonance imaging myocardial tagging. Circulation. 1990;81:1236–1244.

99. Nagel E, Stuber M, Lakatos M, et al. Cardiac rotation and relaxation after anteroseptal myocardial infarction. Coron Artery Dis. 2000;10:261–267.

100. Kroeker CA, Tyberg JV, Beyar R. Effects of ischemia on left ventricular apex rotation. An experimental study in anesthetized dogs. Circulation. 1995;92:3539–3548.

101. Paetsch I, Foell D, Kaluza A, et al. Magnetic resonance stress tagging in ischemic heart disease. Am J Physiol Heart Circ Physiol. 2005;288:H2708–H2714.

102. Sensky PR, Jivan A, Hudson NM, et al. Coronary artery disease: combined stress MR imaging protocol—one stop evaluation of myocardial perfusion and function. Radiology. 2000;215:608–614.

103. Plein S, Ridgway JP, Jones TR, et al. Coronary artery disease: assessment with a comprehensive MR imaging protocol—initial results. Radiology. 2002;225:300–307.

104. Chiu CW, So NM, Lam WW, et al. Combined first-pass perfusion and viability study of MR imaging in patients with non-ST segment-elevation acute coronary syndromes: feasibility study. Radiology. 2003;226:717–722.

105. Kwong RY, Schussheim AE, Rekhraj S, et al. Detecting acute coronary syndrome in the emergency department with cardiac magnetic resonance imaging. Circulation. 2003;107:531–537.

106. Moon JC, de Arenaza DP, Elkington AG, et al. The pathologic basis of Q-wave and non-Q-wave myocardial infarction: a cardiovascular magnetic resonance study. J Am Coll Cardiol. 2004;44:554–560.

107. Finn AV, Antman EM. Images in clinical medicine: isolated right ventricular infarction. N Engl J Med. 2003;349:1636.

108. Wagner A, Mahrholdt H, Holly TA, et al. Contrast enhanced MRI and routine single photon emission computed tomography (SPECT) perfusion imaging for detection of subendocardial myocardial infarcts: an imaging study. Lancet. 2003;361:374–379.

109. Choi KM, Kim RJ, Gubernikoff G, et al. Transmural extent of acute myocardial infarction predicts long term improvement in contractile function. Circulation. 2001;104:1101–1107.

110. Mahrholdt H, Wagner A, Holly TA, et al. Reproducibility of chronic infarct size measurement by contrast enhanced magnetic resonance imaging. Circulation. 2002;106:2322–2327.

111. Garcia-Dorado D, Oliveras J, Gili J, et al. Analysis of myocardial edema by magnetic resonance imaging early after coronary artery occlusion with or without reperfusion. Cardiovasc Res. 1993;27:1462–1469.

112. Abdel-Aty H, Zagrosek A, Schulz-Menger J, et al. Delayed enhancement and T2-weighted cardiovascular magnetic resonance imaging differentiate acute from chronic myocardial infarction. Circulation. 2004;109:2411–2416.

113. Bellenger NG, Rajappan K, Rahman SL, *et al.* Effects of carvedilol on left ventricular remodeling in chronic stable heart failure: a cardiovascular magnetic resonance study. *Heart.* 2004;90:760–764.

114. Schulman SP, Weiss JL, Becker LC, *et al.* Effect of early enalapril therapy on left ventricular function and structure in acute myocardial infarction. *Am J Cardiol.* 1995;76:764–770.

115. Foster RE, Johnson DB, Barilla F, *et al.* Changes in left ventricular mass and volumes in patients receiving angiotensin-converting enzyme inhibitor therapy for left ventricular dysfunction after Q-wave myocardial infarction. *Am Heart J.* 1998;136:269–275.

116. Sakuma H, Koskenvuo JW, Niemi P, *et al.* Assessment of coronary flow reserve using fast velocity encoded cine MR imaging: validation study using positron emission tomography. *Am J Roentgenol.* 2000;165:1029–1033.

117. Clarke GD, Eckels R, Chaney C, *et al.* Measurements of absolute epicardial coronary artery flow and flow reserve with breath-hold cine phase-contrast magnetic resonance imaging. *Circulation.* 1995;91:2627–2634.

118. Sakuma H, Saeed M, Takeda K, *et al.* Quantification of coronary artery volume flow rate using fast velocity encoded cine MR imaging. *Am J Roentgenol.* 1997;168:1363–1367.

119. Nagel E, Thouet T, Klein C, *et al.* Non-invasive determination of coronary blood flow velocity with cardiovascular magnetic resonance in patients after stent deployment. *Circulation.* 2003;107:1738–1743.

120. Al-Saadi N, Nagel E, Gross M, *et al.* Non-invasive detection of myocardial ischemia from perfusion reserve based on cardiovascular magnetic resonance. *Circulation.* 2000;101:1379–1383.

121. Nagel E, Klein C, Paetsch I, *et al.* Magnetic resonance perfusion measurements for the non-invasive detection of coronary artery disease. *Circulation.* 2003;108:432–437.

122. Al-Saadi N, Nagel E, Gross M, *et al.* Improvement of myocardial perfusion reserve early after coronary intervention: assessment with cardiac magnetic resonance imaging. *J Am Coll Cardiol.* 2000;36:1557–1564.

123. Lauerma K, Virtanen KS, Sipila L, *et al.* Multislice MRI assessment of myocardial perfusion in patients with single-vessel proximal left anterior descending coronary artery disease before and after revascularization. *Circulation.* 1997;96:2859–2867.

124. Rehwald WG, Fieno DS, Chen EL, *et al.* Myocardial magnetic resonance imaging contrast agent concentrations after reversible and irreversible ischemic injury. *Circulation.* 2002;105:224–229.

125. Ingkanisorn WP, Rhoads KL, Aletras AH, *et al.* Gadolinium delayed enhancement cardiovascular magnetic resonance correlates with clinical measures of myocardial infarction. *J Am Coll Cardiol.* 2004;43:2253–2259.

126. Steuer J, Bjerner T, Duvernoy O, *et al.* Visualisation and quantification of perioperative myocardial infarction after coronary artery bypass surgery with contrast enhanced magnetic resonance imaging. *Eur Heart J.* 2004;25:1293–1299.

127. Ricciardi JM, Wu E, Davidson CJ, *et al.* Visualization of discrete micro-infarction after percutaneous coronary intervention associated with mild creatine kinase-MB elevation. *Circulation.* 2001;103:2780–2783.

128. Gallegos RP, Swingen C, Xu XJ, *et al.* Infarct extent by MRI correlates with peak serum troponin level in the canine model. *J Surg Res.* 2004;120:266–271.

129. Kim RJ, Wu E, Rafael A, *et al.* The use of contrast enhanced magnetic resonance imaging to identify reversible myocardial dysfunction. *N Engl J Med.* 2000;343:1445–1453.

130. Weiss CR, Aletras AH, London JF, *et al.* Stunned, infarcted, and normal myocardium in dogs: simultaneous differentiation by using gadolinium enhanced cine MR imaging with magnetization transfer contrast. *Radiology.* 2003;226:723–730.

131. Wassmuth R, Erdbruegger U, Leritzsch S, *et al.* Magnetic resonance imaging for monitoring cardiac function and tissue characterization in anthracyclines therapy. *Circulation.* 2000;102:809–810.

132. McCrohon JA, Moon JC, Prasad SK, *et al.* Differentiation of heart failure related to dilated cardiomyopathy and coronary artery disease using gadolinium enhanced cardiovascular magnetic resonance. *Circulation.* 2003;108:54–59.

133. Manning WJ, Li W, Edelman RR. A preliminary report comparing magnetic resonance coronary angiography with conventional angiography. *N Engl J Med.* 1993;328:828–832.

134. Post JC, van Rossum AC, Hofman MB, *et al.* Three-dimensional respiratory-gated MR angiography of coronary arteries: comparison with conventional coronary angiography. *Am J Roentgenol.* 1996;166:1399–1404.

135. Van Geuns RJ, Wielopolski PA, de Bruin HG, *et al.* MR coronary angiography with breath-hold targeted volumes: preliminary clinical results. *Radiology.* 2000;217:270–277.

136. Huber A, Nikolaou K, Gonschior P, *et al.* Navigator echo-based respiratory gating for three-dimensional MR coronary angiography: results from healthy volunteers and patients with proximal coronary artery stenoses. *Am J Roentgenol.* 1999;173:95–101.

137. Kim WY, Danias PG, Stuber M, *et al.* Coronary magnetic resonance angiography for the detection

of coronary stenoses. *N Engl J Med.* 2001;345:1863–1869.

138. Langerak SE, Vliegen HW, de Roos A, *et al.* Detection of vein graft disease using high resolution magnetic resonance angiography. *Circulation.* 2002;105:328–333.

139. Stuber M, Botnar RM, Kissinger KV, *et al.* Freebreathing black blood coronary MR angiography: initial results. *Radiology.* 2001;219:278–283.

140. Stuber M, Botnar RM, Spuentrup E, *et al.* Threedimensional high resolution fast spin-echo coronary magnetic resonance angiography. *Magn Reson Med.* 2001;45:206–211.

141. Fayad ZA, Fuster V, Fallon JT, *et al.* Non-invasive *in vivo* human coronary artery lumen and wall imaging using black blood magnetic resonance imaging. *Circulation.* 2000;102:506–510.

142. Sodickson DK, Manning WJ. Simultaneous acquisition of spatial harmonics (SMASH)—fast imaging with radiofrequency coil arrays. *Magn Reson Med.* 1997;38:591–603.

143. Pruessmann KP, Weiger M, Scheidegger MB, *et al.* SENSE: sensitivity encoding for fast MRI. *Magn Reson Med.* 1999;42:952–962.

144. Stuber M, Botnar RM, Danias PG, *et al.* Contrast agent-enhanced, free-breathing, three-dimensional coronary magnetic resonance angiography. *J Magn Reson Imaging.* 1999;10:790–799.

145. Li D, Dolan B, Walovitch RC, *et al.* Three-dimensional MR imaging of coronary arteries using an intravascular contrast agent. *Magn Reson Med.* 1998;39:1014–1018.

146. Stuber M, Botnar RM, Fischer SE, *et al.* Preliminary report on *in vivo* coronary MRA at 3 Tesla in humans. *Magn Reson Med.* 2002;48:425–429.

147. Nayak KS, Cunningham CH, Santos JM, *et al.* Real time cardiac MRI at 3 Tesla. *Magn Reson Med.* 2004;51:655–660.

148. Peters DC, Korosec FR, Grist TM, *et al.* Undersampled projection reconstruction applied to MR angiography. *Magn Reson Med.* 2000;43:91–101.

149. Larson AC, Simonetti OP, Li D. Coronary MRA with 3D undersampled projection reconstruction TrueFISP. *Magn Reson Med.* 2002;48:594–601.

150. Bornert P, Stuber M, Botnar RM, *et al.* Direct comparison of 3D spiral vs Cartesian gradient-echo coronary magnetic resonance angiography. *Magn Reson Med.* 2001;46:789–794.

151. Taylor AM, Keegan J, Jhooti P, *et al.* A comparison between segmented k-space FLASH and interleaved spiral MR coronary angiography sequences. *J Magn Reson Imaging.* 2000;11:394–400.

152. Taylor AM, Thorne SA, Rubens MB, *et al.* Coronary artery imaging in grown up congenital heart disease: complementary role of magnetic resonance and X-ray coronary angiography. *Circulation.* 2000;101:1670–1678.

153. McConnell MV, Ganz P, Selwyn AP, *et al.* Identification of anomalous coronary arteries and their anatomic course by magnetic resonance coronary angiography. *Circulation.* 1995;92:3158–3162.

154. Post JC, van Rossum AC, Bronzwaer JG, *et al.* Magnetic resonance angiography of anomalous coronary arteries: a new gold standard for delineating the proximal course? *Circulation.* 1995;92:3163–3171.

155. Drory Y, Turetz Y, Hiss Y, *et al.* Sudden unexpected death in persons less than 40 years of age. *Am J Cardiol.* 1991;68:1388–1392.

156. Kasper EK, Agema WR, Hutchins GM, *et al.* The causes of dilated cardiomyopathy: a clinicopathologic review of 673 consecutive patients. *J Am Coll Cardiol.* 1994;23:586–590.

157. Liu PP, Mason JW. Advances in the understanding of myocarditis. *Circulation.* 2001;104:1076–1082.

158. Laissy JP, Messin B, Varenne O, *et al.* MRI of acute myocarditis: a comprehensive approach based on various imaging sequences. *Chest.* 2002;22:1638–1648.

159. Friedrich MG, Strohm O, Schulz-Menger J, *et al.* Contrast media-enhanced magnetic resonance imaging visualizes myocardial changes in the course of viral myocarditis. *Circulation.* 1998;97:1802–1809.

160. Yasuda T, Palacios IF, Dec GW, *et al.* Indium 111-monoclonal antimyosin antibody imaging in the diagnosis of acute myocarditis. *Circulation.* 1987;76:306–311.

161. Morguet AJ, Munz DL, Kreuzer H, *et al.* Scintigraphic detection of inflammatory heart disease. *Eur J Nucl Med.* 1994;21:666–674.

162. Davis MJ, Ward DE. How can myocarditis be diagnosed and should it be treated? *Br Heart J.* 1992;68:346–347.

163. Mason JW, O'Connell JB, Herskowitz A, *et al.* A clinical trial of immunosuppressive therapy for myocarditis: the myocarditis treatment trial investigators. *N Engl J Med.* 1995;333:269–275.

164. Alpert JS, Cheitlin M. Update in cardiology: myocarditis. *Ann Intern Med.* 1996;125:40–46.

165. Brown CA, O'Connell JB. Implications of the myocarditis treatment trial for clinical practice. *Curr Opin Cardiol.* 1996;11:332–336.

166. Sasse-Klaassen S, Probst S, Gerull B, *et al.* Novel gene locus for autosomal dominant left ventricular non-compaction maps to chromosome 11p15. *Circulation.* 2004;109:2720–2723.

167. Hermida-Prieto M, Monserrat L, Castro-Beiras A, *et al.* Familial dilated cardiomyopathy and isolated left ventricular non-compaction associated with lamin A/C gene mutations. *Am J Cardiol.* 2004;94:50–54.

168. Foo TK, Stanley DW, Castillo E, *et al.* Myocardial viability: breath-hold 3D MR imaging of delayed hyperenhancement with variable sampling in time. *Radiology.* 2004;230 (3): 845–851.

169. Selvanayagam JB, Kardos A, Francis JM, *et al.* Value of delayed-enhancement cardiovascular magnetic resonance imaging in predicting myocardial viability after surgical revascularization. *Circulation.* 2004;110 (12): 1535–1541.

170. Schinkel AF, Poldermans D, Rizzello V, *et al.* Why do patients with ischemic cardiomyopathy and a substantial amount of viable myocardium not always recover in function after revascularization? *J Thorac Cardiovasc Surg.* 2004;127 (2): 385–390.

171. Chalil S, Stegemann B, Muhyaldeen SA, *et al.* Effect of posterolateral left ventricular scar on mortality and morbidity following cardiac resynchronization therapy. *Pacing Clin Electrophysiol.* 2007;30 (10): 1201–1209.

172. Codreanu A, Odille F, Aliot E, *et al.* Electroanatomic characterization of post-infarct scars comparison with 3-dimensional myocardial scar reconstruction based on magnetic resonance imaging. *J Am Coll Cardiol.* 2008;52 (10): 839–842.

173. Bleeker GB, Kaandorp TA, Lamb HJ, *et al.* Effect of posterolateral scar tissue on clinical and echocardiographic improvement after cardiac resynchronization therapy. *Circulation.* 2006;113 (7): 969–976.

174. Ichida F, Tsubata S, Bowles KR, *et al.* Novel gene mutations in patients with left ventricular non-compaction or Barth syndrome. *Circulation.* 2001;103:1256–1263.

175. Oechslin EN, Attenhofer Jost CH, Rojas JR, *et al.* Long term follow-up of 34 adults with isolated left ventricular non-compaction: a distinct cardiomyopathy with poor prognosis. *J Am Coll Cardiol.* 2000;36:493–500.

176. Ritter M, Oechslin E, Sutsch G, *et al.* Isolated noncompaction of the myocardium in adults. *Mayo Clin Proc.* 1997;72:26–31.

177. Pignatelli RH, McMahon CJ, Dreyer WJ, *et al.* Clinical characterization of left ventricular non-compaction in children. A relatively common form of cardiomyopathy. *Circulation.* 2003;108:2672–2678.

178. Agmon Y, Connolly HM, Olson LJ, *et al.* Non-compaction of the ventricular myocardium. *J Am Soc Echocardiogr.* 1999;12:859–863.

179. Chin TK, Perloff JK, Williams RG, *et al.* Isolated non-compaction of left ventricular myocardium. A study of eight cases. *Circulation.* 1990;82:507–513.

180. Stollberger C, Finsterer J. Left ventricular hypertrabeculation/non-compaction. *J Am Soc Echocardiogr.* 2004;17:91–100.

181. Tamborini G, Pepi M, Celeste F, *et al.* Incidence and characteristics of left ventricular false tendons and trabeculations in the normal and pathologic heart by second harmonic echocardiography. *J Am Soc Echocardiogr.* 2004;17:367–374.

182. Zagrosek A, Wassmuth R, Abdel-Aty H, Rudolph A, Dietz R, Schulz-Menger J. Relation between myocardial edema and myocardial mass during the acute and convalescent phase of myocarditis–a CMR study. *J Cardiovasc Magn Reson.* 2008;10 (1): 19.

183. Assomull RG, Lyne JC, Keenan N, *et al.* The role of cardiovascular magnetic resonance in patients presenting with chest pain, raised troponin, and unobstructed coronary arteries. *Eur Heart J.* 2007;28 (10): 1242–1249.

184. Chung T, Yiannikas J, Lee LC, *et al.* Isolated noncompaction involving the left ventricular apex in adults. *Am J Cardiol.* 2004;94:1214–1216.

185. Hamamichi Y, Ichida F, Hashimoto I, *et al.* Isolated non-compaction of the ventricular myocardium: ultrafast computed tomography and magnetic resonance imaging. *Int J Cardiovasc Imaging.* 2001;17:305–314.

186. Korcyk D, Edwards CC, Armstrong G, *et al.* Contrast enhanced cardiac magnetic resonance in a patient with familial isolated ventricular non-compaction. *J Cardiovasc Magn Reson.* 2004;6:569–576.

187. Soler R, Rodriguez E, Monserrat L, *et al.* MRI of subendocardial perfusion deficits in isolated left ventricular non-compaction. *J Comput Assist Tomogr.* 2002;26:373–375.

188. Wu KC, Weiss RG, Thiemann DR, *et al.* Late gadolinium enhancement by cardiovascular magnetic resonance heralds an adverse prognosis in nonischemic cardiomyopathy. *J Am Coll Cardiol.* 2008;51(25): 2414–2421.

189. McCrohon JA, Richmond DR, Pennell DJ, *et al.* Isolated non-compaction of the myocardium. A rarity or missed diagnosis? *Circulation.* 2002;106:e22–e23.

190. Maron BJ, Bonow RO, Cannon RO, *et al.* Hypertrophic cardiomyopathy: interrelations of clinical manifestations, pathophysiology, and therapy. *N Engl J Med.* 1987;316:780–789.

191. Wigle ED, Rakowski H, Kimball BP, *et al.* Hypertrophic cardiomyopathy. Clinical spectrum and treatment. *Circulation.* 1995;92:1680–1692.

192. Spirito P, Seidman CE, McKenna WJ, *et al.* The management of hypertrophic cardiomyopathy. *N Engl J Med.* 1997;336:775–785.

193. Varnava AM, Elliott PM, Mahon N, *et al.* Relation between myocyte disarray and outcome in hypertrophic cardiomyopathy. *Am J Cardiol.* 2001;88:275–279.

194. Richard P, Charron P, Carrier L, *et al.* Hypertrophic cardiomyopathy. Distribution of disease genes, spectrum of mutations, and implications for a molecular diagnosis strategy. *Circulation.* 2003;107:2227–2232.

195. Maron BJ, Shen WK, Link MS, et al. Efficacy of implantable cardioverter-defibrillators for the prevention of sudden death in patients with hypertrophic cardiomyopathy. N Engl J Med. 2000;342:365–373.

196. Park JH, Kim YM, Chung JW, et al. MR imaging of hypertrophic cardiomyopathy. Radiology. 1992;185:441–446.

197. Sardanelli F, Molinari G, Petillo A, et al. MRI in hypertrophic cardiomyopathy: a morphofunctional study. J comput Assist Tomogr. 1993;17:862–872.

198. Arrive L, Assayag P, Russ G, et al. MRI and cine MRI of asymmetric septal hypertrophic cardiomyopathy. J Comput Assist Tomogr. 1994;18:376–382.

199. Amano Y, Takayama M, Amano M, et al. MRI of cardiac morphology and function after percutaneous transluminal septal myocardial ablation for hypertrophic obstructive cardiomyopathy. Am J Roentgenol. 2004;182:523–527.

200. Webb JG, Sasson Z, Rakowski H, et al. Apical hypertrophic cardiomyopathy: clinical follow-up and diagnostic correlates. J Am Coll Cardiol. 1990;15:83–90.

201. Suzuki J, Watanabe F, Takenaka K, et al. New subtype of apical hypertrophic cardiomyopathy identified with nuclear magnetic resonance imaging as an underlying cause of markedly inverted T waves. J Am Coll Cardiol. 1993;22:1175–1181.

202. Olivotto I, Maron MS, Autore C, et al. Assessment and significance of left ventricular mass by cardiovascular magnetic resonance in hypertrophic cardiomyopathy. J Am Coll Cardiol. 2008;52:559–566.

203. Young AA, Kramer CM, Ferrari VA, et al. Threedimensional left ventricular deformation in hypertrophic cardiomyopathy. Circulation. 1994;90:854–867.

204. Sipola P, Lauerma K, Husso-Saastamoien M, et al. First-pass MR imaging in the assessment of perfusion impairment in patients with hypertrophic cardiomyopathy and the Asp 175 Asn mutation of the alpha-tropomyosin gene. Radiology. 2003;226:129–137.

205. Choudhury L, Mahrholdt H, Wagner A, et al. Myocardial scarring in asymptomatic or mildly symptomatic patients with hypertrophic cardiomyopathy. J Am Coll Cardiol. 2002;40:2156–2164.

206. Basso C, Thiene G, Corrado D, et al. Hypertrophic cardiomyopathy and sudden death in the young: pathologic evidence of myocardial ischemia. Hum Pathol. 2000;8:988–998.

207. Teraoka K, Hirano M, Ookubo H, et al. Delayed contrast enhancement of MRI in hypertrophic cardiomyopathy. Magn Reson Imaging. 2004;2:155–161.

208. Adabag AS, Maron BJ, Appelbaum E, et al. Occurrence and frequency of arrhythmias in hypertrophic cardiomyopathy in relation to delayed enhancement on cardiovascular magnetic resonance. J Am Coll Cardiol. 2008;51:1369–1374.

209. Maron MS, Finley JJ, Bos JM, et al. Prevalence, clinical significance, and natural history of left ventricular apical aneurysms in hypertrophic cardiomyopathy. Circulation. 2008;118:1541–1549.

210. Tiso N, Stephan DA, Nava A, et al. Identification of mutations in the cardiac ryanodine receptor gene in families affected with arrhythmogenic right ventricular cardiomyopathy type 2 (ARVD2). Hum Mol Genet. 2001;10:189–194.

211. Rampazzo A, Nava A, Malacrida S, et al. Mutation in human desmoplakin domain binding to plakoglobin causes a dominant form of arrhythmogenic right ventricular cardiomyopathy. Am J Hum Genet. 2002;71:1200–1206.

212. Thiene G, Nava A, Corrado D, et al. Right ventricular cardiomyopathy and sudden death in young people. N Engl J Med. 1988;318:129–133.

213. Fontaine G, Fontaliran F, Frank R. Arrhythmogenic right ventricular cardiomyopathies: clinical forms and main differential diagnoses. Circulation. 1998;97:1532–1535.

214. Richardson P, McKenna W, Bristow M, et al. Report of the 1995 World Health Organization/International Society and Federation of cardiology task force on the definition and classification of cardiomyopathies. Circulation. 1996;93:841–842.

215. McKenna WJ, Thiene G, Nava A, Fontaliran F, Blomstrom-Lundqvist C, Fontaine G. Camerini on behalf of the working group myocardial and pericardial disease of the European society of cardiology and of the scientific council on cardiomyopathies of the International society and federation of cardiology, supported by the Schoepfer association. Diagnosis of Arrhythmogenic right ventricular dysplasia/cardiomyopathy. Br Heart J. 1994;71:215–218.

216. Basso C, Thiene G, Corrado D, et al. Arrhythmogenic right ventricular cardiomyopathy: dysplasia, dystrophy, or myocarditis? Circulation. 1996;94:983–991.

217. Burke AP, Farb A, Tashko G, et al. Arrhythmogenic right ventricular cardiomyopathy and fatty replacement of the right ventricular myocardium: are they different diseases? Circulation. 1998;97:1571–1580.

218. Carlson MD, White RD, Trohman RG, et al. Right ventricular outflow tract ventricular tachycardia: detection of previously unrecognized anatomic abnormalities using cine-magnetic resonance imaging. J Am Coll Cardiol. 1994;24:720–727.

219. Proclemer A, Basadonna PT, Slavich GA, et al. Cardiac magnetic resonance imaging findings in patients with right ventricular outflow tract premature contractions. Eur Heart J. 1997;18:2002–2010.

220. Castillo E, Tandri H, Rene Rodriguez ER, *et al.* Arrhyth-mogenic right ventricular dysplasia: *ex vivo* and *in vivo* fat detection with black blood MR imaging. *Radiology.* 2004;232:38–48.

221. Auffermann W, Wichter T, Breithardt G, *et al.* Arrhythmogenic right ventricular disease: MR imaging vs angiography. *Am J Roentgenol.* 1993;161:549–555.

222. Appleton CP, Hatle LK, Popp RL. Relation of transmitral flow velocity patterns to left ventricular diastolic function: new insights from a combined hemodynamic and Doppler echocardiographic study. *J Am Coll Cardiol.* 1988;12:426–440.

223. Kayser H, Schalij M, Van Der Wall E, *et al.* Biventricular function in patients with non-ischemic right ventricular tachyarrhythmias assessed with MR imaging. *Am J Roentgenol.* 1997;159:995–999.

224. Talreja DR, Edwards WD, Danielson GK, *et al.* Constrictive pericarditis in 26 patients with histologically normal pericardial thickness. *Circulation.* 2003;108:1852–1857.

225. Masui T, Finck S, Higgins CB. Constrictive pericarditis and restrictive cardiomyopathy: evaluation with MR imaging. *Radiology.* 1992;182:369–373.

226. Fattori R, Rocchi G, Celletti F, *et al.* Contribution of magnetic resonance imaging in the differential diagnosis of cardiac amyloidosis and symmetric hypertrophic cardiomyopathy. *Heart J.* 1998;136:824–830.

227. Mana J. Nuclear imaging: gallium-67, 201 thallium, ^{18}T-labeled fluoro-2 deoxy-D glucose position emission tomography. *Clin Chest Med.* 1997;18:799–811.

228. Kinney E, Caldwell J. Do thallium myocardial perfusion scan abnormalities predict survival in sarcoid patients without cardiac symptoms? *Angiology.* 1990:41:573–576.

229. Uemura A, Morimoto S, Hiramitsu S, *et al.* Histologic diagnostic rate of cardiac sarcoidosis: evaluation of endocardial biopsies. *Am Heart J.* 1999;138:299–302.

230. Chandra M, Silverman ME, Oshinski J, *et al.* Diagnosis of cardiac sarcoidosis aided by MRI. *Chest.* 1996;110:562–565.

231. Matsuki M, Matsuo M. MR findings of myocardial sarcoidosis. *Clin Radiol.* 2000;55:323–325.

232. Serra JJ, Monte GU, Mello ES, *et al.* Cardiac sarcoidosis evaluated by delayed enhanced magnetic resonance imaging. *Circulation.* 2003;107:e188–e189.

233. Nemeth MA, Muthupillai R, Wilson JM, *et al.* Cardiac sarcoidosis detected by delayed hyperenhancement magnetic resonance imaging. *Tex Heart Inst J.* 2004;31:99–102.

234. Vignaux O, Dhote R, Duboc D, *et al.* Clinical significance of myocardial magnetic resonance abnormalities in patients with sarcoidosis: a 1-year follow-up study. *Chest.* 2002;122:1895–1901.

235. Shimida J, Shimida K, Sakane T, *et al.* Diagnosis of sarcoidosis and evaluation of the effects of steroid therapy by gadolinium-DTPA enhanced magnetic resonance imaging. *Am J Med.* 2001;110:525–527.

236. Paz H, McCormick D, Kutalek S, *et al.* The automatic implantable defibrillator prophylaxis in cardiac sarcoidosis. *Chest.* 1994;106:1603–1607.

237. Mooij CF, de Wit CJ, Graham DA, Powell AJ, Geva T. Reproducibility of MRI measurements of right ventricular size and function in patients with normal and dilated ventricles. *J Magn Reson Imaging.* 2008;28 (1): 67–73.

238. Oosterhof T, van Straten A, Vliegen HW, *et al.* Preoperative thresholds for pulmonary valve replacement in patients with corrected tetralogy of Fallot using cardiovascular magnetic resonance. *Circulation.* 2007;116 (5): 545–551.

239. Meadows J, Powell AJ, Geva T, Dorfman A, Gauvreau K, Rhodes J. Cardiac magnetic resonance imaging correlates of exercise capacity in patients with surgically repaired tetralogy of Fallot. *Am J Cardiol.* 2007;100 (9): 1446–1450.

240. Babu-Narayan SV, Kilner PJ, Li W, *et al.* Ventricular fibrosis suggested by cardiovascular magnetic resonance in adults with repaired tetralogy of fallot and its relationship to adverse markers of clinical outcome. *Circulation.* 2006;113 (3): 405–413.

241. Mohrs OK, Petersen SE, Voigtlaender T, *et al.* Time-resolved contrast-enhanced MR angiography of the thorax in adults with congenital heart disease. *AJR Am J Roentgenol.* 2006;187 (4): 1107–1114.

242. Pettersen E, Helle-Valle T, Edvardsen T, *et al.* Contraction pattern of the systemic right ventricle shift from longitudinal to circumferential shortening and absent global ventricular torsion. *J Am Coll Cardiol.* 2007;49 (25): 2450–2456.

243. Pettersen E, Lindberg H, Smith HJ, *et al.* Left ventricular function in patients with transposition of the great arteries operated with atrial switch. *Pediatr Cardiol.* 2008;29 (3): 597–603.

244. Riehle TJ, Oshinski JN, Brummer ME, *et al.* Velocity-encoded magnetic resonance image assessment of regional aortic flow in coarctation patients. *Ann Thorac Surg.* 2006;81 (3): 1002–1007.

245. Didier D, Saint-Martin C, Lapierre C, *et al.* Coarctation of the aorta: pre and postoperative evaluation with MRI and MR angiography; correlation with echocardiography and surgery. *Int J Cardiovasc Imaging.* 2006;22 (3–4): 457–475.

246. Nielson JC, Powell AJ, Gauvreau K, Marcus EN, Prakash A, Geva T. Magnetic resonance imaging predictors of coarctation severity. *Circulation.* 2005;111 (5): 622–628.

247. Goo HW, Yang DH, Park IS, *et al.* Time-resolved three-dimensional contrast-enhanced magnetic resonance angiography in patients who have undergone a Fontan operation or bidirectional cavopulmonary connection: initial experience. *J Magn Reson Imaging.* 2007;25 (4): 727–736.

248. Fratz S, Hess J, Schwaiger M, Martinoff S, Stern HC. More accurate quantification of pulmonary blood flow by magnetic resonance imaging than by lung perfusion scintigraphy in patients with fontan circulation. *Circulation.* 2002;106 (12): 1510–1513.

249. Whitehead KK, Pekkan K, Kitajima HD, Paridon SM, Yoganathan AP, Fogel MA. Nonlinear power loss during exercise in single-ventricle patients after the Fontan: insights from computational fluid dynamics. *Circulation.* 2007;116 (Suppl. 11): I165–I171.

250. Gelfand EV, Hughes S, Hauser TH, *et al.* Severity of mitral and aortic regurgitation as assessed by cardiovascular magnetic resonance: optimizing correlation with Doppler echocardiography. *J Cardiovasc Magn Reson.* 2006;8:503–507.

251. Gabriel RS, Kerr AJ, Raffel OC, Stewart RA, Cowan BR, Occleshaw CJ. Mapping of mitral regurgitant defects by cardiovascular magnetic resonance in moderate or severe mitral regurgitation secondary to mitral valve prolapse. *J Cardiovasc Magn Reson.* 2008;10 (1): 16.

252. D'Ancona G, Biondo D, Mamone G, *et al.* Ischemic mitral valve regurgitation in patients with depressed ventricular function: cardiac geometrical and myocardial perfusion evaluation with magnetic resonance imaging. *Eur J Cardiothorac Surg.* 2008;34:964–968.

253. Debl K, Djavidani B, Buchner S, *et al.* Assessment of the anatomic regurgitant orifice in aortic regurgitation: a clinical magnetic resonance imaging study. *Heart.* 2008;94 (3): e8.

254. Yap SC, van Geuns RJ, Meijboom FJ, *et al.* A simplified continuity equation approach to the quantification of stenotic bicuspid aortic valves using velocity-encoded cardiovascular magnetic resonance. *J Cardiovasc Magn Reson.* 2007;9 (6): 899–906.

255. Tanaka K, Makaryus AN, Wolff SD. Correlation of aortic valve area obtained by the velocity-encoded phase contrast continuity method to direct planimetry using cardiovascular magnetic resonance. *J Cardiovasc Magn Reson.* 2007;9 (5): 799–805.

256. Burgstahler C, Kunze M, Löffler C, Gawaz MP, Hombach V, Merkle N. Assessment of left ventricular outflow tract geometry in non-stenotic and stenotic aortic valves by cardiovascular magnetic resonance. *J Cardiovasc Magn Reson.* 2006;8 (6): 825–829.

257. Smith SC, Jr, Dove JT, Jacobs AK, *et al.* ACC/AHA guidelines for percutaneous coronary intervention—executive summary: a report of the American college of cardiology/American heart association task force on practice guidelines (committee to revise the 1993 guidelines for percutaneous transluminal angioplasty) endorsed by the society for cardiac angiography and interventions. *Circulation.* 2001;103:3019–3041.

258. Isjkander S, Iskandrian AE. Risk assessment using single-photon emission computed tomographic technetium-99 m sestamibi imaging. *J Am Coll Cardiol.* 1998;32:57–62.

259. Ladenheim ML, Pollock BH, Rozanski A, *et al.* Extent and severity of myocardial hypoperfusion as predictors of prognosis in patients with suspected coronary artery disease. *J Am Coll Cardiol.* 1986;7:464–471.

260. Hendel RC, Berman DS, Cullom SJ, *et al.* Multicenter clinical trial to evaluate the efficacy of correction for photon attenuation and scatter in SPECT myocardial perfusion imaging. *Circulation.* 1999;99:2742–2749.

261. Taillefer R, De Duey EG, Udelson JE, *et al.* Comparative diagnostic accuracy of Tl-201 and Tc-99 m sestamibi SPECT imaging (perfusion and ECG-gated SPECT) in detecting coronary artery disease in women. *J Am Coll Cardiol.* 1997;29:69–77.

262. Gould KL, Kirkeeide RL, Buchi M. Coronary flow reserve as a physiological measure of stenosis severity. *J AM Coll Cardiol.* 1990;15:459–474.

263. Ellis S, Alderman EL, Cain K, *et al.* Morphology of left anterior descending coronary territory lesions favoring acute occlusion and myocardial infarction: a quantitative angiographic study. *J Am Coll Cardiol.* 1989;13:1481–1491.

264. Ellis S, Alderman EL, Cain K, *et al.* Prediction of risk of anterior myocardial infarction by lesion severity and measurement method of stenoses in the left anterior descending coronary distribution: a CASS registry study. *J Am Coll Cardiol.* 1988;11:908–916.

265. Kim RJ, Feino DS, Parish TB, *et al.* Relationship of MRI delayed contrast enhancement to irreversible injury, infarct age, and contractile function. *Circulation.* 1999;100:1992–2002.

266. Werns SW, Walton JA, Hsia HH, *et al.* Evidence of endothelial dysfunction in angiographically normal coronary arteries of patients with coronary artery disease. *Circulation.* 1989;79:287–291.

267. Uren NG, Melin JA, De Bruyne B, *et al.* Relation between myocardial blood flow and the severity of coronary artery stenosis. *N Engl J Med.* 1994;330:1782–1788.

268. Sambuceti G, Parodi O, Marcassa C, *et al.* Alterations in regulation of myocardial blood flow in one-vessel coronary artery disease determined by positron emission tomography. *Am J Cardiol.* 1993;72:538–543.

269. Di Carli M, Czernin J, Hoh CK, *et al.* Relation among stenosis severity, myocardial blood flow, and flow reserve in patients with coronary disease. *Circulation.* 1995;91:1944–1951.

270. Noeske R, Seifert F, Rhein KH, *et al.* Human cardiac imaging at 3 Tesla using phased array coils. *Magn Reson Med.* 2000;44:978–982.

271. Schwitter J, Nanz D, Kneifel S, *et al.* Assessment of myocardial perfusion in coronary artery disease by magnetic resonance: a comparison with positron emission tomography and coronary angiography. *Circulation.* 2001;103:2230–2235.

272. Walsh EG, Doyle M, Lawson MA, *et al.* Multislice first-pass myocardial perfusion imaging on a conventional clinical scanner. *Magn Reson Med.* 1995;34:39–47.

273. Hartnell G, Cerel A, Kamalesh M, *et al.* Detection of myocardial ischemia: value of combined myocardial perfusion and cine-angiographic MR imaging. *Am J Roentgenol.* 1994;163:1061–1067.

274. Saeed M, Wendland MF, Sakuma H, *et al.* Coronary artery stenosis: detection with contrast enhanced MR imaging in dogs. *Radiology.* 1995;196:79–84.

275. Schwitter J, Saeed M, Wendland MF, *et al.* Assessment of myocardial function and perfusion in a canine model of non-occlusive coronary artery stenosis using fast magnetic resonance imaging. *J Magn Reson Imaging.* 1998;9:101–110.

276. Keijer JT, van Rossum AC, van Eenige MJ, *et al.* Magnetic resonance imaging of regional myocardial perfusion in patients with single vessel coronary disease: quantitative comparison with 201 thallium-SPECT and coronary angiography. *Am Heart J.* 1995;130:93–901.

277. Panting JR, Gatehouse PD, Yang GZ, *et al.* Abnormal subendocardial perfusion in cardiac syndrome X detected by cardiovascular magnetic resonance imaging. *N Engl J Med.* 2002;346:1948–1953.

278. Eichenberger AC, Schuiki E, Kochli VD, *et al.* Ischemic heart disease: assessment with gadolinium enhanced ultrafast MR imaging and dipyridamole stress. *J Magn Reson Imaging.* 1994;4:425–431.

279. Bertschinger KM, Nanz D, Buechi M, *et al.* Magnetic resonance myocardial first-pass perfusion imaging: parameter optimization for signal response and cardiac coverage. *J Magn Reson Imaging.* 2001;14:556–562.

280. Wilke N, Simm C, Zhang J, *et al.* Contrast enhanced first-pass myocardial perfusion imaging: correlation between myocardial blood flow in dogs at rest and during hyperemia. *Magn Reson Med.* 1993;29:485–497.

281. Lombardi M, Jones RA, Westby J, *et al.* Use of the mean transit time of an intravascular contrast agent as an exchange-insensitive index of myocardial perfusion. *J Magn Reson Imaging.* 1999;9:402–408.

282. Klocke FJ, Simonetti OP, Judd RM, *et al.* Limits of detection of regional differences in vasodilated flow in viable myocardium by first-pass magnetic resonance perfusion imaging. *Circulation.* 2001;104:2412–2416.

283. Holland AE, Goldfarb JW, Edelman RR. Diaphragmatic and cardiac motion during suspended breathing: preliminary experience and implications for breath-hold MR imaging. *Radiology.* 1998;209:483–489.

284. McConnell MV, Khasgiwala VC, Savord BJ, *et al.* Prospective adaptive navigator correction for breath-hold MR coronary angiography. *Magn Reson Med.* 1997;37:148–152.

285. Chuang ML, Chen MH, Khasgiwala VC, *et al.* Adaptive correction of imaging plane position in segmented k-space cine cardiac MRI. *J Magn Reson Imaging.* 1997;7:811–814.

286. Di Bella EVR, Parker DL, Sinusas AJ. On the dark rim artifact in dynamic contrast-enhanced MRI myocardial perfusion studies. *Magn Reson Med.* 2005;54:1295–1299.

287. Manning WJ, Atkinson DJ, Grossman W, *et al.* First-pass nuclear magnetic resonance imaging studies using gadolinium-DTPA in patients with coronary artery disease. *J Am Coll Cardiol.* 1991;18:959–965.

288. Matheijssen NA, Louwerenburg HW, van Rugge F, *et al.* Comparison of ultrafast dipyridamole magnetic resonance imaging with dipyridamole sestamibi SPECT for detection of perfusion abnormalities in patients with one-vessel disease: assessment by quantitative model fitting. *Magn Reson Med.* 1996;35:221–228.

289. Larsson HB, Fritz Hansen T, Rostrup E, *et al.* Myocardial perfusion modeling using MRI. *Magn Reson Med.* 1996;35:716–726.

290. Muhling OM, Dickson ME, Zenovich A, *et al.* Quantitative magnetic resonance first-pass perfusion analysis: inter and intra-observer agreement. *J Cardiovasc Magn Reson.* 2001;3:247–256.

291. Wilke N, Jerosch HM, Wang Y, *et al.* Myocardial perfusion reserve: assessment with multisection, quantitative, first-pass MR imaging. *Radiology.* 1997;204:373–384.

292. Slavin GS, Wolff SD, Gupta SN, *et al.* First-pass myocardial perfusion MR imaging with interleaved notched saturation: feasibility study. *Radiology.* 2001;219:258–263.

293. Sakuma H, O'Sullivan M, Lucas J, *et al.* Effect of magnetic susceptibility contrast medium on myocardial signal intensity with fast gradient-recalled echo and spin-echo MR imaging: Initial experience in humans. *Radiology.* 1994;190:161–166.

294. Panting JR, Taylor AM, Gatehouse PD, *et al.* First-pass myocardial perfusion imaging and equilibrium signal changes using the intravascular contrast

agent NC 100150 injection. *J Magn Reson Imaging.* 1999;10:404–410.

295. Ding S, Wolff SD, Epstein FH. Improved coverage in dynamic contrast enhanced cardiac MRI using interleaved gradient-echo EPI. *Magn Reson Med.* 1998;39:514–519.

296. Cullen JH, Horsfield MA, Reek CR, *et al.* A myocardial perfusion reserve index in humans using first-pass contrast enhanced magnetic resonance imaging. *J Am Coll Cardiol.* 1999;33:1386–1394.

297. Weiger M, Pruessmann KP, Boesiger P. Cardiac real time imaging using SENSE. Sensitivity encoding scheme. *Magn Reson Med.* 2000;43:177–184.

298. Cheng ASH, Pegg TJ, Karamitsos TD, *et al.* Cardiovascular magnetic resonance perfusion imaging at 3-Tesla for detection of coronary artery disease. A comparison with 1.5-Tesla. *J Am Coll Cardiol.* 2007;49:2440–2449.

299. Kellman P, Arai A. Imaging sequences for first pass perfusion-A review. *J Cardiovasc Magn Reson.* 2007;9:525–537.

300. Shin T, Hu HH, Valencerina SS, Pohost GM, Nayak KS. 3D first pass myocardial perfusion imaging at 3T: towards complete left ventricular coverage. *Proc Intl Soc Mag Reson Med.* 2008;16.

301. Dharmakumar R, Mangalathu J, Ing Dipl, *et al.* Assessment of regional myocardial oxygenation changes in the presence of coronary artery stenosis with balanced SSFP imaging at 3.0 T: theory and experimental evaluation in canines. *J Magn Reson Imaging.* 2008;27:1037–1045.

302. Poncelet BP, Koelling TM, Schmidt CJ, *et al.* Measurement of human myocardial perfusion by double-gated flow alternating inversion recovery EPI. *Magn Reson Med.* 1999;41:510–519.

303. Zun Z, Wong EC, Nayak KS. Arterial spin labeled myocardium perfusion imaging with background supprresion. *Magn Reson Med.* 2009;62:975–983.

304. Gheorghiade M, Bonow RO. Chronic heart failure in the United States: a manifestation of coronary artery disease. *Circulation.* 1998;97:282–289.

305. Hammermeister KE, DeRouen TA, Dodge HT. Variables predictive of survival in patients with coronary artery disease. Selection by univariate and multivariate analyses from the clinical, electrocardiographic, exercise, arteriographic, and quantitative angiographic evaluations. *Circulation.* 1979;59:421–430.

306. Harris PJ, Harell FE, Lee KL, *et al.* Survival in medically treated coronary artery disease. *Circulation.* 1979;60:1259–1269.

307. Mock MB, Ringqvist I, Fisher LD, *et al.* Survival of medically treated patients in the coronary artery surgery study (CASS) registry. *Circulation.* 1982;66:562–568.

308. Rees G, Bristow JD, Kremkau EL, *et al.* Influence of aortocoronary bypass surgery on left ventricular performance. *N Engl J Med.* 1971;284:1116–1120.

309. Chatterjee K, Swan HJ, Parmley WW, *et al.* Influence of direct myocardial revascularization on left ventricular asynergy and function in patients with coronary heart disease: with and without previous myocardial infarction. *Circulation.* 1973;47:276–286.

310. Horn HR, Teichholz LE, Cohn PF, *et al.* Augmentation of left ventricular contraction pattern in coronary artery disease by an inotropic catecholamine: the epinephrine ventriculogram. *Circulation.* 1974;49:1063–1071.

311. Cohn PF, Gorlin R, Herman MV, *et al.* Relation between contractile reserve and prognosis in patients with coronary artery disease and a depressed ejection fraction. *Circulation.* 1975;51:414–420.

312. Diamond GA, Forrester JS, de Luz PL, *et al.* Postextrasystolic potentiation of ischemic myocardium by atrial stimulation. *Am Heart J.* 1978;95:204–209.

313. Rahimtoola SH. The hibernating myocardium. *Am Heart J.* 1989;117:211–221.

314. Heyndrickx GR, Millard RW, McRitchie RJ, *et al.* Regional myocardial functional and electrophysiological alterations after brief coronary artery occlusion in conscious dogs. *J Clin Invest.* 1975;56:978–985.

315. Braunwald E, Kloner RA. The stunned myocardium: prolonged, postischemic ventricular dysfunction. *Circulation.* 1982;66:1146–1149.

316. Kloner RA, Bolli R, Marban E, *et al.* Medical and cellular implications of stunning, hibernation and preconditioning: an NHLBI workshop. *Circulation.* 1998;97:1848–1867.

317. Bolli R. Mechanism of myocardial stunning. *Physiol Rev.* 1999;79:609–634.

318. Kusuoka H, Marban E. Cellular mechanisms of myocardial stunning. *Annu Rev Physiol.* 1992;54:243–256.

319. Anselmi M, Golia G, Cicoira M, *et al.* Prognostic value of detection of myocardial viability using low dose dobutamine echocardiography in infarcted patients. *Am J Cardiol.* 1998;81:21G–28G.

320. Picano E, Sicari R, Landi P, *et al.* Prognostic value of myocardial viability in medically treated patients with global left ventricular dysfunction early after an uncomplicated myocardial infarction: a dobutamine stress echocardiography study. *Circulation.* 1998;98:1078–1084.

321. Previtali M, Fetiveau R, Lanzarini L, *et al.* Prognostic value of myocardial viability and ischemia detected by dobutamine stress echocardiography early after myocardial infarction treated with thrombolysis. *J Am Coll Cardiol.* 1998;32:380–386.

322. Allman KC, Shaw LJ, Hachamovitch R, *et al.* Myocardial viability testing and impact of revascularization on prognosis in patients with coronary artery disease and left ventricular dysfunction: a meta-analysis. *J Am Coll Cardiol.* 2002;39:1151–1158.

323. Schwarz ER, Schaper J, von Dahl J, *et al.* Myocyte degeneration and cell death in hibernating human myocardium. *J Am Coll Cardiol.* 1996;27:1577–1585.

324. Nagel E, Lehmkuhl HB, Bocksch W, *et al.* Non-invasive diagnosis of ischemia-induced wall motion abnormalities with the use of high dose dobutamine stress MRI: comparison with dobutamine stress echocardiography. *Circulation.* 1999;99:763–770.

325. Hoffman R, Lethen H, Marwick T, *et al.* Analysis of interinstitutional observer agreement in interpretation of dobutamine stress echocardiograms. *J Am Coll Cardiol.* 1996;27:330–336.

326. Dubnow MH, Burchell HB, Titus JL. Postinfarction ventricular aneurysm. A clinicomorphologic and electrocardiographic study of 80 cases. *Am Heart J.* 1965;70:753–760.

327. Baer FM, Smolarz K, Jungehulsing M, *et al.* Chronic myocardial infarction: assessment of morphology, function, and perfusion by gradient echo magnetic resonance imaging and 99 m Tc-methoxy-isobutyl-isonitrile SPECT. *Am heart J.* 1992;123:636–645.

328. Baer FM, Voth E, Schneider CA, *et al.* Comparison of low-dose dobutamine-gradient-echo magnetic resonance imaging and positron emission tomography with [^{18}F] fluorodeoxyglucose in patients with chronic coronary artery disease. A functional and morphological approach to the detection of residual myocardial viability. *Circulation.* 1995;91:1006–1015.

329. Dendale P, Franken PR, Waldman GJ, *et al.* Low dosage dobutamine magnetic resonance imaging as an alternative to echocardiography in the detection of viable myocardium after acute infarction. *Am Heart J.* 1995;130:134–140.

330. Sandstede JJ, Bertsch G, Beer M. Detection of myocardial viability by low dose dobutamine cine MR imaging. *Magn Reson Imaging* 1999;17:1437–1443.

331. Dendale P, Franken PR, Block P, *et al.* Contrast enhanced and functional magnetic resonance imaging for the detection of viable myocardium after infarction. *Am Heart J.* 1998;135:875–880.

332. Baer FM, Voth E, La Rosee K, *et al.* Comparison of low dose dobutamine transesophageal echocardiography and dobutamine magnetic resonance imaging for detection of residual myocardial viability. *Am J Cardiol.* 1996;78:415–419.

333. Zoghbi WA, Barasch E. Dobutamine MRI: a serious contender in pharmacological stress imaging? *Circulation.* 1999;99:730–732.

334. Beller GA. Comparison of ^{201}Tl scintigraphy and low dose dobutamine echocardiography for the noninvasive assessment of myocardial viability. *Circulation.* 1996;94:2681–2684.

335. Bonow RO. Identification of viable myocardium. *Circulation.* 1996;94:2674–2680.

336. Perone-Filardi P, Pace L, Prastaro M, *et al.* Assessment of myocardial viability in patients with chronic coronary artery disease. Rest-4-hour-24-hour 201 T$_l$ tomography versus dobutamine echocardiography. *Circulation.* 1996;94:2712–2719.

337. Ausma J, Schaart G, Thone F, *et al.* Chronic ischemic viable myocardium in man: aspects of dedifferentiation. *Cardiovasc Pathol.* 1995;4:29–37.

338. De Roos A, Doornbos J, Van Der Wall E, *et al.* MR imaging of acute myocardial infarction: value of Gd-DTPA. *Am J Roentgenol.* 1998;150:531–534.

339. De Roos A, van Rossum AC, Van Der Wall E, *et al.* Reperfused and non-reperfused myocardial infarction: diagnostic potential of Gd-DTPA enhanced MR imaging. *Radiology.* 1989;172:717–720.

340. Yokota C, Nonogi H, Miyazaki S, *et al.* Gadolinium enhanced magnetic resonance imaging in acute myocardial infarction. *Am J Cardiol.* 1995;75:577–581.

341. Edelman RR, Wallner B, Singer A, *et al.* Segmented turbo-FLASH: method for breath-hold MR imaging of the liver with flexible contrast. *Radiology.* 1990;177:515–521.

342. Simonetti OP, Kim RJ, Fieno DS, *et al.* An improved MR imaging technique for the visualization of myocardial infarction. *Radiology.* 2001;218:215–223.

343. Eichstaedt HW, Felix R, Danne O, *et al.* Imaging of acute myocardial infarction by magnetic resonance tomography (MRT) using the paramagnetic relaxation substance gadolinium-DTPA. *Cardiovasc Drugs Ther.* 1989;3:779–788.

344. Lima JA, Judd RM, Bazille A, *et al.* Regional heterogeneity of human myocardial infarcts demonstrated by contrast enhanced MRI. Potential mechanisms. *Circulation.* 1995;92:1117–1125.

345. Van Rossum AC, Visser FC, van Eenige MJ, *et al.* Value of gadolinium-diethylene-triamine pentaacetic acid dynamics in magnetic resonance imaging of acute myocardial infarction with occluded and reperfused coronary arteries after thrombolysis. *Am J Cardiol.* 1990;65:845–851.

346. Wu E, Judd RM, Vargas JD, *et al.* Visualization of presence, location, and transmural extent of healed Q-wave and non-Q wave myocardial infarction. *Lancet.* 2001;357:21–28.

347. Schinkel AFL, Poldermans D, Vanoverschelde JLJ, *et al.* Incidence of recovery of contractile function following

revascularization in patients with ischemic left ventricular dysfunction. *Am J Cardiol.* 2004;93:14–17.

348. Al-Mohammed A, Mahy IR, Norton MY, *et al.* Prevalence of hibernating myocardium in patients with severely impaired ischemic left ventricles. *Heart.* 1998;80:559–564.

349. Auerbach MA, Schoder H, Gambhir SS, *et al.* Prevalence of myocardial viability as detected by positron emission tomography in patients with ischemic cardiomyopathy. *Circulation.* 1999;99:2921–2926.

350. Schinkel AFL, Bax JJ, Sozzi FB, *et al.* prevalence of myocardial viability assesses by single photon emission computed tomography in patients with chronic ischemic left ventricular dysfunction. *Heart.* 2002;88:125–130.

351. Cleland JG, Pennell DJ, Ray SG, *et al.* Myocardial viability as a determinant of the ejection fraction response to carvedilol in patients with heart failure (CHRISTMAS trial): randomized controlled trail. *Lancet.* 2003;362:14–21.

352. Bax JJ, Poldermans D, Elhendy A, Boersma E, Rahimtoola SH. Sensitivity, specificity and predictive accuracies of various non invasive techniques for detecting hibernating myocardium. *Curr Probl Cardiol.* 2001;26:142–186.

353. Bax JJ, Visser FC, Poldermans D, *et al.* Relationship between preoperative viability and postoperative improvement in LVEF and heart failure symptoms. *J Nucl Med.* 2001;42:79–86.

354. Dicarli MF, Asgarzadie F, Schelbert HR, *et al.* Quantitative relation between myocardial viability and improvement in heart failure symptoms after revascularization in patients with ischemic cardiomyopathy. *Circulation.* 1995;92:3436–3444.

355. Marwick TH, Zuchowski C, Lauer MS, Secknus MA, Williams MJ, Lytle BW. Functional status and quality of life in patients with heart failure undergoing coronary artery bypass surgery after assessment of myocardial viability. *J Am Coll Cardiol.* 1999;33:750–758.

356. Mule J, Bax JJ, Zingone B, *et al.* The beneficial effect of revascularization on jeopardized myocardium:reverse remodeling and improved long-term prognosis. *Eur J Cardiothorac Surg.* 2002;22:426–430.

357. Rohatgi R, Epstein S, Henriquez J, *et al.* Utility of positron emission tomography in predicting cardiac events and survival in patients with coronary artery disease and severe left ventricular dysfunction. *Am J cardiol.* 2001;87:1096–1099.

358. Kaandorp TA, Lamb HJ, Van Der Wall EE, de Roos A, Bax JJ. Cardiovascular MR to assess myocardial viability in chronic ischemic LV dysfunction. *Heart.* 2005;91:1359–1365.

359. Bove CM, DiMaria JM, Voros S, Conaway MR, Kramer CM. Dobutamine response and myocardial infarct transmurality: functional improvement after coronary bypass grafting-initial experience. *Radiology.* 2006;240:835–841.

360. Schvartzman PR, Srichai MB, Grimm RA, *et al.* Nonstress delayed—enhancement magnetic resonance imaging of the myocardium predicts improvement of function after revascularization for chronic ischemic heart disease with left ventricular dysfunction. *Am Heart J.* 2003;146:535–541.

361. Selvanayagam JB, Jerosch-Herold M, Porto I, *et al.* Resting myocardial blood flow is impaired in hibernating myocardium: a magnetic resonance study of quantitative perfusion assessment. *Circulation.* 2005;112:3289–3296.

362. Carmichael BB, Setser RM, Stillman AE, *et al.* Effects of surgical ventricular restoration on left ventricular function: dynamic MR imaging. *Radiology.* 2006;241:710–717.

363. Jennings RB, Schaper J, Hill ML, *et al.* Effect of reperfusion late in the phase of reversible ischemic injury. Changes in cell volume, electrolytes, metabolites and ultrastructure. *Circ Res.* 1985;56:262–278.

364. Whalen DA, Hamilton DG, Ganote CE, *et al.* Effect of a transient period of ischemia on myocardial cells. I. effects on cell volume regulation. *Am J Pathol.* 1974;74:381–397.

365. Koenig SH, Spiller M, Brown RD, 3rd, *et al.* Relaxation of water protons in the intra and extracellular regions of blood containing Gd (DTPA). *Magn Reson Med.* 1986;3:791–795.

366. Rochitte CE, Lima JA, Bluemke DA, *et al.* Magnitude and time course of microvascular obstruction and tissue injury after acute myocardial infarction. *Circulation.* 1998;98:1000–1114.

367. Judd RM, Lugo-Olivieri CH, Arai M, *et al.* Physiological basis of myocardial contrast enhancement in fast magnetic resonance images of two-day-old reperfused canine infarcts. *Circulation.* 1995;92:1902–1910.

368. Hillenbrand HB, Kim RJ, Parker MA, *et al.* Early assessment of myocardial salvage by contrast enhanced magnetic resonance imaging. *Circulation.* 2000;102:1678–1683.

369. Lieberman AN, Weiss JL, Jugdutt BI, *et al.* Twodimensional echocardiogarphy and infarct size: relationship of regional wall motion and thickening to the extent of myocardial infarction in the dog. *Circulation.* 1981;63:739–746.

370. Force T, Kemper A, Perkins L, *et al.* Overestimation of infarct size by quantitative two-dimensional echocardiography: the role of tethering and of analytic procedures. *Circulation.* 1986;73:1360–1368.

371. Armstrong WF. "Hibernating" myocardium: asleep or part dead? *J Am Coll Cardiol*. 1996;28:530–535.

372. Weiss JL, Bulkley BH, Hutchins GM, *et al*. Twodimensional echocardiographic recognition of myocardial injury in man: comparison with postmortem studies. *Circulation*. 1981;63:401–408.

373. Mahrholdt H, Wagner A, Choi K, *et al*. Contrast MRI detects subendocardial infarcts in regions of normal wall motion. *Circulation*. 2001;104 (Suppl. 2): 341.

374. Kuikka J, Yang J, Kilainen H. Physical performance of Siemens E.Cam gamma camera. *Nucl Med Commun*. 1998;19:457–462.

375. Garvin AA, James J, Garcia EV. Myocardial perfusion imaging using single-photon emission computed tomography. *Am J Card Imaging*. 1994;8:189–198.

376. Kannel WB, Abbott RD. Incidence and prognosis of unrecognized myocardial infarction. An update on the Framingham study. *N Engl J Med*. 1984;311:1144–1147.

377. Sigurdsson E, Thorgeirsson G, Sigvaldason H, *et al*. Unrecognized myocardial infarction: epidemiology, clinical characteristics, and the prognostic role of angina pectoris. The Reykjavik study. *Ann Intern Med*. 1995;122:96–102.

378. Nadelmann J, Frishman WH, Ooi WL. Prevalence, incidence and prognosis of recognized and unrecognized myocardial infarction in persons aged 75 years or older: the Bronx aging study. *Am J Cardiol*. 1990;66:533–537.

379. Kim H, Wu E, Meyers SN, *et al*. Prognostic significance of unrecognized myocardial infarction detected by contrast enhanced MRI. *Circulation*. 2002;106:11–38.

380. Neubauer S, Horn M, Cramer M, *et al*. Myocardial phosphocreaine-to-ATP ratio is a predictor of mortality in patients with dilated cardiomyopathy. *Circulation*. 1997;96:2190–2196.

381. Neubauer S, Krahe T, Schindler R, *et al*. 31P magnetic resonance spectroscopy in dilated cardiomyopathy and coronary artery disease. Altered cardiac high-energy phosphate metabolism in heart failure. *Circulation*. 1992;86:1810–1818.

382. Walpoth BH, Mueller MF, Celik B, *et al*. Assessment of cardiac rejection by MR-imaging and MR spectroscopy. *Eur J Cardiothorac Surg*. 1998;14:426–430.

383. Jung W-I, Sieverding L, Breuer J, *et al*. 31P NMR spectroscopy detects metabolic abnormalities in asymptomatic patienst with hypertrophic cardiomyopathy. *Circulation*. 1998;97:2538–2542.

384. Weiss RG, Bottomley PA, Hardy CJ, *et al*. Regional myocardial metabolism of high energy phosphates during isometric exercise in patients with coronary artery disease. *N Engl J Med*. 1990;323:1593–1600.

385. Buchthal SD, den Hollander JA, Merz CN, *et al*. Abnormal myocardial phosphorus-31 nuclear magnetic resonance spectroscopy in women with chest pain but normal coronary angiograms. *N Engl J Med*. 2000;23:829–835.

386. Johnson BD, Shaw CJ, Buchthal SD, *et al*. Prognosis in women with myocardial ischema in the absence of obstructive coronary disease: results from the National institute of health-national heart, lung, blood institute—sponsored women's ischemia syndrome evaluation (WISE). *Circulation*. 2004;109:2993–2999.

387. Crilley JG, Boehm EA, Rajagopalan B, *et al*. Magnetic resonance spectroscopy evidence of abnormal cardiac energetics in Xp21 muscular dystrophy. *J Am Col Cardiol*. 2000;36:1953–1958.

388. Van Der Meer RW, Doornbos J, Kozerke S, *et al*. Metabolic imaging of myocardial triglyceride content: reproducibility of 1 H Mr soectroscopy with respiratory navigator gating in volunteers. *Radiology*. 2007;245:251–257.

CHAPTER 9

MSCT Coronary Imaging

Koen Nieman

Erasmus Medical Center, Rotterdam, The Netherlands

Introduction

Over the recent years we have witnessed rapid technical advancement of multislice, or multidetector-row spiral computed tomography (MSCT), with current technology capable of practically motion-free imaging of the heart, allowing detailed visualization of the coronary arteries. With technical innovation ongoing, the role of cardiac computed tomography (CT) in cardiovascular medicine is being developed.

Data Acquisition and Evaluation

Multislice Spiral CT

The fundamental difference between spiral CT and previously used conventional CT is the absence of a physical connection between the rotating and stationary scanner elements. So-called slip-ring technology allows transfer of energy and data between the rotating tube-detector and the stationary unit without cables that necessitate unwinding after a few scanner rotations. Continuous rotation allows continuous data acquisition, which was crucial for the development of cardiac CT. While conventional, sequential CT scanners apply a step-and-shoot approach, spiral CT allows continuous table advancement and data acquisition. From the table's perspective the path of the rotating elements has the shape of a helix or spiral, hence the name spiral or helical CT. By expanding the number of detector rows coverage speed could be improved significantly. While a 4-slice cardiac CT scan

required up to 40 seconds, current 64-slice CT acquisitions can be completed in less than 10 seconds, a much more comfortable breath-hold duration.

ECG-Synchronization

The width of the combined detector rows is insufficient to cover the heart at once. Although this is likely to change in the near future, current scanners require several scanner rotations during several heart cycles to scan the entire heart (Figure 9.1). In order to create a comprehensible CT angiogram the acquisition or reconstruction of images needs to be synchronized to the heart cycle. During the spiral CT scan the electrocardiogram (ECG) trace is recorded, based on which data acquired during corresponding phases of consecutive heart cycles is gathered to reconstruct iso-cardiophasic images. By scanning each (table) position for the time of at least one heart cycle (by consecutive detectors) the CT angiogram can be reconstructed at any time point within the cardiac cycle. This requires a table advancement that is much slower compared to nongated applications.

Temporal Resolution

More important than the duration of the total scan is the time needed to acquire (data for) a single image. The temporal resolution, comparable to the shutter time of a camera, needs to be as short as possible to avoid motion blurring of the images. The fundamental temporal resolution of CT is determined by the rotation speed, the image reconstruction algorithm, and the number of tube-detector units on the scanner. Standard partial scan reconstruction algorithms require approximately half of a rotation of projection data to create an

Cardiac CT, PET and MR, 2nd edition. Edited by Vasken Dilsizian and Gerry Pohost. © 2010 Blackwell Publishing Ltd.

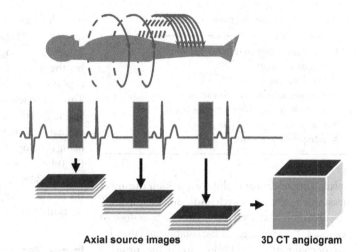

Axial source images   **3D CT angiogram**

Figure 9.1 ECG-gated image reconstruction. Overlapping data is acquired during a spiral CT scan. Using the recorded ECG, images are reconstructed from phase-consistent data acquired during each consecutive heart cycle. Together the reconstructed images from several heart cycles become a complete 3D data set of the heart during a single phase of contraction.

image, so the temporal resolution is about half of the rotation time of the scanner. Alternatively, so-called multisegmental reconstruction algorithms combine scan data from consecutive heart cycles to reconstruct images. Theoretically, the temporal resolution would be a fraction of the number of cycles combined (generally between two and four). In reality the effective temporal resolution is shortened to a lesser magnitude, depending on the heart rate in relation to the scanner rotation time. Another limitation of multisegmental reconstruction algorithms is the requirement that each table position is to be scanned during at least two or more heart cycles. For this reason these they are generally only applied in case of a fast heart rate. In slower heart rates the table speed would need to be decreased, which would result in longer scan times and higher radiation exposure. Depending on the rotation speed currently available single-source CT scanners offer a temporal resolution between 165 and 200 ms, with a variable improvement at fast heart rates using multisegmental reconstruction algorithms. To improve the relative temporal resolution modification of the heart rate by beta-blockers is common practice, and essential in patients with a faster heart rate. Dual-source CT scanners are equipped with two tube-detector units mounted at an angular offset of 90°. Instead of a 180° rotation dual-source can acquire the same number of projections from a 90° rotation, which improved the temporal resolution by a factor of two (83 ms) independent of the heart rate. In the vast majority of patients current CT technology allows virtually motion-free

imaging of the coronary arteries during phases of the heart cycle where the displacement of the heart is small, i.e., the mid-diastolic phase just before atrial contraction and/or the end-systolic phase.

Acquisition Protocol

CT angiography requires intravenous injection of an iodine contrast medium to differentiate the blood from the surrounding tissues. A small test bolus can be injected to determine the time interval between injection and contrast enhancement. Alternatively bolus tracking can be applied, in which case the entire contrast bolus is injected and the scan is automatically initiated as soon as contrast medium is detected in the aortic root. The patient moves in a supine position through the scanner gantry during continuous data acquisition and ECG recording. The total scan time is approximately 10 seconds depending on the number of detector rows on the scanner, the width of the individual detectors and the selected table speed. In patients with a faster heart rate some scanners allow a faster table advancement speed to shorten the scan and reduce radiation exposure. During the scan the patient needs to hold his breath and remain motionless to avoid gross displacement of the heart.

Radiation Exposure

CT cannot be performed without exposing the patient to roentgen radiation, which is potential harmful. The radiation dose of a cardiac scan exceeds that of non-ECG-gated CT scans. ECG-gated spiral CT requires multiple sampling to ensure

Table 9.1   Dose-reduction measures.

Tube current reduction (in small patients)
Tube voltage reduction
Tighter scan ranges
Table speed adjusted to the heart rate
ECG-triggered roentgen tube modulation
Prospectively triggered CT angiography
Anatomic tube modulation

availability of data at each table position during at least one entire heart cycle. Additional contributing factors to the relatively high radiation dose of cardiac CT are the need for fast rotation and thin detector collimation, and the location of the coronary arteries deep inside the chest. The actual radiation dose a patient receives during a given examination varies substantially, and is determined by the scanner type, patient characteristics (body size) and the scan protocol. Over the years the radiation dose of cardiac CT has increased with the development of more powerful CT scanners. Without dose saving measures the dose of a 64-slice CT coronary angiogram varies between 8 and 20 mSv [1–4].

Simple measures to reduce the radiation exposure include narrowing of the scan range, lowering of the tube voltage, and lowering of the tube current, particularly in smaller patients (Table 9.1) [1,5]. In patients with a regular heart rhythm ECG-triggered tube modulation is an effective means

to reduce total dose, without sacrificing image quality [1] (Figure 9.2). Recently, sequential CT scanning is being revisited. Prospectively triggered by the ECG, image acquisition (and radiation exposure) is minimized to the phase of interest. This approach significantly reduces patient dose, although effects on image quality need further evaluation. Anatomic tube current modulation is being developed for cardiac imaging, which allows the tube current to decrease based on the overall roentgen absorption of the scanned body section or the rotational angle. Adaptable table speed reduces oversampling in patients with a fast heart rate.

Image Reconstruction

As mentioned before images are reconstructed after acquisition of the data, using the recorded ECG to create a phase-consistent CT angiogram. Several phases can be reconstructed to find the best data set, although for low heart rates good image quality can usually be found in the mid-diastolic phase. Spiral CT allows reconstruction of overlapping images with a variable individual thickness. Depending on the width of the individual detectors the reconstructed slice width is between 0.6 and 0.8 mm. By overlapping reconstruction of slices, which improves the thru-plane image quality, the total number of images in a single CT angiogram is approximately 300. Depending on the size of the reconstructed field of view in the in-plane

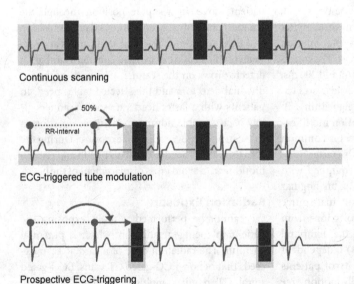

Continuous scanning

ECG-triggered tube modulation

Prospective ECG-triggering

Figure 9.2 ECG-triggered tube modulation. Originally, tube output would be continuous during the data acquisition. Using ECG-triggered tube modulation the roentgen tube output can be alternated during the heart cycle. Based on the previous heart cycles the anticipated phase for reconstruction is predicted, at which time the tube output is elevated to the nominal level. For the remaining of the cycle the tube current is maintained at a very low level. For prospectively ECG-triggered, sequential CT imaging the table is stationary during data acquisition. After each consecutive acquisition the table moves to the next position, which generally requires the time of two heart cycles, during which time no roentgen is emitted.

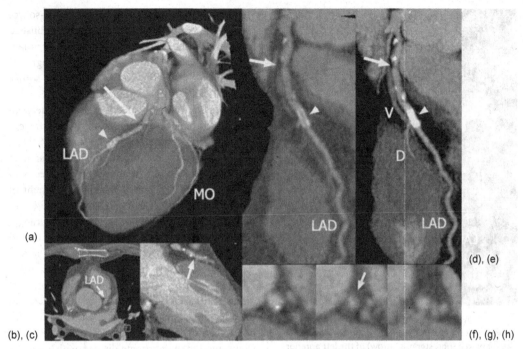

Figure 9.3 Image postprocessing. Use of different postprocessing tools in the same data set, which shows a stent in the left anterior descending coronary artery (LAD), as well as multiple (calcified) lesions in the proximal LAD (d and e). A complete 3D reconstruction of the heart (a) shows a significant lesion in the LAD (arrow) and the high-density stent (arrow head). Only a small section of the LAD can be visualized on a single axial slice (b), while multiplanar reformations can be created to demonstrate a longer section of the vessel (c). Curved multiplanar reformations (d) and maximum intensity projections (e) can be used to show the entire vessel in a single image. Panels (f–h) show cross-sections of the LAD at the proximal reference, the stenosis and the distal reference level, respectively. D, diagonal branch; MO, marginal branch; V, cardiac vein.

resolution will be 0.6 mm × 0.6 mm under optimal conditions.

Image Processing and Analysis

To facilitate the evaluation of the large numbers of CT images postprocessing tools have been developed (Figure 9.3). Cross-sectional images through the CT angiogram can be created in any position or orientation. These multiplanar reformations (MPR) can be flat cross-sectional planes, or they can be created along the (tortuous) course of a vessel to demonstrate the entire course of that vessel in a single image. Thin-slab maximum intensity projections (MIP) are 2D displays of the highest attenuation values, usually contrast medium, calcium or metal, within a given slab. It provides greater overview of the vessel with better contrast between the lumen and the surrounding tissues. Because of the higher attenuation of metal and calcium, MIP is less effective in case of stented or severely calcified vessels. These postprocessing tools can be very helpful in combination with the axial source images, to assess the coronary lumen and detect coronary artery disease. Although not intended for the initial coronary evaluation three-dimensional (3D) volume-rendered images are an attractive means to summarize and communicate findings.

Coronary Lumenography

Detection of Coronary Stenosis

With ongoing technical development the diagnostic performance of CT with respect to the detection and (semi-)quantification of obstructive coronary artery disease is steadily improving (Figures 9.4 and 9.5). Although more advanced CT

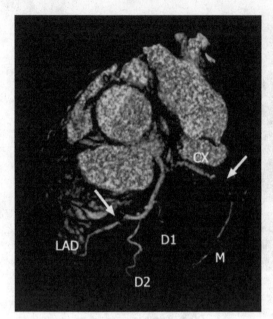

Figure 9.4 Two-vessel disease. A three-dimensional reconstruction of an MSCT coronary angiogram of a patient with a short stenosis (arrow) in the left anterior descending coronary artery (LAD), and a long, more severe lesion (arrow) in the left circumflex coronary artery (CX). Marginal branch (M), first and second marginal branch (D1 and D2).

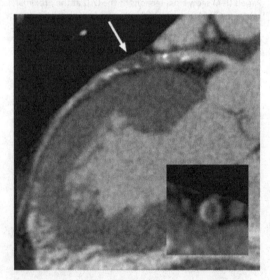

Figure 9.5 Coronary occlusion. CT shows an occluded left anterior descending coronary artery (arrow). Both calcifications as well as material with low roentgen attenuation, presumably thrombus, can be seen. Considering the length of the occlusion, opacification of the distal vessel is likely the result of collateral filling. The insert shows the cross-sectional view of the occluded vessel segment.

technology, 320-slice CT and 128-slice dual-source CT, has become available the latest published literature on the diagnostic accuracy of coronary CT in comparison with conventional angiography concerns 64-slice CT [2–4,6,7] and dual-source (64-slice) CT [8–10]. In studies comparing 64-slice CT with conventional angiography the need to exclude coronary segments due to insufficient image quality ranges between 0 and 12% [11], which is a significant improvement compared to the high exclusion rate of up to 30% reported with earlier 4-slice CT [12–14]. For the assessment of individual coronary segments, the sensitivity to detect significant coronary artery stenosis ranges between 64 and 99%, the specificity between 84 and 98%, with pooled average sensitivity of 87% and specificity of 96%. The positive predictive value is lower: approximately 80%. Calcified coronary disease causes blooming artifacts, which increases the apparent stenosis severity of a lesion. In order not to miss any lesions investigators, as well as clinicians, tend to overestimate disease, which may be another explanation for the high number of false-positive readings in most of the mentioned studies before. The negative predictive value of CT has been consistently high in all studies, with a pooled average of 98%. Because normal segments usually outnumber stenosed ones, the sensitivity to detect individuals with at least one coronary stenosis is better at the expense of the specificity. The negative predictive value remains high at approximately 95%. Single and dual-source CT studies have shown similar performance, with the difference that the dual-source examinations were performed without additional beta-blockers [8–10].

Generally, the confidence and accuracy to assess stenosis is better in larger branches and in the absence of extensive coronary calcification (Figure 9.6). Additionally, obesity decreases the signal to noise and the ability to assess coronary obstruction. An irregular heart rate, in particular atrial fibrillation, causes discontinuity between the consecutive acquisitions and negatively affects interpretation of the images. As discussed previously image quality is better in patients with a low heart rate, for single-source CT preferably below 60–65/minute.

The ability to quantify coronary stenosis severity has been modest in comparison with quantitative (invasive) coronary angiography, particularly

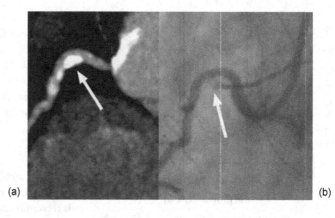

Figure 9.6 Calcified lesion in the proximal RCA. Calcified proximal right coronary artery (arrow) by MSCT (a). The size of the calcified plaque suggests luminal narrowing, which could not be confirmed by conventional coronary angiography (b).

(a)

(b)

in unselected populations [7]. Causes for the quantitative discrepancy between CT and invasive angiography include the limited spatial resolution of CT and the blooming artifacts of calcified lesion, but it is also a consequence of the principle differences between the 2D projection images by catheter angiography and 3D images and vessel area measurements by CT.

Clinical Applications

Due to its high spatial and temporal resolution conventional catheter angiography remains the reference standard for the visualization of the coronary arteries. Catheter angiography involves an invasive procedure with rare but potentially severe risks. This is one of the reasons why stress tests are used in the majority of patients to identify individuals with obstructive coronary artery disease. Noninvasive coronary angiography by CT offers a potential alternative somewhere between ischemia inducing tests and invasive coronary angiography. Over the recent years potential applications of coronary CT have been investigated, and results have lead to the first guidelines and appropriateness criteria on the use of cardiac CT in clinical practice (Table 9.2) [15,16].

CT has a high negative predictive value, which allows reliable exclusion of coronary artery disease. The certainty to exclude significant ischemic heart disease in a patient with no or minimal atherosclerosis on CT scan of sufficient quality is very high. On the other hand the positive predictive value of CT is lower, often a result of limited spatial resolution particularly in the presence of calcified

plaque. CT is an anatomic technique that shows morphologic stenosis but does not inform about the hemodynamic consequences of the lesion. Particularly in case of moderately stenosis the decision to revascularize is based on the presence of objective myocardial ischemia. Analysis of the pre- and post-test probability of a population of 254 patients presenting with chest pain showed that CTA was most useful in patients with a low-to-intermediate probability, particularly to exclude the presence of significant obstruction (Figure 9.7) [17]. The contribution of CTA in patients with a high pretest probability CT is modest, as obstructive or nonobstructive atherosclerosis will often both be present. Functional testing and invasive angiography will be a more sensible approach in the majority of patients with a high-probablity. In patients with a low probability the use of CT is debatable, in

Table 9.2 Appropriate indications for coronary CT angiography.

Chest pain evaluation in patients with an intermediate pretest probability, an uninterpretable ECG and unable to exercise
Chest pain evaluation after an uninterpretable or equivocal stress test
Coronary evaluation in new onset heart failure
Suspected coronary anomalies in symptomatic patients
Acute chest pain evaluation, an intermediate pretest probability, no ECG changes and serial enzymes negative

Uncertain and inappropriate indications not listed.

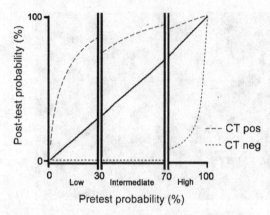

Figure 9.7 Diagnostic value of CT coronary angiography. Pretest and post-test probability of significant coronary artery disease after CT coronary angiography, confirmed by catheter coronary angiography. In the low-to-intermediate pretest probability group CT virtually excludes significant coronary artery disease, while a positive CT scan increases the probability of coronary artery disease to 68 and 88% for low and intermediate pretest probability patients. (Adapted from Meijboom et al. [17].)

part related to the radiation exposure. Therefore coronary CT seems most reasonable in patients with an intermediate-probability of stenosis. Particularly patients at low-intermediate probability with nonconclusive stress test results, in whom an invasive angiography would be necessary to exclude coronary artery disease, CT is a sensible option. At this time, CT angiography is not recommended in the absence of (atypical) symptoms.

While assessment of chest pain will be the most frequent application of cardiac CTA, there are a number of additional emerging applications of this technique. Because of the excellent 3D imaging qualities CT is very effective for demonstration of abnormal coronary (or cardiac) morphology.

A number of studies suggest that CTA could be useful in the emergency department for the assessment of patients with acute chest pain, to rule out an acute coronary syndrome [18,19]. Patients without coronary plaque, or in whom significant coronary obstruction can be excluded, are very unlikely to have myocardial ischemia. CT is not recommended in patients with ECG changes or elevated enzymes, in whom (immediate) coronary catheterization is indicated. Neither is cardiac CT recommended in patients at low risk, in whom suspicion of an acute coronary syndrome is very low.

However, in those patients with at intermediate risk without ECG changes and with negative myocardial biomarkers, CT can be useful to exclude a cardiovascular event. The so-called triple-rule-out of the most life-threatening conditions causing acute chest pain: acute coronary syndrome, pulmonary embolism and aortic dissection, can be done with a single CT scan but has practical disadvantages. Given the fact that clinical investigation will usually direct suspicion toward one (or none) of the conditions mentioned above, dedicated imaging of the most likely responsible vasculature is recommended.

In patients who need to undergo valvular surgery CT angiography can be an alternative to conventional catheter angiography to exclude coronary artery disease. In one study of 70 patients planned for aortic valve and mitral valve surgery CT detected all 18 patients with obstructive coronary artery disease and excluded significant coronary artery disease in 48/52 patients [20].

In patients with new congestive heart failure without history of ischemic heart disease a small number is still caused by unrecognized coronary artery disease. Since coronary artery disease is one of the few treatable causes of congestive heart failure coronary angiography is performed in the majority of the patients. However, in (younger) patients with lower probability of atherosclerotic disease CT can offer an alternative to exclude an ischemic cause in heart failure.

Rather than a substitute for diagnostic angiography, CT angiography can provide valuable, additional information in patients undergoing complex percutaneous coronary intervention, including chronic total occlusion, bifurcation lesions, and ostial disease.

Contrary to established functional test such as nuclear imaging there is few data on the prognostic value of coronary CT. Intuitively, the cardiovascular risk of someone without CT evidence of coronary atherosclerosis is much lower than someone with extensive (obstructing) plaque. Min et al. investigated the prognostic value of coronary CT angiography over 15 months in a large population and found that the extent and localization of obstructive and nonobstructive coronary disease predictive for all-cause mortality [21]. Patients with a normal CT scan had a very good prognosis.

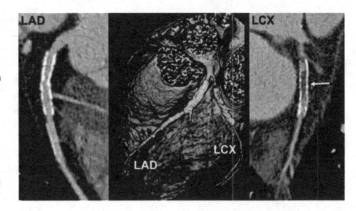

Figure 9.8 **MSCT stent imaging.** Two patent stents in the left anterior descending coronary artery (LAD). The different intensity of the stent struts on CT suggests they are stents of a different type. A septal branch is preserved after stenting. A third stent has been implanted in the left circumflex branch (LCX). The low-density material within the stent suggests occlusion (arrow). Distally the LCX is opacified, likely due by collateral supply.

Imaging of Stents

The high roentgen attenuation of the metal in standard coronary stents causes artifacts that complicate evaluation of the coronary lumen within the stent, particular close to the stent struts. The magnitude of these artifacts vary depending on the material and the stent design, i.e., the strut thickness [22]. The effect on visualization of the in-stent lumen is most severe in smaller stent [23]. Comparative studies have shown a very reasonable accuracy for in-stent stenosis in comparison to conventional angiography, although a substantial number of stent were excluded because of insufficient image quality [24–26]. Accuracy is better in larger stent and is more accurate for detection of occlusion compared to stenosis [27]. Guidelines discourage CT angiography after coronary stenting [15]. On an individual basis CT can be considered to rule out severe obstruction of stents in larger proximal coronary branches of bypass grafts [28]. Even more than in nonstented patients acquisition of high-quality data, with application of dedicated convolution filters for image reconstruction is recommended to achieve interpretable image quality (Figure 9.8).

Graft Imaging

Because of their large diameter, limited calcification and relative immobility bypass grafts, and particularly saphenous vein grafts, are well visualized by CT, although surgical material may cause artifacts (Figure 9.9). Even with earlier generations of CT graft occlusion or patency can be demonstrated with very good accuracy. Current CT technology detects graft occlusion, as well as significant stenosis with an accuracy of approximately 95% (Table 9.3)

[19–33]. However, ischemic symptoms in patients after bypass surgery can be caused by obstruction of bypass grafts, or by progression of disease in the native coronary arteries. Longer after surgery obstruction of the nongrafted coronary arteries or distal coronary run-offs is even more likely than graft failure to be the cause of recurrent complaints [34]. Therefore, evaluation cannot be limited to the

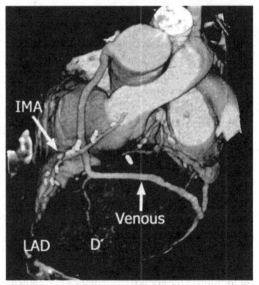

Figure 9.9 **Graft imaging.** Three-dimensional reconstruction of a CT angiogram of a patient with a left internal mammary artery graft (IMA) connected to the middle segment of the left anterior descending coronary artery (LAD) and a venous graft from the ascending aorta with an anastomosis to a diagonal branch (D), a posterolateral branch and a posterior descending branch (not shown). While the grafts are well visualized, assessment of the native coronary arteries, particularly the LAD, is more complicated.

Table 9.3   Diagnostic performance of MSCT to detect significant bypass graft disease.

	N	Excl. (%)	Sens. (%)	Spec. (%)	PPV (%)	NPV (%)
Pache et al. [24]	31	6	98	89	90	98
Malagutti et al. [25]	52	0	99	96	95	99
Ropers et al. [26]	50	0	100	94	76	100
Meyer et al. [27]	138	0	97	97	93	99
Onuma et al. [28]	54	2	100	91	74	100

Number of patients (N), exclusion rate (Excl.), sensitivity (Sens.), specificity (Spec.), positive predictive value (PPV) and negative predictive value (NPV) to detect >50% luminal obstruction.

bypass grafts but should include the coronary arteries as well. The latter however proves to be more complicated due to the diffuse coronary degeneration and excessive presence of coronary calcification [35]. Although results have improved using contemporary technology: sensitivity and specificity of approximately 90%, diagnostic performance is still inferior to the published results in patients without previous bypass graft surgery [30,31,33].

Because of the chronic nature of atherosclerotic disease in these patients luminal obstruction may be diffuse and extensive. Occluded grafts may exist for years without causing symptoms because of maintained coronary flow or development of collateral vessels [36]. Even more than in nonsurgical patients, functional information concerning the presence and localization of ischemic myocardium is important to identify the culprit coronary or graft lesion. As a consequence CT is often not conclusive in patients presenting with symptoms late after surgery. It can be of use in specific situations when one is (exclusively) interested in the condition of the bypass grafts. CT imaging of the grafts (combined with LV CT angiography) can be performed prior to catheterization to shorten the time spent in the catheterization laboratory and save on contrast medium use (not radiation dose), particularly when the location of the grafts is challenging or unknown.

Imaging of Coronary Atherosclerosis

Coronary Calcium

Because of the roentgen attenuating properties of calcium in comparison to other tissues, calcium can be imaged without the need for contrast medium. While most clinical data has been gathered using electron-beam CT, calcium imaging can be performed with MSCT using either prospectively ECG-triggered scanning or retrospectively ECG-gated image reconstruction [37,38]. Finding calcium is evidence of coronary atherosclerosis. Most patients with flow-limiting disease have a positive calcium score. In symptomatic patients the positive predictive value of a positive calcium score for the presence of coronary stenosis is about 50%, without symptoms much lower. The absence of coronary calcium does not exclude the presence (noncalcified) atherosclerosis, although severe coronary artery disease will be unlikely in this case.

The (semi-)quantitative amount of coronary calcium is a surrogate measure for the total coronary plaque burden. Several studies have show that the coronary calcium score [39] predicts adverse coronary events independently of conventional risk factors [40–44]. The St Francis Heart Study showed that the calcium score outperformed the Framingham Risk Score for the prediction of coronary events [41]. According to published guidelines calcium scoring is reasonable to better classify patients at an intermediate risk of cardiovascular events [45]. Patients with an Agatston score below 100 have a annular CV risk well below 1% and can be considered low-risk. Those with a score >400 have a CV risk equal to for instance diabetics and are entitled to more intensive preventive treatment. Whether this will reduce their risk, and whether calcium scoring as such improves clinical outcome still needs to be established.

Contrast-Enhanced Plaque Imaging

On contrast-enhanced CT scans noncalcified plaque components can be identified in addition

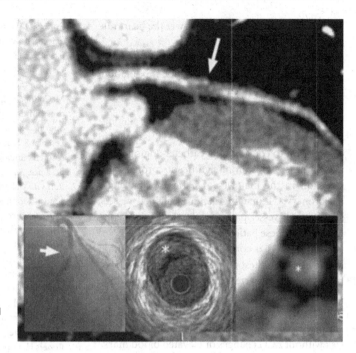

Figure 9.10 Plaque imaging. Left anterior descending coronary artery with a significant stenosis (arrow), mostly consisting of noncalcified material. The inserts show the corresponding conventional coronary angiogram, the IVUS image with the plaque (*), and the MSCT cross-sectional view of the lesion, confirming the presence of the plaque (*).

to calcified ones (Figure 9.10). In comparative studies with IVUS CT detects most of the plaque in the proximal coronary vessels, particularly when some calcium is present [46,47]. Because the outer vessel wall is poorly defined, with user-dependent measurements affected by display settings, plaque quantification remains difficult [48,49]. Measured CT attenuation (Hounsfield units) within plaques has been compared with histology and IVUS [48,50–53]. Calcified plaques have a significantly higher attenuation than noncalcified plaques (Figure 9.11). Differentiation of lipid-rich and fibrous plaque, or hypo- and hyperechodense plaques has proven to be more difficult. Lipid-rich plaques have significantly lower attenuation values, but with significant overlap with measured values in fibrous plaques, particularly between studies. Similar to IVUS studies, CT has shown that culprit plaques in patients with an acute coronary syndrome tend to be larger with positive vessel remodeling and contain less calcium, although with a more spotty distribution and more low-density plaque in comparison to stable coronary plaques [54–58]. Although CT is not able to identify high-risk or rupture-prone lesion, assessment of plaque burden by contrast-enhanced CT may have prognostic value [21].

Summary

- ECG-gated multislice CT allows noninvasive visualization of the heart and coronary arteries.

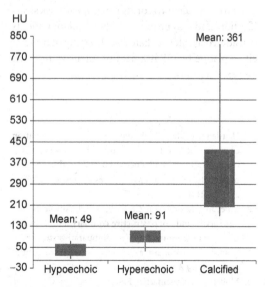

Figure 9.11 Plaque characterization. Measured plaque attenuation (in Hounsfield Units) of coronary plaques categorized by IVUS as hypoechoic ("lipid-rich"), hyperechoic ("fibrotic") or calcific. (Adapted from Leber et al. [47].)

Beta-blockers are often used to lower the heart rate and minimize motion artifacts.

• Measures to reduce the radiation dose of cardiac CT include: ECG-triggered tube modulation, anatomic tube modulation, variable table feed and prospective ECG-triggered CT scanning.

• The diagnostic accuracy of coronary angiography using the latest generation CT is good in comparison to conventional catheter angiography, and permits exclusion of significant coronary obstruction in the majority of patients. Challenges in coronary CT imaging include calcified vessels, stents, small vessel pathology, arrhythmia, tachycardia, and obese patients.

• Coronary CT is considered a reasonable option in patients with chest pain, an intermediate probability for coronary artery disease, particularly when exercise tests were unavailable or nonconclusive. Additional accepted indications include suspected coronary anomaly, acute chest pain at intermediate risk without ECG changes or elevated blood markers, new unexplained heart failure.

• Imaging of small coronary stents is often complicated, and generally discouraged. Imaging of grafts is well feasible, although assessment of the native coronary arteries is more complicated after bypass graft surgery.

• Coronary calcium scoring can improve risk stratification, and may be particularly useful for patients considered at intermediate risk. Imaging of noncalcified plaque by CT is a field of intensive research and expectations.

References

1. Hausleiter J, Meyer T, Hadamitzky M, et al. Radiation dose estimates from cardiac multislice computed tomography in daily practice: impact of different scanning protocols on effective dose estimates. *Circulation.* 2006;113:1305–1310.

2. Leber AW, Knez A, von Ziegler F, et al. Quantification of obstructive and nonobstructive coronary lesions by 64-slice computed tomography: a comparative study with quantitative coronary angiography and intravascular ultrasound. *J Am Coll Cardiol.* 2005;46:147–154.

3. Mollet NR, Cademartiri F, van Mieghem CA, et al. High-resolution spiral computed tomography coronary angiography in patients referred for diagnostic conventional coronary angiography. *Circulation.* 2005;112:2318–2323.

4. Ropers D, Rixe J, Anders K, et al. Usefulness of multidetector row spiral computed tomography with 64- × 0.6-mm collimation and 330-ms rotation for the noninvasive detection of significant coronary artery stenoses. *Am J Cardiol.* 2006;97:343–348.

5. McCollough C, Bruesewitz M, Kofler J. CT dose reduction and dose management tools: overview of available options. *RadioGraphics.* 2006;26:503–512.

6. Leschka S, Alkadhi H, Plass A, et al. Accuracy of MSCT coronary angiography with 64-slice technology: first experience. *Eur Heart J.* 2005;26:1482–1487.

7. Raff GL, Gallagher MJ, O'Neill WW, Goldstein JA. Diagnostic accuracy of noninvasive coronary angiography using 64-slice spiral computed tomography. *J Am Coll Cardiol.* 2005;46:552–557.

8. Weustink AC, Meijboom WB, Mollet NR, et al. Reliable high-speed coronary computed tomography in symptomatic patients. *J Am Coll Cardiol.* 2007;50:786–794.

9. Leber AW, Johnson T, Becker A, et al. Diagnostic accuracy of dual-source multi-slice CT-coronary angiography in patients with an intermediate pretest likelihood for coronary artery disease. *Eur Heart J.* 2007;28:2354–2360.

10. Ropers U, Ropers D, Pflederer T, et al. Influence of heart rate on the diagnostic accuracy of dual-source computed tomography coronary angiography. *J Am Coll Cardiol.* 2007;50:2393–2398.

11. Hamon M, Biondi-Zoccai GG, Malagutti P, et al. Diagnostic performance of multislice spiral computed tomography of coronary arteries as compared with conventional invasive coronary angiography: a meta-analysis. *J Am Coll Cardiol.* 2006;48:1896–1910.

12. Nieman K, Oudkerk M, Rensing BJ, et al. Coronary angiography with multi-slice computed tomography. *Lancet.* 2001;357:599–603.

13. Achenbach S, Giesler T, Ropers D, et al. Detection of coronary artery stenoses by contrast-enhanced, retrospectively electrocardiographically-gated, multislice spiral computed tomography. *Circulation.* 2001;103:2535–2538.

14. Knez A, Becker CR, Leber A, et al. Usefulness of multislice spiral computed tomography angiography for determination of coronary artery stenoses. *Am J Cardiol.* 2001;88:1191–1194.

15. Budoff MJ, Achenbach S, Blumenthal RS, et al. Assessment of coronary artery disease by cardiac computed tomography: a scientific statement from the American heart association committee on cardiovascular imaging and intervention, council on cardiovascular radiology and intervention, and committee on cardiac imaging, council on clinical cardiology. *Circulation.* 2006;114:1761–1791.

16. Hendel RC, Patel MR, Kramer CM, et al. ACCF/ACR/SCCT/SCMR/ASNC/NASCI/SCAI/SIR 2006

appropriateness criteria for cardiac computed tomography and cardiac magnetic resonance imaging. A report of the American college of cardiology foundation quality strategic directions committee appropriateness criteria working group. *J Am Coll Cardiol.* 2006;48:1475–1497.

17. Meijboom WB, van Mieghem CA, Mollet NR, *et al.* 64-slice computed tomography coronary angiography in patients with high, intermediate, or low pretest probability of significant coronary artery disease. *J Am Coll Cardiol.* 2007;50:1469–1475.

18. Hoffmann U, Nagurney JT, Moselewski F, *et al.* Coronary multidetector computed tomography in the assessment of patients with acute chest pain. *Circulation.* 2006;114:2251–2260.

19. Gallagher MJ, Ross MA, Raff GL, Goldstein JA, O'Neill WW, O'Neil B. The diagnostic accuracy of 64-slice computed tomography coronary angiography compared with stress nuclear imaging in emergency department low-risk chest pain patients. *Ann Emerg Med.* 2007;49:125–136.

20. Meijboom WB, Mollet NR, Van Mieghem CA, *et al.* Preoperative computed tomography coronary angiography to detect significant coronary artery disease in patients referred for cardiac valve surgery. *J Am Coll Cardiol.* 2006;48:1658–1665.

21. Min JK, Shaw LJ, Devereux RB, *et al.* Prognostic value of multidetector coronary computed tomographic angiography for prediction of all-cause mortality. *J Am Coll Cardiol.* 2007;50:1161–1170.

22. Maintz D, Seifarth H, Raupach R, *et al.* 64-slice multidetector coronary CT angiography: in vitro evaluation of 68 different stents. *Eur Radiol.* 2006;16:818–826.

23. Nieman K, Cademartiri F, Raaijmakers R, Pattynama P, de Feyter P. Noninvasive angiographic evaluation of coronary stents with multi-slice spiral computed tomography. *Herz.* 2003;28:136–142.

24. Gilard M, Cornily JC, Pennec PY, *et al.* Assessment of coronary artery stents by 16 slice computed tomography. *Heart.* 2006;92:58–61.

25. Cademartiri F, Schuijf JD, Pugliese F, *et al.* Usefulness of 64-slice multislice computed tomography coronary angiography to assess in-stent restenosis. *J Am Coll Cardiol.* 2007;49:2204–2210.

26. Rixe J, Achenbach S, Ropers D, *et al.* Assessment of coronary artery stent restenosis by 64-slice multi-detector computed tomography. *Eur Heart J.* 2006;27:2567–2572.

27. Pugliese F, Weustink AC, Van Mieghem C, *et al.* Dual-source coronary computed tomography angiography for detecting in-stent restenosis. *Heart.* 2008;94:848–854.

28. Van Mieghem CA, Cademartiri F, Mollet NR, *et al.* Multislice spiral computed tomography for the evaluation of stent patency after left main coronary artery stenting: a comparison with conventional coronary angiography and intravascular ultrasound. *Circulation.* 2006;114:645–653.

29. Pache G, Saueressig U, Frydrychowicz A, *et al.* Initial experience with 64-slice cardiac CT: non-invasive visualization of coronary artery bypass grafts. *Eur Heart J.* 2006;27:976–980.

30. Malagutti P, Nieman K, Meijboom WB, *et al.* Use of 64-slice CT in symptomatic patients after coronary bypass surgery: evaluation of grafts and coronary arteries. *Eur Heart J.* 2007;28:1879–1885.

31. Ropers D, Pohle FK, Kuettner A, *et al.* Diagnostic accuracy of noninvasive coronary angiography in patients after bypass surgery using 64-slice spiral computed tomography with 330-ms gantry rotation. *Circulation.* 2006;114:2334–2341.

32. Meyer TS, Martinoff S, Hadamitzky M, *et al.* Improved noninvasive assessment of coronary artery bypass grafts with 64-slice computed tomographic angiography in an unselected patient population. *J Am Coll Cardiol.* 2007;49:946–950.

33. Onuma Y, Tanabe K, Chihara R, *et al.* Evaluation of coronary artery bypass grafts and native coronary arteries using 64-slice multidetector computed tomography. *Am Heart J.* 2007;154:519–526.

34. Alderman EL, Kip KE, Whitlow PL, *et al.* Bypass angioplasty revascularization investigation. Native coronary disease progression exceeds failed revascularization as cause of angina after five years in the bypass angioplasty revascularization investigation (BARI). *J Am Coll Cardiol.* 2004;44:766–774.

35. Nieman K, Pattynama PM, Rensing BJ, Van Geuns RJ, De Feyter PJ. Evaluation of patients after coronary artery bypass surgery: CT angiographic assessment of grafts and coronary arteries, *Radiology.* 2003;229:749–756.

36. Bryan AJ, Angelini GD. The biology of saphenous vein occlusion: etiology and strategies for prevention. *Curr Opin Cardiol.* 1994;9:641–649.

37. Becker CR, Kleffel T, Crispin A, *et al.* Coronary artery calcium measurement: agreement of multirow detector and electron beam CT. *AJR Am J Roentgenol.* 2001;176:1295–1298.

38. Horiguchi J, Nakanishi T, Ito K. Quantification of coronary artery calcium using multidetector CT and a retrospective ECG-gating reconstruction algorithm. *AJR Am J Roentgenol.* 2001;177:1429–1435.

39. Agatston AS, Janowitz WR, Hildner FJ, Zusmer NR, Viamonte M, Jr, Detrano R. Quantification of coronary artery calcium using ultrafast computed tomography. *J Am Coll Cardiol.* 1990;15:827–832.

40. Taylor AJ, Bindeman J, Feuerstein I, Cao F, Brazaitis M, O'Malley PG. Coronary calcium independently predicts incident premature coronary heart disease over measured cardiovascular risk factors: mean three-year

outcomes in the prospective army coronary calcium (PACC) project. *J Am Coll Cardiol.* 2005;46:807–814.

41. Arad Y, Goodman KJ, Roth M, Newstein D, Guerci AD. Coronary calcification, coronary disease risk factors, C-reactive protein, and atherosclerotic cardiovascular disease events: the St. Francis Heart Study. *J Am Coll Cardiol.* 2005;46:158–165.

42. Greenland P, LaBree L, Azen SP, Doherty TM, Detrano RC. Coronary artery calcium score combined with Framingham score for risk prediction in asymptomatic individuals. *JAMA.* 2004;291:210–215.

43. Kondos GT, Hoff JA, Sevrukov A, *et al.* Electron-beam tomography coronary artery calcium and cardiac events: a 37-month follow-up of 5635 initially asymptomatic low- to intermediate-risk adults. *Circulation.* 2003;107:2571–2576.

44. Vliegenthart R, Oudkerk M, Hofman A, *et al.* Coronary calcification improves cardiovascular risk prediction in the elderly. *Circulation.* 2005;112:572–577.

45. Greenland P, Bonow RO, Brundage BH, *et al.* ACCF/AHA 2007 clinical expert consensus document on coronary artery calcium scoring by computed tomography in global cardiovascular risk assessment and in evaluation of patients with chest pain: a report of the American college of cardiology foundation clinical expert consensus task force (ACCF/AHA Writing Committee to Update the 2000 Expert Consensus Document on Electron Beam Computed Tomography). *Circulation.* 2007;115:402–426.

46. Achenbach S, Moselewski F, Ropers D, *et al.* Detection of calcified and noncalcified coronary atherosclerotic plaque by contrast-enhanced, submillimeter multidetector spiral computed tomography: a segment-based comparison with intravascular ultrasound. *Circulation.* 2004;109:14–17.

47. Leber AW, Knez A, Becker A, *et al.* Accuracy of multidetector spiral computed tomography in identifying and differentiating the composition of coronary atherosclerotic plaques: a comparative study with intracoronary ultrasound. *J Am Coll Cardiol.* 2004;43:1241–1247.

48. Leber AW, Becker A, Knez A, *et al.* Accuracy of 64-slice computed tomography to classify and quantify plaque volumes in the proximal coronary system: a comparative study using intravascular ultrasound. *J Am Coll Cardiol.* 2006;47:672–677.

49. Moselewski F, Ropers D, Pohle K, *et al.* Comparison of measurement of cross-sectional coronary atherosclerotic plaque and vessel areas by 16-slice multidetector computed tomography versus intravascular ultrasound. *Am J Cardiol.* 2004;94:1294–1297.

50. Schroeder S, Kopp AF, Baumbach A, *et al.* Imaging of noncalcified coronary plaques using helical CT with retrospective ECG gating. *AJR Am J Roentgenol.* 2000; 175:423–424.

51. Schroeder S, Kopp AF, Baumbach A, *et al.* Noninvasive detection and evaluation of atherosclerotic coronary plaques with multislice computed tomography. *J Am Coll Cardiol.* 2001;37:1430–1435.

52. Schroeder S, Kuettner A, Leitritz M, *et al.* Reliability of differentiating human coronary plaque morphology using contrast-enhanced multislice spiral computed tomography: a comparison with histology. *J Comput Assist Tomogr.* 2004;28:449–454.

53. Pohle K, Achenbach S, MacNeill B, *et al.* Characterization of non-calcified coronary atherosclerotic plaque by multi-detector row CT: comparison to IVUS. *Atherosclerosis.* 2007;190:174–180.

54. Leber AW, Knez A, White CW, *et al.* Composition of coronary atherosclerotic plaques in patients with acute myocardial infarction and stable angina pectoris determined by contrast-enhanced multislice computed tomography. *Am J Cardiol.* 2003;91:714–718.

55. Inoue F, Sato Y, Matsumoto N, Tani S, Uchiyama T. Evaluation of plaque texture by means of multislice computed tomography in patients with acute coronary syndrome and stable angina. *Circ J.* 2004;68:840–844.

56. Hoffmann U, Moselewski F, Nieman K, *et al.* Noninvasive assessment of plaque morphology and composition in culprit and stable lesions in acute coronary syndrome and stable lesions in stable angina by multidetector computed tomography. *J Am Coll Cardiol.* 2006;47:1655–1662.

57. Schuijf JD, Beck T, Burgstahler C, *et al.* Differences in plaque composition and distribution in stable coronary artery disease versus acute coronary syndromes; noninvasive evaluation with multi-slice computed tomography. *Acute Card Care.* 2007;9:48–53.

58. Motoyama S, Kondo T, Sarai M, *et al.* Multislice computed tomographic characteristics of coronary lesions in acute coronary syndromes. *J Am Coll Cardiol.* 2007;50:319–326.

CHAPTER 10

Multislice Cardiac Tomography: Myocardial Function, Perfusion, and Viability

Raymond T. Yan[1], Richard T. George[2] & Joao A.C. Lima[2]
[1] Johns Hopkins Hospital, Baltimore, MD, USA
[2] Johns Hopkins University, Baltimore, MD, USA

Multidetector computed tomography (MDCT) is a rapidly evolving technology with increasing applications in the noninvasive evaluation of cardiovascular disease. The utility of the current generation 64-slice MDCT scanners for defining the anatomical extent of coronary artery disease (CAD) has been demonstrated in various single [1]. and multicenter [2] studies which revealed good sensitivity and specificity for identifying significant coronary stenosis compared to invasive angiography. However, it is well recognized that the physiological impact of CAD on myocardial function, perfusion and viability are of unique clinical significance beyond the degree of luminal obstruction in the prognostication and therapeutic decision on revascularization of patients with CAD [3,4]. Indeed, the rapid technological advancement of MDCT with improved spatial and temporal resolution as well as axial body coverage has afforded MDCT the potential towards a more comprehensive anatomical and functional evaluation of atherosclerotic disease. This chapter aims to review the physiological and technical basics of MDCT in the evaluation of cardiac function, myocardial perfusion and viability.

Cardiac CT, PET and MR, 2nd edition. Edited by Vasken Dilsizian and Gerry Pohost. © 2010 Blackwell Publishing Ltd.

Technical Consideration and Imaging Acquisition

Tissue Contrast

In cardiac CT, the use of iodinated contrast agent is necessary to achieve adequate tissue contrast to delineate cardiac chambers from the myocardium for functional assessment. The facts that iodinated agents are mostly intravascular during first pass circulation and that X-ray attenuation as measured in Houndsfield units (HU) is directly proportional to the iodine concentration in tissue make iodinated contrast an ideal tracer for quantifying myocardial perfusion [5]. The pharmacokinetics of iodinated agent, characterized by relative exclusion from intracellular spaces of living myocytes and increasing re-distribution and accumulation into extracellular space of infarcted myocardium, supports its potential to mediate delayed contrast enhancement for viability assessment [6].

With the use of the modern 16–64 slices MDCT scanners, tissue contrast required for the above objectives in general can be accomplished with the use of a single bolus of 50–120 mL of iodinated contrast administered at 3–6 mL/second according to the patient body weight. The precise bolus geometry should be tailored to achieve the highest tissue contrast (opacification) selectively in the area of interest for the shortest duration dictated by the imaging time using the least volume of contrast to minimize the risk of iodine toxicity and contrast reactions.

To this end, there has been extensive research into the optimal delivery of contrast for MDCT coronary angiography. For the purpose of functional evaluation of the left ventricle (LV), the optimal timing of image acquisition with respect to contrast delivery is largely identical to that for coronary angiography, which is the circulation time for optimizing contrast enhancement in the systemic circulation [7]. The circulation time can vary between 20 and 60 seconds across individuals and is a function of heart rate, blood volume and cardiac output. The two standard techniques of test bolus and bolus tracking supported by most current generation of MDCT scanners can be used to optimize timing of contrast delivery for functional studies. Both strategies employ low-radiation un-gated sequential transaxial imaging of a prespecified region of interest in either the left ventricular cavity or the ascending/descending aorta during contrast administration [8]. In the test-bolus method, the actual peak can be predetermined with a small injection (~10 cc) of contrast at 5–7 mL/second followed by saline. Whereas in bolus-tracking, the full-dose contrast is delivered and volumetric scanning is automatically triggered when a preset HU threshold is reached in the region of interest. With contrast injection at a nominal rate of 3–6 mL/second, adequate opacification for imaging left-sided structures is achieved after the circulation time is reached and is maintained during contrast administration and up to approximately half the circulation time beyond completion of contrast injection. The use of saline chaser and exponentially decelerated contrast injection protocol can prolong the imaging time without necessarily increasing the total amount of contrast [9]. With the advent of 256–320 slices MDCT offering complete heart coverage and thus a drastically shorter acquisition time, the volume of contrast can be further reduced while the proper timing of contrast delivery becomes paradoxically more stringent.

Cardiac Gating and Image Acquisition

With the heart under constant cardiac and respiratory motion, acquisition of volumetric data must be performed with breath-hold and cardiac gating. There are two approaches to cardiac gating: (1) prospective ECG triggering and (2) retrospective ECG gating [10]. In prospective ECG triggering, X-ray is generated only during a predefined portion of a cardiac cycle (denoted as percentage of R-R interval) during which projection data is acquired. The main advantage is a substantial reduction in radiation dose. However, the technique is highly susceptible to heart rate variability and falls short of capturing data of the entire cardiac cycle necessary for functional analysis. With retrospective ECG gating, current MDCT scanner can be programmed in helical mode for continuous acquisition of projection data with simultaneous ECG recording. Image reconstruction is subsequently performed using single or multisegmental reconstruction for specific time intervals within the cardiac cycles. As every axial position of the heart is captured during the entire cardiac cycle, complete temporal sequence of cardiac images can be reconstructed in cine mode for regional and global myocardial functional assessment.

Radiation Exposure

The total radiation dose of a cardiac examination is largely dictated by its protocol. To permit analysis of regional and global myocardial function, retrospective ECG gating with inherently higher radiation is indispensable. Protocols for myocardial perfusion and viability examinations often necessitate additional image acquisitions postpharmacological stress and for visualizing delayed contrast enhancement, respectively. As such, considerations to minimize radiation are of particular value in the functional applications of MDCT.

Dose modulation is a standard feature on most current generation MDCT scanners which can reduce cumulative radiation exposure with the use of retrospective gating by attenuating the tube current during phases when lower image quality is sufficient for evaluating noncoronary structures [11,12]. With dose modulation, radiation dose is reduced by 30–50% and is most significant at lower heart rates. The feature is most beneficial and applicable for patients with stable R-R interval undergoing coronary angiography in which most diagnostic images are to be reconstructed from only a single or few selected diastolic phases. As multiphasic data reconstruction throughout the cardiac cycle is mandated for ventricular functional analysis, excessively restrictive dose modulation during systole may inadvertently impair image quality and signal-to-noise ratio thereby limiting the accuracy in systolic endocardial and epicardial borders delineations. Therefore, a more conservative approach to dose modulation should be considered in studies intended to provide concomitant functional information. Unlike MDCT coronary angiographic applications which necessitate a 0.5 mm slice thickness for isotropic resolution, MDCT imaging of the myocardium can be adequately performed with thicker slices of 1–4 mm. While functional evaluation of the ventricle without coronary imaging is unlikely to be a popular indication for performing volumetric CT examination, the use of thicker slices in functional MDCT examinations when permissible can bring about substantial savings in radiation dose.

Assessment of Myocardial Function

The use of CT to visualize cardiac function has been shown feasible back in the 1970s with cross-sectional imaging techniques including dynamic spatial reconstructor [13] and electron beam CT [14]. However, none of these techniques has matured to become diagnostic tool for routine clinical use. With the introduction of MDCT, a four-dimensional functional data set is inherently available in every retrospective ECG gated cardiac study without the use of additional contrast material or patient preparation. As such, myocardial function can be readily analyzed as an adjunct to any retrospectively-gated MDCT angiography in the workup of patients with ischemic heart disease.

The accuracy in the evaluation of regional and global myocardial function is largely affected by the subject's heart rate, the temporal resolution and the number of cardiac phases reconstructed for analysis. Because of limited temporal resolution, systolic images obtained at higher heart rates are of lower quality and may impact on endocardial border delineation [15]. Myocardial function can be more reliably determined independent of heart rate only if the study is performed with sufficient temporal resolution. Using standard half-scan image reconstruction, the temporal resolution of modern MDCT scanner is in the order of half its gantry rotation time. More precisely, it is the time for the gantry to rotate 180° plus its fan angle which ranges approximately between 165 and 250 ms. Multiseg-

mental reconstruction is a powerful option that can substantially improve temporal resolution at the expense of slightly increased scan time and radiation exposure. Nevertheless, image acquisition and reconstruction need to be prescribed with consideration of heart rate to ensure the multiphasic axial data set is fundamentally of adequate temporal resolution for functional analysis. Beyond data acquisition, it is also important to reconstruct sufficient cardiac phases when evaluating ventricular function. In general, the number of required cardiac phases multiplied by the temporal resolution should exceed the duration of the R-R interval to ensure the entire cardiac cycle is covered. In most clinical applications, images from practically at least ten (10% increment of the R-R interval) and preferably twenty (at 5% R-R intervals) cardiac phases should be reconstructed so that true end-systole and end-diastole can be accurately identified for quantification. Reconstructing insufficient number of phases may increase the extent to which end-systolic and end-diastolic volumes are respectively over- and underestimated, and accordingly the degree of systematic underestimation of ejection fraction [16]. The reconstruction of closely-spaced cardiac phases to generate complete volume–time curves is of potential value for evaluating diastolic function. The use of volume–time curves may in theory provide more accurate quantification of ejection fraction in patients with ventricular asynergy. However, the incremental value of constructing volume–time curves in routine clinical practice remains undefined and needs to be further studied.

Left Ventricular Global Systolic Function

In the assessment of global left ventricular systolic function, end-diastolic and end-systolic axial data set are first reconstructed which can be reformatted into standardized double oblique imaging planes resembling those adapted by echocardiography and other tomographic modalities. Under these standard imaging planes including two-, three- and four-chambers as well as short-axis views, the left ventricular cavity and most myocardial segments can be examined from two orthogonal perspectives (Figure 10.1). Left ventricular ejection fraction as the most commonly used parameter of global left ventricular systolic function can be calculated from

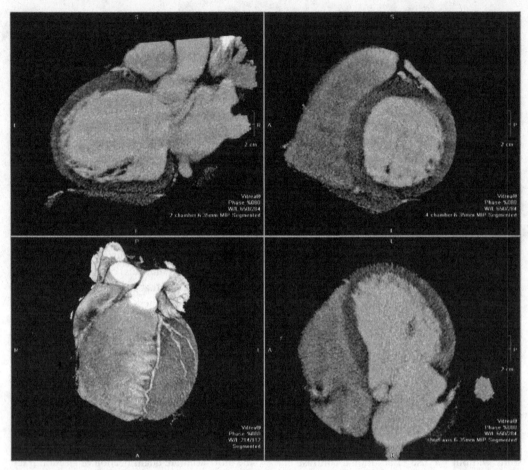

Figure 10.1 Orthogonal cardiac views reconstructed from multiphasic axial image data set (Vitrea Workstation, Vital Images). The standard short-axis view (upper right) and four-chamber view (lower right) are shown.

left ventricular end-diastolic and end-systolic volumes. These ventricular volumes in turn can be calculated semi-automatically from the stack of reformatted 5–8 mm short-axis slices using the Simpson's method, which is the summation of cross-sectional area of the left ventricular cavity (area enclosed endocardial contour) multiplied by the slice thickness across all slices from the base to the apex:

$$LV_{volume}$$
$$= \sum_{\text{Basal slice}}^{\text{Apical slice}} (\text{Area bounded by endocardial contour}$$
$$\times \text{ slice thickness})$$

For more reproducible quantitative measurements, left ventricular papillary muscle and trabeculation are often analyzed as part of the blood pool [17]. In addition, all slices spanning the most apical to the most basal portion of the LV where respectively the cavity and the presence of at least 50% myocardium is visible throughout the entire cardiac cycle should be included. In practice, postprocessing of these image sets can be accomplished semi-automatically with minimal user input using a variety of commercially available three-dimensional (3D) rendering software. With these modern postprocessing packages, the left ventricular long-axis transacting the apex and the mitral valve plane is determined and the endocardial contour at each tomographic level orthogonal to the long-axis is

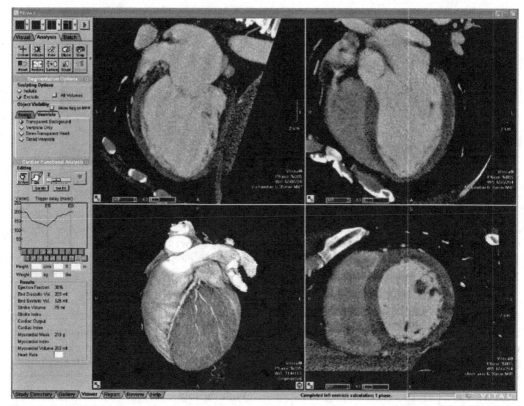

Figure 10.2 Semiautomatic evaluation of left ventricular function on a workstation (Vitrea, Vital Images). Twenty cardiac phases were reconstructed for analysis. Endocardial and epicardial contours on the short-axis images (lower right) were automatically traced for operator verification and correction. The end-diastolic and end-systolic volumes, stroke volume, ejection fraction and cardiac output were automatically determined. On the workstation console, the images can be displayed as a movie cine loop for visual inspection of regional wall motion and global contraction abnormalities. This patient had moderate LV global systolic dysfunction with an ejection fraction of 38%.

automatically traced for operator verification and modification as necessary (Figure 10.2).

Overall, the reproducibility of left ventricular volume and ejection fraction determined by CT has been well-established [18]. Normal ventricular and stroke volumes for adults normalized to body surface area (end-diastolic volume 73 ± 19 mL/m^2, end-systolic volume 24 ± 8 mL/m^2, stroke volume 48 ± 11 mL/m^2) based on electron-beam CT have also been published [19]. More recently, comparisons of left ventricular volume and ejection fraction assessed by CT (largely MDCT) versus other validated imaging modalities including radionuclide angiography, echocardiography and MRI have confirmed excellent correlation across a broad range of values [20–23]. Although left ventricular function can be accurately assessed without

radiation exposure by echocardiography and MRI, volumetric CT can serve as a reliable alternative should there are contraindications to MRI (e.g., claustrophobia, implanted pacemaker or defibrillator) or technical limitations with echocardiography (e.g., suboptimal acoustic window, poor tissue contrast), or particularly when there are discordant functional results or concomitant indications to define coronary anatomy.

Assessment of Regional Left Ventricular Function

In contrast to echocardiography, MDCT has a relatively lower temporal resolution (165–250 ms). However, regional ventricular systolic wall thickening and contractility can be adequately assessed by quantifying the overall systolic displacement of

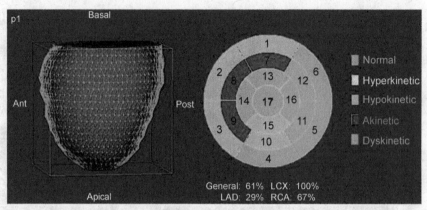

Figure 10.3 Three-dimensional and polar-plot of regional myocardial function. The 17-segment model standardized for tomographic imaging is used. As demonstrated, this patient had an age-undetermined myocardial infarction in the territory supplied by the left-anterior descending coronary artery. Ant, anterior; LAD, left-anterior descending artery; LCX, left circumflex artery; Post, posterior; RCA, right coronary artery.

the endocardial contour relative to the epicardial border using MDCT. The feasibility of regional wall motion assessment based on cine images has been demonstrated in several studies using 16-slice MDCT [20,24,25].

With the reconstruction of cine images in standard orthogonal views, regional ventricular wall motion as conventionally defined by systolic wall thickening can be graded [26] visually as in echocardiography and cardiac MRI on a semi-quantitative five-point scale: normokinetic, hypokinetic, akinetic, dyskinetic and aneurysmal. Supported by virtually all contemporary postprocessing software, regional ventricular wall thickening can be automatically analyzed quantitatively with the results rendered and color-coded for display on polar plots or in three-dimensions (Figure 10.3).

In assessing regional wall motion, it is recommended that the LV be segmented and analyzed according to the 17-segment model standardized for tomographic imaging published by the American Heart Association [27]. This model includes six segments for basal and midventricular short-axis views, four segments for the apical short-axis view, and a separate apical segment in the long-axis orientation. When defined according to this standard 17-segment model, each myocardial segment can be mapped to a coronary artery territory [27]. Complementary to the inherently available angiographic findings of the corresponding coro-

nary artery, analysis of segmental wall motion can provide a more comprehensive insight into both the anatomical and functional state of the different coronary artery territories in one single breath-hold MDCT examination (Figure 10.4).

With the introduction of 256–320 slice MDCT scanners providing whole heart coverage, assessment of ventricular wall motion can be completed during a single acquisition within one heartbeat. The resulting cardiac scan can minimize susceptibility to motion artifacts and eradicate the problem of axial data mis-registration. Furthermore, the advancement in multisegmental reconstruction algorithm can drastically improve temporal resolution to <50 ms. As such, the diagnostic performance of MDCT for regional myocardial function is expected to improve. In recognition of the potential for pharmacological stress myocardial perfusion imaging with MDCT, concomitant assessment of stress-induced augmentation in regional wall thickening on CT may be of value for defining contractile reserve. In contrary to echocardiography and MRI, the prognostic significance of resting or stress-induced regional wall motion abnormalities on MDCT has not been explicitly investigated or established at the present time.

Evaluation of Diastolic Function

As a byproduct of any retrospective ECG gated helical data set, left ventricular volume at any desired

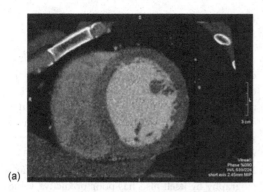

(a)

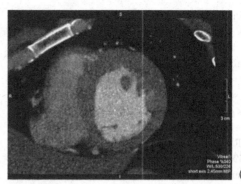

(b)

Figure 10.4 Short-axis end-diastolic (a) and end-systolic (b) images in a patient with inferolateral wall motion abnormalities. Within this same coronary artery territory, the patient also had corresponding perfusion deficits during adenosine infusion as demonstrated by multidetector CT.

phase during the cardiac cycle can be determined. With sufficient cardiac phases reconstructed (5% increment in R-R interval) to interpolate the left ventricular volume–time curve, conventional diastolic functional indices including early and late peak ventricular filling rates as well as time to peak ventricular filling can be well approximated in cases when there is normal sinus rhythm with stable R-R interval. Up to the present time, the use of MDCT to quantify diastolic ventricular hemodynamics has been performed for research purposes. Its validity and appropriateness for routine clinical use remain to be defined.

Assessment of Right Ventricular Systolic Function

With proper acquisition timing and contrast delivery optimized for right ventricular opacification, regional and global right ventricular (RV) systolic function can be selectively examined [23,28,29]. To facilitate right ventricular endocardial border delineation, tailored contrast delivery protocols utilizing a more prolonged or exponentially decelerated injection profile should be used [9]. In normal ventricular-arterial concordance, optimal timing for imaging the right ventricle occurs as the contrast agent transits into the main pulmonary arteries.

In contrary to the LV, the complex geometry of the right ventricle precluded the development and application of reliable geometric models. With the current generation software, the endocardial con-

tours of the right ventricle need to be manually defined. The modified Simpson's method can then be used to calculate right ventricular volumes and ejection fraction based on the manually traced endocardial borders in a similar fashion as for the LV. In comparative studies of MRI and 16-slices MDCT adopting imaging protocols optimized for coronary visualization, RV volumes and ejection fraction as determined respectively by CT and MRI demonstrated excellent correlations [23,29]. With wider multidetector coverage, improved temporal resolution and the use of tailored contrast delivery protocol, it is expected that global RV functional parameters can be reliably determined by contemporary MDCT scanners.

The utility of MDCT to evaluate the right ventricle has been demonstrated for various clinical conditions including selected forms of congenital heart disease [30], pulmonary embolism (PE) [31,32] and arrhythmogenic right ventricular dysplasia (ARVD/C) [33] in which the right heart is preferentially affected. MDCT can provide comparable quantification of RV volumes and ejection fraction as with the use of MRI in patients with tetralogy of Fallot and transposition of great arteries [30]. Although MRI remains the diagnostic modality of choice to quantify RV function, MDCT can serve as an alternative method to assess RV size and function in congenital heart disease patients who may have contraindication to MRI examinations. In patients with confirmed PE, right ventricular dysfunction (RVD) as defined by an increase in right ventricular to left ventricular dimension (RV_D/LV_D) has been shown to be an independent predictor of adverse outcome at 30 days [31] and 3 months [32]. Right ventricular measurements off the reformatted 4-chamber view may be superior to those from the transverse view in identifying high-risk patients with confirmed PE [31]. For PE-related mortality at 3 months, the positive predictive value of $RV_D/LV_D > 1.0$ on 4-chamber view was 10.1% (95% confidence interval [95%CI] = 2.9–17.4%) whereas the negative predictive value of $RV_D/LV_D \leq 1.0$ was 100% (95% CI = 94.3–100%). After adjustment for age, there was a significant graded relationship between RV_D/LV_D and PE-related mortality (Cox regression coefficient 1.55, $p = 0.04$) [32]. As such, incorporating right ventricular assessment into the MDCT diagnostic protocol for PE may refine patient risk stratification.

MRI has been proposed as the gold standard for evaluating the right ventricle in the diagnostic workup of suspected ARVD. In recognition of an increasing number of patients with suspected ARVD having implanted cardioverter-defibrillators, MDCT can serve as a useful alternative to MRI in defining RV abnormalities. Cardiac MDCT has been shown to have a strong potential to detect many qualitative and quantitative abnormalities of the right ventricle in patients with ARVD [33]. Characteristic features including conspicuous RV trabeculation, RV intramyocardial fat, anterior wall scalloping and regional RV wall motion abnormalities can be reliably assessed on MDCT with good inter-observer agreement [33]. MDCT can also accurately quantify RV volumes, RV inlet dimensions and RV outflow tract surface area which were all increased significantly in patients with confirmed ARVD.

In summary, given the radiation dose, contrast requirement and the limited temporal resolution, resorting to MDCT solely for the purpose of evaluating ventricular function when other techniques can be used to provide the same accurate information is not justified at present. On the other hand, information on myocardial function as readily derived from retrospective-gated MDCT studies can serve as a valuable adjuvant to MDCT angiography in providing a more comprehensive and potentially more conclusive workup for patients with cardiovascular disease.

Myocardial Perfusion Imaging by Computed Tomography

Although MDCT angiography can detect subclinical atherosclerosis and coronary obstruction in 3D detail, it is deficient in measuring the physiological impact of epicardial coronary disease on myocardial blood flow (MBF). The degree of luminal stenosis on invasive angiography is known to correlate poorly with coronary reserve and MBF [34]. More recent studies have revealed that MDCT angiography by itself also has poor predictive value for quantifying myocardial ischemia resulting from atherosclerosis [35,36]. However, it has been well-established that myocardial perfusion provides robust incremental prognostic value beyond invasive angiography and that quantification of myocardial ischemia can refine risk stratification and predict benefit from revascularization [3,35]. As such, effort has been directed to combine noninvasive MDCT angiography and radionuclide myocardial perfusion imaging (MPI) with single photon emission computed tomography (SPECT) or positron emission tomography (PET). An approach based on these hybrid systems is feasible but unfavorably incurs more than double the effective radiation dose to patients [37]. There is convincing evidence from recent animal and clinical research that MDCT has the potential for concomitant quantification of myocardial perfusion in conjunction with noninvasive angiography. Such a combined diagnostic approach is of unique clinical value and may have significant diagnostic, prognostic and therapeutic implications in the management of patients with suspected or known ischemic heart disease.

Dynamic Perfusion Imaging with Electron-Beam CT and MDCT

Current MDCT-scanning systems can be programmed to operate in dynamic mode with the table position fixed while all axial locations within the detector coverage are imaged synchronously at the same time. In this dynamic mode, the pharmacokinetics of contrast in the myocardium and the left ventricular blood pool can be possibly traced in real time thereby permitting absolute quantification of myocardial blood flow using various established mathematical models.

The feasibility of myocardial perfusion imaging was reported back in the 1980s using electron-beam CT (EBCT) which functionally operated in "dynamic" mode. Regional myocardial blood flow in dogs at rest and during induced hyperperfusion determined by EBCT had been shown to correlate with microsphere-derived blood flows over a wide range of 0.4–8 mL/min/g [38]. In addition, significant increase in regional flow could be determined from CT measurements between resting and hyperperfusion states. These initial data illustrated the potential of CT for evaluating coronary flow reserve. In subsequent work by Bell *et al.* [39], the use of time–attenuation curve to calculate MBF was first validated in an animal study and when applied to healthy human individuals during basal and adenosine induced vasodilation, changes in MBF with a mean regional perfusion reserve ratio of 2.8 could be measured [39]. Despite the potential of performing MPI with EBCT as demonstrated, the cost and restricted availability of these machines, their limited axial spatial resolution coupled with the rapid advancement in MDCT technology have thus shifted the paradigm of CT MPI to the use of MDCT systems.

Visual and semi-quantitative assessment of first-pass myocardial perfusion can be achieved with dynamical multiphase contrast-enhanced MDCT imaging. Mahnken *et al.* examined various parameters of the time–density curves obtained with 16-slice dynamic MDCT on an occlusive porcine infarction model [40]. The results were contrasted with MRI first-pass perfusion and ultimately triphenyltetrazolin-chloride (TTC) staining. In this study, infarcted myocardium exhibited significant differences in maximum signal intensity, wash-in time and time–attenuation curve upslope compared to the remote territory which allowed the differentiation between hypoperfused and normal myocardium. The time–density curves for MDCT and the time–signal–intensity curve for MRI perfusion also demonstrated identical temporal contrast enhancement pattern. The size of hypoperfused area on MDCT was directly related to but with slight overestimation of (0.7% more of LV sectional area) the extent of myocardial infarction (MI) demonstrated ex-vivo [40]. More recent studies have further demonstrated that first-pass dynamic MDCT can provide an accurate

measurement of MBF using both semi-quantitative and quantitative analytic methods in a canine model of moderate to severe nonocclusive left-anterior descending artery (LAD) stenosis [41]. With the use of 64-slice MDCT, stress dynamic imaging of the LV during adenosine infusion was performed with images reconstructed at 1-second interval for regions of interest in the LAD and remote territories. Based on the time–attenuation curves, myocardial perfusion was analyzed using two up-slope methods (myocardial upslope normalized to (a) LV blood pool upslope and (b) left ventricular maximum attenuation intensity) and a 2-compartmental model-based deconvolution method. The results were compared to microsphere MBF measurements. Myocardial upslope when normalized to both LV parameters showed strong correlations with microsphere-derived MBF (R^2 of 0.87 and 0.92 for normalization to LV upslope and LV maximum attenuation, respectively) and were significantly lower in stenosed versus remote territories. MBF as quantified by the model-based deconvolution method also exhibited a significant correlation with microsphere MBF over the entire range of flows studied ($R^2 = 0.91$, mean difference: 0.45 mL/min/g, $p =$ NS) [41]. These findings illustrated that dynamic MDCT can be successfully implemented for semiquantitative and quantitative evaluation of MBF during pharmacological stress.

At present, the practical implementation of dynamic MDCT for MPI has not been realized in part because of its restricted axial coverage. The commonly-used 64 detectors MDCT scanners span only 32–40 mm coverage along the z-axis and are deficient of covering the entire LV as required for imaging contrast enhancement over time and performing coronary angiography in dynamic mode. Continuous dynamic MDCT MPI also entailed a relatively high radiation exposure and delivery of additional contrast material. However, with the recently introduced state-of-the-art 256–320 detectors MDCT scanners offering complete heart coverage, dynamic MDCT can be potentially performed with prospective ECG gating at relatively lower radiation and contrast doses for concomitant angiographic and myocardial perfusion evaluation during a single examination. The technique has the potential to become a powerful and more comprehensive diagnostic tool for detecting is-chemic myocardium at risk.

Single Arterial Phase Perfusion Imaging with Helical MDCT

With the possible exception of 256–320 detectors MDCT scanners, noninvasive coronary angiography is currently performed with the MDCT scanners operating in helical mode. As the scanner table is constantly transported through the rotating gantry during image acquisition, raw data is acquired in a spiral manner around the patient where different axial positions of the heart are imaged asynchronously at different moment relative to peak contrast enhancement. As a consequence, unlike dynamic MDCT where images are acquired in various fixed slice locations over a predetermined period of time to characterize contrast wash-in and wash-out kinetics, such data needed to construct the traditional time–attenuation curves is not available from helical MDCT. However, there is accumulating evidence that myocardial perfusion can be derived from single arterial phase imaging based on data extracted from routine helical MDCT studies performed for coronary angiography.

With the use of 16-detector helical MDCT, Hoffman *et al.* [42] had utilized a porcine model of acute occlusive nonreperfused MI. It was demonstrated that regions of resting myocardial hypoattenuation (32 ± 9 HU vs 76 ± 17 HU in remote areas) during contrast first-pass circulation corresponded to areas of infarction which also correlated with decrease in microsphere-determined blood flow. In another study by Lardo *et al.* [43] on helical MDCT imaging of a canine model with acute occlusion and reperfusion of the left anterior-descending artery, areas of myocardial hypoenhancement representing reduced myocardial perfusion postinfarction could be detected within the infarction-related artery territory. More recent experimental findings have further illustrated that regional myocardial perfusion under pharmacological stress can be derived from helical MDCT data sets obtained for routine noninvasive angiography. In this study [44], helical MDCT modeling clinical angiography protocol (retrospective gating, gantry rotation time 400 ms, tube voltage 120 kV, tube current 400 mA, short-axis multiplanar reconstruction at 4-mm slice thickness) was performed at

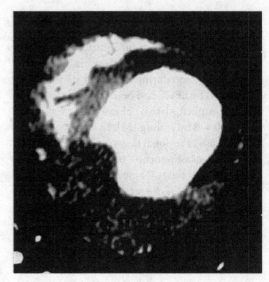

Figure 10.5 Multiplanar reconstruction at mid-ventricular level showing the extent of perfusion deficits (hypoattenuation) in the anteroseptal and anterior walls of a canine model of left-anterior descending artery stenosis. The perfusion deficits can be readily identified visually and on quantitative analysis demonstrated significantly lower Hounsfield Unit.

the end of 5-minutes adenosine infusion (0.14 and 0.21 µg/kg/min) on a canine model of nonocclusive LAD stenosis to capture myocardial perfusion data during first-pass contrast circulation. Perfusion deficits showed marked differences in myocardial signal density compared to remote regions on visual inspection in all and individual experiment (Figure 10.5). On quantitative measurements, myocardial signal density in stenosed and nonstenosed territories measured 92 ± 40 HU and 180 ± 42 HU, respectively ($p = 0.001$ for difference) (Figure 10.6). When myocardial attenuation density is normalized to LV blood pool signal density to permit comparison with microsphere-derived absolute blood flow, there was a significant curvilinear relationship between myocardial signal density ratio and MBF. The relationship was linear up to a maximum flow of 8 mL/g/min which thereafter MDCT measurements would tend to underestimate MBF. For the first time, this study demonstrated that relative differences in first-pass myocardial perfusion under routine adenosine stress could be measured with single arterial phase imaging using helical MDCT protocol designed for noninvasive angiography.

More recently, the potential clinical utility of helical MDCT perfusion imaging has been examined in patients with suspected ischemic heart disease (Figure 10.7). In a pilot study [45] of seven high-risk patients with chest pain and abnormal radionuclide MPI referred for invasive coronary angiography, 64-slice helical MDCT during routine pharmacological stress (adenosine 0.14 μg/kg/min) was performed. Perfusion images were reconstructed along with MDCT angiography. Regional perfusion was defined as normal when there is no detected perfusion defect and the region being concurrently supplied by a coronary artery without significant stenosis on MDCT angiography. Perfusion deficits were defined as myocardial density of one standard deviation below that of normal myocardium (64 ± 27 HU vs 125 ± 26 HU, $p < 0.001$). On a vessel level, the sensitivity and specificity for perfusion defects identifying corresponding coronary stenosis ≥50% was 83 and 100% for MDCT and 67 and 80% for radionuclide MPI, respectively [45]. First-pass adenosine helical MDCT can thus potentially assess the physiological significance of coronary

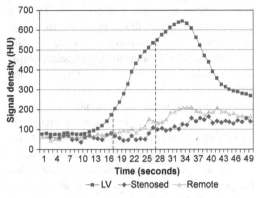

Figure 10.6 In this canine model of left-anterior descending artery stenosis during adenosine infusion, myocardial signal–density curves were constructed for the anterior (stenosed) and inferior (remote) walls. Helical MDCT can be performed to capture regional variations in myocardial perfusion during a single arterial phase of the first-pass contrast enhancement curve at a time point depicted by the vertical line. As illustrated, the area supplied by the stenotic artery exhibited lower X-ray attenuation. LV, left ventricle (Reproduced from George *et al.* [44].)

Figure 10.7 First-pass adenosine-induced stress MDCT myocardial perfusion imaging in a patient with fixed inferior and inferolateral wall perfusion deficits on SPECT. Panels (a) and (c) demonstrated inferior and inferolateral subendocardial perfusion deficits in the mid and distal left ventricle, respectively. Using semi-automated perfusion myocardial function/perfusion software, myocardium with signal density one standard deviation below that of the remote area was color-coded in blue in panels (b) and (d). Invasive coronary angiography (e) revealed a chronically occluded distal right coronary artery with left to right collaterals filling the posterior descending artery (arrows) and posterolateral branches. The standard 17-segment polar plot (panel f) of MDCT-derived myocardial signal densities identified hypoperfused inferior/inferolateral regions as depicted in blue. (Reproduced from George *et al.* [44].)

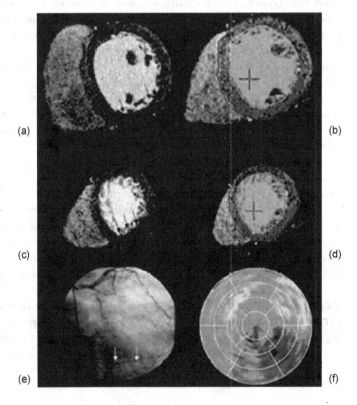

atherosclerosis in patients with chest pain. The very preliminary results in this small pilot study suggested that CT perfusion may be more sensitive and specific than SPECT for identifying impaired perfusion in territories supplied by a significant stenotic artery.

In comparison to nuclear technologies, a distinctive advantage of MDCT for perfusion imaging is its submillimeter isotropic spatial resolution. As reduced subendocardial MBF is the hallmark underlying flow-limiting coronary stenosis, MDCT has the potential to visualize the extent of subendocardial perfusion deficits and delineate transmural gradient in MBF. With this consideration, a recent pilot study was conducted to quantify subendocardial perfusion deficits during adenosine stress in patients with history of chest pain undergoing 64-slice MDCT angiography [46]. MDCT images were reconstructed at 3 mm slice thickness and a 16-segment model of the LV was adapted with each segment further subdivided into subendocardial, mid-myocardial and subepicardial layers. The signal density at each layer was measured to calculate mean transmural attenuation and transmural perfusion ratio (subendocardial to subepicardial) for each segment. Perfusion deficits in territories with a corresponding coronary stenosis (>50%) were found to have significant lower transmural signal density compared to remote areas (106 ± 20 HU vs 127 ± 17 HU, $p = 0.03$ with a mean difference of 21 HU) while their corresponding subendocardial signal density were 94 ± 14 HU and 128 ± 18 HU (mean difference of 34 HU, $p = 0.001$). Moreover, these subendocardial perfusion deficits were visually evident. Importantly, the transmural perfusion ratio was also significantly lower in areas of perfusion deficits in comparison with remote territories (0.77 vs 1.03, $p < 0.0001$) [46]. These findings attest to the potential of helical MDCT to detect the marked subendocardial deficits and transmural differences in perfusion for differentiating ischemic from remote myocardium.

Merits and Limitations of CT Perfusion Imaging

Depending on the precise imaging protocol, the successful incorporation of MDCT perfusion imaging into noninvasive angiographic study would likely entail some increase in radiation exposure and contrast dose. As a temporal resolution of approximately one image per R-R interval is required for establishing a sufficient arterial input function [47] as needed for determining myocardial perfusion, the limited temporal resolution of the present generation MDCT scanners has been a major deterrent hampering the application of MDCT perfusion imaging particularly during stress at increased heart rates. Other CT-specific limitations including beam hardening artifacts caused by contrast material transiting through the right and LVs which may result in hypo- and hyperdense steak artifacts averting reliable extraction of perfusion information. Not withstanding these limitations, MDCT offers several practical and theoretical advantages for perfusion imaging. Compared to radionuclide MPI and MRI, MDCT can provide a substantially higher spatial resolution. The linear relationship between contrast enhancement and iodine concentration over a broad range permits a direct quantification of MBF without the potential need for error-bearing corrections to account for signal intensity saturation as with the use of gadolinium in MRI. Other advantages of MDCT include its ubiquitous availability, shorter examination time and ease of operation with less patient-specific prescription of imaging parameters. The unique potential to integrate noninvasive coronary angiography and perfusion imaging into a single examination for discerning ischemic myocardium at risk may afford MDCT the potential to become a powerful clinical tool for comprehensive work up of known or suspected ischemic heart disease.

MDCT for the Evaluation of Myocardial Viability

In the management of patients with coronary artery disease, reliable distinction between dysfunctional but viable myocardium from nonviable tissue after acute or chronic ischemia has important prognostic and therapeutic implications. With acute ischemia, revascularization procedures such as percutaneous coronary intervention or coronary artery bypass surgery in patients with viable myocardium may lead to improvement in ventricular function [48] and long-term survival [49] whereas revascularization of nonviable myocardium may pose an upfront risk of unnecessary invasive procedures and increased long-term mortality [50]. With LV dysfunction in the setting of chronic ischemia, the presence of myocardial viability can identify subjects with hibernating myocardium who may benefit from improved LV function postrevascularization [51].

In clinical practice, low-dose dobutamine stress echocardiography, SPECT, and PET have been well established for evaluating myocardial viability. In recent years, MRI has been extensively investigated for differentiation between viable and nonviable myocardium using delayed-enhancement MRI (DE-MRI) techniques which can be considered as the current reference standard for detailed viability assessment. The mechanism of delayed hyperenhancement in MRI is ascribed to the accumulation of gadolinium chelates resulting from expanded distribution volume and alterations in wash-in and wash-out kinetics of extravascular contrast agent in the infarcted myocardium [6]. Given the nearly identical kinetics of iodinated contrast agent, contrast-enhanced MDCT (CE-MDCT) is expected to have the potential to visualize infarction and assess viability in the same manner as MRI.

The potential of CT to visualize infarction was first demonstrated back in the 1970s in a series of experimental studies [52]. As confirmed in explanted tissue, acute infarctions were detected on CT as regions of early hypo-enhancement relative to normal myocardium [52]. Regions of low signal on CT in a porcine model of nonreperfused infarction were also shown to exhibit good correlation with TTC-derived infarction. However, infarction or viability assessment based solely on first-pass imaging had important limitations. Specifically, regions of hypo-enhancement may be indicative of under-perfusion as a consequence of an occlusive infarction, acute microvascular obstruction or chronic scar formation. Indeed, it has been suggested in human study that decreased myocardial attenuation on MDCT first-pass imaging may correspond to either infarcted or ischemic but viable myocardium. In a study [53] of 30 patients with known or suspected coronary artery disease, MDCT optimized for coronary imaging as well as MRI stress perfusion and DE-MRI were performed for cross comparison. CT was found to accurately delineate infarction (sensitivity 91%, specificity 79% and accuracy 83%) but systematically underestimated infarction size com-

pared to DE-MRI. Importantly, there was significant overlap in HU between infarcted and viable tissue. Furthermore, areas of hypo-attenuation on images acquired during the arterial phase for coronary imaging cannot reliably distinguish between necrotic and hypoperfused viable tissue [53]. Not withstanding these limitations, increasing number of recent experimental and clinical studies have validated and better characterized the potential of adapting a modified dual-phase early and delayed CE-MDCT imaging protocol for assessing myocardial viability.

Delayed Contrast-Enhanced MDCT

The accuracy of CE-MDCT for quantifying myocardial necrosis, microvascular obstruction and chronic scar was demonstrated by Lardo and his group. In this validation study [43], acute (90 minutes) canine and chronic (8 weeks) porcine models of occlusive reperfused myocardial infarction were evaluated by CE-MDCT with images acquired during first-pass perfusion and every 5 minutes after contrast injection up to 40 minutes (Figure 10.8). Contrast kinetics in the infarcted and remote myocardium was also studied in the acute infarction model. CE-MDCT images were analyzed to define infarct size and microvascular obstruction and the results were compared with postmortem TTC staining and regional microsphere blood flow measurements. On MDCT imaging, both acute and chronic infarctions were identified as myocardial lesions with well-delineated hyper-enhancement of peak signal intensity at 5 minutes after contrast injection. The geometric and spatial extent of myocardial damage can be easily appreciated qualitatively. The mean CT attenuation was significantly higher in the infarcted than remote myocardium both in the acute (261 ± 57 HU vs 134 ± 11 HU) and chronic infarction (181 ± 39 HU vs 97 ± 15 HU) models. Direct comparison of reconstructed slice-matched MDCT and TTC-stained images also revealed excellent correlation in terms of infarction morphology and extent of myocardial injury transmurality (Figure 10.9). In addition, regions with microvascular obstruction could be readily identified as early hypo-enhanced regions which were most prominent early after contrast injection (mean signal of 73 ± 18 HU vs 134 ± 11 HU in normal myocardium). Microsphere-derived MBF

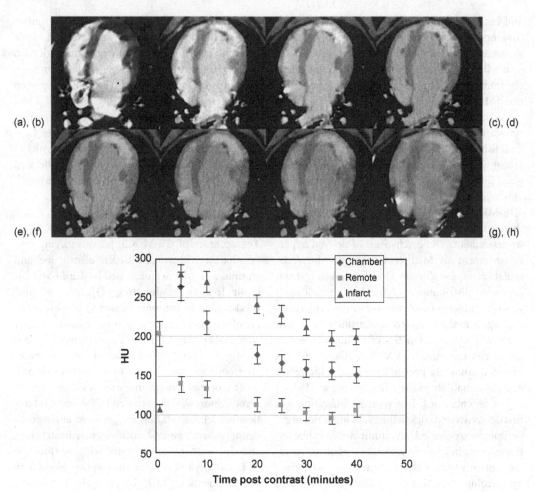

Figure 10.8 A temporal series of images demonstrating postreperfusion iodinated contrast agent kinetics. Image (a) is the first-pass image during contrast injection. The signal density in the infarcted area is substantially lower than that of the remote myocardium and denotes subendocardial microvascular obstruction. Image (b) is obtained at 5-minutes after contrast injection. Of note, the signal density of the myocardial region with damaged tissue is significantly higher than that of the healthy myocardium. Subsequent wash-out of contrast over the next 35 minutes at 5-minute interval is demonstrated in the sequence of images (c) to (h). The plot below illustrated quantitative contrast kinetics for the left ventricular chamber (blood pool), remote and infarcted myocardium after contrast injection. As demonstrated visually and on the quantitative plot, the infarction became well-delineated and reached peak enhancement with strongest contrast differences at 5-minutes. (Reproduced from Lardo *et al.* [43].)

also confirmed decreased myocardial blood flow in these regions of microvascular obstruction [43]. These findings support the potential application of CE-MDCT in defining the spatial extent of irreversible myocardial damage and microvascular obstruction.

Beyond experimental evidence on animal models, late-enhancement MDCT has also been shown to be reliable as DE-MRI in assessing infarction size and viability in human with acute MI. In the study by Mahnken *et al.* [54], 28 patients with acute reperfused MI underwent DE-MRI per usual protocol and 16-MDCT examination with images acquired during the arterial phase and 15 minutes after contrast administration. Compared to normal myocardium, infarcted myocardium had a significant lower CT value (59 ± 17 HU vs 101 ± 15 HU) in the arterial phase but a relatively higher value on

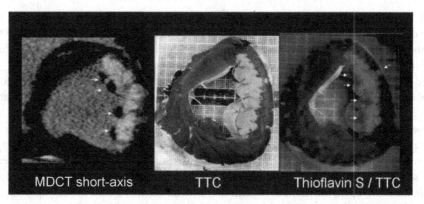

Figure 10.9 **MDCT and histopathologic staining comparison of infarct morphology in a canine model of reperfused myocardial infarction. The reconstructed short-axis MDCT image was taken at 5 minutes after contrast injection and demonstrated a large anterolateral infarct (hyperenhanced region) with discrete endocardial** regions of hypoenhancement (arrows) representing microvascular obstruction. The corresponding TTC and thioflavin stained slices confirm the location, morphology and size of reperfused myocardial infarction and underlying microvascular obstruction. (Reproduced from Lardo *et al.* [43].)

delayed imaging (108 ± 16 HU vs 75 ± 11 HU). Contrast enhancement patterns on DE-MRI and late-enhancement MDCT showed an excellent agreement (kappa score 0.88) while agreement between patterns of DE-MRI and early-perfusion deficits on MDCT was distinctly inferior (kappa 0.64) [54]. This study also proved an excellent agreement but slight systematic overestimation of infarction size as determined by late-enhancement MDCT compared to DE-MRI.

The mechanism and potential utility of CE-MDCT to characterize acute and chronic infarction were evaluated in another study by Gerber *et al.* [55] In his series of work, the time course of contrast enhancement by MDCT was first studied in a porcine nonacute infarction model. The mechanism of contrast enhancement of iodinated agent was also compared to that of gadolinium in ex vivo isolated perfused rabbit hearts. With these experimental results, two groups of patients with acute infarction and chronic ischemic LV dysfunction then underwent first-pass and delayed CE-MRI as well as a dual-stage CE-MDCT examination with image acquisition during the resting arterial phase and at 10 minutes after iodinated contrast injection. In the series of MDCT images of the porcine infarction model, infarcted myocardium demonstrated significantly higher CT signal than the remote region starting 2 minutes and lasting

until 24 minutes after contrast injection. In the isolated perfused rabbit hearts, gadolinium and iodinated agent demonstrated similar wash-in and wash-out rates in the noninfarcted regions as well as the core and peripheral rim of the infarct. The size of bright areas on CE-MDCT measured at 5 minutes after contrast injection also correlated well with infarction size on TTC staining. Among the 37 patients studied, there was an overall moderate concordance (kappa 0.54) in the identification of early hypo-enhanced regions between MDCT and MRI on a segment basis. However, the two techniques were in good agreement in detecting delayed hyperenhanced regions (kappa 0.61). On a patient level, concordance for identification of infarct location was excellent (kappa 0.90). For both the early hypo-enhanced and late hyper-enhanced regions, their corresponding sizes as measured by MDCT and MRI were highly correlated. Consistent with the similar kinetics of iodinated agents and gadolinium as shown, these important results demonstrated that CE-MDCT can characterize acute and chronic infarcts with contrast patterns similar to CE-MRI [55]. Accordingly, hypo-enhanced regions on early MDCT images may reflect microvascular obstruction (the "no-reflow phenomenon") while delayed hyper-enhancement on MDCT analogous to that on DE-MRI may correspond to myocardial necrosis.

In addition to DE-MRI, the clinical value of DE-MDCT in defining viability has also been compared against other imaging modalities. In a study [56] of patients with first acute MI, 64-slice MDCT was performed shortly after invasive coronary angiography without contrast re-injection (mean delay of 24 ± 11 minutes). The extent of hyper-enhancement on MDCT as an indicator of non-viability was compared to viability assessment by low-dose dobutamine echocardiography. MDCT had 98% sensitivity, 94% specificity and 97% accuracy for detecting viable myocardial segments. MDCT performed after invasive coronary angiography for an acute MI may serve as a promising method for early evaluation of myocardial viability [56]. Beyond the acute stage of MI, MDCT can also identify infarcted myocardium in patients with nonacute MI. In a recent report [57] of 101 patients with previous MI, segmental extent of infarcted myocardium as detected by DE-MDCT exhibited good correlation with decreased thallium uptake on SPECT and predicted contractile reserve on dobutamine stress echocardiography. All these observations could place CE-MDCT in a favorable position relative to other current techniques for assessing myocardial viability in patients with coronary artery disease.

As the potential of CE-MDCT for evaluating viability is emerging, concurrent effort to better define its most suitable protocol balancing diagnostic performance, radiation dose and contrast utilization is needed. Higher contrast-to-noise ratio and signal contrast between infarcted and healthy myocardium can be achieved using lower tube voltage at 80 kV [58] which has an added benefit of reducing radiation and thus making the technique more attractive. Although the optimal timing for imaging delayed enhancement has not been robustly defined, delayed MDCT when performed at 5 and 10 minutes after bolus contrast injection apparently performed best in delineating infarction [43,55,59]. Careful selection of contrast bolus geometry may also optimize diagnostic performance. In comparison with the commonly-used pure bolus injection protocol, additional application of a subsequent low-flow contrast material may provide a longer time frame for late imaging and has been shown to enhance signal contrast and image quality for delayed enhancement imaging [60]. Yet, the various technical aspects on how DE-MDCT should be performed remains to be defined before this technique can materialize to become a useful clinical tool.

In summary, the potential of MDCT to evaluate myocardial function, perfusion and viability has been promising. In concert with its unique capability for accurate noninvasive coronary imaging, MDCT has the potential to function as a comprehensive diagnostic tool for noninvasive evaluation of coronary artery disease and its physiological impact on the myocardium. The rapid advancement in MDCT technology in terms of detector coverage, spatial and temporal resolution could bring this closer to reality. Large clinical and prospective studies will be needed to define the diagnostic and prognostic value of integrated MDCT imaging for coronary anatomy, myocardial function, perfusion and viability.

References

1. Vanhoenacker PK, Heijenbrok-Kal MH, Van Heste R, et al. Diagnostic performance of multidetector CT angiography for assessment of coronary artery disease: meta-analysis. *Radiology*. 2007;244:419–428.
2. Miller JM, Rochitte CE, Dewey M, et al. Diagnostic performance of coronary angiography by 64-row CT. *N Engl J Med* 2008;359(22):2324–2336.
3. Iskandrian AS, Chae SC, Heo J, Stanberry CD, Wasserleben V, Cave V. Independent and incremental prognostic value of exercise single-photon emission computed tomographic (SPECT) thallium imaging in coronary artery disease. *J Am Coll Cardiol*. 1993;22:665–670.
4. Hachamovitch R, Hayes SW, Friedman JD, Cohen I, Berman DS. Comparison of the short-term survival benefit associated with revascularization compared with medical therapy in patients with no prior coronary artery disease undergoing stress myocardial perfusion single photon emission computed tomography. *Circulation*. 2003;107:2900–2907.
5. Newhouse JH, Murphy RX, Jr. Tissue distribution of soluble contrast: effect of dose variation and changes with time. *AJR Am J Roentgenol*. 1981;136:463–467.
6. Lima JA, Judd RM, Bazille A, Schulman SP, Atalar E, Zerhouni EA. Regional heterogeneity of human myocardial infarcts demonstrated by contrast-enhanced MRI. Potential mechanisms. *Circulation*. 1995;92:1117–1125.
7. Awai K, Hiraishi K, Hori S. Effect of contrast material injection duration and rate on aortic peak time and peak

enhancement at dynamic CT involving injection protocol with dose tailored to patient weight. *Radiology.* 2004; 230:142–150.

8. Cademartiri F, Nieman K, Van Der Lugt A, *et al.* Intravenous contrast material administration at 16-detector row helical CT coronary angiography: test bolus versus bolus-tracking technique. *Radiology.* 2004;233:817–823.

9. Bae KT, Tran HQ, Heiken JP. Uniform vascular contrast enhancement and reduced contrast medium volume achieved by using exponentially decelerated contrast material injection method. *Radiology.* 2004;231: 732–736.

10. Desjardins B, Kazerooni EA. ECG-gated cardiac CT. *AJR Am J Roentgenol.* 2004;182:993–1010.

11. Jakobs TF, Becker CR, Ohnesorge B, *et al.* Multislice helical CT of the heart with retrospective ECG gating: reduction of radiation exposure by ECG-controlled tube current modulation. *Eur Radiol.* 2002;12:1081–1086.

12. Hundt W, Rust F, Stabler A, Wolff H, Suess C, Reiser M. Dose reduction in multislice computed tomography. *J Comput Assist Tomogr.* 2005;29:140–147.

13. Ritman EL, Robb RA, Johnson SA, *et al.* Quantitative imaging of the structure and function of the heart, lungs, and circulation. *Mayo Clin Proc.* 1978;53:3–11.

14. Lipton MJ, Farmer DW, Killebrew EJ, *et al.* Regional myocardial dysfunction: evaluation of patients with prior myocardial infarction with fast CT. *Radiology.* 1985;157: 735–740.

15. Schroeder S, Kopp AF, Kuettner A, *et al.* Influence of heart rate on vessel visibility in noninvasive coronary angiography using new multislice computed tomography: experience in 94 patients. *Clin Imaging.* 2002;26: 106–111.

16. Yamamuro M, Tadamura E, Kubo S, *et al.* Cardiac functional analysis with multi-detector row CT and segmental reconstruction algorithm: comparison with echocardiography, SPECT, and MR imaging. *Radiology.* 2005; 234:381–390.

17. Papavassiliu T, Kuhl HP, Schroder M, *et al.* Effect of endocardial trabeculae on left ventricular measurements and measurement reproducibility at cardiovascular MR imaging. *Radiology.* 2005;236:57–64.

18. Schmermund A, Rensing BJ, Sheedy PF, Rumberger JA. Reproducibility of right and left ventricular volume measurements by electron-beam CT in patients with congestive heart failure. *Int J Card Imaging.* 1998;14: 201–209.

19. Rumberger JA, Sheedy PF, Breen JF. *Use of Ultrafast (cine) X-ray Computed Tomography in Cardiac and Cardiovascular Imaging.* St Louis: Mosby, 1996, pp. 303–324.

20. Mahnken AH, Koos R, Katoh M, *et al.* Sixteen-slice spiral CT versus MR imaging for the assessment of left ventric-

ular function in acute myocardial infarction. *Eur Radiol.* 2005;15:714–720.

21. Dewey M, Muller M, Teige F, Hamm B. Evaluation of a semiautomatic software tool for left ventricular function analysis with 16-slice computed tomography. *Eur Radiol.* 2006;16:25–31.

22. Heuschmid M, Rothfuss JK, Schroeder S, *et al.* Assessment of left ventricular myocardial function using 16-slice multidetector-row computed tomography: comparison with magnetic resonance imaging and echocardiography. *Eur Radiol.* 2006;16:551–559.

23. Raman SV, Shah M, McCarthy B, Garcia A, Ferketich AK. Multi-detector row cardiac computed tomography accurately quantifies right and left ventricular size and function compared with cardiac magnetic resonance. *Am Heart J.* 2006;151:736–744.

24. Schuijf JD, Bax JJ, Jukema JW, *et al.* Noninvasive evaluation of the coronary arteries with multislice computed tomography in hypertensive patients. *Hypertension.* 2005; 45:227–232.

25. Schuijf JD, Bax JJ, Jukema JW, *et al.* Assessment of left ventricular volumes and ejection fraction with 16-slice multi-slice computed tomography; comparison with 2D-echocardiography. *Int J Cardiol.* 2007;116:201–205.

26. Lawler LP, Ney D, Pannu HK, Fishman EK. Four-dimensional imaging of the heart based on near-isotropic MDCT data sets. *AJR Am J Roentgenol.* 2005;184:774–776.

27. Cerqueira MD, Weissman NJ, Dilsizian V, *et al.* Standardized myocardial segmentation and nomenclature for tomographic imaging of the heart: a statement for healthcare professionals from the Cardiac Imaging Committee of the Council on Clinical Cardiology of the American Heart Association. *Circulation.* 2002;105:539–542.

28. Elgeti T, Lembcke A, Enzweiler CN, Breitwieser C, Hamm B, Kivelitz DE. Comparison of electron beam computed tomography with magnetic resonance imaging in assessment of right ventricular volumes and function. *J Comput Assist Tomogr.* 2004;28:679–685.

29. Koch K, Oellig F, Oberholzer K, *et al.* Assessment of right ventricular function by 16-detector-row CT: comparison with magnetic resonance imaging. *Eur Radiol.* 2005;15: 312–318.

30. Raman SV, Cook SC, McCarthy B, Ferketich AK. Usefulness of multidetector row computed tomography to quantify right ventricular size and function in adults with either tetralogy of Fallot or transposition of the great arteries. *Am J Cardiol.* 2005;95:683–686.

31. Quiroz R, Kucher N, Schoepf UJ, *et al.* Right ventricular enlargement on chest computed tomography: prognostic role in acute pulmonary embolism. *Circulation.* 2004; 109:2401–2404.

32. Van Der Meer RW, Pattynama PM, van Strijen MJ, *et al.* Right ventricular dysfunction and pulmonary obstruction index at helical CT: prediction of clinical outcome during 3-month follow-up in patients with acute pulmonary embolism. *Radiology.* 2005;235:798–803.

33. Bomma C, Dalal D, Tandri H, *et al.* Evolving role of multidetector computed tomography in evaluation of arrhythmogenic right ventricular dysplasia/cardiomyopathy. *Am J Cardiol.* 2007;100:99–105.

34. Uren NG, Melin JA, De Bruyne B, Wijns W, Baudhuin T, Camici PG. Relation between myocardial blood flow and the severity of coronary-artery stenosis. *N Engl J Med.* 1994;330:1782–1788.

35. Hacker M, Jakobs T, Matthiesen F, *et al.* Comparison of spiral multidetector CT angiography and myocardial perfusion imaging in the noninvasive detection of functionally relevant coronary artery lesions: first clinical experiences. *J Nucl Med.* 2005;46:1294–1300.

36. Schuijf JD, Wijns W, Jukema JW, *et al.* Relationship between noninvasive coronary angiography with multislice computed tomography and myocardial perfusion imaging. *J Am Coll Cardiol.* 2006;48:2508–2514.

37. Rispler S, Keidar Z, Ghersin E, *et al.* Integrated single-photon emission computed tomography and computed tomography coronary angiography for the assessment of hemodynamically significant coronary artery lesions. *J Am Coll Cardiol.* 2007;49:1059–1067.

38. Gould RG, Lipton MJ, McNamara MT, Sievers RE, Koshold S, Higgins CB. Measurement of regional myocardial blood flow in dogs by ultrafast CT. *Invest Radiol.* 1988;23:348–353.

39. Bell MR, Lerman LO, Rumberger JA. Validation of minimally invasive measurement of myocardial perfusion using electron beam computed tomography and application in human volunteers. *Heart.* 1999;81:628–635.

40. Mahnken AH, Bruners P, Katoh M, Wildberger JE, Gunther RW, Buecker A. Dynamic multi-section CT imaging in acute myocardial infarction: preliminary animal experience. *Eur Radiol.* 2006;16:746–752.

41. George RT, Jerosch-Herold M, Silva C, *et al.* Quantification of myocardial perfusion using dynamic 64-detector computed tomography. *Invest Radiol.* 2007;42:815–822.

42. Hoffmann U, Millea R, Enzweiler C, *et al.* Acute myocardial infarction: contrast-enhanced multi-detector row CT in a porcine model. *Radiology.* 2004;231:697–701.

43. Lardo AC, Cordeiro MA, Silva C, *et al.* Contrast-enhanced multidetector computed tomography viability imaging after myocardial infarction: characterization of myocyte death, microvascular obstruction, and chronic scar. *Circulation.* 2006;113:394–404.

44. George RT, Silva C, Cordeiro MA, *et al.* Multidetector computed tomography myocardial perfusion imaging during adenosine stress. *J Am Coll Cardiol.* 2006;48:153–160.

45. George RT, Resar J, Silva C, *et al.* Combined computed tomography coronary angiography and perfusion imaging accurately detects the physiological significance of coronary stenoses in patients with chest pain. *Circulation.* 2006;114:691–692.

46. George RT, Lardo AC, Silva C, Bluemke DA, Resar J, Lima JAC. Subendocardial perfusion deficits predict the functional significance of coronary stenoses during adenosine stress multidetector computed tomography in patients with chest pain . *J Am Coll Cardiol.* 2007;49(9):161A.

47. Kroll K, Wilke N, Jerosch-Herold M, *et al.* Modeling regional myocardial flows from residue functions of an intravascular indicator. *Am J Physiol.* 1996;271:H1643–H1655.

48. Alderman EL, Fisher LD, Litwin P, *et al.* Results of coronary artery surgery in patients with poor left ventricular function (CASS). *Circulation.* 1983;68:785–795.

49. Pagley PR, Beller GA, Watson DD, Gimple LW, Ragosta M. Improved outcome after coronary bypass surgery in patients with ischemic cardiomyopathy and residual myocardial viability. *Circulation.* 1997;96:793–800.

50. Bax JJ, Schinkel AF, Boersma E, *et al.* Early versus delayed revascularization in patients with ischemic cardiomyopathy and substantial viability: impact on outcome. *Circulation.* 2003;108(Suppl. 1):II39–II42.

51. Kim RJ, Wu E, Rafael A, *et al.* The use of contrast-enhanced magnetic resonance imaging to identify reversible myocardial dysfunction. *N Engl J Med.* 2000;343:1445–1453.

52. Gray WR, Jr, Parkey RW, Buja LM, *et al.* Computed tomography: in vitro evaluation of myocardial infarction. *Radiology.* 1977;122:511–513.

53. Nikolaou K, Sanz J, Poon M, *et al.* Assessment of myocardial perfusion and viability from routine contrast-enhanced 16-detector-row computed tomography of the heart: preliminary results. *Eur Radiol.* 2005;15:864–871.

54. Mahnken AH, Koos R, Katoh M, *et al.* Assessment of myocardial viability in reperfused acute myocardial infarction using 16-slice computed tomography in comparison to magnetic resonance imaging. *J Am Coll Cardiol.* 2005;45:2042–2047.

55. Gerber BL, Belge B, Legros GJ, *et al.* Characterization of acute and chronic myocardial infarcts by multidetector computed tomography: comparison with contrast-enhanced magnetic resonance. *Circulation.* 2006;113:823–833.

56. Habis M, Capderou A, Ghostine S, *et al.* Acute myocardial infarction early viability assessment by 64-slice computed tomography immediately after coronary

angiography: comparison with low-dose dobutamine echocardiography. *J Am Coll Cardiol.* 2007;49:1178–1185.

57. Chiou KR, Liu CP, Peng NJ, *et al.* Identification and viability assessment of infarcted myocardium with late enhancement multidetector computed tomography: comparison with thallium single photon emission computed tomography and echocardiography. *Am Heart J.* 2008; 155:738–745.

58. Mahnken AH, Bruners P, Muhlenbruch G, *et al.* Low tube voltage improves computed tomography imaging of delayed myocardial contrast enhancement in an experi-

mental acute myocardial infarction model. *Invest Radiol.* 2007;42:123–129.

59. Buecker A, Katoh M, Krombach GA, *et al.* A feasibility study of contrast enhancement of acute myocardial infarction in multislice computed tomography: comparison with magnetic resonance imaging and gross morphology in pigs. *Invest Radiol.* 2005;40:700–704.

60. Brodoefel H, Reimann A, Klumpp B, *et al.* Assessment of myocardial viability in a reperfused porcine model: evaluation of different MSCT contrast protocols in acute and subacute infarct stages in comparison with MRI. *J Comput Assist Tomogr.* 2007;31:290–298.

CHAPTER 11

Cardiac Computed Tomography and Magnetic Resonance for the Evaluation of Acute Chest Pain in the Emergency Department

Eric M. Thorn & Charles S. White
University of Maryland School of Medicine, Baltimore, MD, USA

Introduction

Each year, chest pain accounts for nearly six million visits to emergency departments (ED) in the United States, making this one of the most common presenting complaints [1]. Of these visits, only a minority are caused by the triad of acute coronary syndrome (ACS), aortic dissection, or pulmonary embolism [2]. This makes differentiating the patients who require admission and treatment from those who can be safely discharged a significant challenge for the ED physician. In approximately 2% of patients with acute myocardial infarction and 2% of those with unstable angina the diagnosis is missed and these patients are inappropriately discharged from the ED [3]. Mortality of those patients who are inappropriately discharged is almost double that of those who are admitted [3]. On the other hand, most patients presenting with chest pain, who are admitted to chest pain units and telemetry units, will ultimately be found to have a noncardiac cause for their pain [2]. The admission of these patients, most of whom would have a good prognosis regardless, is a significant financial and opportunity burden on already strained medical systems with limited resources. Additionally, inability to exclude

ACS rapidly in patients with noncardiac pain will expose a certain proportion of them to medical and invasive diagnostic and therapeutic interventions that carry small but significant risks.

Standard Approach to the Diagnosis of Pulmonary Embolism and Aortic Dissection

Developments in multidetector computed tomography (MDCT) and, to a lesser degree, magnetic resonance imaging (MRI) have revolutionized the diagnostic approach toward pulmonary embolism over the past decade. For pulmonary embolism, MDCT has become the diagnostic reference standard. Reported sensitivity and specificity range from 83 to 100% and 89 to 97% respectively [4]. Current technology permits visualization of the pulmonary arteries to a subsegmental level. The use of clinical prediction rules and D-dimer testing allows ED physicians to use MDCT judiciously, forgoing scanning in patients with low likelihood of pulmonary embolism and a negative D-dimer. Using such a strategy limits the number of scans required in suspected pulmonary embolism while maintaining very low rates of subsequent venous thromboembolism or death [5,6]. The use of MDCT for the diagnosis of pulmonary embolism is advantageous in that the study is noninvasive,

Cardiac CT, PET and MR, 2nd edition. Edited by Vasken Dilsizian and Gerry Pohost. © 2010 Blackwell Publishing Ltd.

short in duration, and generally performed in close proximity to the ED. Protocols require the injection of a bolus of iodinated contrast dye through a large bore peripheral intravenous catheter at a rate of approximately 4 mL/second. The scan acquisition is carefully timed using either bolus tracking or a test bolus to maximize enhancement of the pulmonary artery. The scan is generally performed in a diaphragmatic to apical direction during a breath-hold. Reconstruction is typically at a slice thickness of ≤1.25 mm, with better scan quality with narrower collimation and slice thickness [7]. While electrocardiographic gating is not required for the assessment of pulmonary embolism by MDCT, gating does provide certain advantages. First is the ability to evaluate right ventricular size and function [8], an important prognostic marker in acute pulmonary embolism. Second, electrocardiographic gating can improve image quality of the pulmonary arteries, with optimal quality in diastolic reconstructions [9]. Thus, electrocardiographic gating of MDCT scans for the diagnosis of pulmonary embolism may result in improved diagnostic accuracy and certainty.

Technologic improvements in MRI, parallel imaging in particular, have improved spatial and temporal resolution and acquisition times to the point that MRI is now a viable option for the diagnostic evaluation of suspected pulmonary embolism. The most commonly used approaches include either high-resolution or time-resolved three-dimensional (3D) gadolinium contrast enhanced gradient echo pulmonary magnetic resonance angiography (MRA). High-resolution sequences allow for submillimeter pulmonary angiography. On the other hand, time-resolved sequences have less spatial resolution but better temporal resolution. This decreases motion artifact, allows separation of arteries and veins, and allows for imaging of lung perfusion. Using these techniques, reported sensitivities of MRI for the detection of pulmonary embolism are greater than 70% and specificities are greater than 90% [10]. However, while sensitivity of MRA for central, lobar, and segmental arteries is high, the utility of MRA for detection of subsegmental pulmonary emboli is not as good. In a recent study with enough pulmonary emboli to look at anatomic subgroups, the sensitivity for subsegmental pulmonary emboli was only 40%

[11]. Another useful approach to the pulmonary arterial evaluation with MRI is real time steady-state precession two-dimensional (2D) imaging. The acquisition of these images is rapid and does not require contrast administration. Using real time 2D imaging, Kluge et al. reported patient-based sensitivity and specificity of 90 and 98% respectively [12]. The best approach for the use of MRI to diagnose pulmonary embolism may be a combined one that incorporates MRA techniques and real time 2D imaging. Kluge et al. report that such an approach improved patient-based sensitivity to 100% while only marginally decreasing specificity to 93% [12]. Despite these encouraging results, MRI presents a number of limitations. In addition to limited sensitivity for subsegmental emboli, scan times are longer than those of MDCT, availability of MRI scanners to patients in the ED is often limited in terms of proximity and hours of operation, and ability to detect other pulmonary pathology is low. Still, the use of MRI for the detection of pulmonary emboli is an important option for patients who have a contraindication to iodinated contrast dye or in whom radiation exposure related to MDCT is a concern.

In the case of suspected aortic dissection, imaging with either MDCT or MRI is the standard non-invasive diagnostic approach. Though individual studies are small due to the low incidence of aortic dissection, a recent meta-analysis found sensitivities and specificities of MDCT and MRI to be greater than 95% [13]. MDCT is particularly attractive as a diagnostic modality for aortic dissection due to the rapidity with which a scan can be performed and the proximity of scanners to most EDs. These are extremely important considerations given the inherent instability of patients with ascending aortic dissections. MDCT performed for the detection of aortic dissection should start with a noncontrast-enhanced scan to evaluate for the presence of intramural hematoma. Such a hematoma will be apparent as increase in aortic wall thickness with increased radiodensity. In the absence of a dissection flap and false lumen, an intramural hematoma may not be visible following the administration of contrast. Following the nonenhanced scan, iodinated contrast is infused through a large bore peripheral intravenous catheter at a rate of 3–5 mL/second. A bolus tracking technique is used to time the scan for optimal aortic enhancement. Thin slice reconstructed images are then evaluated in the axial orientation with use of other orientations and multiplanar and maximal intensity reconstructions as required. One of the challenges of using MDCT for the diagnosis of aortic dissection is in differentiating motion artifact from true aortic dissection. The aortic root and proximal aorta are particularly susceptible to such artifact due to motion related to the cardiac cycle. For this reason, it may be advantageous to gate MDCT examinations electrocardiographically for the detection of aortic dissection.

For MRI examinations of suspected aortic dissection, a combination of 3D gadolinium contrast enhanced MRA and T_1 weighted black blood spin echo images are primarily used. The MRA allows for full volume visualization of the aortic lumen while the 2D technique allows for visualization of the aortic wall in addition to the lumen. Black blood techniques also allow differentiation of the true and false lumens based on incomplete blood signal suppression due to slow flow or thrombus in the false lumen. In general, MDCT is the preferred modality over MRI for reasons of patient instability, scanner proximity, and speed of examination. However, with improvements MRI including the development of fast spin echo sequences and the rapidity with which a 3D MRA can be performed, the advantage of MDCT over MRI is narrowing. Furthermore, the use of steady-state free precession sequences for 2D imaging may allow for equivalent accuracy to studies done using 3D contrast enhanced MRA [14]. This would be advantageous for the evaluation of patients with acute or chronic kidney disease in whom iodinated and gadolinium-based contrast are relatively contraindicated.

Standard Approach to the Diagnosis of ACS

The term ACS encompasses a spectrum of presentations ranging from unstable angina to ST segment elevation myocardial infarction. These clinical presentations share the common pathophysiology of myocardial ischemia secondary to coronary artery obstruction. The diagnosis of ACS is challenging due to the nonspecific nature of the most common presenting complaint—chest pain. In the case

of pulmonary embolism and aortic dissection, this challenge is largely surmounted by the availability of highly accurate noninvasive imaging tools. Unfortunately, until recently, two characteristics of ACS have limited the diagnostic role of noninvasive imaging in this disease. First, ACS is caused by rupture or erosion of atherosclerotic plaques and subsequent thrombosis within coronary arteries. Prior to the development of cardiac computed tomography (CCT), the small size of these arteries and their motion with the cardiac cycle has prevented accurate anatomic assessment. Second, the process of plaque rupture, thrombosis, and resultant ischemia is a dynamic one, limiting the opportunity for functional imaging to the time of actual symptoms. This makes imaging challenging since the symptoms are by definition transient in cases of ACS that do not require immediate invasive angiography.

Due to these diagnostic challenges and the imperative to avoid inappropriate discharge of patients with ACS, a standard approach to the diagnosis of ACS has evolved that incorporates an initial evaluation followed by a period of prolonged observation. Initial evaluation of patients with chest pain includes the triad of clinical history, electrocardiogram (ECG), and cardiac biomarkers. Patients experience typical ischemic chest pain as pressure or heaviness that may radiate to the arms or neck, occurs with exertion, and improves following usage of sublingual nitroglycerin. However, in ACS, the clinical presentation is often atypical, limiting the sensitivity and specificity of the patient history [15,16]. This is not to say that the clinical history is unimportant. Particular chest pain characteristic may increase or decrease the likelihood of ACS. This information is critical in determining pretest probability for ACS in order to apply Bayesian analysis to the interpretation of the results of subsequent diagnostic testing.

The second component of the initial assessment, the ECG, is diagnostic in the case of ST segment elevation myocardial infarction and occasionally diagnostic for nonST segment elevation myocardial infarction. Often, however, the ECG is nondiagnostic or normal. Pope *et al.* found that 20% of ECGs were normal in the setting of acute myocardial infarction and 37% were normal in the setting of unstable angina [2]. This is likely secondary to the intermittent nature of coronary ischemia and the fact that the lateral and apical territories of the myocardium are inadequately represented by conventional ECG leads [17].

In acute myocardial infarction, cardiac specific biomarkers of necrosis are present in the blood at detectable levels within 2–4 hours following the onset of symptoms. In a meta-analysis, sensitivity of initial biomarkers for acute myocardial infarction ranged from 37 to 49% [18]. For ACS, including unstable angina in which myocardial injury has not occurred, sensitivity of initial markers decreased to 16–19% [18]. Even when positive, the presence of biomarker elevation only confirms the presence of myocardial injury, not the presence of ACS. [18] Elevation of cardiac biomarkers can be seen in myocarditis, pericarditis, pulmonary embolism, sepsis, heart failure, or other conditions resulting in ischemia, hemodynamic imbalance, or inflammation [19]. Because of the limitations of the initial evaluation for diagnosing ACS, a period of observation is required to improve diagnostic sensitivity. The rationale for this is that with time, even if not detected initially, biomarkers will eventually be detectable in patients with acute myocardial infarction. In the meta-analysis referenced above, sensitivity of cardiac biomarkers for myocardial infarction increased to 79–93% when serial measurements were performed [18]. Higher sensitivity is found with longer durations between tests, with a recommendation from the American College of Cardiology and American Heart Association for repeat testing 8–12 hours after the initial lab draw [20].

The foremost advantage of this standard approach to the evaluation of patients with chest pain is that it allows for diagnosis of ACS with high sensitivity. Following initial evaluation and observation, ED physicians hospitalize more than 90% of patients with ACS [21]. However, this diagnostic accuracy comes at a cost. The high sensitivity of the current diagnostic strategy for ACS is achieved by using a very low threshold for admission and treatment. A large proportion of those patients hospitalized with chest pain do not have ACS. This represents a significant allocation of financial and logistical resources for the care of patients who ultimately are at very low risk of experiencing a morbid or mortal event. Additionally, these low risk patients bear a personal cost in that some of them will be exposed to diagnostic and therapeutic

interventions including anticoagulants, antiplatelet agents, and cardiac catheterization. These represent finite but significant sources of iatrogenic risk that is not appropriately balanced by individual benefit in the cases of these low risk patients. Beyond the risk of experiencing adverse health consequences, these patients with noncardiac chest pain who undergo hospitalization or prolonged observation also bear the costs of inconvenience, lost work, and anxiety.

There is a need for strategies for the evaluation of chest pain patients that preserve high diagnostic sensitivity while simultaneously reducing the burden of the current strategy born by patients and society. A useful addition to the current strategy for the evaluation of chest pain would be highly accurate, expeditious, relatively inexpensive, and safe to patients. The addition of noninvasive cardiac imaging modalities to the current approach to ACS has the potential to achieve all of these goals.

Noninvasive Imaging in the Evaluation of ACS

To date, the most widely used noninvasive imaging modalities for the evaluation of possible ACS include the chest radiograph, transthoracic echocardiography, and radionuclide perfusion imaging. The chest radiograph is most commonly the first imaging modality used in the evaluation of the chest pain patient. This allows rapid diagnosis of noncardiac causes of chest pain such as pneumonia, pneumothorax, or rib fracture. However, while identification of coronary artery calcification is sometimes possible, such detection is neither sensitive nor specific for ACS [22,23]. The most common roles of echocardiography and radionuclide perfusion imaging are as modalities for stratification of patients subsequent to observation and a negative serial biomarker evaluation. Given the limitations of cardiac biomarker assessment in the presence of acute coronary ischemia without necrosis, these imaging modalities are important adjuncts allowing identification of high-risk patients with obstructive coronary disease. This improvement in diagnostic sensitivity using stress testing comes at the cost of prolongation of patient stays and additional financial burden.

An alternative approach to the use of echocardiography and radionuclide perfusion imaging is that of acute chest pain imaging. Chest pain resulting from myocardial ischemia is the end result of a series of pathophysiologic events including the development of perfusion mismatches leading to abnormalities of diastolic and systolic myocardial function [24]. When imaging is employed during episodes of ischemia, identification of these abnormalities that occur upstream from the clinical presentation of chest pain identify the pain as being ischemic in etiology. Studies investigating the accuracy of resting echocardiography in patients presenting with acute chest pain are difficult to apply in clinical practice due to variability in the populations studied in terms of overall risk, variability in the endpoints evaluated, and the fact that most of these studies were performed over a decade ago and did not take advantage of newer technologies. Though some studies have demonstrated a high negative predictive value of resting echocardiography for detection of myocardial infarction, when unstable angina is included as an endpoint, negative predictive value is substantially lower [25]. This limitation can be attributed to multiple factors. Ischemia in ACS is dynamic. While myocardial stunning can result in persistence of wall motion abnormalities [26], the absence of wall motion abnormalities does not imply that a chest pain episode was not due to myocardial ischemia if the pain is not present at the time of imaging. If the territory of ischemia or infarction is small, a segmental wall motion abnormality may not be present [27]. In addition, there are logistical limitations to the use of rest echocardiography in the ED. Transthoracic echocardiography is very operator dependent and requires highly trained personnel for study acquisition and interpretation. Technologic advances such as the use of microbubble echocontrast for enhanced endomyocardial border definition [28,29], perfusion assessment [30,31], or molecular imaging [32] may ultimately overcome some of the challenges to the use of echocardiography for the assessment of acute chest pain. At this time however, none of these advances are positioned to become clinical diagnostic options in most EDs.

Radionuclide perfusion imaging with single-photon emission computed tomography (SPECT) at the time of presentation takes advantage of the fact that ischemic chest pain episodes are preceded by and correspond to relative deficits in myocardial perfusion. The myocardium takes up Technetium-99m-based perfusion tracers injected during chest pain based on relative flow and viability of myocytes. Since Technetium-99m-based tracers do not redistribute, imaging 45–60 minutes following injection reflects the pathophysiologic conditions present at the time of injection. When used for the evaluation of symptomatic patients with nondiagnostic findings on ECG, this technique has a very high sensitivity for acute myocardial infarction, ranging from 99 to 100% across multiple single-center observational studies [33]. In multicenter, randomized comparison with the standard ACS evaluation approach, the use of Technetium-99m acute chest pain perfusion imaging had equivalent diagnostic accuracy for acute myocardial infarction and unstable angina [34]. However, the rest perfusion-based strategy was significantly more effective at identifying low risk non-ACS patients, reducing hospitalizations of patients without ACS from 52 to 42%. Other reports suggest that a rest radionuclide imaging strategy would reduce hospital length of stays and angiography rates as well [35]. Thus, despite the additive cost of the imaging study itself, a radionuclide SPECT-based strategy meaningfully reduces financial costs and utilization of limited hospital resources. Unfortunately, similar to the case of rest echocardiography, widespread implementation of rest SPECT imaging has not occurred. This is likely secondary to the significant logistic commitment involved requiring availability of the radionuclide tracer, a physician or technician to inject it, a SPECT camera with a technician to perform the imaging, and a nuclear cardiologist or radiologist to interpret the images.

Computed Tomographic Calcium Scoring for the Evaluation of Acute Chest Pain

The progression of coronary atherosclerosis is marked by calcification of atherosclerotic plaques [36]. Electrocardiographic gated CCT can detect and quantify this calcification. The presence of coronary calcification on CCT is pathognomonic for the presence of atherosclerosis. The extent of such calcification correlates with both extent of atherosclerosis [37] and the presence of obstructive stenoses [38]. In symptomatic patients undergoing angiography for clinical indications, the sensitivity of the presence of any coronary calcium for a stenosis >50% is 95–99% [39]. Beyond correlation with anatomic coronary disease, calcium detected by CCT in symptomatic and asymptomatic patients is predictive of nonfatal myocardial infarction, cardiovascular death, and all-cause mortality [40–42].

As a tool for the evaluation of acute chest pain patients, CCT calcium scoring is limited in that it is not able to identify the presence of an unstable plaque or myocardial ischemia or infarction. However, the ability to identify the presence or absence of atherosclerotic plaque has potential to allow for identification of the subgroup of noncardiac chest pain patients presenting to the ED who are very likely to have no coronary disease and thus, by definition, are at minimal risk for ACS. To date, the use of CCT calcium scoring in acute chest pain patients has been investigated in four single-center studies (Table 11.1) [43–46]. Each of these studies excluding that of Esteves *et al.* enrolled patients presenting to the ED with chest pain and a non-diagnostic ECG who did not have a prior history of coronary artery disease. This exclusion is important, as the cutoff value for the determination of a positive test in these studies was the presence of any calcification. Patients with a history of coronary artery disease are expected to have calcium regardless of whether they are in the midst of an ACS and thus the calcium score would not be expected to provide additive information to the clinical history. Despite using different reference standards for the determination of the presence of ACS, these studies each demonstrated relatively high sensitivity with values ranging from 82 to 100%. Specificities on the

other hand were much lower, ranging from 37 to 63%. This is not surprising given that the presence of calcium on CCT is not reflective of underlying ACS, but rather the underlying substrate necessary for ACS to occur. Patients without a history of coronary disease who present to the ED with chest pain have a relatively low prevalence of ACS, and the sample populations in these studies reflect this. As a result, the low specificity of CCT calcium detection for ACS translates into very low positive predictive values.

Given the high sensitivity and low specificity of CCT calcium scoring, its role would appear to be as a screening tool to rapidly exclude the presence of ACS and identify acute chest pain patients whom the ED physician can rapidly discharge. This could result in a substantial reduction in financial costs, resource utilization, and patient risk. It is important then to examine the reasons for the small number of false negatives. In the study by Georgiou *et al.*, the one participant without coronary calcification who had a definite myocardial infarction was young (age 38 years compared to a mean age for the study of 55 years) [45]. In the study by McLaughlin *et al.*, the one participant without coronary calcification who had ACS was a 45-year-old cocaine user [44]. These two cases do not allow for conclusions. However, they suggest that the use of CCT calcium scoring may not be ideal for younger patients who may be more likely to have isolated noncalcified plaque at earlier stages in the development of coronary artery disease or for abusers of cocaine who may be at risk for coronary spasm, intracoronary thrombus formation, noncalcified atherosclerosis, and non-ACS cardiovascular complications [47]. The supposition that younger patients are more likely to have ACS in

Table 11.1   Diagnostic accuracy studies of CCT calcium scoring for the detection of ACS.

Study	N (total)	Reference standard for ACS	Prevalence of ACS	Sensitivity (%)	Specificity (%)	PPV (%)	NPV (%)
Laudon [43]	100	Positive stress test or angiography	14	100	63	30	100
McLaughlin [44]	134	In hospital death, AMI, or revascularization	6	88	37	8	98
Georgiou [45]	138	AMI by biomarkers or ECG	12	82	50	19	95
Esteves [46]	84	Positive stress MPI	15	100	48	26	100

ACS, acute coronary syndrome; AMI, acute myocardial infarction; MPI, myocardial perfusion scan.

the absence of coronary calcification is supported by data from Schmermund *et al.* from a study of 118 ACS patients [48]. They found that the 12 patients without calcification had similar cardiac risk factors to but were on average 12 years younger than those with calcification. Rubinshtein *et al.* made similar observations in a retrospective study of 668 chest pain patients who underwent 64-slice CCT coronary angiography [49]. Of those with an acute presentation, 7% of those with a calcium score of zero had obstructive coronary disease. These patients were younger and more likely to be women. This group also noted that obstructive coronary disease with no or minor calcification tended to be more frequent in acute chest pain presentations compared to stable chest pain presentations. This is consistent with a recent report of the 64-slice CCT coronary angiography results from 40 ACS patients in which only 14% of observed plaques were calcified while 86% were mixed or noncalcified [50]. Figure 11.1 is an example of a patient with a calcium score of zero in whom CCT coronary angiography revealed a significant stenosis.

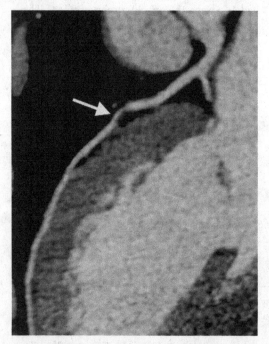

Figure 11.1 Example of a significant left anterior descending coronary artery stenosis in a patient with a coronary calcium score of zero (yellow arrow).

Due to the small proportion of ACS patients who do not have coronary calcification, if ED physicians are to use CCT calcium scoring for early triage, patient selection will be important. With a properly selected patient population, the high negative predictive value of a CCT calcium scoring based strategy for acute chest pain could allow diagnostic performance equivalent to current standard approaches. However, to achieve such results, it may be necessary to reserve this tool for patients over a certain age, possibly dependent on gender. A potential problem with such a strategy is that the increase in coronary calcification seen with age will likely minimize the number of patients who have no calcification and thus will minimize the benefit of CCT calcium scoring for this patient population. At this point, the use of CCT calcium scoring for acute chest pain requires validation in larger, multicenter trials before it can be implemented clinically.

Beyond the potential cost benefits of a CCT calcium scoring based strategy for acute chest pain, this strategy may have value in determination of long-term prognosis. Georgiou *et al.* followed 192 patients who were admitted to the ED with chest pain and did not experience a cardiac event during the admission [51]. Over an average follow-up of 50 months, the absence of coronary artery calcium was associated with a very low annualized event rate of <1% (Figure 11.2). In a multivariate analysis, including traditional risk factors, coronary calcium was a strong independent predictor of events.

Computed Tomographic Coronary Angiography for the Evaluation of Acute Chest Pain

Ultimately, the inability of CCT coronary calcium imaging to detect noncalcified coronary plaques means that a more comprehensive approach to the evaluation of acute chest pain patients for ACS is necessary. ACS is typically the result of in situ thrombosis on an underlying ruptured or eroded atherosclerotic plaque [52]. The thrombus that forms results in significant coronary stenosis in 80–90% of ACS [53]. An ideal imaging strategy for the detection of ACS would therefore include assessment for the presence of coronary stenoses and intraluminal thrombi, and characterization of

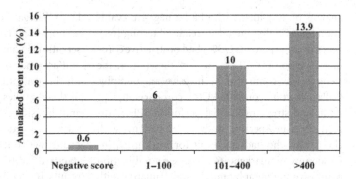

Figure 11.2 Annualized rates for future cardiovascular events by Cox proportional-hazards regression. Patients with scores >400 had an event rate of 58% over the entire study, with an annualized event rate of 13.9%. This was significantly greater than the 0.6% annual event rate of those with scores of zero ($p < 0.001$). (Adapted from Georgiou et al. [51], with permission.)

atherosclerotic plaques. Invasive coronary angiography provides these capabilities. However, due to rare but serious risks to patients, high costs, and high resource requirements, the use of invasive angiography is reserved for patients with a clear diagnosis of ACS and high-risk features on clinical presentation or stress testing [20]. With the advancement of MDCT technology, CCT coronary angiography may offer a noninvasive alternative to coronary angiography that overcomes the limitations of this invasive approach.

The current generation of MDCT scanners has 64–320 detector rows and one or two X-ray sources. These scanners are capable of imaging with isotropic spatial resolution of approximately 0.4 mm and temporal resolutions as low as 83 ms [54]. These parameters are inferior to those of invasive coronary angiography, which has spatial resolution of approximately 0.2 mm and temporal resolution of approximately 5 ms. Despite these inferiorities, CCT coronary angiography is highly accurate for the detection of coronary stenoses. In a meta-analysis of published diagnostic accuracy studies using invasive angiography as a reference standard, Abdulla et al. found the sensitivity and specificity of CCT coronary angiography to be 97.5 and 91% respectively in a per-patient analysis [55]. Most of the studies included in this meta-analysis were performed in populations of patients with stable angina with an intermediate to high prevalence of coronary disease [55]. However, studies including non-ST segment elevation ACS patients have reported similar findings [56–60]. In addition to the capability to detect coronary stenoses, CCT angiography may allow for detection of intraluminal thrombus. In a sample of ACS patients, Dorgelo et al. noted thrombus in 53%

[59]. Criteria used for identification of thrombus included the identification of a filling defect with an intraluminal position, irregular borders, and low density (19.3 ± 7.3 HU) [59]. An advantage of CCT coronary angiography over invasive coronary angiography is that CCT angiography allows visualization of the vessel walls in addition to the lumen. CCT coronary angiography has been used to characterize plaques based on morphology [61,62] and MDCT density [63,64]. With the ability to identify coronary stenoses and intraluminal thrombus and to characterize plaques, CCT coronary angiography can identify the ultimate upstream event in the ischemic cascade, potentially making it a highly sensitive test for the detection of ACS, even compared to resting echocardiography or SPECT.

Due to the insensitivity of serial ECGs and cardiac biomarkers for the detection of unstable angina, the standard approach to the evaluation of ACS typically includes evaluation with a stress ECG test with or without the inclusion of echocardiographic or SPECT imaging. One potential role for CCT coronary angiography would be as an alternative to these diagnostic modalities. Similar to the cases of stress echocardiography and stress myocardial perfusion imaging, CCT coronary angiography has been demonstrated to be superior to exercise treadmill ECG testing in the setting of acute chest pain. Rubinshtein et al. performed a retrospective analysis of 103 consecutive patients with chest pain who had undergone CCT coronary angiography in addition to a standard evaluation including serial ECGs, serial biomarkers, and exercise treadmill testing [65]. They found obstructive coronary disease in 22% of those with a negative treadmill test and 39% of those with a nondiagnostic exercise treadmill test. Bonello et al. reported similar findings in a prospective analysis of 30 patients who had a negative evaluation for ACS that included treadmill testing [66]. Seven of these patients (23%) had obstructive coronary disease on CCT. In each of these cases, the stenosis was confirmed by invasive angiography. Gallagher *et al.* compared CCT coronary angiography and stress myocardial perfusion SPECT directly in a prospective study of 92 patients with chest pain who had ruled out for myocardial infarction by biomarkers [67]. Using a combination of invasive angiography and clinical evaluation with 1-month follow-up as a reference standard, they found comparable sensitivities of 71 and 86% and specificities of 90 and 92% for stress nuclear imaging and CCT respectively. However, this study was limited by wide confidence intervals around these values and the fact that 7 of the 92 patients were not included in the analysis due to technically uninterpretable CCT scans.

In the standard evaluation of acute chest pain, the primary reason for delaying stress testing until after the resolution of pain and completion of serial ECGs and biomarkers is to avoid inappropriately stressing a patient with a not yet detected myocardial infarction. As discussed above, rest echocardiography and myocardial perfusion SPECT protocols are used to avoid the necessity of a period of prolonged observation. However, these techniques are limited by logistical challenges and the fact that the abnormalities that they detect may not be present once a patient's chest pain has resolved. CCT coronary angiography has the advantage of being able to detect the underlying abnormality

in ACS regardless of the presence of symptoms without requiring stress. A number of small observational studies have investigated the feasibility and accuracy of early CCT coronary angiography for the evaluation of possible ACS [65,68–76]. All of these studies are limited by small sample sizes and by single-center enrollment. Furthermore, there is considerable variability in methodological quality with only two studies employing a reference standard for ACS that was fully blinded to the CCT results [68,69]. Moreover, the reference standard employed by most of these studies was a combination of invasive catheterization in high-risk patients and stress testing in low-risk patients. This introduces bias due to the lower sensitivity and specificity of the noninvasive testing. With these limitations in mind, these observational studies of the use of CCT for the evaluation of acute chest pain uniformly demonstrate high sensitivity and specificity for the diagnosis of ACS (Table 11.2.)

Ultimately, no diagnostic strategy used in acute chest pain is 100% accurate. As with other approaches, even under optimal conditions, CCT will miss a small percentage of ACS patients. Furthermore, some patients who present with non-ACS chest pain will go on to develop symptomatic coronary disease. Therefore, the prognostic implications of a negative CCT coronary angiogram are an important consideration. To date, the longest follow-up has been in a study by Rubinshtein *et al.* in which 35 patients were discharged directly from the ED, 15 of whom had normal coronary arteries and 20 of whom had nonobstructive

Table 11.2   Diagnostic accuracy studies of CCT coronary angiography for the detection of ACS.

Study	N (total)	Scanner type	Protocol	Prevalence of ACS (%)	Sensitivity (%)	Specificity (%)	PPV (%)	NPV (%)
Hoffmann [69]	40	16 or 64 slice	Coronary	13	100	74	38	100
Hoffmann [68]	103	64 slice	Coronary	14	100	82	47	100
Johnson [72]	55	64 slice	Triple rule out	7	83	84	38	98
Johnson [71]	109	Dual source	Triple rule out	12	100	100	100	100
Olivetti [73]	31	16 slice	Triple rule out	58	83	100	100	81
Rubinshtein [65]	58	64 slice	Coronary/triple rule out	34	100	92	87	100
Savino [75]	23	64 slice	Triple rule out	35	100	100	100	100
Sato [74]	31	4 or 16 slice	Coronary	71	96	89	96	89
White [76]	69	16 slice	Triple rule out	17	83	96	83	96

atheroma [65]. Of this group of 35 patients, none experienced death or myocardial infarction and three (two with coronary stents already in place) underwent clinically directed invasive coronary angiography. Hoffmann *et al.* followed 73 patients in whom obstructive coronary disease could be definitively ruled out by CCT for 5 months [68]. Incidence of cardiac death, myocardial infarction, or revascularization in this group was 0%. In a series of 54 patients, Hollander *et al.* used CCT as the primary determinant of admission, discharging 46 (85%) immediately from the ED [70]. At 30 days, none of the 54 patients had experienced death or myocardial infarction. Interpretation of these studies is difficult as they are small and observational without a concurrent control group with which to compare event rates. Goldstein *et al.* compared a CCT-based strategy with the standard diagnostic approach for evaluating acute chest pain in a small randomized control trial (Figure 11.3) [77]. In this study, no patient in either group experienced cardiac death, myocardial infarction, or unstable angina over a 6-month follow-up.

This study also found similar diagnostic efficacy between the two diagnostic strategies. In both cases, greater than 90% of patients did not require further cardiovascular testing over the 6-month follow-up. These studies of the prognostic value of a CCT-based strategy suggest that such a strategy will allow identification of patients at very low risk for cardiovascular events. However, larger, multicenter studies are required to validate these findings. In light of the current limited evidence, American College of Cardiology/American Heart Association guidelines support the use of CCT coronary angiography as an alternative to stress testing in patients with suspected ACS with a low or intermediate probability of coronary disease after serial ECG and biomarker testing is negative [20].

To date, diagnosis of ACS in studies of CCT coronary angiography have primarily used the presence of significant coronary stenosis as the positive criterion. The most common cutoff value selected has been a diameter stenosis of greater than 50%. While this standard has resulted in good accuracy, the ability of CCT to identify other characteristics

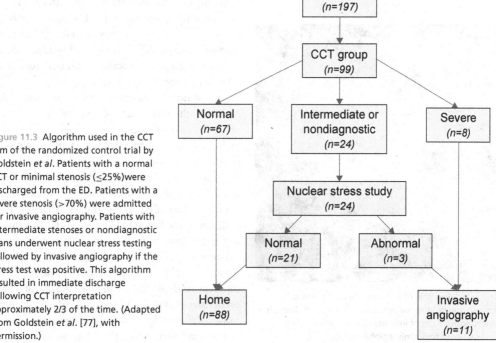

Figure 11.3 Algorithm used in the CCT arm of the randomized control trial by Goldstein *et al.* Patients with a normal CCT or minimal stenosis (≤25%) were discharged from the ED. Patients with a severe stenosis (>70%) were admitted for invasive angiography. Patients with intermediate stenoses or nondiagnostic scans underwent nuclear stress testing followed by invasive angiography if the stress test was positive. This algorithm resulted in immediate discharge following CCT interpretation approximately 2/3 of the time. (Adapted from Goldstein *et al.* [77], with permission.)

of coronary disease and consequences of ischemia may prove to increase sensitivity further. As noted above, CCT has the potential to detect intracoronary thrombus [59] and plaque characteristics. When extent of coronary plaque regardless of the severity of luminal stenosis was added to multivariate logistic regression models consisting of either traditional risk factors or the results of clinical risk assessment, the extent of plaque markedly improved the ability of either model to predict ACS [68]. In a small study including a high proportion of patients with non-ST segment elevation myocardial infarctions (42%) an unstable angina (26%), all of the identified culprit plaques were noncalcified with average densities of 23.5 ± 22.4 HU and 38.4 ± 6.9 HU respectively [74]. CCT also has the ability to identify downstream consequences of coronary obstruction. In some cases of ACS, a resting myocardial perfusion abnormality can be detected as a region of low-density myocardium, typically subendocardial (Figure 11.4) [74,76]. This phenomenon has not been systematically examined for the detection of ACS. However, preliminary evidence suggests that low enhancement of myocardium on CCT has good sensitivity for myocardial infarction [78–80] and correlates with delayed gadolinium enhancement on cardiac magnetic resonance (CMR)

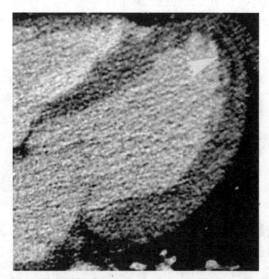

Figure 11.4 Example of a left anterior descending coronary distribution subendocardial infarction. There is a subendocardial rim of low attenuation (arrowhead) corresponding to diminished/absent perfusion.

[81]. Because CCT utilized electrocardiographic gating, left and right ventricular function and segmental wall motion can also be measured with accuracy and reliability comparable to CMR [82]. In a small study of ACS patients, wall motion abnormalities were observed by CCT in 96% and there was 90% concordance with the results of transthoracic echocardiography [57]. Whether the incorporation of additional plaque features, perfusion defects, or functional analysis will improve upon the apparent high accuracy of CCT stenosis detection for the diagnosis of ACS requires further study.

Another important consideration is that CCT coronary angiography allows for the detection of nonatherosclerotic causes of ischemic chest pain (Figure 11.5.) A subset of coronary anomalies have been associated with primary or secondary myocardial ischemia [83]. Along with CMR, CCT is the reference standard for the detection of coronary anomalies [84]. CCT is also proving to have higher sensitivity than invasive angiography for the identification of an intramyocardial course of coronary arteries, so-called myocardial bridging [85]. The clinical implications of this increased detection rate are uncertain. With a prevalence of approximately one in three persons in autopsy studies, it is clear that most cases of myocardial bridging do not result in clinically important chest pain [86]. However, in some cases, myocardial bridges have been implicated as causes of myocardial ischemia, infarction, myocardial stunning, and sudden cardiac death, and they are associated with atherosclerosis proximal to the tunneled segment [86].

In addition to ischemic causes of chest pain, MDCT is the reference standard for the diagnosis of a number of other potential causes of chest pain, including pulmonary embolism, acute aortic syndromes, pleural or pericardial effusions, pulmonary infiltrates, pneumothorax, and hiatal hernia. Dedicated CCT coronary angiography is limited in its ability to detect these noncoronary causes of chest pain due to the limited field of view and the timing of the contrast bolus for optimal coronary artery enhancement. These limitations can be overcome using a so-called "triple rule-out" protocol, a full thoracic field of view scan that allows for comprehensive evaluation for multiple life-threatening causes of chest pain, including ACS, pulmonary embolism, and aortic dissection. The use of the triple

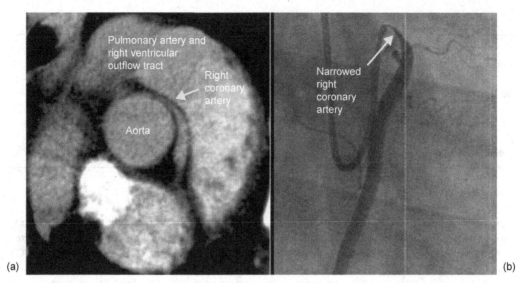

Figure 11.5 CCT (a) and invasive angiogram (b) from a 36-year-old man with atypical chest pain. Anomalous right coronary artery arising from the left coronary cusp and coursing between the right ventricular outflow tract and aortic root. The ostium and the intra-arterial segment are severely narrowed.

rule-out protocol does require certain compromises (Table 11.3). First, due to the longer caudo-cranial field of view, a longer breath-hold of approximately 15–20 seconds is necessary. Scanning is performed in a caudo-cranial direction so that the heart will be scanned early in the breath-hold. Second, to optimally opacify the pulmonary artery as well as the coronary artery, a larger contrast bolus is administered with slightly altered timing. Third, the larger coverage area results in slightly greater radiation doses, with average exposures of 20–30 msv vs 10–15 msv for a dedicated coronary scan. Because

of these compromises, visualization of the coronary arteries may be less optimal than with a dedicated scan.

Despite the disadvantages of the triple rule-out protocol, it may be the optimal approach in chest pain patients since it allows for accurate diagnosis of an array of significant noncoronary pathologies. Overall, approximately 5–10% of CCT scans performed to image the coronaries will contain clinically significant extracardiac findings [87]. When a triple rule-out protocol is employed in patients with acute chest pain, this proportion is frequently

Table 11.3 Sample triple rule-out and dedicated coronary CCT protocols using 64-slice scanner.

Parameter	Triple rule out	Dedicated CCT
kv	120	120
mAs/slice	600–800	600–800
FOV	400	220
Thickness (mm)	0.9	0.9
Increment (mm)	0.4	0.4
Direction of scanning	Caudal to cephalad	Cephalad to caudal
Scan duration (s)	12–15	7–9
Injection protocol	5 mL/s (60 mL contrast) then	5 mL/s (90–120 mL contrast)
	2.5 mL/s (30 mL contrast) then	5 mL/s (30 mL saline)
	2.5 mL/s (30 mL saline)	

Table 11.4   Summary of prevalence findings from triple rule-out studies.

Study	Significant CT findings (%)	Cardiac findings on CT (%)	Noncardiac findings on CT (%)	Pulmonary embolism (%)	Significant aortic disease (%)
White [76]	19	14	4	1	0
Savino [75]	52	43	9	9	0
Schertler [88]	45	8	37	18	8
Johnson [72]	67	22	42	18	13
Johnson [71]	76	40	39	9	13

higher. The reported prevalence of significant non-cardiac findings in this setting has ranged from 4 to 42% (Table 11.4) [71,72,75,76,88]. While the goal of clinically targeted scanning for the specific suspected condition is attractive, pulmonary embolism and aortic dissection are often not suspected when present. Pulmonary embolism is found incidentally on scans performed for evaluation of the coronary arteries in approximately 0.6–1.0% of cases [89,90]. In a prospective study of unselected inpatients, pulmonary embolism was an unsuspected finding on contrast enhanced MDCT in 5.7% of cases [91]. Physicians suspect the correct diagnosis in only 15–43% of patients ultimately diagnosed with aortic dissection [92]. On the other hand, the clinical significance of findings that are clinically unsuspected is not always clear. Many pulmonary emboli detected incidentally are small and subsegmental. [89] Additionally, when pretest probability is low, the proportion of pulmonary emboli and dissections that are detected that are false positives will be higher [93].

There are many theoretic advantages of a CCT-based approach to acute chest pain and the results of small single-center studies are promising regardless of the imaging protocol used. However, future studies will need to address a number of important considerations in addition to diagnostic accuracy. To date, most CCT uses retrospective ECG gating, resulting in substantial radiation exposure, even with the use of dose modulation. Radiation exposure from CCT is comparable to that of a myocardial perfusion SPECT study and clinicians and patients will likely considered this acceptable. However, it is not clear what proportion of patients will still require nuclear stress testing and invasive

cardiac catheterization in addition to CCT resulting in a higher radiation burden. In the randomized trial by Goldstein et al., 24 of 99 patients in the CCT group required nuclear stress testing due to indeterminate CCT findings and 11 required invasive angiography compared to 3 in the standard of care group [77]. Conversely, a CCT-based strategy may result in decreased exposure to medical radiation following discharge if it provides greater diagnostic certainty. In the same trial by Goldstein et al., there was no significant difference in the overall number of invasive angiograms after 6-month follow-up [77]. Cost-effectiveness is another important consideration for the implementation of a CCT-based strategy. Assessment of cost and hospital resource utilization is severely limited in the observational studies performed to date due to variability in patient populations and study sites, and absence of control groups [69,75]. An analysis by Goldstein et al. suggests potential savings with an average ED cost for the CCT-based strategy of $1586 vs $1872, primarily due to reduced length of stay [77]. Other important questions that remain to be answered regarding a CCT-based strategy for acute chest pain include the following. How does this strategy affect referral rates for invasive angiography and revascularization procedures? Is 24-hour CCT service necessary in order to be cost effective and ethical? Are certain patient populations better suited or unsuited for a CCT-based strategy?

Cardiac Magnetic Resonance for the Evaluation of Acute Chest Pain

Whereas CCT-based strategies for the detection of ACS have focused on the detection of anatomic evidence of the upstream cause (i.e., coronary plaque with associated luminal stenosis), CMR-based strategies have sought to take advantage of the ability of CMR to detect multiple downstream components of the ischemic cascade. CMR is the gold standard noninvasive imaging modality for the measurement of cardiac structure and function. Cine sequences produce high contrast-to-noise images that allow detection of segmental wall motion abnormalities due to ischemia [94,95]. Reported sensitivity and specificity of CMR stress testing using either wall motion analysis or gadolinium contrast perfusion imaging are similar or better than reported values for other stress testing modalities [96,97]. T_2-weighted imaging and T_1-weighted delayed gadolinium enhancement imaging allow for detection of both acute and chronic myocardial infarcts [98,99]. As a result of the higher spatial resolution of CMR in comparison to SPECT, smaller, subendocardial infarcts are detected [100]. Additionally, CMR does have the capability for noninvasive coronary angiography. Though, this generally only allows for reliable diagnostic quality imaging of the proximal coronary arteries [101].

Data on the use of CMR in the diagnostic evaluation of patients with acute chest pain is limited to four single-center prospective diagnostic accuracy studies. Reported diagnostic characteristics for individual potential CMR characteristics of ACS are shown in Table 11.5 [102–105]. Of these, adenosine perfusion stress testing is most promising in terms of accuracy. In a study of 135 troponin and ECG negative patients imaged at least 6 hours after the last episode of chest pain, adenosine perfusion alone had 100% sensitivity for the detection of adverse cardiovascular events within a year after the initial chest pain presentation [104]. Of note, the definition of adverse events in this study included interval diagnosis of coronary disease. Specificity in this study was high as well at 93%. While these results are very promising, the use of adenosine stress CMR as a diagnostic and risk stratification test is logistically similar to the use of stress echocardiography or radionuclide imaging for the evaluation of low risk chest pain patients in that it requires a period of observation including negative troponins and ECGs. Still, adenosine CMR perfusion may have a unique role in that it allows for evaluation of other aspects of cardiovascular pathophysiology in a single study and does not expose patients to ionizing radiation. Another important consideration is the underlying risk for ACS in the population being studied. Adenosine CMR perfusion was investigated in another study that included mostly low to intermediate risk patients with suspected or diagnosed ACS who were scheduled to undergo coronary angiography. Sensitivity and specificity of adenosine CMR perfusion in this study were high [102]. However, likely due to the higher prevalence of disease in the participants, negative predictive value in this study was only 59%.

Unlike adenosine CMR perfusion, other aspects of myocardial pathophysiology can be safely imaged by CMR shortly after presentation with acute chest pain. Resting wall motion abnormalities, perfusion defects, and delayed enhancement can all be signs of ongoing or recent myocardial ischemia or infarction. Each of these potential consequences of ACS have been investigated for use in acute chest pain (Figure 11.6) In general, while demonstrating high specificity, the sensitivities of these abnormalities for ACS are low. In the case of resting wall

Table 11.5 Diagnostic performance of individual CMR components in detecting ACS [102–105].

	Resting regional wall motion	Resting perfusion*	Rest–adenosine perfusion	Delayed enhancement	T_2 weighted*	Coronary angiography[†]
Sensitivity (%)	68–85	77	88–100	55—73	69	84
Specificity (%)	75–96	92	83–93	83—97	100	75
PPV (%)	56–93	71	71–96	50—94	100	94
NPV (%)	69–95	94	87–100	42—93	92	50

*Resting perfusion and T_2 weighted imaging only reported in [105].
[†]Coronary angiography only reported in [102].

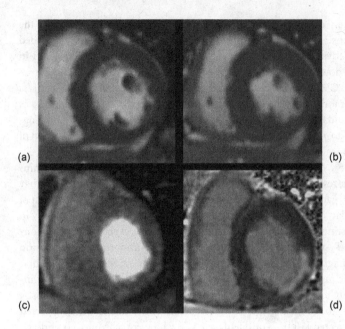

(a)

(b)

(c)

(d)

Figure 11.6 Example of an inferolateral subendocardial myocardial infarction diagnosed by CMR. Still frames of diastolic (a) and systolic (b) short-axis cine images demonstrate a resting wall motion abnormality. Rest perfusion imaging (c) demonstrates a subendocardial rim of low signal intensity indicative of hypoperfusion. Delayed gadolinium enhancement imaging (d) demonstrates subendocardial scar/inflammation in the inferolateral wall.

motion and perfusion imaging, this low sensitivity likely represents that fact that, in the absence of persistent coronary obstruction and myocardial infarction, these are transient abnormalities. As with resting echocardiography and radionuclide SPECT, sensitivity for unstable angina likely decreases as the time since the acute chest pain episode increases [106]. This may explain the higher sensitivity (85%) for regional wall motion reported by Cury *et al.* in a study in which participants were imaged within 3 hours of presentation, a much shorter time frame than the other three studies. The limitation of delayed enhancement for the assessment of acute chest pain is even more pronounced. By definition, the presence of unstable angina precludes myocardial infarction. Thus, of all CMR parameters investigated for the detection of ACS, delayed enhancement is consistently the least sensitive.

Given the diagnostic limitations of any single CMR parameter for the detection of ACS, it appears that optimal diagnostic accuracy requires the combination of multiple parameters. Kwong *et al.* reported a sensitivity of 84% and specificity of 85% by accepting either the presence of a wall motion abnormality or delayed enhancement as representative of the presence of ACS (rest perfusion was used in a supportive fashion to help identify other abnormalities, but was not itself a diagnostic cri-

terion) [103]. One of the limitations of this study was inability to distinguish acute from chronic infarction, decreasing specificity. Additionally, sensitivity of this approach for unstable angina is likely limited for the reasons discussed above. In a study of higher risk patients with suspected or definite ACS, Plein *et al.* found the combination of resting wall motion and delayed enhancement to be less sensitive (77%) than other two-component combinations [102]. T_2 weighted sequences are able to demonstrate myocardial edema in acute myocardial infarction and thus allow differentiate between acute and chronic infarction [98]. In light of this, Cury investigated the utility of T_2 weighted images for the diagnosis of acute chest pain [105]. Consistent with the hypothesis that increased T_2 signal signifies that an event is acute, elevated T_2 signal in acute chest pain patients was 100% specific for ACS. When the criteria of increased T_2 signal and the absence of wall thinning were added to a protocol utilizing segmental wall motion, rest perfusion, and delayed enhancement, the specificity for ACS increased from 85 to 96% [105]. Additionally, the use of T_2 weighted images allowed for the detection of five of nine patients with unstable angina [105].

Despite this promising early data on the use of CMR for the evaluation of patients with acute chest pain, the clinical use of CMR for this purpose faces a number of challenges. Similar to the use of CMR for other purposes, patients with cardiac devices (e.g., pacemakers or implanted defibrillators) and patients with claustrophobia cannot be scanned. Additionally, even when a magnetic resonance scanner with cardiac capabilities is located in proximity to the ED, the scanner must be available for at least 30–60 minutes and the patient must be stable enough to tolerate being in the scanner. Kwong *et al.* report scan durations of 38 ± 12 minutes with patient time away from the ED of 58 ± 10 minutes with a protocol that did not include stress perfusion or coronary imaging [103]. Cury *et al.* were able to improve this to 32 ± 8 minutes despite the addition of T_2 weighted imaging by using an adiabatic 3D technique for the acquisition of delayed enhancement images [105]. Concerns regarding the use of gadolinium in patients with renal disease may also prove to be a significant limitation resulting in the exclusion of some patients and also in the delay of scanning until results of serum creatinine testing can be obtained from the lab. Furthermore, availability of expertise to perform and interpret CMR studies is generally limited to specialized centers.

In light of these challenges, more data will be necessary before the use of CMR in acute chest pain patients can be advocated. To date, only a total of 426 patients at three centers have been studied (including the study by Plein *et al.* which is not a study of ED patients) [102–105]. Future work will need to include larger sample sizes, multiple centers, randomization to CMR versus standard diagnostic strategies, and cost effectiveness analyses. Appropriateness criteria published in 2006 suggest that the appropriateness of the use of adenosine or dobutamine stress CMR for the evaluation of acute chest pain is uncertain [84]. Otherwise, the use of CMR for the evaluation of acute chest pain is not discussed in any major practice guidelines.

Conclusions

The greatest need for highly accurate noninvasive imaging modalities is for the diagnosis of conditions with high morbidity and mortality characterized by nonspecific signs and symptoms. In cardiology, the paradigm conditions for which noninvasive imaging are most useful are the triad of ACS, aortic dissection, and pulmonary embolism. Each of these conditions presents commonly with the symptom of chest pain. MDCT and MRI have clearly defined roles in the evaluation of suspected aortic dissection and pulmonary embolism. To date, the noninvasive modalities of SPECT, and echocardiography have proven useful for the clinical evaluation of acute chest pain when ACS is the chief diagnostic consideration. However, characteristics of CCT, and CMR, make these modalities promising as adjuncts or alternatives to imaging techniques currently in use for the evaluation of ACS.

This promise is supported by a growing number of small, single-center observational studies and a single randomized controlled trial that have documented the high diagnostic accuracy of both CCT and CMR in the setting of acute chest pain. As these technologies become widespread, follow-up of these early studies that includes multicenter investigations, clarification of optimal protocols and diagnostic algorithms, and cost-effectiveness analyses will be critical.

References

1. Nawar EW, Niska RW, Xu J. National Hospital Ambulatory Medical Care Survey: 2005 emergency department summary. *Adv Data*. 2007;(386):1–32.
2. Pope JH, Ruthazer R, Beshansky JR, et al. Clinical features of emergency department patients presenting with symptoms suggestive of acute cardiac ischemia: a multicenter study. *J Thromb Thrombolysis*. 1998;6(1): 63–74.
3. Pope JH, Aufderheide TP, Ruthazer R, et al. Missed diagnoses of acute cardiac ischemia in the emergency department. *N Engl J Med*. 2000;342(16):1163–1170.
4. Remy-Jardin M, Pistolesi M, Goodman LR, et al. Management of suspected acute pulmonary embolism in the era of CT angiography: a statement from the Fleischner Society. *Radiology*. 2007;245(2):315–329.
5. van Belle A, Büller HR, Huisman MV, et al. Effectiveness of managing suspected pulmonary embolism using an algorithm combining clinical probability, D-dimer testing, and computed tomography. *JAMA*. 2006;295(2):172–179.
6. Righini M, Le Gal G, Aujesky D, et al. Diagnosis of pulmonary embolism by multidetector CT alone or combined with venous ultrasonography of the leg: a randomised non-inferiority trial. *Lancet*. 2008;371 (9621):1343–1352.
7. Schoepf UJ, Holzknecht N, Helmberger TK, et al. Subsegmental pulmonary emboli: improved detection

with thin-collimation multi-detector row spiral CT. *Radiology.* 2002;222(2):483–490.

8. Plumhans C, Mühlenbruch G, Rapaee A, *et al.* Assessment of global right ventricular function on 64-MDCT compared with MRI. *AJR Am J Roentgenol.* 2008;190(5):1358–1361.

9. Hofmann LK, Zou KH, Costello P, Schoepf UJ. Electrocardiographically gated 16-section CT of the thorax: cardiac motion suppression. *Radiology.* 2004;233(3): 927–933.

10. Fink C, Ley, S, Schoenberg, SO, Reiser, MF, Kauczor, HU. Magnetic resonance imaging of acute pulmonary embolism. *Eur Radiol.* 2007;17(10):2546–2553.

11. Oudkerk M, van Beek EJ, Wielopolski P, *et al.* Comparison of contrast-enhanced magnetic resonance angiography and conventional pulmonary angiography for the diagnosis of pulmonary embolism: a prospective study. *Lancet.* 2002;359(9318):1643–1647.

12. Kluge A, Luboldt W, Bachmann G. Acute pulmonary embolism to the subsegmental level: diagnostic accuracy of three MRI techniques compared with 16-MDCT. *AJR Am J Roentgenol.* 2006;187(1):W7–14.

13. Shiga T, Wajima Z, Apfel CC, Inoue T, Ohe Y. Diagnostic accuracy of transesophageal echocardiography, helical computed tomography, and magnetic resonance imaging for suspected thoracic aortic dissection: systematic review and meta-analysis. *Arch Intern Med.* 2006;166(13):1350–1356.

14. Gebker R, Gomaa O, Schnackenburg B, Rebakowski J, Fleck E, Nagel E. Comparison of different MRI techniques for the assessment of thoracic aortic pathology: 3D contrast enhanced MR angiography, turbo spin echo and balanced steady state free precession. *Int J Cardiovasc Imaging.* 2007;23(6):747–756.

15. Swap CJ, Nagurney JT. Value and limitations of chest pain history in the evaluation of patients with suspected acute coronary syndromes. *JAMA.* 2005;294(20): 2623–2629.

16. Goodacre S, Locker T, Morris F, Campbell S. How useful are clinical features in the diagnosis of acute, undifferentiated chest pain? *Acad Emerg Med.* 2002;9(3):203–208.

17. Zimetbaum PJ, Josephson ME. Use of the electrocardiogram in acute myocardial infarction. *N Engl J Med.* 2003;348(10):933–940.

18. Balk EM, Ioannidis JP, Salem D, Chew, PW, Lau J. Accuracy of biomarkers to diagnose acute cardiac ischemia in the emergency department: a meta-analysis. *Ann Emerg Med.* 2001;37(5):478–494.

19. Jeremias A, Gibson CM. Narrative review: alternative causes for elevated cardiac troponin levels when acute coronary syndromes are excluded. *Ann Intern Med.* 2005;142(9):786–791.

20. Anderson JL, Adams CD, Antman EM, *et al.* ACC/AHA 2007 guidelines for the management of patients with unstable angina/non-ST-elevation myocardial infarction – executive summary. *J Am Coll Cardiol.* 2007; 50(7):652–726.

21. Pope JH, Selker HP. Acute coronary syndromes in the emergency department: diagnostic characteristics, tests, and challenges. *Cardiol Clin.* 2005;23(4):423–451, v–vi.

22. Souza AS, Bream PR, Elliott LP. Chest film detection of coronary artery calcification. The value of the CAC triangle. *Radiology.* 1978;129(1):7–10.

23. Margolis JR, Chen JT, Kong Y, Peter RH, Behar VS, Kisslo, JA. The diagnostic and prognostic significance of coronary artery calcification. A report of 800 cases. *Radiology.* 1980;137(3):609–616.

24. Nesto RW, Kowalchuk GJ. The ischemic cascade: temporal sequence of hemodynamic, electrocardiographic and symptomatic expressions of ischemia. *Am J Cardiol.* 1987;59(7):23C–30C.

25. Lewis WR. Echocardiography in the evaluation of patients in chest pain units. *Cardiol Clin.* 2005;23(4): 531–539, vii.

26. Camici PG, Prasad SK, Rimoldi OE. Stunning, hibernation, and assessment of myocardial viability. *Circulation.* 2008;117(1):103–114.

27. Lieberman AN, Weiss JL, Jugdutt BI, *et al.* Two-dimensional echocardiography and infarct size: relationship of regional wall motion and thickening to the extent of myocardial infarction in the dog. *Circulation.* 1981;63(4):739–746.

28. Rainbird AJ, Mulvagh SL, Oh JK, *et al.* Contrast dobutamine stress echocardiography: clinical practice assessment in 300 consecutive patients. *J Am Soc Echocardiogr.* 2001;14(5):378–385.

29. Rinkevich D, Kaul S, Wang XQ, *et al.* Regional left ventricular perfusion and function in patients presenting to the emergency department with chest pain and no ST-segment elevation. *Eur Heart J.* 2005;26(16):1606–1611.

30. Korosoglou G, Labadze N, Hansen A, *et al.* Usefulness of real-time myocardial perfusion imaging in the evaluation of patients with first time chest pain. *Am J Cardiol.* 2004;94(10):1225–1231.

31. Kaul S, Senior R, Firschke C, *et al.* Incremental value of cardiac imaging in patients presenting to the emergency department with chest pain and without ST-segment elevation: a multicenter study. *Am Heart J.* 2004;148(1):129–136.

32. Kaufmann BA, Lewis C, Xie A, Mirza-Mohd A, Lindner JR. Detection of recent myocardial ischaemia by molecular imaging of P-selectin with targeted contrast echocardiography. *Eur Heart J.* 2007;28(16):2011–2017.

33. Wackers FJ, Brown KA, Heller GV, *et al.* American Society of Nuclear Cardiology position statement on

radionuclide imaging in patients with suspected acute ischemic syndromes in the emergency department or chest pain center. *J Nucl Cardiol.* 2002;9(2):246–250.

34. Udelson JE, Beshansky JR, Ballin DS, *et al.* Myocardial perfusion imaging for evaluation and triage of patients with suspected acute cardiac ischemia: a randomized controlled trial. *JAMA.* 2002;288(21):2693–2700.

35. Kontos MC, Tatum JL. Imaging in the evaluation of the patient with suspected acute coronary syndrome. *Semin Nucl Med.* 2003;33(4):246–258.

36. Ross R. The pathogenesis of atherosclerosis: a perspective for the 1990s. *Nature.* 1993;362(6423):801–809.

37. Rumberger JA, Simons DB, Fitzpatrick LA, Sheedy PF, Schwartz RS. Coronary artery calcium area by electron-beam computed tomography and coronary atherosclerotic plaque area. A histopathologic correlative study. *Circulation.* 1995;92(8):2157–2162.

38. Rumberger JA, Sheedy PF, Breen JF, Schwartz RS. Electron beam computed tomographic coronary calcium score cutpoints and severity of associated angiographic lumen stenosis. *J Am Coll Cardiol.* 1997;29(7): 1542–1548.

39. Budoff MJ, Diamond GA, Raggi P, *et al.* Continuous probabilistic prediction of angiographically significant coronary artery disease using electron beam tomography. *Circulation.* 2002;105(15):1791–1796.

40. Detrano R, Hsiai T, Wang S, *et al.* Prognostic value of coronary calcification and angiographic stenoses in patients undergoing coronary angiography. *J Am Coll Cardiol.* 1996;27(2):285–290.

41. Budoff MJ, Achenbach S, Blumenthal RS, *et al.* Assessment of coronary artery disease by cardiac computed tomography: a scientific statement from the American Heart Association Committee on Cardiovascular Imaging and Intervention, Council on Cardiovascular Radiology and Intervention, and Committee on Cardiac Imaging, Council on Clinical Cardiology. *Circulation.* 2006;114(16):1761–1791.

42. Budoff MJ, Shaw LJ, Liu ST, *et al.* Long-term prognosis associated with coronary calcification: observations from a registry of 25,253 patients. *J Am Coll Cardiol.* 2007;49(18):1860–1870.

43. Laudon DA, Vukov LF, Breen JF, Rumberger JA, Wollan PC, Sheedy PF, 2nd. Use of electron-beam computed tomography in the evaluation of chest pain patients in the emergency department. *Ann Emerg Med.* 1999;33(1):15–21.

44. McLaughlin VV, Balogh T, Rich S. Utility of electron beam computed tomography to stratify patients presenting to the emergency room with chest pain. *Am J Cardiol.* 1999;84(3):327–328.

45. Georgiou D, Budoff MJ, Bleiweis MS, *et al.* A new approach for screening patients with chest pain

in the emergency department using fast computed-tomography. *Circulation.* 1993;88(4):15–15.

46. Esteves FP, Sanyal R, Santana CA, Shaw L, Raggi P. Potential impact of noncontrast computed tomography as gatekeeper for myocardial perfusion positron emission tomography in patients admitted to the chest pain unit. *Am J Cardiol.* 2008;101(2):149–152.

47. Lange RA, Hillis LD. Cardiovascular complications of cocaine use. *N Engl J Med.* 2001;345(5):351–358.

48. Schmermund A, Baumgart D, Görge G, *et al.* Coronary artery calcium in acute coronary syndromes – a comparative study of electron-beam computed tomography, coronary angiography, and intracoronary ultrasound in survivors of acute myocardial infarction and unstable angina. *Circulation.* 1997;96(5):1461–1469.

49. Rubinshtein R, Gaspar T, Halon DA, Goldstein J, Peled N, Lewis BS, *et al.* Prevalence and extent of obstructive coronary artery disease in patients with zero or low calcium score undergoing 64-slice cardiac multidetector computed tomography for evaluation of a chest pain syndrome. *Am J Cardiol.* 2007;99(4):472–475.

50. Henneman MM, Schuijf JD, Pundziute G, *et al.* Noninvasive evaluation with multislice computed tomography in suspected acute coronary syndrome: plaque morphology on multislice computed tomography versus coronary calcium score. *J Am Coll Cardiol.* 2008; 52(3):216–222.

51. Georgiou D, Budoff MJ, Kaufer E, *et al.* Screening patients with chest pain in the emergency department using electron beam tomography: a follow-up study. *J Am Coll Cardiol.* 2001;38(1):105–110.

52. Mizuno K, Satomura K, Miyamoto A, *et al.* Angioscopic evaluation of coronary-artery thrombi in acute coronary syndromes. *N Engl J Med.* 1992;326(5):287–291.

53. Roe MT, Harrington RA, Prosper DM, *et al.* Clinical and therapeutic profile of patients presenting with acute coronary syndromes who do not have significant coronary artery disease. The Platelet Glycoprotein IIb/IIIa in Unstable Angina: Receptor Suppression Using Integrilin Therapy (PURSUIT) Trial Investigators. *Circulation.* 2000;102(10):1101–1106.

54. Bluemke DA, Achenbach S, Budoff M, *et al.* Noninvasive coronary artery imaging. magnetic resonance angiography and multidetector computed tomography angiography. a scientific statement from the American Heart Association Committee on cardiovascular imaging and intervention of the council on cardiovascular radiology and intervention, and the councils on clinical cardiology and cardiovascular disease in the young. *Circulation.* 2008;118(5):586–606.

55. Abdulla J, Abildstrom SZ, Gotzsche O, Christensen E, Kober L, Torp-Pedersen C. 64-multislice detector computed tomography coronary angiography as potential

alternative to conventional coronary angiography: a systematic review and meta-analysis. *Eur Heart J.* 2007;28 (24):3042–3050.

56. Leschka S, Alkadhi H, Plass A, *et al.* Accuracy of MDCT coronary angiography with 64-slice technology: first experience. *Eur Heart J.* 2005;26(15):1482–1487.

57. Dirksen MS, Jukema JW, Bax JJ, *et al.* Cardiac multidetector-row computed tomography in patients with unstable angina. *Am J Cardiol.* 2005;95(4):457–461.

58. Meijboom WB, Mollet NR, Van Mieghem CA, *et al.* 64-slice CT coronary angiography in patients with non-ST elevation acute coronary syndrome. *Heart.* 2007;93(11):1386–1392.

59. Dorgelo J, Willems TP, Geluk CA, van Ooijen PMA, Zijlstra F, Oudkerk M. Multidetector computed tomography-guided treatment strategy in patients with non-ST elevation acute coronary syndromes: a pilot study. *Eur Radiol.* 2005;15(4):708–713.

60. Tsai IC, Lee T, Lee WL, *et al.* Use of 40-detector row computed tomography before catheter coronary angiography to select early conservative versus early invasive treatment for patients with low-risk acute coronary syndrome. *J Comp Assist Tomogr.* 2007;31(2):258–264.

61. Achenbach S, Ropers D, Hoffmann U, *et al.* Assessment of coronary remodeling in stenotic and non-stenotic coronary atherosclerotic lesions by multidetector spiral computed tomography. *J Am Coll Cardiol.* 2004;43(5):842–847.

62. Moselewski F, Ropers D, Pohle K, *et al.* Comparison of measurement of cross-sectional coronary atherosclerotic plaque and vessel areas by 16-slice multidetector computed tomography versus intravascular ultrasound. *Am J Cardiol.* 2004;94(10):1294–1297.

63. Achenbach S, Moselewski F, Ropers D, *et al.* Detection of calcified and noncalcified coronary atherosclerotic plaque by contrast-enhanced, submillimeter multidetector spiral computed tomography – a segment-based comparison with intravascular ultrasound. *Circulation.* 2004;109(1):14–17.

64. Leber AW, Knez A, Becker A, *et al.* Accuracy of multidetector spiral computed tomography in identifying and differentiating the composition of coronary atherosclerotic plaques: a comparative study with intracoronary ultrasound. *J Am Coll Cardiol.* 2004;43(7):1241–1247.

65. Rubinshtein R, Halon DA, Gaspar T, *et al.* Usefulness of 64-slice cardiac computed tomographic angiography for diagnosing acute coronary syndromes and predicting clinical outcome in emergency department patients with chest pain of uncertain origin. *Circulation.* 2007;115(13):1762–1768.

66. Bonello L, Armero S, Jacquier A, *et al.* Non-invasive coronary angiography for patients with acute atypical chest pain discharged after negative screening including maximal negative treadmill stress test. A prospective study. *Int J Cardiol.* 2009;134(1):140–143.

67. Gallagher MJ, Raff GL. Use of multislice CT for the evaluation of emergency room patients with chest pain: the so-called "triple rule-out". *Catheter Cardiovasc Interv.* 2008;71(1):92–99.

68. Hoffmann U, Nagurney JT, Moselewski F, *et al.* Coronary multidetector computed tomography in the assessment of patients with acute chest pain. *Circulation.* 2006;114(21):2251–2260.

69. Hoffmann U, Pena AJ, Moselewski F, *et al.* MDCT in early triage of patients with acute chest pain. *AJR Am J Roentgenol.* 2006;187(5):1240–1247.

70. Hollander JE, Litt HI, Chase M, Brown AM, Kim W, Baxt WG. Computed tomography coronary angiography for rapid disposition of low-risk emergency department patients with chest pain syndromes. *Acad Emerg Med.* 2007;14(2):112–116.

71. Johnson TRC, Nikolaou K, Becker A, *et al.* Dual-source CT for chest pain assessment. *Eur Radiol.* 2008; 18(4):773–780.

72. Johnson TRC, Nikolaou K, Wintersperger BJ, *et al.* ECG-gated 64-MDCT angiography in the differential diagnosis of acute chest pain. *Am J Roentgenol.* 2007; 188(1):76–82.

73. Olivetti L, Mazza G, Volpi D, Costa F, Ferrari O, Pirelli S, *et al.* Multislice CT in emergency room management of patients with chest pain and medium-low probability of acute coronary syndrome. *Radiol Med (Torino).* 2006;111(8):1054–1063.

74. Sato Y, Matsumoto N, Ichikawa M, *et al.* Efficacy of multislice computed tomography for the detection of acute coronary syndrome in the emergency department. *Circ J.* 2005;69(9):1047–1051.

75. Savino G, Herzog C, Costello P, Schoepf UJ, *et al.* 64 slice cardiovascular CT in the emergency department: concepts and first experiences. *Radiol Med (Torino).* 2006;111(4):481–496.

76. White CS, Kuo D, Kelemen M, *et al.* Chest pain evaluation in the emergency department: can MDCT provide a comprehensive evaluation? *AJR Am J Roentgenol.* 2005;185(2):533–540.

77. Goldstein JA, Gallagher MJ, O'Neill WW, Ross MA, O'Neil BJ, Raff GL. A randomized controlled trial of multi-slice coronary computed tomography for evaluation of acute chest pain. *J Am Coll Cardiol.* 2007;49(8):863–871.

78. Gosalia A, Haramati LB, Sheth MP, Spindola-Franco H. CT detection of acute myocardial infarction. *AJR Am J Roentgenol.* 2004;182(6):1563–1566.

79. Doherty PW, Lipton MJ, Berninger WH, Skioldebrand CG, Carlsson E, Redington RW. Detection and quantitation of myocardial infarction in vivo

using transmission computed tomography. *Circulation.* 1981;63(3):597–606.

80. Cury RC, Nieman K, Shapiro MD, *et al.* Comprehensive assessment of myocardial perfusion defects, regional wall motion, and left ventricular function by using 64-section multidetector CT. *Radiology.* 2008;248(2): 466–475.

81. Gerber BL, Belger B, Legros GJ, *et al.* Characterization of acute and chronic myocardial infarcts by multidetector computed tomography: comparison with contrast-enhanced magnetic resonance. *Circulation.* 2006;113(6):823–833.

82. Dewey M, Müller M, Eddicks S, *et al.* Evaluation of global and regional left ventricular function with 16-slice computed tomography, biplane cineventriculography, and two-dimensional transthoracic echocardiography: comparison with magnetic resonance imaging. *J Am Coll Cardiol.* 2006;48(10):2034–2044.

83. Angelini, P. Coronary artery anomalies: an entity in search of an identity. *Circulation.* 2007;115(10):1296–1305.

84. Hendel RC, Patel MR, Kramer CM, *et al.* ACCF/ACR/SCCT/SCMR/ASNC/NASCI/SCAI/SIR 2006 appropriateness criteria for cardiac computed tomography and cardiac magnetic resonance imaging: a report of the American College of Cardiology Foundation Quality Strategic Directions Committee Appropriateness Criteria Working Group, American College of Radiology, Society of Cardiovascular Computed Tomography, Society for Cardiovascular Magnetic Resonance, American Society of Nuclear Cardiology, North American Society for Cardiac Imaging, Society for Cardiovascular Angiography and Interventions, and Society of Interventional Radiology. *J Am Coll Cardiol.* 2006;48(7):1475–1497.

85. Leschka S, Koepfli P, Husmann L, *et al.* Myocardial bridging: depiction rate and morphology at CT coronary angiography—comparison with conventional coronary angiography. *Radiology.* 2008;246(3):754–762.

86. Mohlenkamp S, Hort W, Ge J, Erbel R. Update on myocardial bridging. *Circulation.* 2002;106(20):2616–2622.

87. Sosnouski D, Bonsall RP, Mayer FB, Ravenel JG, *et al.* Extracardiac findings at cardiac CT: a practical approach. *J Thorac Imaging.* 2007;22(1):77–85.

88. Schertler T, Scheffel H, Frauenfelder T, *et al.* Dual-source computed tomography in patients with acute chest pain: feasibility and image quality. *Eur Radiol.* 2007;17(12):3179–3188.

89. Haller S, Kaiser C, Buser P, Bongartz G, Bremerich J, *et al.* Coronary artery imaging with contrast-enhanced MDCT: extracardiac findings. *AJR Am J Roentgenol.* 2006;187(1):105–110.

90. Patel S, Woodrow A, Bogot N, *et al.* Non-coronary findings on 16-row multidetector CT coronary angiography. *Am J Roentgenol.* 2005;184(4):3–3.

91. Ritchie G, McGurk S, McCreath C, Graham C, Murchison JT, *et al.* Prospective evaluation of unsuspected pulmonary embolism on contrast enhanced multidetector CT (MDCT) scanning. *Thorax.* 2007;62(6): 536–540.

92. Klompas M. Does this patient have an acute thoracic aortic dissection? *JAMA.* 2002;287(17):2262–2272.

93. Barbant SD, Eisenberg MJ, and Schiller NB. The diagnostic value of imaging techniques for aortic dissection. *Am Heart J.* 1992;124(2):541–543.

94. Nagel E, Lehmkuhl HB, Bocksch W, *et al.* Noninvasive diagnosis of ischemia-induced wall motion abnormalities with the use of high-dose dobutamine stress MRI: comparison with dobutamine stress echocardiography. *Circulation.* 1999;99(6):763–770.

95. Hundley WG, Hamilton CA, Thomas MS, *et al.* Utility of fast cine magnetic resonance imaging and display for the detection of myocardial ischemia in patients not well suited for second harmonic stress echocardiography. *Circulation.* 1999;100(16):1697–1702.

96. Nandalur KR, Dwamena BA, Choudhri AF, Nandalur MR, Carlos RC. Diagnostic performance of stress cardiac magnetic resonance imaging in the detection of coronary artery disease: a meta-analysis. *J Am Coll Cardiol.* 2007;50(14):1343–1353.

97. Schwitter J, Wacker CM, van Rossum AC, *et al.* MR-IMPACT: comparison of perfusion-cardiac magnetic resonance with single-photon emission computed tomography for the detection of coronary artery disease in a multicentre, multivendor, randomized trial. *Eur Heart J.* 2008;29(4):480–489.

98. Abdel-Aty H, Zagrosek A, Schulz-Menger J, *et al.* Delayed enhancement and T_2-weighted cardiovascular magnetic resonance imaging differentiate acute from chronic myocardial infarction. *Circulation.* 2004; 109(20):2411–2416.

99. Wu E, Judd RM, Vargas JD, Klocke FJ, Bonow RO, Kim RJ, *et al.* Visualisation of presence, location, and transmural extent of healed Q-wave and non-Q-wave myocardial infarction. *Lancet.* 2001;357(9249): 21–28.

100. Wagner A, Mahrholdt H, Holly TA, *et al.* Contrast-enhanced MRI and routine single photon emission computed tomography (SPECT) perfusion imaging for detection of subendocardial myocardial infarcts: an imaging study. *Lancet.* 2003;361(9355):374–379.

101. Dewey M, Teige F, Schnapauff D, *et al.* Noninvasive detection of coronary artery stenoses with multislice computed tomography or magnetic resonance imaging. *Ann Intern Med.* 2006;145(6):407–415.

102. Plein S, Greenwood JP, Ridgway JP, Cranny G, Ball SG, Sivananthan MU, et al. Assessment of non-ST-segment elevation acute coronary syndromes with cardiac magnetic resonance imaging. *J Am Coll Cardiol.* 2004;44(11):2173–2181.

103. Kwong RY, Schussheim AE, Rekhraj S, et al. Detecting acute coronary syndrome in the emergency department with cardiac magnetic resonance imaging. *Circulation.* 2003;107(4):531–537.

104. Ingkanisorn WP, Kwong RY, Bohme NS, et al. Prognosis of negative adenosine stress magnetic resonance in patients presenting to an emergency department with chest pain. *J Am Coll Cardiol.* 2006;47(7):1427–1432.

105. Cury RC, Shash K, Nagurney JT, et al. Cardiac magnetic resonance with T_2-weighted imaging improves detection of patients with acute coronary syndrome in the emergency department. *Circulation.* 2008;118(8): 837–844.

106. Fram DB, Azar RR, Ahlberg AW, et al. Duration of abnormal SPECT myocardial perfusion imaging following resolution of acute ischemia: an angioplasty model. *J Am Coll Cardiol.* 2003;41(3):452–459.

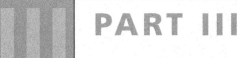

PART III

Concurrent Noninvasive Assessment of Coronary Anatomy, Physiology, and Myocellular Integrity

CHAPTER 12

PET and MRI in Cardiac Imaging

Stephan G. Nekolla[1] *& Antti Saraste*[2]
[1]Technischen Universität München, Munich, Germany
[2]Klinikum rechts der Isar der TU München, Munich, Germany

Introduction

Magnetic resonance imaging (MRI) and positron emission tomography (PET) were developed in the early to mid seventies [1,2]. Since their development, however, they have taken very different paths with respect to their transition from research systems into successful diagnostic tools.

Without any doubt, the clinical use of computerized tomography (CT) and MRI surpasses PET by far. However, the introduction of combined PET/CT devices around the year 2000 [3,4], together with a change in the reimbursement policy in the USA, resulted in an increased interest in the use of PET. Within 3 years, PET/CT scanner sales rose from 0 to 85% of all sales [5]. These devices combine high sensitivity of PET for imaging biological processes with the capability of CT to assess anatomy in detail.

Although primarily driven by oncological applications, there are several emerging applications where multimodality imaging can provide incremental value in cardiology. As reviewed elsewhere each of these modalities has distinct, well-documented cardiovascular applications in research and clinical routine [6,7]. For PET in particular, there has been increase in the clinical utilization of cardiac PET with [82]Rubidium [8], a generator based radioisotope which does not require an on-site cyclotron and exhibits a fast radioactive decay for assessment of coronary artery disease (CAD). In the light of the fact that the number of planar and tomographic nuclear myocardial perfusion examinations approaches 10 million per year, it is understandable that not only other modalities such as MRI, CT, and ultrasound imaging target this market, but also PET.

The success of combined PET/CT devices in oncological research, as well as clinical applications, clearly demonstrates the advantage of combined assessment of morphological and specific functional parameters. Unfortunately, the combination of MRI and PET is not only technically more challenging (fortunately there is evidence of the successful development of an integrated hybrid system of MRI and PET [9]). More importantly were in the past, however, the logistical and political hurdles. PET and CT in oncology, have a long tradition to perform both studies sequentially—even prior to the advent of hybrid systems. For cardiac imaging, this was only rarely the case and if so, only in academic centers. Even with 64 slice CT systems available in hybrid PET/CT tomographs, the combined an acquisition is not performed routinely. Consequently, there is hardly data available on the benefit of a combined acquisition of CT angiography and PET perfusion and/or metabolism. The primary reasons for this are the high radiation dose and the total costs of the examination. When looking into the foremost scenarios for hybrid PET/CT in cardiac imaging, very fast perfusion protocols dominate where the CT component is used for attenuation correction and to some extent for the assessment of coronary calcifications. Thus, the clinical reality of hybrid cardiac imaging appears to be not that bright. But compared to CT, cardiac MRI has other established cardiac

Cardiac CT, PET and MR, 2nd edition. Edited by Vasken Dilsizian and Gerry Pohost. © 2010 Blackwell Publishing Ltd.

applications to offer—including evaluation of cardiac structure, assessment of ventricular function, and detection of myocardial infarction. And in addition to contributing to the existing applications, combination of high-resolution anatomic MRI images with high sensitivity of PET for detection of molecular targets may help to extend these modalities into new applications, such as atherosclerotic plaque characterization, imaging of stem cells and evaluation of angiogenesis.

This review summarizes the experience from comparative studies using parallel PET and MRI in different cardiac applications. Often one modality has been used as the reference for validation of the other. Potential benefits of combining information from these techniques are discussed in present as well as emerging cardiac applications. In two methodological sections, software-based co-registration solutions and their limitations are discussed. Finally, the current status of hardware-based solutions is summarized.

Perfusion Studies

Assessment of myocardial perfusion plays an important role in the diagnostic work-up of patients with suspected coronary artery disease (CAD) as well as in the assessment of prognosis and guiding therapy in patients with established CAD [10]. The available evidence indicates that myocardial perfusion PET provides the most accurate noninvasive means of diagnosing obstructive CAD with sensitivity and specificity of about 90% [10]. PET appears superior to conventional nuclear imaging techniques especially in the obese patients and those undergoing pharmacological stress. It allows diagnosis of myocardial ischemia by showing a reversible reduction of myocardial tracer uptake at peak exercise or pharmacological stress as compared to rest in the myocardial regions supplied by stenotic coronary arteries. Recent evidence also indicates the usefulness of PET for determining prognosis [11,12]. The unique feature of PET is that myocardial perfusion and perfusion reserve can be quantified in absolute terms using mathematical modeling of the tracer kinetics. ^{13}N-labeled ammonia and ^{15}O-labelled water have been well validated for this purpose in experimental studies using microspheres as well as in CAD patients [13,14]. The potential of the generator-produced potassium

analog [82]Rb still remains under investigation [15]. The quantification of myocardial blood flow and coronary flow reserve is of diagnostic importance particularly in those patients with extensive, multivessel CAD [6,10]. It also allows evaluation of very early changes in coronary vasoreactivity and the progression or regression of CAD [6].

Manning and colleagues demonstrated in the early 1990s that dynamic MR imaging of the first-pass signal changes in the myocardium after injection of a fast bolus of gadolinium diethylenetriamine pentaacetic acid (Gd-DTPA) was capable of detecting coronary artery stenoses [16]. A meta-analysis of the single center studies including mainly patients with a high prevalence of disease indicated good sensitivity and specificity (0.91 and 0.81, respectively) of stress perfusion MRI in the diagnosis of CAD [17]. Recently, a randomized, prospective multicenter trial involving 234 patients carried out in experienced centers demonstrated that diagnostic accuracy of myocardial perfusion MRI with pharmacological stress was comparable to that of SPECT (areas under the ROC curve 0.86 and 0.75, respectively) for detection of significant coronary stenosis defined as >50% stenosis [18].

But myocardial perfusion MRI relies on semiquantitative measurements. Only few studies have directly correlated the MRI derived flow against quantitative PET data in humans. One study compared ^{13}N-ammonia PET and MRI, using a pixelwise upslope parameter of the signal intensity curve during contrast media passage as flow index. This study, performed on 18 healthy subjects and 48 CAD patients, revealed a good correlation between the number of pathological segments per patient (PET coronary flow reserve (CFR) threshold: 1.65, MRI threshold: derived from mean upslope values in rest and stress studies individually) and high accuracy when implementing PET as reference in a receiver operating characteristic (ROC) analysis (sensitivity 91%, specificity 94%) [19]. In a similar study, it was found that the MRI CFR was significantly underestimated. MRI threshold for the pathological CFR was very low being 1.3 as compared PET (2.5) [20]. Finally, we can only briefly list the controversially discussed limitations of first pass perfusion MRI: (a) the direct assessment of the arterial input function is a problem, (b) the low extraction of Gd-DTPA during high myocardial blood

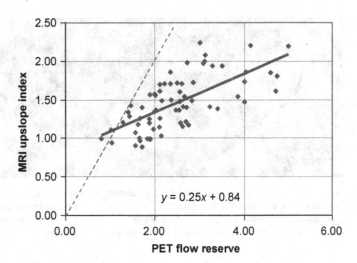

Figure 12.1 Correlation between myocardial flow reserve as assessed with dynamic ^{13}N-ammonia versus semiquantitative flow reserve index from dynamic MRI imaging with Gd-DTPA bolus injection (upslope stress divided by upslope rest study). Although one appreciates that the correlation is good, the significant underestimation of the flow reserve is demonstrated as well. (Figure modified with permission from: Ibrahim et al.[20])

flows with substantial "roll off" as is known from SPECT (Figure 12.1). (c) Modeling of the myocardial kinetics of Gd-DTPA is hampered by its rapid diffusion into the extracellular space. (d) The overall spatial coverage of the left ventricle, as well as the actual slice thickness, is limited to only 3–5 slices.

Currently, more studies are needed to fully understand the potential of MRI perfusion imaging in detection of CAD in comparison to nuclear imaging techniques whereas PET provides reliable CFR values with only a modest radiation low dose. Due to the dynamic nature of perfusion changes, hybrid scanners allowing acquisition of either first-pass signal or the uptake of PET perfusion tracers together with other parameters of interest within very short time frame or even simultaneously may provide interesting possibilities not only for research purposes.

Viability Imaging and Tissue Characterization

Ischemic myocardium that is dysfunctional, but viable has the potential for recovery of contractile function after revascularization [21]. Evaluation of myocardial glucose utilization with ^{18}F-fluorodeoxyglucose (FDG) and positron emission tomography (PET) is considered as the most reliable tool to assess myocardial viability [22]. Its quantitative nature allows assessment of the amount of viable tissue as a continuum from fully viable, through partially viable in the areas of partial

infarction, to non-viable scar. Contrast-enhanced magnetic resonance imaging (MRI) appears to be a promising alternative capable of visualizing transmural distribution of viable and infarcted myocardium with excellent spatial resolution [23]. Contrast-enhanced MRI of myocardial infarction is based on delayed-enhancement technique using inversion-recovery prepared T1 weighed gradient-echo pulse sequences after intravenous administration of Gd-DTPA. Infarcted myocardium appears enhanced relative to normal myocardium when imaged after a delay (typically 5–20 minutes) from intravenous contrast injection due to different washout kinetics [21].

The comparison of delayed-enhancement (or contrast enhancement) MRI with ^{18}F-FDG PET and ^{13}N ammonia (NH$_3$) in 31 patients with ischemic heart failure revealed that the spatial location and extent of infarct scar as delineated by delayed enhancement correlated very well with the non-viable segments from PET [24] (Figure 12.2). The main source of difference between the methods was related to the presence of non-transmural enhancement in regions that were viable by PET. This is likely explained by higher spatial resolution of MRI compared with nuclear imaging methods that makes delayed-enhancement suitable to detect small areas of subendocardial infarcts. A combination of MRI and PET would clearly improve the physiological specificity of this measurement.

An improved contractile performance is commonly considered as the gold-standard for

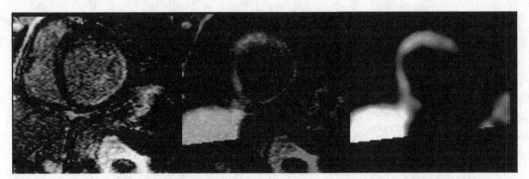

Figure 12.2 Co-visualization of an MRI late enhancement image with ^{13}N-ammonia PET flow data. The subendocardial enhancement pattern in the MRI is matched with a reduced ^{13}N-ammonia uptake because of partial volume effects as well as reduced myocardial blood flow. Because of the limited spatial resolution of PET, however, these effects cannot be separated. (Figure modified with permission from [24].)

assessing myocardial viability, although benefits of revascularization do not appear to be limited to improved function. In the initial study by Kim *et al.* it was shown that in 41 patients with chronic ischemic heart disease dysfunctional segments with less than 25% of delayed enhancement were likely to recover after complete revascularization [25]. In contrast, segments with more than 50% of delayed-enhancement had low probability (<10%) of functional improvement. Comparable positive predictive values (73%) for functional recovery 6 months after revascularization were found for the lack of delayed-enhancement (cut-off value less than 50% scar transmurality) and the presence of preserved ^{18}F-FDG uptake (cut-off value more than 50% of normal myocardium) as assessed by PET as a reference method to detect viable versus nonviable myocardium [26]. A recent meta-analysis of diagnostic studies indicated higher sensitivity for ^{18}F-FDG PET than delayed enhancement MRI (92% vs 84%) in predicting functional recovery upon revascularization while specificities were comparable (63%) [22]. Relatively low specificity of the techniques indicates that a substantial percentage of segments that are classified as viable by the imaging techniques do not improve after revascularization. Although there is limited data on their combined use, adjunctive PET and MRI markers of viability, such as reduced diastolic wall thickness, lack of contractile response to inotropic stimulation with low dose of dobutamine, preserved epicardial rim of viable myocardium, and preserved perfusion have been proposed to help to refine the classification of dysfunctional segments as clinically viable or nonviable. [27–31].

In addition to improved detection of viability, multimodal imaging approaches could contribute to clarify the complex pathophysiological basis underlying the left ventricular dysfunction in ischemic heart failure. The term myocardial "stunning" describes prolonged postischemic contractile depression despite restoration of adequate perfusion after a brief ischemic insult [32]. The term myocardial "hibernation" is used to describe more persistent form of reversible contractile dysfunction due to coronary artery disease. The mechanisms of myocardial hibernation are still incompletely understood: the classic definition of hibernation postulated that myocardial function is reduced to match chronic and severe reduction of resting myocardial blood flow. More recent evidence has shown that resting perfusion is not always significantly reduced in areas of hibernating myocardium. Instead, repetitive stunning caused by repeated ischemic episodes may result in chronic dysfunction. Consistent with this, a study combining MRI and ^{13}N ammonia PET demonstrated that myocardial perfusion was reduced in proportion to increasing transmural extent of delayed enhancement in the dysfunctional segments providing evidence of stunning as the underlying mechanism [30]. Thus, reversible myocardial dysfunction in a patient with chronic ischemic heart disease (IHD) is likely to present an admixture of stunned and hibernating tissue jeopardized by various degree of ischemia. An example of the complexity is presented in Figure 12.3 where

Figure 12.3 Co-registered ^{18}F-FGD and ceMRI in a rat model of occlusion/reperfusion [33]. Myocardial images of ^{18}F-FDG PET and ceMRI from a rat with coronary occlusion (20 minutes), which was followed by reperfusion. ^{18}F-FDG was administrated under a fasting condition 24 hours after coronary reperfusion. Increased ^{18}F-FDG uptake is seen (arrow), corresponding to the area of delayed enhancement on ceMRI (arrow).

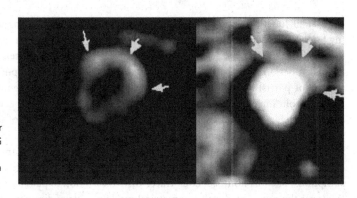

the presence of transmural delayed enhancement is associated with normal ^{18}F-FDG uptake after ischemia reperfusion in a rat [33,34]. In this case, ^{18}F-FDG uptake may be related to the presence of inflammation or metabolically active, stunned myocardium in the MI area or its border zone.

Non-invasive detection of viable myocardium in chronic left ventricular dysfunction associated with coronary artery disease (CAD) has important clinical implications for treatment of patients. Although limited by the lack of large randomized clinical trials, a meta-analysis of retrospective data indicates that such patients are also at substantial risk of death, which can be effectively reduced by successful revascularization [35]. Furthermore, preoperative assessment of viability may identify patients who are at low risk for serious perioperative complications [36]. Thus, discrimination between viable dysfunctional myocardium from scar permits selection of patients who are most likely to benefit most from revascularization allowing others to avoid the risks associated with revascularization when they are unlikely to benefit. The prognostic significance of myocardial scars detected by delayed-enhancement is currently under investigation [37]. Among 159 patients with clinical suspicion of CAD but without a history of MI, the presence of even small amounts of delayed enhancement was associated with high risk of major adverse clinical events (hazard ratio 8.29 for death, acute myocardial infarction or unstable angina pectoris, hospitalization for heart failure, and life-threatening arrhythmias requiring defibrillation) and cardiac death (hazard ratio 10.9) during follow-up of 16 months [37]. It is important to emphasize, that delayed-enhancement MRI is specific for either acute myocardial infarction or scar of old

infarction, but not for hibernating myocardium: plain infarct size carries well established prognostic value that is also expected to apply to MRI. But in contrast, the prognostic value of PET relies on the relative comparison of flow and glucose uptake (mismatch), which has been shown experimentally and clinically to reflect viable, but jeopardized myocardium. Several studies have indicated that there is an association between PET "mismatch" and adverse clinical outcome [35]. There is a need for prospective clinical trials comparing measures of infarction and either hibernation or stunning obtained with the use of MRI and PET, to obtain prognostic data to better understand whether they provide complementary clinical value.

Assessment of Regional and Global Function

MRI is a highly accurate and reproducible method to determine the basic parameters used to characterize cardiac function, such as ventricular volumes, ventricular mass, ejection fraction and regional wall thickening by delineating the exact endo- and epicardial contours. Thus, the high reproducibility makes MRI an attractive tool for serial examinations [38]. Determination of LV function is essential for the diagnosis of heart failure and its prognostic value is well established. Therefore, combination of LV function measured with MRI with any other imaging parameter is likely to provide incremental information. Moreover, some measures used for evaluation of heart failure therapies, such as efficiency of cardiac work, combine PET acquisitions of myocardial oxidative metabolism by the clearance kinetics of ^{11}C-acetate with the assessment of ventricular function that could be ideally done using hybrid PET/MRI tomograph [39].

In contrast to MRI, the determination of left ventricular function in gated PET studies is based on the use of partial volume effects. As the effective spatial resolution in clinical cardiac PET scans is approximately 6–10 mm FWHM (full width at half maximum), changes in wall thickness can be estimated as changes in regional count rates during cardiac contraction. Using algorithm dependent assumptions, such as homogeneous tracer distribution over the myocardial wall, geometrical models can be adjusted to the count profiles over the myocardial wall and estimates of endo- and epicardial borders can be made. This approach has been extensively implemented and validated in SPECT imaging, which is associated with lower spatial resolution than PET [40,41]. Because of the substantial use of myocardial perfusion scintigraphy in clinical routine, these algorithms were soon available on a commercial basis, providing a high degree of reproducibility and automated data analysis. Results from MRI and several PET tracers were extensively correlated [41–44] and can be summarized that due to its comparatively lower spatial resolution, the accuracy of the assessment of global and regional left ventricular function in SPECT or PET studies is limited when compared with MRI. However, the presence of excellent tissue contrast allows the use of fully automated analysis packages, avoiding time consuming manual or computer assisted definitions of endo- and epicardial contours.

Molecular Imaging

High sensitivity and the wide variety of potential probes make PET an attractive modality for molecular imaging where the concentrations of potential tracers fall in the subpicomolar range. However, a high resolution anatomical reference is often necessary.

Coronary Angiography and Vessel Wall Imaging

Given the better spatial resolution (approx. 0.4 mm in CT vs 0.8 mm in MRI) and thus, better diagnostic accuracy MSCT appears to be the preferred technique for non-invasive coronary angiography at present. However, technical advances in non-invasive coronary angiography by MRI have been rapid and it has potential to become a valuable diagnostic tool for detection of CAD in the future [45]. In a multicenter, single-vendor trial of 3D coronary MR angiography in 109 patients sensitivity, specificity and negative predictive values were 93, 58, and 81%, respectively for detection of >50% diameter stenosis of proximal and middle segments of coronary arteries using quantitative coronary angiography as the reference [46]. Notably, 16% of segments were of non-diagnostic quality. In addition to patency of the vascular lumen, MRI is capable of directly detecting atherosclerotic plaques and identification of their structural components, such as fibrous cap, necrotic core, calcification and intraplaque hemorrhage in proton weighed anatomical images [47]. Although the small dimensions of the coronary artery walls make their evaluation challenging, there are reports indicating the feasibility of visualization of an increased coronary artery wall thickness in patients with atherosclerosis using black-blood pulse sequences [48,49]. Molecular imaging may provide an opportunity to enhance contrast in plaque imaging by combining high sensitivity of PET to demonstrate accumulation of a specific contrast agent with MRI characterization of the morphology of individual plaques.

Macrophages are the target of many molecular imaging approaches of atherosclerosis, because inflammation is a key pathophysiological process throughout the progression of atherosclerosis [50]. Among several anatomical features, such as severe luminal obstruction, thin fibrous cap and large lipid core, the presence of active inflammation is a major feature of the rupture prone, so-called vulnerable plaques [50]. Sudden rupture of an atherosclerotic plaque that can happen even in the absence of significant luminal stenosis is a major cause of acute coronary events (myocardial infarction, unstable angina pectoris or sudden cardiac death). Therefore, non-invasive imaging of vascular inflammation might lead to better assessment of individuals at risk for acute coronary events, such as myocardial infarction. Moreover, detection of inflammation in the subclinical phase of atherosclerosis might help to refine estimates of the cardiovascular risk of an individual. Rudd *et al.* first demonstrated in humans that ^{18}F-FDG accumulation in the atherosclerotic carotid artery can be visualized in PET images [51]. ^{18}F-FDG is a glucose analog that is taken up by the metabolically active macrophages in the atherosclerotic lesions [52,53]. Recent studies provide evidence that the arterial ^{18}F-FDG signal is highly reproducible and thus, provides a highly reproducible measure of vascular inflammation [53]. However, ^{18}F-FDG is a relatively non-specific marker of metabolic activity and thus, there is interest in developing tracers for both PET and MRI that would allow more specific for identification of the vulnerable atherosclerotic plaques. Targets of such tracers may include specific macrophage receptors, protease activity, angiogenesis, and apoptosis as reviewed elsewhere [54]. In addition to providing an essential anatomical reference of plaque burden, MRI of the vessel wall could provide a means to do partial volume corrections of the PET signal and thus, facilitate its quantification [55].

Sympathetic Nervous System

This system plays an important role in regulating cardiac performance to meet changing circulatory demands by increasing heart rate and force of cardiac contraction. Several PET tracers, such as catecholamine analog ^{11}C labeled meta-hydroxyephedrine (HED) and tracers of beta-adrenoceptors can be used to visualize global and local defects in myocardial sympathetic innervation caused by various cardiac diseases, such as IHD, heart failure and arrythmogenic disorders [56]. Initial studies indicate that these defects are related to worse outcome of heart failure patients and thus, innervation imaging might provide prognostic information as well as guide in selection of therapies [57]. The combination of PET and MRI might facilitate risk stratification by allowing immediate combination of innervation studies with left ventricular function, which is currently the major prognostic indicator and criterion for therapy selection [58]. Moreover, it might facilitate focusing the studies into the myocardial areas of interest, such as the viable border zone of myocardial infarction which provides substrate of ventricular tachycardia [59].

Cell and Gene Therapies

Stem cell transplantation is a promising therapeutic option for heart diseases related to cardiomyocyte death, in particular acute myocardial infarction and subsequent heart failure. Randomized clinical trials have demonstrated improvements in left ventricular function (ejection fraction improvement in the range of 3–9%) and probably smaller infarct sizes after intracoronary injection of bone-marrow derived cells in the diseased coronary artery after an acute myocardial infarction [60]. Direct visualization of stem cells by imaging methods may provide novel insights in the number of cells surviving in the heart and help validating novel regenerative cell therapies non-invasively [61]. Radionuclides, such as ^{111}Indium-oxine, ^{99m}Technetium-exametazime or ^{18}F-FDG can be used to directly label stem cells for direct visualization of the stem cells in the infracted myocardium after intravenous administration. Reporter gene imaging is based on transfection of stem cells prior to their implantation with genes that are not normally expressed in the heart, and that encode protein products that mediate accumulation of a radiolabeled reporter probe. After application, cells can then be detected by an intravenously administered, radiolabeled or optical reporter probe, which is specific for the reporter gene and which accumulates in the transduced therapeutic cells. This approach can be performed repeatedly over a long period of time, because it is not limited by radioactive decay. Reporter gene PET imaging has been shown to be feasible for visualization of the survival of stem cells in experimental models of myocardial infarction. However, its feasibility in patient studies of stem cell treatment still remains to be tested in the future. An example of imaging of myocardial expression of the reporter gene herpesviral thymidine kinase (HSV1-tk) using ^{124}Iodine-2'-Fluoro-2-deoxy-5-iodo-1-β-D-arabinofuranosyluracil (^{124}I-FIAU) as the probe is shown in Figure 12.4 [62]. In this study, reporter gene imaging was used to assess delivery of adenoviral gene therapy after intramyocardial injection. The elevated FIAU retention during the first 30 minutes after injection was located in the myocardium by co-registration with ^{13}N-ammonia flow signal and MRI. Merging with the MRI image shows detailed visualization of the location of the reporter gene expression. Combination of reporter gene signal of PET with MRI is also attractive, because accurate evaluation of left ventricular function and myocardial infarct size are important

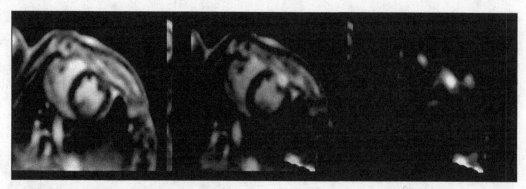

Figure 12.4　Co-registration and fusion display in PET "hot spot" imaging using Iodine-124 2'-Fluoro-2'-deoxy-5-iodo-1-β-D-arabinofuranosyluracil (^{124}I-FIAU) as marker of gene expression in a pig model. Without anatomical reference, the tracer uptake is impossible to locate. For this display, a PET flow tracer study was aligned to the MRI and the co-registration matrix was subsequently applied to the FIAU data. (Figure reproduced with permission from [62].)

surrogate endpoints for evaluation of cardiac cell therapies.

Angiogenesis

Formation of new capillaries from pre-existing vasculature, known as angiogenesis, occurs in response to ischemia and inflammation being part of the healing process after an ischemic tissue injury. RGD peptides can be radiolabeled to produce a PET tracer ^{18}F Galacto-RGD that allows noninvasive imaging of expression of $\alpha_v\beta_3$ integrin, a cell-membrane glycoprotein receptor that is highly expressed in the endothelium of angiogenic vessels [63,64]. Recent studies have provided evidence that ^{18}F Galacto-RGD accumulate in ischemically injured myocardium and the uptake can be visualized by PET imaging in the area of myocardial infarct scar [65]. Since expression of $\alpha_v\beta_3$ integrin reflect regional myocardial responses to injury, imaging of its expression might be useful for monitoring the effectiveness of various therapies aimed at improving the healing of myocardium after injury. An example of this type of very specific imaging in conjunction with high resolution MRI imaging is shown in Figure 12.5 [66]. ^{18}F-Galakto-RGD was used to assess integrin expression in a patient who had an acute myocardial infarction and successful revascularization 2 weeks earlier. In this case, delayed-enhancement signal allowed exact localization of the ^{18}F-Galakto-RGD uptake into the region of myocardial infaction.

Software Approaches for Cardiac MRI and PET Co-Registration and Fusion

In order to combine MRI and PET, the resulting image data from the two independent modalities must be combined in a single computer environment, aligned in the spatial domain, and analyzed. There has been substantial success in the implementation of a standardized image format (DICOM) and communication mechanisms in recent years. The first step towards technically combining MRI and PET image data has been greatly facilitated by the elimination of the previously experienced problems caused by various data formats and computer platforms, and limited computing resources. Despite this achievement, cardiac studies typically provide two additional challenges. Firstly, routine gated acquisitions performed in MRI are also possible in PET. Thus, the three spatial dimensions must be supplemented with a time dimension (this yields 4D data). Secondly, the highly varying acquisition times between PET and MRI are problematic. MRI scans are typically performed in a few seconds during breath-holds and PET scans have a minimum scan duration of five minutes. In addition, despite heart phased resolved data acquisition in PET, the effect of breathing motion is essentially ignored in all scanner systems and results in motional blurring. This creates the challenge of data co-registration of only one particular breathing state (MRI) with a mean breathing motion position (PET).

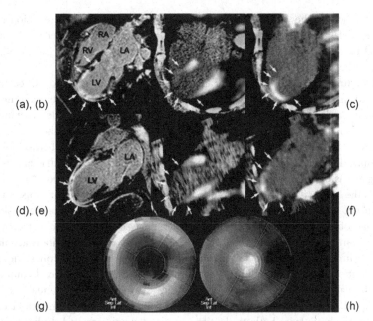

(a), (b)

(c)

(d), (e)

(f)

(g)

(h)

Figure 12.5 Integration of ceMRI and PET perfusion and a_vb_3 integrin expression in a patient 2 weeks after myocardial infarction [66]. (a and d) ceMRI with delayed enhancement (arrows) extending from the anterior wall to the apical region in the four- (a) and two-chamber (d) view. (b and e) Identically reproduced location and geometry with severely reduced myocardial blood flow using ^{13}N-ammonia, corresponding to the regions of delayed enhancement by ceMRI (arrows). (c and f) Focal ^{18}F-RGD signal co-localized to the infarcted area. (g) Polar map of myocardial blood flow assessed by ^{13}N-ammonia indicating severely reduced flow in the distal LAD-perfused region. (h) Co-localized ^{18}F-RGD signal corresponding to the regions of severely reduced ^{13}N-ammonia flow signal, reflecting the extent the of a_vb_3 expression within the infarcted area.

Practical Co-Registration

The methodological complexity described above is rarely, if at all, accounted for in validation studies or in studies incorporating both modalities. In most cases, mapping of the regional properties, such as wall motion or contrast media uptake in the left ventricle, is performed according to a standard model suggested by the American Heart Association [67]. This seventeen-segment model is typically filled out with the qualitative or quantitative information from both studies on a visual basis and subsequently statistically compared. Slice to slice comparisons are also used, but suffer from a limitation in MRI data acquisition. In contrast to CT and PET, where the complete data volume is sampled isotropically, MRI is in most cases slice based. In other words, arbitrary multiplanar reformatted images can be derived from the isotropic data volume. The foundation for this approach are similar voxel sizes in all spatial dimensions; this does not hold true for many MRI acquisitions, where the in plane resolution is much higher than the slice thickness. Thus, in order to create matching slices, the CT or PET volume must be reformatted to the parameters at which the MR image was acquired. As this is a demanding and time consuming step, the pixel by pixel comparison is rarely found in publications.

Approaches to Cardiac Data Co-Registration

Two major groups of registration algorithms are known today. Feature based techniques identify common structures in both data sets and use, thereafter, an optimization routine to minimize the distance between the common structures as defined by these surfaces can be implemented. Thus, errors in the delineation of the surfaces limit the applicability of this approach. Those errors might stem from mistakes in the manual definition of common morphological elements. Or, if automatic feature extraction methods are used, the two imaging methods delineate inherently non-matching borders. This can be demonstrated by infarcted myocardial tissue, which shows excellent signal intensity in MRI delayed enhancement imaging, whereas normal tissue is blacked. PET perfusion imaging presents the exact opposite situation, in which normal perfused tissue shows significant tracer uptake and infarcted tissue shows little or even no uptake. In cardiac imaging, this poses an especially large problem, because of the limited number of accurate anatomical landmarks in the heart. For example, the rotational symmetry along the heart's long axis is much higher than the conditions found in the brain, making co-registration much more difficult.

The second class of registration algorithms focus on information from the data volumes, thus limiting the need for image segmentation steps. One of the early publications on the subject of MRI and PET co-registration appeared in 1993 [68]. Woods *et al.* used the standard deviation of signal intensity histograms in the brain from both modalities and calculated an optimal co-registration matrix to match MRI and PET. Other statistical properties, such as joint entropy [69] or mutual information [70–72] were investigated as well. The latter technique built the foundation for several commercial co-registration packages. The alignment precision, as found in thoracic image registration, is not yet available from MRI/PET studies, but might be estimated from PET/CT studies. Here, this value was found to be in the order of 2 mm in brain studies [73] and less than 10 mm in oncological studies of the thorax [74,75].

So far, the discussed approaches have used linear registration. This allows translation in all three directions and rotation around three axes. As the heart is located in the thorax, non-linear techniques might apply as well, as substantial deformation occurs over both the breathing and cardiac cycles. Unfortunately, there is only limited data on this subject, even from PET/CT studies. One reason for the sparse number of publications may be the problems inherent in validation studies. Even sophisticated phantom studies fail to describe the complex motion and deformation patterns found in patients [76]. Thus, the practical consequences continue to be unclear, which also holds true for any dual modality acquisitions when not performed simultaneously [77,78]. Interestingly, the displacement found in this hardware approach was in the

order of the linear software fusion (< 10 mm) as mentioned above. However, the misalignment was considered to be modest from a clinical point of view, at least in oncology.

The previously mentioned co-registration of four-dimensional data sets (volume over time or volume over cardiac cycle) remains a challenging issue. Unfortunately, there is very limited data available to demonstrate its feasibility [79]. In this study, we utilized the cardiac analysis framework, "MunichHeart," developed at our institution for a model based approach to this issue. Data from PET acquisitions were analyzed using volumetric data analysis, which is facilitated by the fact that PET, as well as SPECT, data is acquired with near isotropic voxels [80,81]. From static and gated MRI studies, endo- and epicardial contours of the left ventricle were defined manually. Combined with the volume contours of the tracer distribution in static, dynamic or gated studies, this approach allowed the co-registration of the bimodal data sets (Figure 12.6) in a two-step implementation. First, the two sets of contours describing the left ventricle in MRI and PET were matched as closely as possible, based on geometrical constraints. However, as already mentioned, the fundamental difference in imaging physics and physiology requires the assistance of a second step: a final, manual adjustment of the two modalities.

Klein and colleagues implemented a non-uniform, elastic model, described by 12 parameters, and adjusted the PET data within this model. Although this is not a multimodal application in the strictest sense, it shows great promise for this field [82]. Another model-based technique was published, which also integrated the right ventricle and used external markers to integrate data from a third modality, magnetocardiography [83].

Aladl and colleagues [84] described an approach to 4D SPECT-MRI co-registration and fusion, in which the MRI study was segmented, based on regional pixel value changes due to motion, essentially removing any static tissue; they subsequently applied mutual information measures to co-register the data sets. These results were compared to a co-registration performed manually by an expert. The translational differences were found to be in the order of 1 mm with MRI segmentation and 4 mm without it. For the rotational offset, 4°

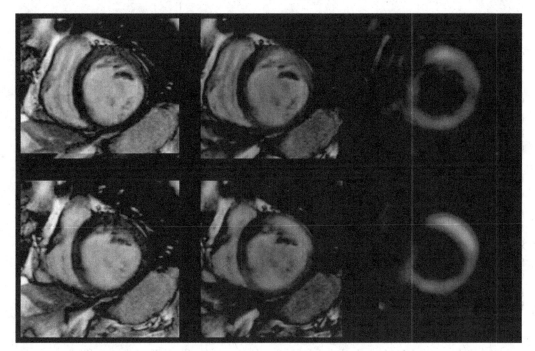

Figure 12.6 Four-dimensional co-registration and fusion of a gated MRI and a gated FDG study in a patient with severe myocardial dysfunction. Only the end-systolic and the end-diastolic frame are displayed. The partial volume dependent FDG uptake is visible in the anterior wall because of the increasing proximity of myocardial wall and papillary muscle during systole.

and 10° respectively were found. Technically, this technique can be applied to PET data as well and offers a high degree of automation.

All methods described so far require a substantial amount of user interaction or computing time. A scalable system, implementing algorithms based on voxel similarity, was developed by Shekhar *et al.* [85,86]. Their system has shown substantial potential, as it makes possible computationally very demanding procedures, which allow even for correction of misalignment between, for example pre- and poststress gated 3D echo data.

From a practical point, the alignment issue is similar to the registration of CT and PET or SPECT studies. As this alignment is a prerequisite for successful correction of photon attenuation, this problem has recently received quite some attention [87,88]. The discussion can be summarized as follows as it has immediate consequences for a potential integrated MRI-PET device: (a) misalignment between emission and transmission data is one of the most significant sources of errors due to the temporal delay between the acquisitions and the non avoidable motion of the patient and (b) the alignment is mostly performed manually as not automated algorithms is available so far for any vendor's system.

Image and Parametric Data Integration

The high complexity of cardiac data acquisition co-registration would ideally require a multimodal integration of both image and parametric information, such as myocardial blood flow, which itself is derived from a series of temporal images. These parametric mapping techniques are common in functional imaging of the brain and were also used in MRI for perfusion and delayed enhancement studies [20]. However, very limited data is available on this issue, which goes beyond the visualization of so-called 4D bimodal data sets (three dimension of space and one comprising the time, e.g., the offsets from the R wave). The work of Mäkela has already been mentioned above [83]. As the authors also added magnetocardiography to their study parameters, the amount of qualitative and quantitative data was even larger, as expected, and an efficient means of data visualization for the interpretation of the data was required. Although significant advances have been made in academic centers (Figure 12.6 [89], Figure 12.2 [90]), complex cardiac data integration is still an ambitious project and commercial solutions have not yet come onto the market.

Limitations of Spatial Co-Registration

Unfortunately, there is little data on the possible accuracy of aligning multimodal data in the chest from MRI and PET studies because of: (a) gross patient motion, (b) thoracic motion, and (c) cardiac motion. The first two types of motion are very challenging, as they occur rather randomly and can produce irregular patterns. However, the availability of PET/CT systems has enabled studies to be conducted in the thorax. Although these limited publications focus primarily on oncological issues, they are briefly summarized here, as they provide a good estimate of the potential limitations.

Osman and co-authors evaluated the incidence of inaccurate lesion detection in 300 patients and found incorrect localizations in the liver/lung border zone in only six examinations [91]. Other studies on respiratory induced motion, which focused more specifically on developing an optimal breathing protocol for the CT portion of the examination, reported displacements between PET and CT ranging between 5 and 20 mm [92,93]. One conclusion of these papers was that co-registration can be achieved in the order of the spatial resolution of the PET system, which is between 6 and 10 mm. The study by Boucher and colleagues measured a mean ± SD motion in axial direction of the apex of the heart of 6.7 ± 3.0 mm (maximal displacement: 11.9 mm) for breathing triggered PET acquisition [94]. This group used a temperature sensitive respiratory gating device installed in a breathing mask. The derived apical motion was calculated from the reconstructed images. One should note that the transmission scan applied was ungated.

These numbers give some idea of the potential motion found in thorax imaging. Although animal models exist, which could serve as a validation platform [95], most research concentrates on retrospective alignment of complete patients. In their review, Mäkela et al. summarized the registration accuracy for intra- and intermodal applications [96]. For MRI intramodal alignment, 1.5–3.0 mm accuracies were reported. With PET-PET co-registration, 1.0–2.5 mm was found and finally, PET-MRI showed 1.95 ± 1.6 mm [97] through the implementation of a rigid heart surface based approach for gated MRI and gated PET and 80 landmarks. A second reference calculated 2.8 ± 0.5 mm using an indirect measure for cardiac data (actually using thorax and lung surfaces for validation) [98].

In summary, patient, thorax and cardiac motion make co-registration of any imaging sequences not acquired simultaneously a major obstacle in inter- and intramodal data acquisition. Significant advances have been made in cardiac software co-registration, yielding accuracies in the range between 1–3 mm. However, essentially none of the publications discussed in the validation and synergetic applications sections used these advanced software algorithms. Thus, major efforts are necessary to link the cardiological users with the image postprocessing specialists in order to create user friendly applications, which will extract maximal information from multimodal studies.

Combined Imaging in Hardware

All previous results and discussions were based on separate examinations in the two modalities, MRI and PET. From a logistical and patient comfort point of view, this procedure is clearly suboptimal. The success of combined PET/CT devices is proof that more efficient methods can be obtained; certainly they are required. Even if the measurements cannot be performed simultaneously but only sequentially (as in PET/CT), the improvement in the solving of logistical problems and the gains in comfort for the patient will be significant. However, the absolute hardware costs, as well as cost efficiency, must be considered. This short review will provide basic insights into the technological challenges and the potential solution. For a more detailed description see review from Pichler et al. [99].

Technical Challenges

The basic aim of PET is the detection of high-energy photons resulting from an annihilation event during the decay of a positron emitting isotope. This isotope is typically bound to a pharmaceutical with the advantage that the concentration of these substances can be in the pico to femto molar range. The high energy photon (minimum 511 keV) is typically stopped by, and detected in, a detector crystal, where it is absorbed. After a short time, the particular atom emits a lower energy photon. This photon is detected by a photomultiplier tube, which is available in almost all PET scanners. In the photomultiplier, the photon releases an electron, which, in turn, is amplified at a high voltage cascade. Unfortunately, free electrons in the vacuum of the tube are displaced by even the smallest magnetic fields (approximately 1–10 mT), rendering the usual technique of photon detection and amplification in MR systems completely useless. For this reason, even the sequential approach of combining hardware in close proximity, as found in PET/CT systems is technically not feasible in PET/MRI.

Use of Large Magnetic Fields to Increase Spatial Resolution

Before discussing possible solutions, an interesting strategy, (which was discussed in the nineties) based on theoretical considerations and simulations should be mentioned here. As described above, a positron is emitted during the decay of a radioisotope bound to the radiopharmaceutical. Depending on the actual isotope, the positron is emitted with substantial energy (examples of isotopes with special relevance in cardiac imaging: ^{18}F Emax = 0.64 MeV; ^{11}C Emax = 0.97 MeV; ^{13}N Emax = 1.2 MeV; ^{15}O Emax = 1.74 MeV, and ^{82}Rb Emax = 3.15 MeV). This energy allows it to travel several millimeters through water or biological substances before it forms the so-called positronium with an electron, and before it finally annihilates with the emission of two 511-keV photons. This means that the spatial location of the emitting radioisotope does not coincide with the detected location of the annihilation. A large magnetic field, however, could force the positron on a circular path perpendicular to the magnetic field because of the Lorenz force, effectively improving the spatial resolution of a PET scanner. Following up on simulation studies by Iida *et al.* [100], Hammer and colleagues implemented an experimental set up, where 4-m long optical light guides transported the photons to an

area without disrupting magnetic fields [101–103]. Using ^{68}Ge (Emax = 1.90 MeV), they showed a clear improvement of spatial resolution at five Tesla (T) field strength and the full width at half maximum (FWHM) decreased by a factor of 1.42. They also concluded that the effect of using lower energy positron-emitters, such as ^{22}Na (Emax = 0.55 MeV) should have little or no effect. At least for the widely used ^{82}Rb in a hypothetical 3T system, a certain gain in spatial resolution can be anticipated.

MR Spectroscopy and PET

Two years later, the next step from improvements of the spatial resolution of PET experiments in high magnetic fields towards the combination of the two modalities was performed at Guy's hospital in London, UK. A "minimal" PET scanner, consisting of a pair of electronically coupled sodium-iodine (NaI) detectors, was integrated within a 9.4T wide bore spectroscopy system [104]. Again, long light guides were used to transfer the postannihilation photons to detectors outside of the main magnetic fields. This kind of PET system is not capable of acquiring image data, but is used at several PET centers to study the pharmacokinetics of various radiotracers in isolated rat or mouse heart models. This approach allowed the first simultaneous measurements of time resolved ^{31}P and ^{13}C spectra during ^{18}F-FDG metabolic studies of isolated rat hearts. The temporal resolution was 15s in both modalities.

Through a collaborative effort between the London group and the UCLA School of Medicine, the two coupled scintillation detectors were replaced by a miniature PET scanner [105]. Based on the UCLA group's micro-PET system [106], a single ring lutetium oxyorthosilicate (LSO) system with 72 crystals (2 mm × 2 mm × 25 mm) was built and inserted in a 7.3 cm bore, 9.4 T MR device. Once again, 4-m long optical fibers were used to transfer the scintillation photons to an external detection system. The disadvantage of long fibers, which attenuate the light output from the scintillators, was partly offset by the use of LSO, which shows a significantly higher light yield compared to other PET detectors' materials. With this system, which is essentially a one-slice PET tomograph, a spatial PET resolution of 2 mm FWHM with an axial field-of-view of 25 mm was achieved inside and outside the magnetic field. Using an isolated rat heart model, simultaneous PET FDG images and ^{31}P spectra were acquired, thus demonstrating the feasibility of dual modality data acquisition. The operation of the PET subsystem within the MR led to a 30% degradation of the ^{31}P line, which could not be improved with the shim coils. However, the authors concluded that such degradation would not cause significant problems in biological MR experiments.

In a subsequent study by Garlick et al. ^{31}P spectroscopy and ^{18}F-FDG PET imaging was combined [107]. The authors were able to demonstrate that there is a differential effect of the uptake of the two glucose analogs, ^{18}F 2-fluoro-2-deoxyglucose (as a standard PET tracer) and 2-deoxyglucose (DG), in a model of regional ischemia. Thus, the two modalities were able to trace two different glucose analogs, which are mutually exclusive to PET or MR in the very same physiological model. Very recently, the same group reported further findings, using ^{19}F spectroscopy [108], and was able to highlight the complex nature of FDG metabolism and the potential consequences in PET imaging. Although this was a pure NMR spectroscopy study, it clearly showed the potential for synergetic effects in basic research with hypothetical consequences for clinical routine examinations.

Simultaneous MRI and PET Imaging

The next step of MRI/PET imaging is the generation of MR images not only to accompany PET data, but to be acquired at the same time as the PET data is measured. This research focuses on preclinical applications, because the smaller dimensions make the design of hardware easier and the use of high resolution CT in small animals is still limited due to its high radiation dose.

A modified PET system, based on the device described above consisted of forty-eight $2 \times 2 \times 10$ mm^3 LSO crystals forming a 38-mm diameter ring. This modular scanner was inserted in 0.2T vertical field open MRI system [106]. The coupling to the photo multiplier tubes was again achieved with 4-m long optical fibers. Using a 2D FLASH sequence, a cylindrical phantom with seven 1-mm holes and a 5-mm separation, filled with a FDG and NiCl2 solution was acquired without visible artifacts.

In 1999, Slates and colleagues [109] utilized the setup as presented above in a series of imaging experiments in different MR scanners (0.2, 1.5, 4.7 and 9.4T) and with a variety of MR image sequences, using a dedicated phantom and biological material (an orange). Susceptibility artifacts from the LSO scintillators and the optical fibers in the MR images were not observed. Other limitations, such as interactions with the scanners' magnetic field or electromagnetic interference with the PET acquisition, were not detected using various sequences (T_1 as well as T_2 spin echo, turbo spin echo and gradient echo). Although these results proved the feasibility of this concept, several limitations were observed. Because of the one-ring concept and the optical fiber readout, the PET scanner showed an overall limited performance, as well as a very small field of view, when compared to dedicated small animal PET systems. In a review article, published in 2002, Paul Marsden and colleagues outlined the concept of a successor imaging device [110]. However, no further studies have been released so far. Although the concept of an optical readout is intriguing, the sensitivity of such an approach will always be limited because of substantial photon attenuation over long fiber optics.

The most recent advances are based on concepts of integrated detectors utilizing avalanche photodiodes for a complete, multi-ring PET animal scanner which are insensitive or high magnetic fields [111–113]. In 2006, Pichler et al. reported on the integration of a high-resolution, APD based PET scanner with a 7-T MRI system for animal research [114]. This device, which again used optical fibers, showed its capability for simultaneous MRI and PET acquisitions in ex vivo mouse experiments [115]. The next generation of a hybrid MR/PET system featured an compact PET insert which was capable of PET acquisitions with simultaneous MR imaging or spectroscopy [9,116]. Besides developments in research institutions, a first commercial solution with a 3T whole body MRI and a PET insert suitable for imaging the human brain and an axial field-of-view of 18 cm was recently presented [99,117].

However, these devices have not been applied in cardiac imaging—but as no principal technical limitations can be anticipated, first preclinical results are expected soon.

Conclusion

This overview has discussed the wide range of applications in which MRI and PET acquisitions have been used in the same patients. Unfortunately, but understandably, validation studies represented the majority of the examples. Within the validation studies, one modality attempted to replace another in situations where there were potential clinical applications. This strategy is a result of cost pressures, clinical logistics and overall efficiency. However, it was also demonstrated that while the two modalities each had unique strengths, they were also able to complement each other extremely well.

There have been major achievements in software-based co-registration in the past. However, the application of these techniques and tools to a widespread use has not yet occurred.

Finally, whether a hybrid MRI/PET system will repeat the clinical success of PET/CT is still an open question where the answer will strongly be influenced by cost efficiency considerations.

Acknowledgments

The authors thank Axel Martinez Möller for critically reading the manuscript. Dr. Saraste received financial assistance through EC-FP6-project DiMI (LSHBCT-2005-512146) and Finnish Foundation for Cardiovascular Research.

References

1. Lauterbur PC. Image formation by induced local interactions. Examples employing nuclear magnetic resonance. *Nature.* 1973 16 March;242:190–191.
2. Ter-Pogossian MM, Phelps ME, Hoffman EJ, Mullani NA. A positron-emission transaxial tomograph for nuclear imaging (PETT). *Radiology.* 1975;114(1):89–98.
3. Beyer T, Townsend DW, Brun T, *et al.* A combined PET/CT scanner for clinical oncology. *J Nucl Med.* 2000;41(8):1369–1379.
4. Townsend DW. A combined PET/CT scanner: the choices. *J Nucl Med.* 2001;42(3):533–534.
5. Phelps ME. Comments and perspectices. *J Nucl Med.* 2004;45:1601–1603.
6. Schwaiger M, Melin J. Cardiological applications of nuclear medicine. *Lancet.* 1999;354(9179):661–666.
7. Pohost GM, Hung L, Doyle M. Clinical use of cardiovascular magnetic resonance. *Circulation.* 2003;108(6): 647–653.
8. Selwyn AP, Allan RM, L'Abbate A, *et al.* Relation between regional myocardial uptake of rubidium-82 and perfusion: absolute reduction of cation uptake in ischemia. *Am J Cardiol.* 1982;50(1):112–121.
9. Judenhofer MS, Wehrl HF, Newport DF, *et al.* Simultaneous PET-MRI: a new approach for functional and morphological imaging. *Nat Med.* 2008;14(4):459–465.
10. Klocke FJ, Baird MG, Lorell BH, *et al.* ACC/AHA/ASNC guidelines for the clinical use of cardiac radionuclide imaging–executive summary: a report of the American college of cardiology/American heart association task force on practice guidelines (ACC/AHA/ASNC Committee to Revise the 1995 Guidelines for the Clinical Use of Cardiac Radionuclide Imaging). *J Am Coll Cardiol.* 2003;42(7):1318–1333.
11. Yoshinaga K, Chow BJ, Williams K, *et al.* What is the prognostic value of myocardial perfusion imaging using rubidium-82 positron emission tomography? *J Am Coll Cardiol.* 2006;48(5):1029–1039.
12. Marwick TH, Shan K, Patel S, Go RT, Lauer MS. Incremental value of rubidium-82 positron emission tomography for prognostic assessment of known or suspected coronary artery disease. *Am J Cardiol.* 1997;80(7): 865–870.
13. Sawada S, Muzik O, Beanlands RS, Wolfe E, Hutchins GD, Schwaiger M. Interobserver and interstudy variability of myocardial blood flow and flow-reserve measurements with nitrogen 13 ammonia-labeled positron emission tomography. *J Nucl Cardiol.* 1995;2(5): 413–422.
14. Kaufmann PA, Gnecchi-Ruscone T, Yap JT, Rimoldi O, Camici PG. Assessment of the reproducibility of baseline and hyperemic myocardial blood flow measurements with 15 O-labeled water and PET. *J Nucl Med.* 1999;40(11):1848–1856.
15. El Fakhri G, Sitek A, Guerin B, Kijewski MF, Di Carli MF, Moore SC. Quantitative dynamic cardiac 82Rb PET using generalized factor and compartment analyses. *J Nucl Med.* 2005;46(8):1264–1271.
16. Manning WJ, Atkinson DJ, Grossman W, Paulin S, Edelman RR. First-pass nuclear magnetic resonance imaging studies using gadolinium-DTPA in patients with coronary artery disease. *J Am Coll Cardiol.* 1991;18(4): 959–965.
17. Nandalur KR, Dwamena BA, Choudhri AF, Nandalur MR, Carlos RC. Diagnostic performance of stress cardiac magnetic resonance imaging in the detection of coronary artery disease: a meta-analysis. *J Am Coll Cardiol.* 2007;50(14):1343–1353.
18. Schwitter J, Wacker CM, van Rossum AC, *et al.* MR-IMPACT: comparison of perfusion-cardiac magnetic resonance with single-photon emission computed tomography for the detection of coronary artery disease in

a multicentre, multivendor, randomized trial. *Eur Heart J.* 2008;29(4):480–489.

19. Schwitter J, DeMarco T, Kneifel S, *et al.* Magnetic resonance-based assessment of global coronary flow and flow reserve and its relation to left ventricular functional parameters: a comparison with positron emission tomography. *Circulation.* 2000;101(23):2696–2702.

20. Ibrahim T, Nekolla SG, Schreiber K, *et al.* Assessment of coronary flow reserve: comparison between contrast-enhanced magnetic resonance imaging and positron emission tomography. *J Am Coll Cardiol.* 2002;39(5):864–870.

21. Klein C, Nekolla SG, Balbach T, *et al.* The influence of myocardial blood flow and volume of distribution on late Gd-DTPA kinetics in ischemic heart failure. *J Magn Reson Imaging.* 2004;20(4):588–593.

22. Schinkel AF, Poldermans D, Elhendy A, Bax JJ. Assessment of myocardial viability in patients with heart failure. *J Nucl Med.* 2007;48(7):1135–1146.

23. Kim RJ, Fieno DS, Parrish TB, *et al.* Relationship of MRI delayed contrast enhancement to irreversible injury, infarct age, and contractile function. *Circulation.* 1999;100(19):1992–2002.

24. Klein C, Nekolla SG, Bengel FM, *et al.* Assessment of myocardial viability with contrast-enhanced magnetic resonance imaging: comparison with positron emission tomography. *Circulation.* 2002;105(2):162–167.

25. Kim RJ, Wu E, Rafael A, *et al.* The use of contrast-enhanced magnetic resonance imaging to identify reversible myocardial dysfunction. *N Engl J Med.* 2000;343(20):1445–1453.

26. Kuhl HP, Lipke CS, Krombach GA, *et al.* Assessment of reversible myocardial dysfunction in chronic ischaemic heart disease: comparison of contrast-enhanced cardiovascular magnetic resonance and a combined positron emission tomography-single photon emission computed tomography imaging protocol. *Eur Heart J.* 2006;27(7):846–853.

27. Perrone-Filardi P, Bacharach SL, Dilsizian V, *et al.* Metabolic evidence of viable myocardium in regions with reduced wall thickness and absent wall thickening in patients with chronic ischemic left ventricular dysfunction. *J Am Coll Cardiol.* 1992;20(1):161–168.

28. Baer FM, Voth E, Schneider CA, Theissen P, Schicha H, Sechtem U. Comparison of low-dose dobutamine-gradient-echo magnetic resonance imaging and positron emission tomography with [18F]fluorodeoxyglucose in patients with chronic coronary artery disease. A functional and morphological approach to the detection of residual myocardial viability. *Circulation.* 1995;91(4):1006–1015.

29. Gerber BL, Rochitte CE, Bluemke DA, *et al.* Relation between Gd-DTPA contrast enhancement and regional inotropic response in the periphery and center of myocardial infarction. *Circulation.* 2001;104(9):998–1004.

30. Schmidt M, Voth E, Schneider CA, *et al.* F-18-FDG uptake is a reliable predictory of functional recovery of akinetic but viable infarct regions as defined by magnetic resonance imaging before and after revascularization. *Magn Reson Imaging.* 2004;22(2):229–236.

31. Knuesel PR, Nanz D, Wyss C, *et al.* Characterization of dysfunctional myocardium by positron emission tomography and magnetic resonance: relation to functional outcome after revascularization. *Circulation.* 2003;108(9):1095–1100.

32. Wijns W, Vatner SF, Camici PG. Hibernating myocardium. *N Engl J Med.* 1998;339(3):173–181.

33. Higuchi T, Nekolla SG, Jankaukas A, *et al.* Characterization of normal and infarcted rat myocardium using a combination of small-animal PET and clinical MRI. *J Nucl Med.* 2007;48(2):288–294.

34. Thomas D, Bal H, Arkles J, *et al.* Noninvasive assessment of myocardial viability in a small animal model: comparison of MRI, SPECT, and PET. *Magn Reson Med.* 2008;59(2):252–259.

35. Allman KC, Shaw LJ, Hachamovitch R, Udelson JE. Myocardial viability testing and impact of revascularization on prognosis in patients with coronary artery disease and left ventricular dysfunction: a meta-analysis. *J Am Coll Cardiol.* 2002;39(7):1151–1158.

36. Haas F, Haehnel CJ, Picker W, *et al.* Preoperative positron emission tomographic viability assessment and perioperative and postoperative risk in patients with advanced ischemic heart disease. *J Am Coll Cardiol.* 1997;30(7):1693–1700.

37. Kwong RY, Chan AK, Brown KA, *et al.* Impact of unrecognized myocardial scar detected by cardiac magnetic resonance imaging on event-free survival in patients presenting with signs or symptoms of coronary artery disease. *Circulation.* 2006;113(23):2733–2743.

38. Bellenger NG, Davies LC, Francis JM, Coats AJ, Pennell DJ. Reduction in sample size for studies of remodeling in heart failure by the use of cardiovascular magnetic resonance. *J Cardiovasc Magn Reson.* 2000;2(4):271–278.

39. Bengel FM, Lehnert J, Ibrahim T, *et al.* Cardiac oxidative metabolism, function, and metabolic performance in mild hyperthyroidism: a noninvasive study using positron emission tomography and magnetic resonance imaging. *Thyroid.* 2003;13(5):471–477.

40. Germano G, Kavanagh PB, Su HT, *et al.* Automatic reorientation of three-dimensional, transaxial myocardial perfusion SPECT images. *J Nucl Med.* 1995;36(6):1107–1114.

41. Germano G, Kiat H, Kavanagh PB, *et al.* Automatic quantification of ejection fraction from gated

myocardial perfusion SPECT. *J Nucl Med*. 1995;36(11): 2138–2147.

42. Khorsand A, Graf S, Frank H, *et al*. Model-based analysis of electrocardiography-gated cardiac (18)F-FDG PET images to assess left ventricular geometry and contractile function. *J Nucl Med*. 2003;44(11):1741–1746.

43. Schaefer WM, Lipke CS, Nowak B, *et al*. Validation of an evaluation routine for left ventricular volumes, ejection fraction and wall motion from gated cardiac FDG PET: a comparison with cardiac magnetic resonance imaging. *Eur J Nucl Med Mol Imaging*. 2003;30(4):545–553.

44. Schaefer WM, Lipke CS, Nowak B, *et al*. Validation of QGS and 4D-MSPECT for quantification of left ventricular volumes and ejection fraction from gated 18F-FDG PET: comparison with cardiac MRI. *J Nucl Med*. 2004;45(1):74–79.

45. Bluemke DA, Achenbach S, Budoff M, *et al*. Noninvasive coronary artery imaging. Magnetic resonance angiography and multidetector computed tomography angiography. A scientific statement from the American Heart Association Committee on Cardiovascular Imaging and Intervention of the Council on Cardiovascular Radiology and Intervention, and the Councils on Clinical Cardiology and Cardiovascular Disease in the Young. *Circulation*. 2008;118(5):586–606.

46. Kim WY, Danias PG, Stuber M, *et al*. Coronary magnetic resonance angiography for the detection of coronary stenoses. *N Engl J Med*. 2001;345(26):1863–1869.

47. Yuan C, Mitsumori LM, Beach KW, Maravilla KR. Carotid atherosclerotic plaque: noninvasive MR characterization and identification of vulnerable lesions. *Radiology*. 2001;221(2):285–299.

48. Fayad ZA, Fuster V, Fallon JT, *et al*. Noninvasive in vivo human coronary artery lumen and wall imaging using black-blood magnetic resonance imaging. *Circulation*. 2000;102(5):506–510.

49. Kim WY, Stuber M, Bornert P, Kissinger KV, Manning WJ, Botnar RM. Three-dimensional black-blood cardiac magnetic resonance coronary vessel wall imaging detects positive arterial remodeling in patients with nonsignificant coronary artery disease. *Circulation*. 2002;106(3):296–299.

50. Libby P. Inflammation in atherosclerosis. *Nature*. 2002;420(6917):868–874.

51. Rudd JH, Warburton EA, Fryer TD, *et al*. Imaging atherosclerotic plaque inflammation with [18F]-fluorodeoxyglucose positron emission tomography. *Circulation*. 2002;105(23):2708–2711.

52. Tawakol A, Migrino RQ, Bashian GG, *et al*. In vivo 18F-fluorodeoxyglucose positron emission tomography imaging provides a noninvasive measure of carotid plaque inflammation in patients. *J Am Coll Cardiol*. 2006;48(9):1818–1824.

53. Rudd JH, Myers KS, Bansilal S, *et al*. Atherosclerosis inflammation imaging with 18F-FDG PET: carotid, iliac, and femoral uptake reproducibility, quantification methods, and recommendations. *J Nucl Med*. 2008;49(6):871–878.

54. Sanz J, Fayad ZA. Imaging of atherosclerotic cardiovascular disease. *Nature*. 2008;451(7181):953–957.

55. Davies JR, Rudd JH, Fryer TD, *et al*. Identification of culprit lesions after transient ischemic attack by combined 18F fluorodeoxyglucose positron-emission tomography and high-resolution magnetic resonance imaging. *Stroke*. 2005;36(12):2642–2647.

56. Bengel FM, Schwaiger M. Assessment of cardiac sympathetic neuronal function using PET imaging. *J Nucl Cardiol*. 2004;11(5):603–616.

57. Verberne HJ, Brewster LM, Somsen GA, van Eck-Smit BL. Prognostic value of myocardial 123I-metaiodobenzylguanidine (MIBG) parameters in patients with heart failure: a systematic review. *Eur Heart J*. 2008;29(9):1147–1159.

58. Swedberg K, Cleland J, Dargie H, *et al*. Guidelines for the diagnosis and treatment of chronic heart failure: executive summary (update 2005): The task force for the diagnosis and treatment of chronic heart failure of the European society of cardiology. *Eur Heart J*. 2005;26(11):1115–1140.

59. Sasano T, Abraham MR, Chang KC, *et al*. Abnormal sympathetic innervation of viable myocardium and the substrate of ventricular tachycardia after myocardial infarction. *J Am Coll Cardiol*. 2008;51(23):2266–2275.

60. Beeres SL, Zeppenfeld K, Bax JJ, *et al*. Electrophysiological and arrhythmogenic effects of intramyocardial bone marrow cell injection in patients with chronic ischemic heart disease. *Heart Rhythm*. 2007;4(3):257–265.

61. Zhang SJ, Wu JC. Comparison of imaging techniques for tracking cardiac stem cell therapy. *J Nucl Med*. 2007;48(12):1916–1919.

62. Bengel FM, Anton M, Richter T, *et al*. Noninvasive imaging of transgene expression by use of positron emission tomography in a pig model of myocardial gene transfer. *Circulation*. 2003;108(17):2127–2133.

63. Haubner R, Weber WA, Beer AJ, *et al*. Noninvasive visualization of the activated alphavbeta3 integrin in cancer patients by positron emission tomography and [18F]Galacto-RGD. *PLoS Med*. 2005;2(3):e70.

64. Beer AJ, Haubner R, Goebel M, *et al*. Biodistribution and pharmacokinetics of the alphavbeta3-selective tracer 18F-galacto-RGD in cancer patients. *J Nucl Med*. 2005;46(8):1333–1341.

65. Higuchi T, Bengel FM, Seidl S, *et al*. Assessment of alphavbeta3 integrin expression after myocardial infarction by positron emission tomography. *Cardiovasc Res*. 2008;78(2):395–403.

66. Makowski MR, Ebersberger U, Nekolla S, Schwaiger M. In vivo molecular imaging of angiogenesis, targeting $\alpha_v\beta_3$ integrin expression, in a patient after acute myocardial infarction. *Eur Heart J.* 2008;29(18):2201.

67. Cerqueira MD, Weissman NJ, Dilsizian V, *et al.* Standardized myocardial segmentation and nomenclature for tomographic imaging of the heart. A statement for healthcare professionals from the cardiac imaging committee of the council on clinical cardiology of the American heart association. *Int J Cardiovasc Imaging.* 2002;18(1):539–542.

68. Woods RP, Mazziotta JC, Cherry SR. MRI-PET registration with automated algorithm. *J Comput Assist Tomogr.* 1993;17(4):536–546.

69. Hill DL, Hawkes DJ, Gleeson MJ, *et al.* Accurate frameless registration of MR and CT images of the head: applications in planning surgery and radiation therapy. *Radiology.* 1994;191(2):447–454.

70. Wells WM, 3rd, Viola P, Atsumi H, Nakajima S, Kikinis R. Multi-modal volume registration by maximization of mutual information. *Med Image Anal.* 1996;1(1): 35–51.

71. Maes F, Collignon A, Vandermeulen D, Marchal G, Suetens P. Multimodality image registration by maximization of mutual information. *IEEE Trans Med Imaging.* 1997;16(2):187–198.

72. Pluim JP, Maintz JB, Viergever MA. Mutual-information-based registration of medical images: a survey. *IEEE Trans Med Imaging.* 2003;22(8):986–1004.

73. West J, Fitzpatrick JM, Wang MY, *et al.* Comparison and evaluation of retrospective intermodality brain image registration techniques. *J Comput Assist Tomogr.* 1997;21(4):554–566.

74. Skalski J, Wahl RL, Meyer CR. Comparison of mutual information-based warping accuracy for fusing body CT and PET by 2 methods: CT mapped onto PET emission scan versus CT mapped onto PET transmission scan. *J Nucl Med.* 2002;43(9):1184–1187.

75. Slomka PJ, Dey D, Przetak C, Aladl UE, Baum RP. Automated 3-dimensional registration of stand-alone (18)F-FDG whole-body PET with CT. *J Nucl Med.* 2003;44(7):1156–1167.

76. Visser JJ, Sokole EB, Verberne HJ, *et al.* A realistic 3-D gated cardiac phantom for quality control of gated myocardial perfusion SPET: the Amsterdam gated (AGATE) cardiac phantom. *Eur J Nucl Med Mol Imaging.* 2004;31(2):222–228.

77. Goerres GW, Kamel E, Heidelberg TN, Schwitter MR, Burger C, von Schulthess GK. PET-CT image co-registration in the thorax: influence of respiration. *Eur J Nucl Med Mol Imaging.* 2002;29(3):351–360.

78. Nakamoto Y, Tatsumi M, Cohade C, Osman M, Marshall LT, Wahl RL. Accuracy of image fusion of normal upper abdominal organs visualized with PET/CT. *Eur J Nucl Med Mol Imaging.* 2003;30(4):597–602.

79. Nekolla SG, Ibrahim T, Balbach T, Klein C. Co-registration and fusion of cardiac MRI and PET studies. In: Marzullo P (ed.) *Understanding Cardiac Imaging Techniques: From Basic Pathology to Image Fusion.* Amsterdam: IOS Press, 2001.

80. Nekolla SG, Miethaner C, Nguyen N, Ziegler SI, Schwaiger M. Reproducibility of polar map generation and assessment of defect severity and extent assessment in myocardial perfusion imaging using positron emission tomography. *Eur J Nucl Med.* 1998;25(9):1313–1321.

81. Hattori N, Bengel FM, Mehilli J, *et al.* Global and regional functional measurements with gated FDG PET in comparison with left ventriculography. *Eur J Nucl Med.* 2001;28(2):221–229.

82. Klein GJ, Huesman RH. Four-dimensional processing of deformable cardiac PET data. *Med Image Anal.* 2002;6(1):29–46.

83. Makela T, Pham QC, Clarysse P, *et al.* A 3-D model-based registration approach for the PET, MR and MCG cardiac data fusion. *Med Image Anal.* 2003;7(3): 377–389.

84. Aladl UE, Hurwitz GA, Dey D, Levin D, Drangova M, Slomka PJ. Automated image registration of gated cardiac single-photon emission computed tomography and magnetic resonance imaging. *J Magn Reson Imaging.* 2004;19(3):283–290.

85. Shekhar R, Zagrodsky V, Castro-Pareja CR, Walimbe V, Jagadeesh JM. High-speed registration of three- and four-dimensional medical images by using voxel similarity. *Radiographics.* 2003;23(6):1673–1681.

86. Shekhar R, Walimbe V, Raja S, *et al.* Automated 3-dimensional elastic registration of whole-body PET and CT from separate or combined scanners. *J Nucl Med.* 2005;46(9):1488–1496.

87. Martinez-Moller A, Souvatzoglou M, Navab N, Schwaiger M, Nekolla SG. Artifacts from misaligned CT in cardiac perfusion PET/CT studies: frequency, effects, and potential solutions. *J Nucl Med.* 2007;48(2):188–193.

88. Gould KL, Pan T, Loghin C, Johnson NP, Guha A, Sdringola S. Frequent diagnostic errors in cardiac PET/CT due to misregistration of CT attenuation and emission PET images: a definitive analysis of causes, consequences, and corrections. *J Nucl Med.* 2007;48(7):1112–1121.

89. Schwaiger M, Ziegler S, Nekolla SG. PET/CT: challenge for nuclear cardiology. *J Nucl Med.* 2005;46(10):1664–1678.

90. Schroeder S, Achenbach S, Bengel F, *et al.* Cardiac computed tomography: indications, applications,

limitations, and training requirements: report of a writing group deployed by the working group nuclear cardiology and cardiac CT of the European society of cardiology and the European council of nuclear cardiology. *Eur Heart J.* 2008;29(4):531–556.

91. Osman MM, Cohade C, Nakamoto Y, Marshall LT, Leal JP, Wahl RL. Clinically significant inaccurate localization of lesions with PET/CT: frequency in 300 patients. *J Nucl Med.* 2003;44(2):240–243.

92. Goerres GW, Kamel E, Seifert B, *et al.* Accuracy of image coregistration of pulmonary lesions in patients with non-small cell lung cancer using an integrated PET/CT system. *J Nucl Med.* 2002;43(11): 1469–1475.

93. Goerres GW, Burger C, Kamel E, *et al.* Respiration-induced attenuation artifact at PET/CT: technical considerations. *Radiology.* 2003;226(3):906–910.

94. Boucher L, Rodrigue S, Lecomte R, Benard F. Respiratory gating for 3-dimensional PET of the thorax: feasibility and initial results. *J Nucl Med.* 2004;45(2): 214–219.

95. Casali C, Obadia JF, Canet E, *et al.* Design of an isolated pig heart preparation for positron emission tomography and magnetic resonance imaging. *Invest Radiol.* 1997;32(11):713–720.

96. Makela T, Clarysse P, Sipila O, *et al.* A review of cardiac image registration methods. *IEEE Trans Med Imaging.* 2002;21(9):1011–1121.

97. Sinha S, Sinha U, Czernin J, Porenta G, Schelbert HR. Noninvasive assessment of myocardial perfusion and metabolism: feasibility of registering gated MR and PET images. *AJR Am J Roentgenol.* 1995;164(2): 301–307.

98. Mäkela TJCP, Lötjönen J, *et al.* A new method for the registration of cardiac PET and MR images using deformable model based segmentation of the main thorax structures. In: MA NWaV (ed.) *4th International Conference on Medical Image Computing and Computer Assisted Intervention (MICCAI 01).* Berlin, Heidelberg: Springer-Verlag, 2001, pp. 557–564.

99. Pichler BJ, Wehrl HF, Kolb A, Judenhofer MS. Positron emission tomography/magnetic resonance imaging: the next generation of multimodality imaging? *Semin Nucl Med.* 2008;38(3):199–208.

100. Iida H, Kanno I, Miura S, Murakami M, Takahashi K, Uemura K. A simulation study of a method to reduce positron-annihilation spread distributions using a strong magnetic-field in positron emission tomography. *IEEE Trans Nucl Sci.* 1986;33:597–600.

101. Hammer BE, Christensen NL, Heil BG. Use of a magnetic field to increase the spatial resolution of positron emission tomography. *Med Phys.* 1994;21(12): 1917–1920.

102. Christensen NL, Hammer BE, Heil BG, Fetterly K. Positron emission tomography within a magnetic field using photomultiplier tubes and lightguides. *Phys Med Biol.* 1995;40(4):691–697.

103. Raylman RR, Hammer, BE, Christensen NL. Combined MRI-PET scanner: a Monte Carlo evaluation of the improvements in PET resolution due to the effects of a static homogeneous magnetic field. *IEEE Trans Nucl Sci.* 1996;43:2406–2412.

104. Buchanan M, Marsden PK, Mielke CH, Garlick PB. A system to obtain radiotracer uptake data simultaneously with NMR spectra in a high field magnet. *IEEE Trans Nucl Sci.* 1996;43:2044–2048.

105. Garlick PB, Marsden PK, Cave AC, *et al.* PET and NMR dual acquisition (PANDA): applications to isolated, perfused rat hearts. *NMR Biomed.* 1997;10(3): 138–142.

106. Shao Y, Cherry SR, Farahani K, *et al.* Simultaneous PET and MR imaging. *Phys Med Biol.* 1997;42(10): 1965–1970.

107. Garlick PB, Medina RA, Southworth R, Marsden PK. Differential uptake of FDG and DG during post-ischaemic reperfusion in the isolated, perfused rat heart. *Eur J Nucl Med.* 1999;26(10): 1353–1358.

108. Southworth R, Parry CR, Parkes HG, Medina RA, Garlick PB. Tissue-specific differences in 2-fluoro-2-deoxyglucose metabolism beyond FDG-6-P: a 19F NMR spectroscopy study in the rat. *NMR Biomed.* 2003;16(8):494–502.

109. Slates RB, Farahani K, Shao Y, *et al.* A study of artefacts in simultaneous PET and MR imaging using a prototype MR compatible PET scanner. *Phys Med Biol.* 1999;44(8):2015–2027.

110. Marsden PK, Strul D, Keevil SF, Williams SC, Cash D. Simultaneous PET and NMR. *Br J Radiol.* 2002;75:Spec No:S53–S59.

111. Pichler B, Lorenz E, Mirzoyan R, *et al.* [Readout of lutetium oxyorthosilicate crystals with avalanche photodiodes for high resolution positron emission tomography]. *Biomed Tech (Berl).* 1997;42(Suppl): 37–38.

112. Ziegler SI, Pichler BJ, Boening G, *et al.* A prototype high-resolution animal positron tomograph with avalanche photodiode arrays and LSO crystals. *Eur J Nucl Med.* 2001;28(2):136–143.

113. Pichler BJ, Swann BK, Rochelle J, Nutt RE, Cherry SR, Siegel SB. Lutetium oxyorthosilicate block detector readout by avalanche photodiode arrays for high resolution animal PET. *Phys Med Biol.* 2004;49(18): 4305–4319.

114. Pichler BJ, Judenhofer MS, Catana C, *et al.* Performance test of an LSO-APD detector in a 7-T MRI scanner

for simultaneous PET/MRI. *J Nucl Med.* 2006;47(4): 639–647.

115. Catana C, Wu Y, Judenhofer MS, Qi J, Pichler BJ, Cherry SR. Simultaneous acquisition of multislice PET and MR images: initial results with a MR-compatible PET scanner. *J Nucl Med.* 2006;47(12):1968–1976.

116. Judenhofer MS, Catana C, Swann BK, *et al.* PET/MR images acquired with a compact MR-compatible PET detector in a 7-T magnet. *Radiology.* 2007;244(3): 807–814.

117. Pichler B, Wehrl H, Judenhofer M. Latest advances in molecular imaging instrumentation. *J Nucl Med.* 2008;49(Suppl. 6):5S–23S.

CHAPTER 13

PET and CT Imaging

Marcelo F. Di Carli

Brigham and Women's Hospital, Harvard Medical School, Boston, MA, USA

The introduction and dissemination of new imaging technology provides the potential for enhancing our understanding of pathophysiology (e.g., atherosclerosis, myocardial dysfunction), diagnosis and risk prediction, as well as newer ways to guide management and monitor therapeutic responses. In this context, the integration of nuclear medicine cameras with multidetector computed tomography (CT) scanners (e.g., PET-CT) provides a unique opportunity to delineate cardiac and vascular anatomic abnormalities, and their physiologic consequences in a single setting. For the evaluation of the patient with known or suspected coronary artery disease (CAD), it allows detection and quantification of the burden of the extent of calcified and noncalcified plaques (coronary artery calcium and coronary angiography), quantification of vascular reactivity and endothelial health, identification of flow-limiting coronary stenoses, and assessment of myocardial viability. In addition, by integrating the detailed anatomic information from CT with the high sensitivity of positron emission tomography (PET) to evaluate targeted molecular and cellular abnormalities, hybrid PET/CT imaging may play a key role in shaping the future of molecular diagnostics and therapeutics. The discussion that follows will review potential clinical applications of hybrid PET/CT imaging in cardiovascular disease.

Rationale for integrating PET and CT

For many decades, CT and PET imaging have followed separate and distinct developmental pathways. Both modalities have their strengths; CT scanners image cardiac and coronary anatomy with high spatial resolution, whereas PET imaging can identify a functional abnormality in, for example, myocardial perfusion, metabolism, or receptors. While it may seem that, in many cases, it would be equally effective to view separately acquired CT and nuclear images for a given patient on adjacent computer displays, with or without software registration, experience over the past 10 years with commercial PET/CT scanners has highlighted the superiority of the hybrid technology for improved detection and staging of cancer. However, the concept of applying dual-modality imaging to the evaluation of patients with known or suspected cardiovascular disease is relatively new and not without controversy. In thinking about the potentially complementary aspects of dual-modality imaging, one must necessarily begin by reviewing the strengths and limitations of single-modality approaches.

PET Myocardial Perfusion Imaging

PET myocardial perfusion imaging provides a robust approach to diagnosing obstructive CAD, quantify the magnitude of myocardium at risk, assess the extent of tissue viability, and guide therapeutic management (i.e., selection of patients for revascularization). The average weighted sensitivity for detecting at least one coronary artery with >50% stenosis is 90% (range, 83–100%), whereas the average specificity is 89% (range, 73–100%). The corresponding average positive and negative predictive values are 94% (range, 80–100%) and 73% (range, 36–100%) respectively, and the overall diagnostic accuracy is 90% (range, 84–98%) [1].

Cardiac CT, PET and MR, 2nd edition. Edited by Vasken Dilsizian and Gerry Pohost. © 2010 Blackwell Publishing Ltd.

As with single-photon emission computed tomography (SPECT), a recognized limitation of this approach is that it often uncovers only coronary territories supplied by the most severe stenosis and, consequently, it is relatively insensitive to accurately delineate the extent of obstructive angiographic CAD especially in the setting of multivessel CAD [2]. Recent evidence suggests that two quantitative approaches may be able to help mitigate this limitation, at least in part. One of them relates to PET's unique ability to assess left ventricular function at rest and during peak stress (as opposed to post-stress with SPECT) [2]. The available data suggest that in normal subjects, left ventricular ejection fraction (LVEF) increases during peak vasodilator stress [2]. In patients with obstructive CAD, however, the change in LVEF (from baseline to peak stress) is inversely related to the extent of obstructive angiographic CAD. Indeed, patients with multivessel or left main disease show a frank drop in LVEF during peak stress even in the absence of apparent perfusion defects. In contrast, those without significant CAD or with one-vessel disease show a normal increase in LVEF. Consequently, the diagnostic sensitivity of gated PET for correctly ascertaining the presence of multivessel disease increases from 50 to 79% [2].

The second approach is based on the ability of PET to enable absolute measurements of myocardial blood flow (in mL/min/g) and coronary vasodilator reserve. Absolute estimates of coronary vasodilator reserve correlate inversely with the severity of coronary artery stenosis [3–6]. In patients with so-called "balanced" ischemia or diffuse CAD, measurements of coronary vasodilator reserve uncover areas of myocardium at risk that would generally be missed by performing only relative assessments of myocardial perfusion [7], thereby improving ascertainment of multivessel CAD. It is important to point out, however, that neither approach has been tested in prospective clinical trials.

Another limitation of the PET (and SPECT) myocardial perfusion imaging approach is that it fails to describe the presence and extent of subclinical atherosclerosis [8,9]. This is not unexpected since the myocardial perfusion imaging method is designed and targeted on the identification of flow-limiting stenoses. This is potentially important especially in patient subgroups with intermediate–high clinical risk in whom there may be extensive subclinical CAD, and may explain, at least in part, the limitations of perfusion imaging alone to identify low-risk patients among those with high clinical risk (e.g., diabetes, end-stage renal disease) [10].

Cardiac CT

Using state-of-the-art technology in carefully selected patients, it is possible to obtain high-quality images of the coronary arteries. The available evidence suggest that on a per patient basis, the average weighted sensitivity for detecting at least one coronary artery with >50% stenosis is 94% (range, 75–100%), whereas the average specificity is 77% (range, 49–100%) [11]. The corresponding average positive and negative predictive values are 84% (range, 50–100%) and 87% (range, 35–100%) respectively, and the overall diagnostic accuracy is 89% (range, 68–100%).

Two multicenter, single-vendor trials evaluating the diagnostic accuracy of coronary CT angiography using MDCT-64 technology (CCTA-64) have been completed and recently published [12,13]. The results of these two studies confirm the robustness of CCTA-64 for complete visualization of the coronary tree. The Assessment by Coronary Computed Tomographic Angiography of Individuals Undergoing Invasive Coronary Angiography (ACCURACY) trial enrolled 230 patients with a disease prevalence of 25%. On a patient-based model, the sensitivity, specificity, and positive and negative predictive values to detect ≥50% were 95, 83, 64, and 99%, respectively, and for ≥70% stenosis the reported numbers were 94, 83, 48, 99%, respectively. The study reported no differences in sensitivity and specificity for nonobese compared with obese subjects, whereas calcium scores ≥400 reduced specificity significantly. The Coronary Artery Evaluation Using 64-Row Multidetector Computed Tomography Angiography (CorE 64) trial [13] enrolled 291 patients with a disease prevalence of 56% and provides additional evidence that is somewhat discordant to the ACCURACY trial and to initial results from single center studies. The CorE 64 study excluded patients with calcium scores >600. On a per patient basis, the sensitivity for detecting at least one coronary artery with ≥50% stenosis was 85%, considerably lower than in single center studies and in the ACCURACY trial using similar technology, whereas the specificity was 90%, higher than previously reported. The corresponding average positive and negative predictive values were 91% and 83%, respectively, surprisingly different than most previous studies. On a per vessel basis, the reported sensitivity for detecting coronary arteries with ≥50% stenosis was 75%, whereas the specificity was 93%. The corresponding positive and negative predictive values were 82 and 89%, respectively.

Except for the ACCURACY study, these reported accuracies of CCTA to date should be interpreted in light of the relatively narrow range of CAD likelihood in patients examined (i.e., high or intermediate–high), as evidenced by the high prevalence of obstructive CAD in these series (56–62%) [11,13]. Further, results are generally limited to relatively large vessel sizes (≥1.5 mm), excluding the results of smaller or uninterpretable vessels (generally distal vessels and side branches), the inclusion of which lowers sensitivity. An ongoing problem with CT is that high-density objects such as calcified coronary plaques and stent struts limit its ability to accurately delineate the degree of coronary luminal narrowing [14,15]. Of note, the Core 64 trial excluded patients with high calcium scores (>600) [13].

From a clinical perspective, a normal CCTA is helpful as it effectively excludes the presence of obstructive CAD and the need for further testing, defines a low clinical risk, and makes management decisions straightforward. Because of its limited accuracy to define stenosis severity and predict flow-limiting disease [16,17], however, abnormal CCTA results are more problematic to interpret and to use as the basis for defining the potential need of invasive coronary angiography and myocardial revascularization.

Dual-Modality Imaging Protocols

CT Scans

Patient positioning is performed with a CT scout image or topogram. This is followed by a low-dose CT scan covering the heart region. It is important to understand that acquisition parameters for CT-based transmission imaging vary with the detector configuration of the CT scanner (e.g., 8, 16, 64 slices) and clinical protocol [18,19]. However, the general scan settings utilized in most clinics for CT transmission imaging, independent of the manufacturer, include (1) a slow rotation speed (e.g., 1 second/revolution), combined with a relatively high pitch (e.g., 0.5–0.6:1), (2) a nongated scan, (3) a high tube potential (e.g., 140 kVp) and a low tube current (~10–20 mA), and (4) a CT acquisition obtained during tidal expiration breath-hold or shallow breathing.

It is also possible to use a prospectively gated CT scan, in which the X-ray tube is "turned on" only during the end-diastolic phase of the cardiac cycle- typically 75–80% of the R-R interval) with higher tube current (~250 mA) acquired during (preferably) an expiratory breath-hold. This gated CT scan can be used for attenuation correction and for quantification of coronary calcium score. This approach is more challenging because it tends to result in more frequent misalignment between the transmission (breath-hold) and emission (free-breathing) images, thereby requiring dedicated software for re-alignment of the two data sets before reconstruction of the PET images. The gated protocol also results in higher radiation dose to the patient compared to the nongated scan (~0.4–0.6 mSv vs. ~1.6 mSv for a 64 slice PET/CT scanner, respectively).

In selected patients, it is also possible to obtain a CCTA immediately following the assessment of myocardial perfusion. In order to perform a CCTA, a 16- or, preferably, a 64-detector CT scanner is required to cover the heart rapidly enough so as to prevent artifacts. In patients undergoing a hybrid study (myocardial perfusion PET + CCTA), there is general agreement that the CCTA should be performed after the PET scan. This sequence avoids potential interference of oral and/or intravenous beta blockers used for heart rate control in preparation for the CCTA exam with the maximal hyperemic or heart rate responses during vasodilator- and dobutamine-stress, respectively. The CCTA imaging protocol has been discussed in detail elsewhere [20]. With appropriate training and experience, the integrated protocol can be completed in approximately 30 minutes.

Emission Scans

For ^{82}Rubidium, approximately the same dose (40–60 mCi) is injected for both the rest and stress myocardial perfusion studies. For ^{13}N-ammonia, the general trend is to use a lower activity for the rest images (~10 mCi) and a higher activity for the stress images (~30 mCi). Ideally, the doses of the radiotracers should also be adjusted according to the size of the patient and, importantly, the type of PET data acquisition (i.e., 2-D vs. 3-D mode). The low-dose/high-dose protocol is faster (than same dose protocols for rest and stress) as it does not require waiting for decay of N-13 to background levels before a second dose can be administered. However, large patients may require relatively large doses for both the rest and stress studies (analogous to the 2-day Tc-99m SPECT protocol). Some laboratories perform stress imaging first, as a normal scan may avoid the need for rest imaging. The downside of "stress-only" imaging is that there will be no opportunity to obtain rest and stress LVEF or myocardial blood flow and coronary vasodilator reserve, thereby limiting the ability to identify patients with extensive CAD and "balanced" ischemia, as discussed below.

There are several ways in which the emission images can be acquired. These include:

1 *ECG gated imaging*: This is a common clinical approach. Imaging begins 90–120 seconds after ^{82}Rubidium injection, or 3–5 minutes after ^{13}N-ammonia injection, to allow for clearance of radioactivity from the lungs and blood pool; the scan duration is approximately 5 or 20 minutes, respectively, for ^{82}Rubidium or ^{13}N-ammonia. The number of gated frames is usually set to 8 or 16, with rejection of ectopic beats outside of the acceptance window.

2 *Multiframe or dynamic imaging*: Imaging begins with the bolus (short infusion) of ^{82}Rubidium or ^{13}N-ammonia and continues for 7–8 minutes or 20 minutes, respectively. The advantage of this approach is that it allows quantification of myocardial blood flow (in mL/min/g), e.g., by fitting regional tissue and blood time-activity curves (TAC) to a suitable kinetic model (refs). However, its main disadvantage is that one needs to perform a separate radionuclide injection to obtain ECG-gated images from which to assess cardiac function, especially when using ^{82}Rubidium. Using ^{13}N-ammonia, one can acquire a short multiframe or dynamic scan

(4 minutes) that can be followed with a separate ~15-minute ECG gated scan to assess myocardial perfusion and LVEF, without the need of an additional radionuclide injection owing to its longer physical half-life (~10 minutes). To measure the LV blood TAC noninvasively, one must acquire many dynamic PET image frames while the tracer bolus passes through the right ventricle, the lungs, and the LV. During this interval, it is common for a relatively large amount of activity (~20–30 mCi) to be located entirely within the PET scanner's axial field-of-view. Because of possible count-rate limitations under such conditions, particularly in 3D (septa-less) scan mode, great care must be taken to ensure the accuracy of the PET system's corrections for random- and scatter-coincidences, and dead-time. Although quantitative inaccuracies seen at high count rates may be mitigated by injecting less activity to begin with, this could yield too much image noise in the later (tissue) phase of the dynamic study, so a careful compromise needs to be determined for each given PET system and scan mode.

3 *List mode imaging*: This is the ideal approach and, based on technological advances in modern PET/Ct scanners, is rapidly becoming standard practice because a single injection and data acquisition allows multiple image reconstructions (i.e., summed, ECG gated, and multiframe or dynamic) for a comprehensive physiologic examination of the heart (Figure 13.1). With this approach, image acquisition commences with the bolus injection of the radionuclide and continues for 7–8 minutes or 20 minutes for ^{82}Rubidium and ^{13}N-ammonia, respectively. List-mode imaging requires significant computer power to perform the multiple reconstructions, especially for the 3D image acquisition mode.

Stress testing can be performed with pharmacologic means (e.g., adenosine, dipyridamole, regadenoson, or dobutamine)- most common, or with exercise [21]. The latter is easier with ^{13}N-ammonia (half-life ~10 minutes) than with ^{82}Rubidium (half-life 76 seconds).

Clinical Applications of Hybrid PET/CT Imaging

Attenuation Correction

As discussed above, one of the most basic uses of CT in hybrid PET/CT imaging is for patient positioning and attenuation correction. Attenuation

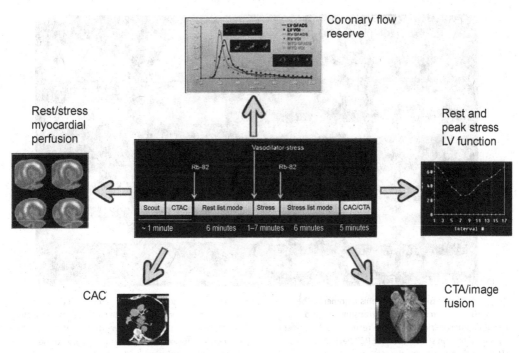

Coronary flow reserve

Rest/stress myocardial perfusion

Rest and peak stress LV function

CAC

CTA/image fusion

Figure 13.1 Comprehensive cardiac PET/CT protocol for delineation of the extent of anatomic abnormalities and their functional consequence. CAC, coronary artery calcium; CTA, computed tomography angiography; CTAC, computed tomographic based attenuation correction; LV, left ventricle.

correction errors leading to artifacts have been reported in 30–60% of cases with both SPECT/CT and PET/CT [22,23] (Figure 13.2). These artifacts are usually related to misalignments between the emission and CT transmission data sets caused by patient, cardiac, and/or respiratory motion [23,24], leading to regional defects and frequent in-homogeneity in quantitative tracer distribution [25]. Proper quality control and availability of registration software is crucial before interpretation of hybrid PET/CT images.

Localization of Targeted Molecular Imaging Agents

An emerging advantage of dual-modality imaging relates to the ability of CT to provide an anatomic roadmap that is critical for localization of targeted imaging agents. This has proven useful in both clinical and research applications in oncology imaging. For cardiovascular imaging, dual-modality approaches may be especially useful for imaging of atherosclerosis, where the CT can help delineate plaques and the localization of the tar-

geted imaging probe in relation to those plaques [26] (Figure 13.3). The proposed integration between PET and MRI may expand the possibilities for characterization of both myocardial tissue and vasculature [27].

Integrating Calcium Scoring with Myocardial Perfusion Imaging

There is growing, consistent evidence that coronary artery calcium (CAC) scores are generally predictive of a higher likelihood of ischemia (reflecting obstructive CAD) on myocardial perfusion imaging, and the available data supports the concept of a threshold phenomenon governing this relationship [28–31] (Figure 13.4). Indeed, the frequency of myocardial ischemia increases significantly with increasing CAC scores, especially among patients with CAC ≥400 [28,29,31]. A recent study reported that a CAC score ≥709 increased the sensitivity of SPECT MPI for detecting patients with obstructive CAD despite normal regional perfusion [32], probably reflecting the ability of the CAC score to uncover the presence of extensive

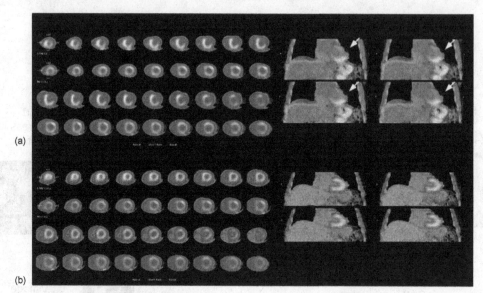

Figure 13.2 Transmission-emission misalignment. The top panel (a) shows the misaligned CT transmission and [82]Rubidium images (right), and the resulting anterolateral perfusion defect on stress-rest [82]Rb PET (left). The perfusion defect results from applying incorrect attenuation coefficients during tomographic reconstruction to the area of the LV myocardium overlaying on the lung field on the CT transmission scan (arrows). The lower panel (b) shows the correction of the emission–transmission misalignment (right), and the resulting normal perfusion study. (Reproduced from Di Carli *et al.* [1].)

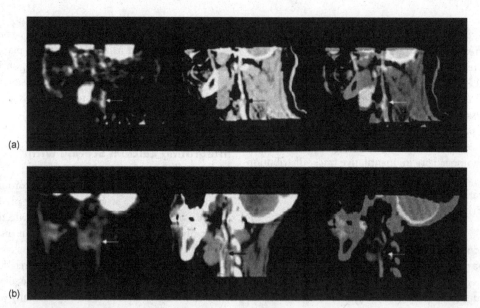

Figure 13.3 The upper row (a) (from left to right) shows PET, contrast CT, and co-registered PET/CT images in the sagittal plane, from a 63-year-old man who had experienced two episodes of left-sided hemiparesis. Angiography demonstrated stenosis of the proximal right internal carotid artery; this was confirmed on the CT image (black arrow). The white arrows show [18]FDG uptake at the level of the plaque in the carotid artery. As expected, there was high [18]FDG uptake in the brain, jaw muscles, and facial soft tissues. The lower row (b) (from left to right) demonstrates a low level of [18]FDG uptake in an asymptomatic carotid stenosis. The black arrow highlights the stenosis on the CT angiogram, and the white arrows demonstrate minimal [18]FDG accumulation at this site on the [18]FDGPET and co-registered PET/CT images. (Reproduced from Rudd *et al.* [26].)

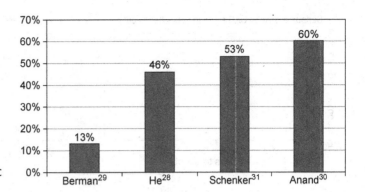

Figure 13.4 Frequency of inducible ischemia by myocardial perfusion imaging in patients with Agatston CAC score ≥400.

atherosclerosis in selected patients with balanced ischemia. Given the fact that CAC scores are not specific markers of obstructive CAD [33], however, one should be cautious in considering integrating this information into management decisions regarding coronary angiography, especially in patients with normal perfusion imaging. Conversely, CAC scores <400, especially in symptomatic patients with intermediate likelihood of CAD, may be less effective in excluding CAD especially in young subjects and women [34]. In a recent study of symptomatic patients with intermediate likelihood of CAD, the absence of CAC only afforded a NPV of 84% to exclude ischemia [31].

The potential to acquire and quantify rest and stress myocardial perfusion, and non-contrast CT scan for CAC scoring from a single hybrid PET/CT study may offer a unique opportunity to expand the prognostic value of stress nuclear imaging. The rationale for this integrated approach is predicated on the fact that the perfusion imaging approach is designed to uncover only obstructive atherosclerosis and, thus, insensitive for detecting subclinical disease. The CAC score, reflecting the anatomic extent of atherosclerosis [35], may offer an opportunity to improve the conventional models for risk assessment using nuclear imaging alone (especially in patients with normal perfusion), a finding that may serve as a more rational basis for personalizing the intensity and goals of medical therapy in a more cost-effective manner. For example, recent data suggest that quantification of CAC scores at the time of stress PET imaging using a hybrid imaging approach can enhance risk predictions in patients with suspected CAD [31]. In a consecutive series of 621 patients undergoing stress PET imaging and CAC scoring in the same clinical setting, risk ad-

justed analysis demonstrated that for any degree of perfusion abnormality there was a stepwise increase in adverse events (death and myocardial infarction or MI) with increasing CAC scores. This finding was observed in patients with and without evidence of ischemia on PET MPI. Indeed, the annualized event rate in patients with normal PET MPI and no CAC was substantially lower than among those with normal PET MPI and a CAC ≥1000 (Figure 13.5). Likewise, the annualized event rate in patients with ischemia on PET MPI and no CAC was lower than among those with ischemia and a CAC ≥1000. While CT coronary angiography as an adjunct to perfusion imaging could expand the opportunities to identify patients with noncalcified plaques at greater risk of adverse cardiovascular events, it is unclear how much added prognostic information there is in the contrast CT scan over the simple CAC scan [36].

Integrating CT Coronary Angiography and Myocardial Perfusion Imaging for Diagnosis and Management of CAD

One of the most compelling arguments supporting a potential clinical role of dual-modality imaging is its potential ability for optimizing and individualizing management decisions. While CCTA is an excellent method to exclude CAD, its ability to accurately assess the degree of luminal narrowing as a surrogate for physiologic significance is only modest. Indeed, recent data from multiple laboratories using either sequential (computed tomography angiography or CTA followed by SPECT) [8, 37–39] or hybrid imaging (SPECT/CT or PET/CT) [9,40–42] suggest that the positive predictive value of CCTA for identifying coronary stenoses producing objective evidence of stress-induced ischemia is

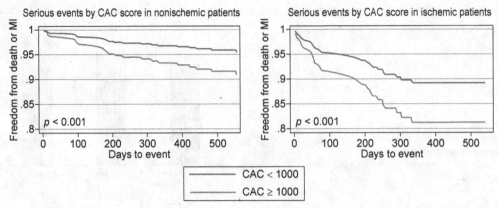

Figure 13.5 Adjusted survival curves for freedom from death or MI adjusted for age, sex, symptoms, and conventional CAD risk factors in patients without ischemia (top panel) and with ischemia (lower panel) by level of coronary artery calcium score. CAC, coronary artery calcium; MI, myocardial infarction. (Reproduced from Schenker et al. [31].)

suboptimal (Figures 13.6 and 13.7). The importance of stress perfusion imaging in the integrated strategy is the ability of noninvasive estimates of jeopardized myocardium to identify which patients may benefit from revascularization—that is differentiating high-risk patients with extensive scar versus those with extensive ischemia. The advantages of this approach are clear—avoidance of unnecessary

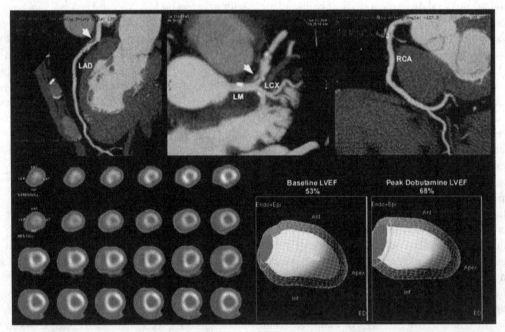

Figure 13.6 Integrated PET/CTA study. The CTA images demonstrate a noncalcified plaque (arrow) in the proximal LAD with 50–70% stenosis. However, the rest and peak dobutamine stress myocardial perfusion PET study (lower left panel) demonstrates only minimal inferoapical ischemia. In addition, LVEF was normal at rest and demonstrated a normal rise during peak dobutamine stress. LAD, left anterior descending artery; LCX, left circumflex; LM, left main; LVEF, left-ventricular ejection fraction; RCA, right coronary artery. (Reproduced from Di Carli and Hachamovitch [11].)

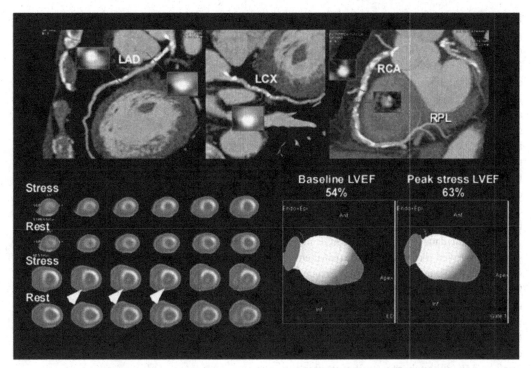

Figure 13.7 Integrated PET/CTA study. There is extensive calcified plaque burden throughout the coronary arteries. The left anterior descending and circumflex coronary arteries shows severe calcified plaque in their proximal and mid segments. The dominant right coronary artery shows multiple calcified plaques, with a severe predominantly noncalcified plaque in its mid segment. However, the rest and peak adenosine stress myocardial perfusion PET study (lower left panel) demonstrates only moderate ischemia in the inferior wall (arrows). In addition, LVEF was normal at rest and demonstrated a normal rise during peak stress, effectively excluding the presence of flow-limiting three-vessel CAD. LAD, left anterior descending artery; LCX, left circumflex; LVEF, left-ventricular ejection fraction; RCA, right coronary artery; RPL, right posterolateral branch. (Reproduced from Di Carli and Hachamovitch [11].)

catheterizations that expose patients to risk and the potential for associated cost savings [43].

The value of ischemia information for optimizing clinical decision-making has been demonstrated by multiple studies, and remains standard care for decisions regarding revascularization in patients with stable coronary syndromes. The nonrandomized Coronary Artery Surgery Study (CASS) registry reported that surgical revascularization in patients with CAD improved survival only among those with three-vessel disease with severe ischemia on exercise stress testing, while medical therapy was a superior initial therapy in patients without this finding [44]. A recent study in 10,627 diagnostic patients followed up after stress SPECT compared post-scan cardiac mortality with revascularization versus medical therapy using multivariable model-ing with adjustment for a propensity score. In the setting of little or no evidence of ischemia (<10% total myocardium), patients undergoing medical therapy enjoyed a survival benefit compared to patients treated with revascularization. Conversely, revascularized patients had enhanced survival benefit over patients undergoing medical therapy when moderate to severe ischemia was present (>10% total myocardium). This survival benefit, as measured by lives saved per 100 treated, increased with increasing extent and severity of ischemia, and was particularly striking in higher-risk patients (elderly and women, especially diabetics).

This approach of physiology-based patient assessment identifying which patients may benefit from revascularization versus medical therapy alone was recently reinforced by the results of the

FAME (Fractional Flow Reserve versus Angiography for Multivessel Evaluation) randomized trial demonstrating that guiding PCI by means of physiologic data (fractional flow reserve) was associated with a significantly lower incidence of major adverse cardiac events compared with routine angiography-guided PCI in patients with multivessel disease [45]. This concept is also supported by the results of the DEFER trial which investigated the use of a FFR-based approach to the management of CAD, revealing that stenting in the absence of a functionally significant stenosis was not associated with improved outcomes compared to medical management of these lesions [46].

More recent data from the COURAGE nuclear substudy revealed that regardless of treatment assignment, the magnitude of residual ischemia on follow-up perfusion imaging was proportional to the risk of death or MI. Although underpowered, these preliminary observations showed that in patients with a ≥5% reduction in ischemia after randomization to either arm had a reduced rate of death or MI (although not significant after risk-adjustment) [47].

Together, these data suggest that by identifying which patients have sufficient ischemia to merit revascularization, stress perfusion imaging may play a significant role in the selection of patients for catheterization within a strategy based on identification of patient benefit (Figure 13.7). From the discussion above, this physiologic data would have greater clinical impact than coronary anatomy for decisions regarding revascularization. In patients with multivessel CAD, the value of dual-modality imaging would allow better localization of the culprit stenosis and may offer a more targeted approach to revascularization.

Challenges, Opportunities, and Unresolved Issues for PET/CT Imaging

Although intellectually appealing, the concept of a hybrid imaging approach in general and PET/CT in particular is the subject of considerable debate within the cardiovascular imaging community. While it offers potential unique opportunities as discussed above, there are also significant challenges and unresolved issues that one must consider.

Access to Myocardial Perfusion PET/CT Imaging

The expense associated with either the purchase of an [82]Strontium/[82]Rubidium generator or running of the cyclotron for ^{13}N-ammonia production limits access to cardiac PET or PET/CT imaging, despite the widespread use and availability of PET/CT in oncology. This is the main reason why PET MPI represents a small fraction of all myocardial perfusion studies performed in the US. The new development of an [18]Fluorine-based PET radiopharmaceutical for myocardial perfusion imaging, which has recently entered clinical trials, will likely change this as it would allow unit dose distribution similar to FDG, thereby reducing high fixed expenses associated with cardiac PET imaging. Beyond the economic implications of this new radiotracer, there may be other advantages related to improvement in image quality and a superior flow-tissue extraction relationship compared with existing flow tracers that may improve detection of obstructive CAD.

Single Setting Dual-Modality PET/CT Versus Sequential Imaging

First, the cost of hybrid scanners integrating PET with advanced CT technology (64 slice CT) is considerably high making it difficult to develop a justifiable business model for both the practice and hospital settings in the absence of accepted clinical indications. We first must develop the evidence that would support which patients benefit from same setting dual-modality testing from both a diagnostic and prognostic perspectives. As discussed above, there is some evidence that assessment CAC scores in combination with stress nuclear imaging may offer an opportunity to improve risk assessment especially in symptomatic patients without prior CAD [31]. However, evaluation of CAC can be achieved without the need of advanced multidetector CT technology (i.e., 64-slice MDCT). For patients with equivocal stress nuclear test results, CT coronary angiography can be performed as a sequential test in a different scanner. Conversely, stress nuclear imaging is often used as a follow-up of patients with abnormal CTA studies to define hemodynamic significance of coronary stenosis. In such cases of sequential testing, the two data sets can be registered and fused off-line for interpretation and reporting [38,48,49]. Thus, the specific impact of hybrid imaging on treatment strategy and subsequently on outcome remains to be determined in prospective and long-term studies.

Radiation Dosimetry

The potential diagnostic appeal of a dual-modality approach must also be weighed against the challenges that it poses with regards to the added radiation dose to patients. This is a key issue as conventional spiral CCTA protocols using retrospective ECG-gating have been shown to be associated with high total radiation doses between 9.4 and 21.4 mSv [50,51]. However, this is changing rapidly. New low dose CCTA acquisition protocols with prospective electrocardiogram (ECG)-triggering have recently been introduced and shown to offer a significant reduction in radiation dose to an average of 2.1 mSv in selected patients (although more realistic numbers would be in the 5–7 mSv range) [52–54] at maintained accuracy [53], making this technique most suitable for hybrid imaging. Hybrid imaging with prospectively triggered CTA in conjunction with a stress only PET protocol may offer a significant reduction in dose as it has been shown for SPECT [53].

Conclusions

Innovation in noninvasive cardiovascular imaging is rapidly advancing our ability to image in great detail the structure and function in the heart and vasculature, and hybrid PET/CT and SPECT/CT represent clear examples of this innovation. By providing concurrent quantitative information about myocardial perfusion and metabolism with coronary and cardiac anatomy, hybrid imaging offers the opportunity for a comprehensive noninvasive evaluation of the burden of atherosclerosis and its physiologic consequences in the coronary arteries and the myocardium. This integrated platform for assessing anatomy and biology offers a great potential for translating advances in molecularly targeted imaging into humans. The goals of future investigation will be to refine these technologies, establish standard protocols for image acquisition and interpretation, address the issue of cost-effectiveness, and validate a range of clinical applications in large-scale clinical trials.

References

1. Di Carli MF, Dorbala S, Meserve J, El Fakhri G, Sitek A, Moore SC. Clinical myocardial perfusion PET/CT. *J Nucl Med.* 2007;48(5):783–793.
2. Dorbala S, Vangala D, Sampson U, Limaye A, Kwong R, Di Carli MF. Value of vasodilator left ventricular ejection fraction reserve in evaluating the magnitude of myocardium at risk and the extent of angiographic coronary artery disease: a 82Rb PET/CT study. *J Nucl Med.* 2007; 48(3):349–358.
3. Di Carli M, Czernin J, Hoh CK, *et al.* Relation among stenosis severity, myocardial blood flow, and flow reserve in patients with coronary artery disease. *Circulation.* 1995;91(7):1944–1951.
4. Uren NG, Melin JA, De Bruyne B, Wijns W, Baudhuin T, Camici PG. Relation between myocardial blood flow and the severity of coronary- artery stenosis. *N Engl J Med.* 1994;330(25):1782–1788.
5. Beanlands RS, Muzik O, Melon P, *et al.* Noninvasive quantification of regional myocardial flow reserve in patients with coronary atherosclerosis using nitrogen-13 ammonia positron emission tomography. Determination of extent of altered vascular reactivity. *J Am Coll Cardiol.* 1995;26(6):1465–1475.
6. Anagnostopoulos C, Almonacid A, El Fakhri G, *et al.* Quantitative relationship between coronary vasodilator reserve assessed by 82Rb PET imaging and coronary artery stenosis severity. *Eur J Nucl Med Mol Imaging.* 2008;35(9):1593–1601.
7. Parkash R, deKemp RA, Ruddy Td T, *et al.* Potential utility of rubidium 82 PET quantification in patients with 3-vessel coronary artery disease. *J Nucl Cardiol.* 2004; 11(4):440–449.
8. Schuijf JD, Wijns W, Jukema JW, *et al.* Relationship between noninvasive coronary angiography with multi-slice computed tomography and myocardial perfusion imaging. *J Am Coll Cardiol.* 2006;48(12):2508–2514.
9. Di Carli MF, Dorbala S, Curillova Z, *et al.* Relationship between CT coronary angiography and stress perfusion imaging in patients with suspected ischemic heart disease assessed by integrated PET-CT imaging. *J Nucl Cardiol.* 2007;14(6):799–809.
10. Shaw LJ, Iskandrian AE. Prognostic value of gated myocardial perfusion SPECT. *J Nucl Cardiol.* 2004;11(2): 171–185.
11. Di Carli MF, Hachamovitch R. New technology for noninvasive evaluation of coronary artery disease. *Circulation.* 2007;115(11):1464–1480.
12. Budoff MJ, Dowe D, Jollis JG, *et al.* Diagnostic performance of 64-multidetector row coronary computed tomographic angiography for evaluation of coronary artery stenosis in individuals without known coronary

artery disease: results from the prospective multicenter ACCURACY (Assessment by Coronary Computed Tomographic Angiography of Individuals Undergoing Invasive Coronary Angiography) trial. *J Am Coll Cardiol.* 2008;52(21):1724–1732.

13. Miller JM, Rochitte CE, Dewey M, *et al.* Diagnostic performance of coronary angiography by 64-row CT. *N Engl J Med.* 2008;359(22):2324–2336.

14. Hoffmann U, Moselewski F, Cury RC, *et al.* Predictive value of 16-slice multidetector spiral computed tomography to detect significant obstructive coronary artery disease in patients at high risk for coronary artery disease: patient-versus segment-based analysis. *Circulation.* 2004;110(17):2638–2643.

15. Mollet NR, Cademartiri F, Krestin GP, *et al.* Improved diagnostic accuracy with 16-row multi-slice computed tomography coronary angiography. *J Am Coll Cardiol.* 2005;45(1):128–132.

16. Leber AW, Becker A, Knez A, *et al.* Accuracy of 64-slice computed tomography to classify and quantify plaque volumes in the proximal coronary system: a comparative study using intravascular ultrasound. *J Am Coll Cardiol.* 2006;47(3):672–677.

17. Raff GL, Gallagher MJ, O'Neill WW, Goldstein JA. Diagnostic accuracy of noninvasive coronary angiography using 64-slice spiral computed tomography. *J Am Coll Cardiol.* 2005;46(3):552–557.

18. Gould KL, Pan T, Loghin C, Johnson NP, Sdringola S. Reducing radiation dose in rest-stress cardiac PET/CT by single poststress cine CT for attenuation correction: quantitative validation. *J Nucl Med.* 2008;49(5):738–745.

19. Lautamaki R, Brown TL, Merrill J, Bengel FM. CT-based attenuation correction in (82)Rb-myocardial perfusion PET-CT: incidence of misalignment and effect on regional tracer distribution. *Eur J Nucl Med Mol Imaging.* 2008;35(2):305–310.

20. Hoffmann U, Ferencik M, Cury RC, Pena AJ. Coronary CT angiography. *J Nucl Med.* 2006;47(5):797–806.

21. Chow BJ, Beanlands RS, Lee A, *et al.* Treadmill exercise produces larger perfusion defects than dipyridamole stress N-13 ammonia positron emission tomography. *J Am Coll Cardiol.* 2006;47(2):411–416.

22. Goetze S, Wahl RL. Prevalence of misregistration between SPECT and CT for attenuation-corrected myocardial perfusion SPECT. *J Nucl Cardiol.* 2007;14(2):200–206.

23. Gould KL, Pan T, Loghin C, Johnson NP, Guha A, Sdringola S. Frequent diagnostic errors in cardiac PET/CT due to misregistration of CT attenuation and emission PET images: a definitive analysis of causes, consequences, and corrections. *J Nucl Med.* 2007;48(7):1112–1121.

24. McQuaid SJ, Hutton BF. Sources of attenuation-correction artefacts in cardiac PET/CT and SPECT/CT. *Eur J Nucl Med Mol Imaging.* 2008;35(6):1117–1123.

25. Slomka PJ, Le Meunier L, Hayes SW, *et al.* Comparison of myocardial perfusion 82Rb PET performed with CT- and transmission CT-based attenuation correction. *J Nucl Med.* 2008;49(12):1992–1998.

26. Rudd JH, Warburton EA, Fryer TD, *et al.* Imaging atherosclerotic plaque inflammation with [18F]-fluorodeoxyglucose positron emission tomography. *Circulation.* 2002;105(23):2708–2711.

27. Judenhofer MS, Wehrl HF, Newport DF, *et al.* Simultaneous PET-MRI: a new approach for functional and morphological imaging. *Nat Med.* 2008;14(4):459–465.

28. He ZX, Hedrick TD, Pratt CM, *et al.* Severity of coronary artery calcification by electron beam computed tomography predicts silent myocardial ischemia. *Circulation.* 2000;101:244–251.

29. Berman DS, Wong ND, Gransar H, *et al.* Relationship between stress-induced myocardial ischemia and atherosclerosis measured by coronary calcium tomography. *J Am Coll Cardiol.* 2004;44:923–930.

30. Anand DV, Lim E, Raval U, Lipkin D, Lahiri A. Prevalence of silent myocardial ischemia in asymptomatic individuals with subclinical atherosclerosis detected by electron beam tomography. *J Nucl Cardiol.* 2004;11:450–457.

31. Schenker MP, Dorbala S, Hong EC, *et al.* Interrelation of coronary calcification, myocardial ischemia, and outcomes in patients with intermediate likelihood of coronary artery disease: a combined positron emission tomography/computed tomography study. *Circulation.* 2008;117(13):1693–1700.

32. Schepis T, Gaemperli O, Koepfli P, *et al.* Added value of coronary artery calcium score as an adjunct to gated SPECT for the evaluation of coronary artery disease in an intermediate-risk population. *J Nucl Med.* 2007;48(9):1424–1430.

33. Nallamothu BK, Saint S, Bielak LF, *et al.* Electron-beam computed tomography in the diagnosis of coronary artery disease: a meta-analysis. *Arch Intern Med.* 2001;161(6):833–838.

34. Knez A, Becker A, Leber A, *et al.* Relation of coronary calcium scores by electron beam tomography to obstructive disease in 2,115 symptomatic patients. *Am J Cardiol.* 2004;93(9):1150–1152.

35. Sangiorgi G, Rumberger JA, Severson A, *et al.* Arterial calcification and not lumen stenosis is highly correlated with atherosclerotic plaque burden in humans: a histologic study of 723 coronary artery segments using nondecalcifying methodology. *J Am Coll Cardiol.* 1998;31(1):126–133.

36. Mahmarian JJ. Computed tomography coronary angiography as an anatomic basis for risk stratification: deja vu or something new? *J Am Coll Cardiol.* 2007;50(12):1171–1173.

37. Hacker M, Jakobs T, Matthiesen F, *et al.* Comparison of spiral multidetector CT angiography and myocardial perfusion imaging in the noninvasive detection of functionally relevant coronary artery lesions: first clinical experiences. *J Nucl Med.* 2005;46(8):1294–1300.

38. Gaemperli O, Schepis T, Kalff V, *et al.* Validation of a new cardiac image fusion software for three-dimensional integration of myocardial perfusion SPECT and stand-alone 64-slice CT angiography. *Eur J Nucl Med Mol Imaging.* 2007;34(7):1097–1106.

39. Gaemperli O, Schepis T, Valenta I, *et al.* Cardiac image fusion from stand-alone SPECT and CT: clinical experience. *J Nucl Med.* 2007;48(5):696–703.

40. Rispler S, Roguin A, Keidar Z, *et al.* Integrated SPECT/CT for the assessment of hemodynamically significant coronary artery lesions. *J Am Coll Cardiol.* 2006;47:115A.

41. Malkerneker D, Brenner R, Martin WH, *et al.* CT-based attenuation correction versus prone imaging to decrease equivocal interpretations of rest/stress Tc-99m tetrofosmin SPECT MPI. *J Nucl Cardiol.* 2007;14(3):314–323.

42. Hacker M, Jakobs T, Hack N, *et al.* Combined use of 64-slice computed tomography angiography and gated myocardial perfusion SPECT for the detection of functionally relevant coronary artery stenoses. First results in a clinical setting concerning patients with stable angina. *Nuklearmedizin.* 2007;46(1):29–35.

43. Shaw LJ, Hachamovitch R, Berman DS, *et al.* The economic consequences of available diagnostic and prognostic strategies for the evaluation of stable angina patients: an observational assessment of the value of precatheterization ischemia. Economics of Noninvasive Diagnosis (END) Multicenter Study Group. *J Am Coll Cardiol.* 1999;33(3):661–669.

44. Weiner DA, Ryan TJ, McCabe CH, *et al.* The role of exercise testing in identifying patients with improved survival after coronary artery bypass surgery. *J Am Coll Cardiol.* 1986;8(4):741–748.

45. Tonino PA, De Bruyne B, Pijls NH, *et al.* Fractional flow reserve versus angiography for guiding percutaneous coronary intervention. N Engl J Med. 2009;360:213–224.

46. Pijls NH, van Schaardenburgh P, Manoharan G, *et al.* Percutaneous coronary intervention of functionally non-significant stenosis: 5-year follow-up of the DEFER Study. *J Am Coll Cardiol* 2007;49:2105–11.

47. Shaw LJ, Berman DS, Maron DJ, *et al.* Optimal medical therapy with or without percutaneous coronary intervention to reduce ischemic burden: results from the Clinical Outcomes Utilizing Revascularization and Aggressive Drug Evaluation (COURAGE) trial nuclear substudy. *Circulation.* 2008;117(10):1283–1291.

48. Santana CA, Garcia EV, Faber TL, *et al.* Diagnostic performance of fusion of myocardial perfusion imaging (MPI) and computed tomography coronary angiography. *J Nucl Cardiol.* 2009.

49. Slomka PJ. Software approach to merging molecular with anatomic information. *J Nucl Med.* 2004; 45 Suppl. 1:36S–45S.

50. Mollet NR, Cademartiri F, de Feyter PJ. Non-invasive multislice CT coronary imaging. *Heart.* 2005;91(3):401–407.

51. Hausleiter J, Meyer T, Hadamitzky M, *et al.* Radiation dose estimates from cardiac multislice computed tomography in daily practice: impact of different scanning protocols on effective dose estimates. *Circulation.* 2006;113(10):1305–1310.

52. Husmann L, Wiegand M, Valenta I, *et al.* Diagnostic accuracy of myocardial perfusion imaging with single photon emission computed tomography and positron emission tomography: a comparison with coronary angiography. *Int J Cardiovasc Imaging.* 2008;24(5):511–518.

53. Herzog BA, Husmann L, Landmesser U, Kaufmann PA. Low-dose computed tomography coronary angiography and myocardial perfusion imaging: cardiac hybrid imaging below 3mSv. *Eur Heart J.* 2008;29:3037–3042.

54. Javadi M, Mahesh M, McBride G, *et al.* Lowering radiation dose for integrated assessment of coronary morphology and physiology: first experience with step-and-shoot CT angiography in a rubidium 82 PET-CT protocol. *J Nucl Cardiol.* 2008;15(6):783–790.

CHAPTER 14

Image-Guided Electrophysiology Mapping and Ablation

Timm-Michael L. Dickfeld

University of Maryland School of Medicine, Baltimore, MD, USA

Introduction to Electrophysiology and Imaging

After the development of intracardiac recording and pacing catheters in the 1940s and 1950s enabled the characterization of various arrhythmias, the first curative atrioventricular (AV) node ablations in the early 1980s ushered electrophysiology (EP) in a new era of therapeutic applications [1,2]. While originally high-current DC shocks were used, this was quickly replaced by catheter-based radio-frequency ablation (RFA), which allowed to more sophistically titrate and target the radio-frequency (RF) delivery [3]. Due to its low risk and high success rate RFA emerged in the 1980s and 1990s as the first-line treatment for a variety of supraventricular tachycardias including atrial flutter, AV reentrant tachycardia, and AV nodal reentry tachycardia. However, a similarly successful catheter-based ablation strategy remained elusive for more complex arrhythmias such as atrial fibrillation or ventricular tachycardia.

Fortunately, simultaneous improvements in understanding the arrhythmia mechanisms and the development of advanced mapping tools have enabled novel treatment approaches for these arrhythmias over the last 10 to 15 years. As many of these approaches are anatomically based cardiac imaging has been increasingly utilized to assist in procedure planning, guidance and follow-up.

The landmark study by Haissaguerre *et al.* describing pulmonary vein triggers as a frequent initiator of atrial fibrillation allowed the first targeted ablation strategies. Initially, triggers sites within the proximal pulmonary veins were directly targeted with RFA [4]. However, this approach was abandoned due to a high rate of pulmonary vein stenoses [5]. Modified ablation strategies were developed, which aimed either at isolating the pulmonary veins at their ostia (ostial segmental approach) [6] or employed left atrial circumferential ablation lines encircling the left and right pulmonary veins [7]. As these approaches require a detailed knowledge of the anatomy of the left atrium and the pulmonary veins, the limited armamentarium of imaging technologies became evident. Fluoroscopy was widely available, but provided only a poor visualization of soft tissue. Prolonged procedure times exposed the patient and medical staff to significant ionizing radiation. Three-dimensional (3D) mapping systems had become available in the mid-1990s, which allowed the real-time display of a catheter tip within a mathematically reconstructed cardiac chamber (Figure 14.1a) [8]. However, they lacked the anatomic detail desired for these complex ablation procedures. Cardiac imaging was increasingly employed to provide this information. Preprocedural computed tomography (CT) and magnetic resonance (MR) imaging to characterize the individual left atrial and pulmonary vein anatomy became standard-of-care in many arrhythmia centers and allowed a tailored, patient-specific ablation approach. Detailed anatomic information gained from cardiac imaging was made available

Cardiac CT, PET and MR, 2nd edition. Edited by Vasken Dilsizian and Gerry Pohost. © 2010 Blackwell Publishing Ltd.

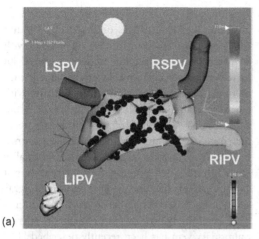

(a)

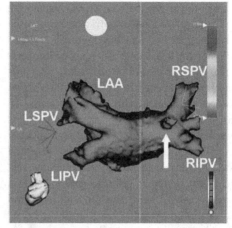

(b)

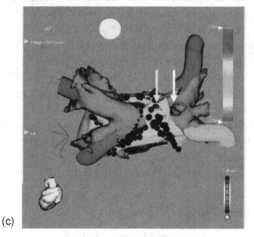

(c)

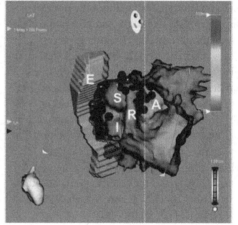

(d)

Figure 14.1 Image Integration for Atrial fibrillation ablation. (a) Electroanatomic shell of left atrium (turquoise) shown in posterior-anterior orientation reconstructed from multiple endocardial recording sites (white dots). Left superior pulmonary vein, (LSPV), left inferior pulmonary vein (LIPV), right superior pulmonary vein (RSPV), and right inferior pulmonary vein (RIPV) represented as blue, purple, red, and green tube, respectively. Individual ablation sites marked by brown points on electroanatomical shell. (b) CT-derived, high-resolution reconstruction of the left atrium demonstrating anatomical details all four pulmonary veins, pulmonary vein branches, and left atrial appendage (LAA). CT reconstruction demonstrates existence of an additional right superior-posterior roof vein (white arrow), which was not evident from electroanatomic shell. (c) Registration and fusion of electroanatomic map and CT-derived model of the left atrium. Based on the preprocedural knowledge and simultaneous display of the right roof vein (white arrow) circumferential lesions set around the right pulmonary veins (yellow arrow) was placed closer to the left sided veins to avoid ablation inside the roof vein, which can lead to pulmonary vein stenosis. (d) Clipping of the left atrium allows "fly-through" visualization from inside the CT derived left atrial reconstruction into the left superior pulmonary vein (S), left inferior pulmonary vein (I) and left atrial appendage (A). This allows the anatomic assessment of the width/length of the ridge (R) between the left superior pulmonary vein and left atrial appendage which is part of the circumferential ablation strategy. Note the simultaneous display of the esophagus (E) extracted from the CT data set.

during the ablation procedure by integrating the CT and MR images with 3D mapping systems (Figures 14.1b–d). Finally, cardiac imaging was increasingly used in the detection of procedural complications and postprocedural patient care.

With the growing experience and available commercial imaging tools new applications are being developed to facilitate also ventricular tachycardia ablations. MRI, PET, and CT are all well validated to provide detailed information about the cardiac anatomy or the myocardial scar, which is usually the target for substrate-guided ventricular tachycardia ablations. Current software developments are aiming at exporting this detailed 3D imaging information into the actual ablation procedure and provide anatomic guidance for patients with recurrent episodes of ventricular tachycardia.

An emerging application of cardiac imaging is the visualization of atrial or ventricular ablation lesions using MRI or CT. This has the potential to assess the discrepancies between intended versus actual ablation lines, delineate gaps in ablation sets and provide a road map for additional and repeat ablation procedures. Additionally, the temporal evolution of the ablation lesions can provide a more profound understanding of temporary inflammation versus long-term scar and gain insight into procedural failure and long-term success.

A very exciting field is the use of real-time imaging for electrophysiolgical procedures, which is currently being evaluated in animal and preliminary human studies. Employing either MRI or CT catheter navigation and ablation can be guided under direct visualization of the ablation tip in relation to the surrounding anatomy. This novel imaging paradigm has the potential for direct confirmation of the exact anatomic location, catheter-tissue contact, lesion visualization and early detection of complications.

Specific Applications

Atrial Fibrillation Ablation

Preablation Imaging
Preprocedural imaging is routinely performed to delineate the left atrial and pulmonary vein anatomy in many centers. CT is more commonly used due to its wide availability, consistent imaging quality and high spatial resolution (up to <1 mm^3). Depending on the local expertise, some centers prefer contrast-enhanced MRI to minimize ionizing radiation and the risk of contrast-induced nephropathy. Multiple studies have validated a significant variability in left atrial and pulmonary vein anatomy, which may influence the individual ablation strategies. Wongcharoen et al. reported in patients with paroxysmal atrial fibrillation a significantly larger orifice and neck of the left atrial

appendage (LAA) as well as a more inferior LAA position [9]. Septal ridges occurred in 32% and roof pouches were seen in 15% of patients with atrial fibrillation. The same authors reported an increased left atrial isthmus length and a tendency to more medial-isthmus ridges in patients with paroxysmal atrial fibrillation [10]. Kato et al. found a remarkable variability of the pulmonary veins with up to 38% demonstrating abnormal anatomical patterns [11]. Most common single abnormality was a common left pulmonary vein truncus, but 21% of patients had one or more additional right-sided pulmonary vein. Other unusual PV patterns such as additional roof veins or common inferior pulmonary vein has been recently described [12]. MRI studies confirmed an oval shape of the pulmonary vein ostia with the largest diameter in the cranio-caudal orientation [11]. Additionally, dynamic changes of the pulmonary vein os occur during the cardiac cycle (decrease of up to 33% during atrial systole) [13] or during respiration (splaying and diameter decrease of up to 2.6 mm with inspiration) [14]. These findings can be used to optimize imaging protocols (e.g., expiratory acquisition) or individualize the ablation approach (e.g., singular ablation circle in common left ostia).

Peri-Ablation Imaging

Three-Dimensional Mapping Systems
The advent of 3D mapping systems in the mid-1990s has facilitated a wide range of complex ablation procedures [8].

Using mostly electromagnetic fields or impedance measurements of electrical currents, they function similar to global positioning system (GPS) technology using triangulation algorithms [15,16]. The exact catheter position is calculated in real-time up to 100 times per second and displayed as a moving icon on a live monitor in the procedure room. To create a cardiac chamber a roving catheter is moved sequentially along the endocardial surface. Based on the specific 3D location information an electroanatomic shell is mathematically reconstructed which approximates the actual cardiac anatomy. The catheter motion is displayed in relation to the created chamber and enables the electrophysiologist to navigate to defined morphological targets, return to specific anatomic locations and mark ablation locations. A careful and exact anatomical reconstruction is important to minimize complications such as an ablation in the pulmonary veins (resulting in PV stenosis), left atrial appendage (perforation), or esophagus (atrio-esophageal fistula) and avoid gaps in the ablation lines (treatment failure) [17,18]. The accuracy of these 3D mapping systems is in the range of 1–4 mm and has been shown to reduce the amount of fluoroscopy time by 82% for atrial flutter [19] and 49% for atrial fibrillation [20].

Image Integration

While 3D mapping systems represent a significant improvement over sole fluoroscopic guidance, the mathematical reconstruction derived from multiple endocardial recordings can only incompletely represent the complex true cardiac anatomy (Figures 14.1a and b). This let to the development of image integration strategies in early 2000 [21,22]. Image integration refers to a process, in which the detailed 3D anatomy from CT or MRI is extracted and superimposed on the shell created from catheter recordings. For this application an accurate registration (alignment of the CT/MRI derived data set with the catheter-created shell) is critical. In a first step a contrast-enhanced CT or MRI is acquired using axial slices or 3D volume. This data set is uploaded into the 3D mapping system. Using proprietary imaging processing software the left atrium and pulmonary veins are reconstructed from the CT or MRI scan, segmented and exported as a 3D rendered model (Figure 14.1b) [15,16,23]. After creation of the endocardial shell with a roving catheter registration of the 3D anatomic model is performed Figures 14.1c and d). Several corresponding, well-defined anatomic landmarks are selected on the catheter-derived shell and the CT/MRI derived 3D model (such as pulmonary vein ostia) are used for this process. Depending on the mapping system additional proprietary algorithms exist that can either adjust the 3D model position to achieve the minimal average error between the shell and 3D model points (surface registration) or will adjust points of the catheter-derived map to fit into the 3D anatomic model (dynamic registration) [15,16]. The resulting registration accuracies have been reported in the range of 2–3 mm, which enables a clinical useful application [15,16,23].

After successful registration the 3D mapping system displays the catheter tip location and orientation in real-time in relation to the complex cardiac anatomy and allows the accurate placement of anatomically targeted lesions. The use of "clipping planes" allows the creation of endoscopic views from the left atrium onto the pulmonary veins (Figure 14.1d). Additional relevant anatomic structures such as the esophagus can be integrated in the 3D anatomic map.

While CT and MRI have both been successfully used for left atrial reconstruction with similar registration quality, CT allows a slightly superior visualization of pulmonary vein anatomy [24]. Increasing left atrial size and left atrial volume (>110 mL) are independent predictors of decreased registration accuracy [25]. To minimize inherent differences between imaged volume and catheter-derived chamber decreased time intervals between scan and procedure, end-diastolic image acquisition and end-expiratory scan time have been proposed [14]. Changes in cardiac rhythm, such as atrial fibrillation versus sinus rhythm during image acquisition and procedure do not appear to significantly effect the registration accuracy [26].

The obvious advantages of image integration have let to a rapid implementation of this technology. However, despite its widespread use only limited data exist to validate its clinical superiority. Single-center, nonrandomized, retrospective trials showed a reduction in fluoroscopy time of 21% and a decrease of recurrences of atrial fibrillation/atrial tachycardia of 20–28% [27,28]. Larger, prospective randomized-trials are currently being conducted.

Most recently, a new software module has been introduced that uses multiple 2D intracardiac ultrasound slices to define the endocardial contours to which CT and MRI reconstructions can be registered. By avoiding deforming chamber anatomy by catheter pressure and minimizing catheter mapping prior to image registration, a more accurate registration and decreased procedure times might be possible.

Post-Ablation Imaging

Complications

Cardiac Imaging has played a substantial role in detection and follow-up of postprocedural

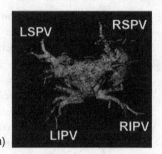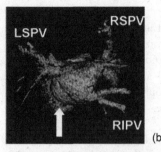

Figure 14.2 Pulmonary Vein Stenosis after atrial fibrillation ablation. (a) Preprocedural 3D CT-derived reconstruction in posterior-anterior view demonstrates typical pulmonary vein anatomy with left superior pulmonary vein (LSPV), left inferior pulmonary vein (LIPV), right superior pulmonary vein (RSPV), and right inferior pulmonary vein (RIPV). (b) Post-procedural CT performed 3 months after atrial fibrillation ablation for increasing shortness of breath demonstrates complete occlusion of left inferior pulmonary vein as consequence of intrapulmonary vein lesions required to achieve complete vein isolation.

complications. The insights gained have led to changes in procedural methods and ablation techniques.

Pulmonary Vein Stenosis: After the description of pulmonary vein triggers as a cause of atrial fibrillation, a direct approach targeting these triggers directly was used by most centers in the late 1990s [4,29]. Early studies using TEE demonstrated an incidence of pulmonary vein stenosis as high as 42% based on pulmonary vein velocities of 120 ± 12 cm/second [5]. With the transition to ablate outside of the pulmonary vein, reduction of power delivery, and the adjunct use of intracardiac ultrasound, the incidence pulmonary vein stenosis has been significantly decreased. CT and MRI provide comparable sensitivity for follow-up (Figure 14.2). Studies suggest that these changes in ablation strategy have reduced the incidence of pulmonary vein stenosis to <10%, which might further decrease with operator experience to as low as 1% [17,29]. Symptomatic pulmonary vein stenosis requiring interventional therapy is frequently characterized by a >75% lumen reduction by CT/MRI and a >80% reduction in pulmonary perfusion determined with V/Q scanning [17]. Long-term follow-up in all patients has been recommended by some centers, but most commonly cardiac imaging is employed in selected patients presenting with clinical symptoms suggestive of pulmonary vein stenosis [30].

Cardiac Perforation: Cardiac perforation with tamponade has been described in up to 6% of patients after atrial fibrillation ablation as a result of its technical complexity and the use of anticoagulation during the procedure. While mostly detected in the peri-procedural period with transthoracic or intracardiac ultrasound, cardiac effusions without hemodynamic compromise have been documented in regular follow-up scans using CT or MRI.

Thrombo-Embolic Complications: The reported incidence of thrombo-embolism is between 0 and 7% [30]. They are thought to be due to development of thrombus on stationary sheaths or left atrially placed catheters, char formation on the ablation tip or the ablation site, or disruption of thrombus previously present in the left atrium. Diagnosis is readily made upon clinical suspicion using CT and/or MRI and allowing lytic therapy if detected early (Figure 14.3). Using diffusion-weighted MRI sequences, which can detect early cerebral ischemia >30 minutes, an incidence of up to 10% of cerebral, subclinical thrombo-embolic events were seen [31].

Additionally, air embolus can be caused by introducing air through the transseptal sheath, via the open-irrigation catheter, or as a paradoxical embolus after transseptal access. If MRI or CT scans are obtained promptly before rapid absorption multiple serpiginous hypodensities, which represent air in the cerebral vasculature, can be detected with or without acute infarction [30].

Atrio-Esophageal Fistula: A rare, but significant complication is the occurrence of an atrio-esophageal fistula after atrial fibrillation ablation. While its exact incidence is unclear it has been estimated as <0.25% [30]. Due to the close proximity

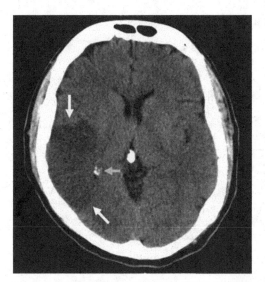

Figure 14.3 Thrombo-embolic Embolism. MRI performed for left-sided hemi-neglect and hypoesthesia immediately following an atrial fibrillation ablation demonstrates right parietal hypoperfusion due to embolic occlusion of right middle cerebral artery (white arrows). Additional coincidental finding of choroid plexus marked by gray arrow.

of the esophagus to the posterior left atrial wall, RFA can result in direct temperature-related damage of the esophageal mucosa or interrupt its blood supply. CT studies have shown that the distance between left atrium and the esophagus is only 4.4 ± 1.2 mm and a temperature increase of ≥2°C can frequently observed during ablations on the posterior wall [32]. The mean thicknesses of the posterior left atrium and the anterior esophageal walls were reported as 2.2+/−0.9 and 3.6+/−1.7 mm, respectively [33]. Significant lateral movement of the esophagus occurs during the atrial fibrillation procedure resulting in a ≥2 cm lateral shift in 67% of patients during conscious sedation [34]. Administration of oral contrast material and placement of intraesophageal temperature probes have been used to minimize this risk. CT or MRI are the preferred diagnostic tools if an atrio-esophageal fistula is suspected. Frequently air can be seen at the site of the fistula or within the cardiac chambers. Peripheral embolization to brain or kidneys is commonly seen [35]. While atrio-esophageal fistulas carry a very high mortality and if survived frequently result in long-term thrombo-embolic sequela early diagnosis is critical as successful surgeries have been reported [18].

Structural and Hemodynamic Effects of Atrial Fibrillation Ablations

Atrial fibrillation results in structural and electrical remodeling leading ultimately to left atrial dilatation. MRI and CT have been used to assess the effect of atrial fibrillation ablation on the left atrium size and function. Lemola *et al.* found that the left atrial volume decreased by 15 ± 16% 4 months after circumferential left atrial ablation [36]. Similarly, Verma *et al.* reported a decrease of the end-diastolic left atrial surface (−11%) and volume (−15%) 6 months after atrial fibrillation ablation using electro-beam CT [37]. Tsao *et al.* used magnetic resonance angiography images to assess left atrial volume 12 months after RFA for paroxysmal atrial fibrillation. Patients with no recurrence of atrial fibrillation showed a borderline reduction of the left atrial volume (62 mL to 57 ms), while patients with recurrence demonstrated a significant further left atrial dilatation (61–79 mL) [38].

Less consistent results are available in regard to the left atrial transport function. While the left atrial ejection fraction improved from 17 ± 6 to 22 ± 5% 6 months after antral ablation [37], Wylie *et al.* reported a significant decrease in left atrial ejection fraction (−14%) as well as left atrial volume (−15%) after 48 days [39].

Ventricular Tachycardia Ablation

Ablation of ventricular tachycardia (VT) is the next emerging frontier in EP. Over the last decades the number of patients with cardiomyopathy has substantially increased due to a higher incidence of coronary artery disease and improved pharmacological and interventional treatments of ischemic and nonischemic heart failure [40,41]. At the same time, multiple studies have demonstrated a significant survival benefit for implantable cardiac defibrillators (ICD) in these patient groups with systolic heart failure [42,43]. As the number of ICD patients grew, this resulted in an increasing number of patients with frequent and appropriate ICD therapy [42].

While antiarrhythmic medications are commonly prescribed as a first line treatment, their use is frequently limited by its side effects and decreasing long-term efficacy. In these patients, RFA has been used as an effective treatment

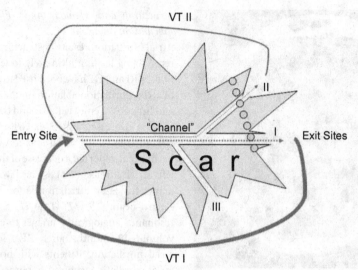

Figure 14.4 Scar-mediated ventricular tachycardia. Myocardial scar (blue) frequently presents a heterogeneous 3D structure with complex borders and intersecting channels of surviving myocardium ("Channel"). Electrical wave fronts can enter the network of surviving channels (entry site), travers the scar ("Channel") and exit into the normal myocardium (Exit sites I, II, and III). If the wave front can progress through the surrounding, normal myocardium and reenter into the entry site an reentrant loop has been established supporting sustained, monomorphic ventricular tachycardia (VT I). Placement of an ablation lesion at the Exit site I would eliminate VT I. However, the electrical wave front could still propagate through Exit site II resulting in a different ventricular tachycardia (VT II). Based on electrophysiological maneuvers and electrocardiograms empiric linear ablation lines (yellow, dotted line) are created dissecting channels I and II, which eliminate the clinical tachycardias (VT I and II).

strategy to decrease the ventricular arrhythmia burden and number of ICD shocks [44–46].

More recently, studies have suggested that a more aggressive approach in ablation of ventricular tachycardia might be justified. Reddy *et al.* demonstrated that by performing VT ablation prior to the implantation of an ICD for secondary prevention appropriate ICD therapy could be reduced from 33 to 12% ($p = 0.007$) over a 22.5 ± 5.5 months follow-up [47].

Myocardial Scar and VT

Myocardial scar usually acts as the substrate for reentrant ventricular tachycardia and is present in the majority of patients with ischemic and nonischemic cardiomyopathy [48]. Pathological studies were able to demonstrate complex "channels" of surviving myocardium within the scar itself [49,50]. During reentrant ventricular tachycardia an electrical wave front enters and traverses the myocardial scar via a network of such electrically conducting channels [46]. After exiting the scar, it depolarizes the rest of the ventricle and

returns to the original entry site, repeating the cycle (Figure 14.4). This concept of entry sites, slowly conducting channels and exit sites has been successfully validated in post-MI patients during clinical electrophysiological studies [45,46].

Of special interest is the border zone between scar and healthy myocardium. This border zone contains the exit sites, from which electricity spreads to the rest of the ventricle. Indeed, in patients with ischemic VT 68% of successful ablation sites were located in the border zone, while 18% were in the scar, 4% in normal myocardium and 10% on the epicardial surface [51]. Histological and imaging studies have shown that patients with scar-mediated ventricular tachycardia frequently present with nontransmural or nonhomogenous necrosis, which results in formation of complex endocardial, epicardial, and lateral border zones [49,50,52]. Such irregular extensions and isolated islets could potentially be visualized with cardiac imaging and used to define individual ablation strategies based on pre-procedural knowledge of the complex, 3D VT substrate.

Ventricular Tachycardia Ablations

A comprehensive characterization of scar-mediated ventricular tachycardia is possible in patients with stable monomorphic VT. Targeted ablation at the site of the slowly conducting isthmus has been able to successfully eliminate ventricular tachycardia in about 70–80% of patients during a 1- to 3-year follow-up period [45,46].

However, specific reentrant loops cannot be defined in up to ~90% of ventricular tachycardias as they are not hemodynamically tolerated and/or alternate between multiple reentrant pathways [44]. These arrhythmias are frequently treated using a "substrate-guided" ablation approach.

Goal of this strategy is the empiric interruption of the slowly conducting channels implicated in maintaining the tachycardia. Using the 12-lead ECG morphology of the clinical ventricular tachycardia, stored intracardiac electrograms from the ICD and pacing at different endocardial locations the exit site(s) of the ventricular tachycardia can approximated. Linear ablation lesions are created along the scar border to cauterize the surviving myocardial fibers that form the anatomic reentrant loops within the scar (Figure 14.4, yellow line) [51,53]. The same result can frequently be achieved in an alternative and supplemental approach in which linear lesions are placed from the scar center to the healthy surrounding myocardium or adjacent electrical barriers [44]. The clinical success rate of these substrate-guided approaches has been reported to be ~75% [44].

Scar Characterization

Voltage Mapping

The current "gold standard" of defining myocardial scar is based on endocardial bipolar voltage recordings. Using a 3D mapping system a roving mapping catheter is moved sequentially along the endocardial surface of the left ventricle. Assuming that the voltage amplitude will be lower on scarred myocardium due to a paucity of alive cells, a tiered classification with >1.5 mV for normal myocardium, 0.5–1.5 mV for abnormal myocardium and <0.5 mV for scar is generally accepted for defining scar and its border zone in the left ventricle [44].

These clinical criteria derive from several animal and patients studies correlating bipolar endocardial voltage recordings to areas of previous myocardial infarction.

Gepstein *et al.* found in canines a significantly lower bipolar amplitude in the histopathologically defined infracted area (2.3 ± 0.2 mV) than in the noninfarcted area (4.0 ± 0.7 mV to 10.2 ± 1.5 mV) or in controls (10.3 ± 1.3 mV) [54]. In a pig model Callans *et al.* demonstrated a decrease of bipolar endocardial voltage from control animals or areas remote from scar (5.2 ± 2.2 mV and 5.1 ± 2.1 mV, respectively) to border zone (2.8 ± 0.9) and infarcted areas (1.2 ± 0.5) as defined by pathology and intracardiac ultrasound. Infarct size by pathology correlated well with the area defined by bipolar amplitude of ≤1 mV ($r = 0.98$) [55]. This was confirmed in human studies, which found bipolar voltages of 5.8 ± 1.0 mV in the left ventricle of 12 healthy control patients. In 12 patients with prior myocardial infarction bipolar voltage in the area of previous myocardial infarction as assessed by echocardiography was 1.4 ± 0.7 mV compared to 4.5 ± 1.1 mV in noninfarcted segments [56].

Voltage measurements are displayed color-coded in the 3D mapping system and allow targeted ablations at the electrical defined scar border (Figures 14.5 and 14.6a). However, a purely voltage-based scar characterization has several limitations. A single endocardial voltage recording is unable to adequately represent the complex 3D scar anatomy and to differentiate between different degrees of endocardial and epicardial scar components. Low voltage recordings may rather represent intermittent or suboptimal catheter contact than true wall pathology. Additionally, the spatial resolution of voltage mapping is limited by the distance between the recording electrodes, which is ≥5 mm in the frequently used catheter systems. Finally, high-resolution voltage mapping prolongs the procedure time frequently by as much as 1–2 hours. While decreased mapping density in areas not thought to participate in the tachycardia may reduce mapping time, localized scar areas might be overlooked.

Cardiac Imaging

Therefore, several cardiac imaging strategies have been employed to supply additional scar characterization.

Magnetic Resonance Imaging: Delayed enhanced magnetic resonance imaging (MRI) has been well

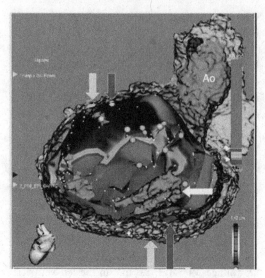

Figure 14.5   Fusion of CT reconstruction of left ventricular anatomy and voltage map. Left lateral wall has been removed for better visualization of the inferior, anterior, and septal wall. Registered 3D reconstruction of contrast-enhanced CT demonstrates high-resolution endocardial (blue) and epicardial (turquoise) left ventricular surface, papillary muscle (white arrow) and aorta (Ao). Normal myocardial wall thickness represented as distance between endo- and epicardium is seen along the inferior wall (lower turquoise and blue arrow). However, marked wall thinning is seen along the anterior wall (upper turquoise and blue arrow). Voltage map confirmed normal myocardium (>1.5 mV, purple color) along the inferior wall. Voltage-defined scar was demonstrated in the area of wall thinning (<0.5 mV, red color).

established to accurately characterize the location and extent of myocardial scar [57,58]. Hypoperfusion with resulting hypoenhancement is seen in about 50% of patients [59]. Due to the different wash-in and wash-out kinetics delayed enhancement is seen 5–25 minutes after contrast injection [57–59]. In animal studies gadolinium is found in an increased concentration up to 20 minutes after injection in areas of myocardial necrosis/fibrosis [60].

Recently, the importance of delayed enhancement on magnetic resonance imaging for further risk stratification has been recognized.

Kwong et al. examined 195 patients without previous myocardial infarction and assessed the occurrence of major adverse cardiac events and cardiac mortality. The presence of delayed enhancement resulted in a hazard ratio of 8.3 and 10.9, respectively [61].

Bello et al. performed contrast-enhanced MRI in 48 patients undergoing electrophysiological testing. Infarct mass and surface area assessed with delayed enhancement were a better predictor of inducibility of monomorphic ventricular tachycardia than left ventricular ejection fraction. Patients with monomorphic ventricular tachycardia had larger infarcts than noninducible patients (49 ± 5 g vs 28 ± 5 g) [62].

Nazarian et al. demonstrated that in patients with nonischemic cardiomyopathy nontransmural scar with a transmurality of 25–75% as diagnosed with contrast-enhanced MRI was significantly predictive of inducible ventricular tachycardia [63].

Furthermore, MRI may allow to characterize the anatomic substrate of ventricular arrhythmias. Yan et al. showed that a larger-than-median peri-infarct zone (defined as delayed enhancement from two to three standard deviations above the normal myocardial segment) was an independent predictor of all cause-mortality (hazard ratio 1.42) and cardiovascular mortality (hazard ratio 1.49) [64].

Similarly, Schmidt et al. demonstrated that tissue heterogeneity (defined as <50% of maximum signal intensity) at the infarct periphery was strongly associated with inducibility for monomorphic ventricular tachycardia (noninducible versus inducible 13 ± 9 vs 19 ± 8 g) [65]. Such an infarct definition as <50% of maximum signal intensity may avoid the overestimation of infarct size which has been reported with a intensity cutoff of two standard deviations [65].

Ashikaga et al. assessed ventricular arrhythmias using MRI, epicardial sock electrodes, and endocardial mapping in a chronic infarct model in swine. The investigators demonstrated that the reentry isthmus was characterized by a relatively small volume of viable myocardium bound by the scar tissue at the infarct border zone or over the infarct. MRI was able to identify spatial complex scar structures at the isthmus sites [52]. This could potentially enable the prospective identification of ablation targets for unmappable ventricular arrhythmias.

However, substrate assessment using MRI is still limited in most patients presenting with ICD shocks for ventricular tachycardia as the presence of a defibrillator is still considered a contraindication

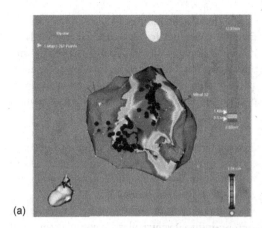
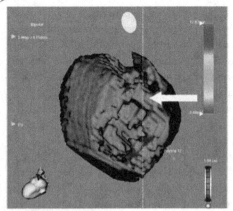

(a)

(b)

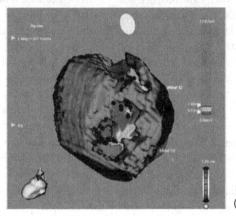

(c)

Figure 14.6 Integration of 3D PET-Derived scar for ventricular tachycardia ablation. (a) Voltage map of the left ventricle in left lateral view. Endocardial voltages are represented color-coded ranging from red (scar with <0.5 mV) to yellow-blue (border zone with 0.5–1.5 mV) to purple (normal myocardium with >1.5 mV). A continuous area of scar is seen along the basal lateral wall (red). (b) 3D scar map reconstruction from fluorodeoxyglucose-PET displays scar (in this binary display form) scar as absent wall segments ("hole") in the corresponding lateral wall segments. Note a "bridge-like" area of metabolically alive myocardium can be seen in the lateral basal wall segment (white arrow). (c) After successful registration of the voltage map and 3D PET-derived scar map, the bridge of metabolically alive tissue can be seen traversing in the middle of the presumingly homogeneous voltage-defined myocardial scar. Such surviving channels, which may function as conducting channels, would not have been suspected from the endocardial voltage map alone.

[66]. Additionally, metal artifacts from the ICD significantly impact the imaging quality. Recently, nephrogenic systemic fibrosis has also been reported after gadolinium administration in patients with renal insufficiency [67].

Computed Tomography: Multidetector CT (MDCT) has the ability to provide high-resolution information about the cardiac anatomy, contractility, and potentially the myocardial scar.

First-pass CT images can display morphological changes characteristic for areas of myocardial infarction/scar such as wall thinning, aneurysms, and intramyocardial calcifications (Figure 14.5). Human studies found a significant difference in wall thickness (4.1 ± 2 mm vs 10.5 ± 3.8 mm) in chronic infarction compared to normal myocardium. However, ~20% of wall segments showed no significant wall thinning despite old infarct age [68]. Similarly, Nieman *et al.* reported a reduced wall thickness to <5 mm in ~50% of patients with infarcts >12 months old while no significant reduction could be seen with infarcts <7 days old [69].

Additionally, MDCT is able to detect regional changes in contractility observed with myocardial scarring. In a study of 39 patients 82% agreement was found in segmental, graded contractility when comparing echocardiography and MDCT. In the area of the left anterior descending artery and left circumflex artery sensitivity and specificity were 78, 93% and 85, 100%, respectively [70].

More recently first-pass perfusion defects and delayed enhanced CT has been studied for imaging of myocardial scar.

Gerber *et al.* showed in a series of 20 patients a moderately good concordance of early hypoenhanced regions (92%, $\kappa = 0.54$) and late hyperenhanced regions (82%, $\kappa = 0.61$) between contrast-enhanced CT and MRI. Concordance between delayed enhanced MDCT and MRI was seen in acute infarcts (11 days) in 84% and in chronic infarcts (>6 months) in 81%. Absolute sizes of early hypoenhanced (6 ± 16 versus 7 ± 16 g) and late hyperenhanced (36 ± 34 vs 31 ± 40 g) regions were similar on CT and MR and were highly correlated ($r = 0.93$ and $r = 0.89$, respectively). However, hypoenhancement was more frequently observed in acute myocardial infarction (69%) than in chronic infarcts (33%) [71].

Mahnken *et al.* documented the ability to visualize (reperfused) myocardial infarction in 28 patients. Eighty-four percent of wall segments with early hypoperfusion on MDCT displayed delayed enhancement on MRI [72]. A good correlation was found between delayed enhanced MRI (31.2 ± 22.5%) when compared with early-phase CT (24.5 ± 18.3%, $\kappa = 0.635$) and delayed enhanced CT (33.3 ± 23.8%, $\kappa = 0.878$) [72]. In acute infarcts (5 days after reperfusion) delayed MDCT and delayed MRI correlated in 93% [72].

Nieman *et al.* compared prospectively delayed enhanced MRI and CT in regard to infarct size after acute reperfused myocardial infarction in 21 patients. While delayed enhancement could be seen in all patients using MRI, it could only be detected in 73% of CT images. Contrast-to-noise ratio was significantly better with MRI, but early hypoenhancement and delayed hyperenhancement correlated well between MRI and CT [73].

However, CT imaging still suffers from low contrast between infarct and blood pool when compared to MRI. Further protocol optimizations are still required (optimal contrast application, optimal delay for image acquisition) to improve contrast.

Additionally, nephrotoxic effects of CT contrast material continues to be a concern, especially as many cardiomyopathy/ICD patients present with underlying renal dysfunction. Furthermore, metal artifacts from the ICD system can significantly impact on the interpretability of the high-resolution CT data sets.

Positron Emission Tomography: Given various tracers and imaging protocols PET has been used to study the role of ischemia, hibernation, and innervation for arrhythmogenesis.

In patients with previous myocardial infarction, exercise-induced ventricular arrhythmias appeared to be triggered by transient ischemia occurring within a partially necrotic area containing large amounts of viable myocardium [74]. Krause *et al.* demonstrated that segments with perfusion/metabolism mismatch were present in 94% of patients with ventricular arrhythmias versus 64% without [75]. In an animal study of myocardial infarction Sasano *et al.* showed that a significantly larger perfusion/innervation mismatch measured with 13N-ammonia and 11C-epinephrine in animals with inducible ventricular tachycardia (10 ± 4% vs 4 ± 2%) [76]. These findings lead to the PARAPET study, a prospective, observational trial, which will assess if hibernating myocardium or inhomogeneity of sympathetic innervation measured with PET can predict sudden cardiac death or cardiovascular mortality [77].

Of significant interest for electrophysiologists is the ability of PET to define myocardial scar. Different from delayed enhanced MRI and CT, which rather provide a morphological substrate assessment, PET allows a metabolic characterization of the myocardial scar and its border zone. It is widely applicable in the VT/ICD patient population as ICD safety; metal artifacts or nephrotoxicity is not of clinical concern.

Quantitative and qualitative PET scar imaging is usually performed by incorporating a radioactive tracer isotope into a metabolically active molecule, such as fluorodeoxyglucose (FDG). FDG is taken up by viable myocardial cells, but is absent in nonviable cells forming myocardial scar. Regional blood flow and sarcolemmal integrity (as reflected by the Na-K-ATPase transport system) can be assessed by a preprocedural rest-redistribution thallium scan or rubidium PET. A comparison of both data sets provides insight into the relation between regional blood flow and FDG metabolism, and can define myocardial regions as scarred (FDG:blood flow match pattern), diseased/hibernating/stunned (FDG:blood flow mismatch pattern) or normal.

Scar characterization using PET imaging has been clinically established, extensively validated [78,79], and its prognostic value has been demonstrated for cardiac interventions and cardiac surgery [80,81].

In animal studies infarct size assessed with FDG PET correlated well with the necropsy findings ($r = 0.89$ to 0.96) [82,83]. Studies involving humans undergoing heart transplantation found a correlation of $r = 0.65$ to 0.94 when comparing PET images to explanted myocardial preparations [82,84]. Similarly, a comparison between FDG PET and contrast-enhanced MRI in patients with an ischemic cardiomyopathy demonstrated a correlation of $r = -0.86$ [85]. Accordingly, in human studies FDG PET defined scar demonstrated a significantly decreased unipolar, endocardial voltage compared to normal myocardium (6.5 ± 2.6 mV vs 11.0 ± 3.6 mV [86] and 4.8 ± 2.1 mV vs 10.9 ± 3.7 mV [87]).

Only recently has PET imaging been used to guide and facilitate the ventricular tachycardia ablations.

A good correlation was found between PET-derived metabolic scar maps and endocardial voltage maps in 14 patients undergoing VT ablation ($r = 0.89$, $p < 0.05$). Additionally, 3D scar reconstructions were successfully registered in ten patients with a commercial mapping system with an acceptable registration error of 3.7 ± 0.7 mm. Scar size, location, and border zone accurately predicted high-resolution voltage map findings ($r = 0.87$; $p < 0.05$). After integration of metabolic maps relevant information was available during the procedure. Low voltage recordings within wall segment displaying preserved metabolic activity were shown rather to be due to suboptimal catheter contact than actual myocardial wall disease. Integrated scar maps revealed metabolically active channels within the myocardial scar, which were not detected by voltage mapping (Figure 14.6). Moreover, PET/CT maps correctly predicted non-

transmural epicardial scar that was confirmed with epicardial mapping despite normal endocardial map [88].

Multimodality Imaging: An attractive approach is the combination of PET with either CT or MRI (Figures 14.7a and b). While PET provides the metabolic differentiation between normal, hibernating, and scarred myocardium detailed anatomic information can be obtained from MDCT or MRI with a spatial resolution of ≤1 mm or 2–3 mm, respectively. Fusing both data sets can enable a synergistic metabolic and morphological evaluation, which extends beyond what each imaging technique can offer as a stand-alone technology, which has been successfully validated in many oncological and radiological applications. New elastic algorithms are able to register PET with CT or MR images from separate scanners fast and with an accuracy on par with manual elastic registration performed by human experts using up to 32 anatomic landmarks [89].

Image Integration of Scar Map: Both currently available commercial 3D mapping systems enable the integration of CT and MR images [16,23,24]. However, the "paper-thin" surface reconstruction used to assess PV anatomy and location for atrial fibrillation ablation is not well suited for ventricular tachycardia ablations. Several changes will have to be implemented to take advantage of the additional information that cardiac imaging can provide for VT ablations (Figure 14.8).

Three-Dimensional Volume Display: A more advanced 3D volume display is required that allows morphologically correct representation of endocardial and epicardial surface as well as a simultaneous embedded 3D display of the scar substrate. This allows to assess local wall thickness and the transmural extent as well as delineation of endocardial and epicardial scar components.

Differential Substrate Representation: Given the increasing body of evidence of that border zones are implicated in arrhythmogenesis and represent potential ablation sites [51,64,65] a differential display of the scar area derived from PET, CT, or MRI is desirable. Areas felt to represent border zone [64,65] could be color-coded versus areas of dense scar. A similar display would allow the additional identification of hibernating or ischemic myocardium.

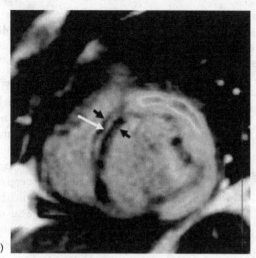
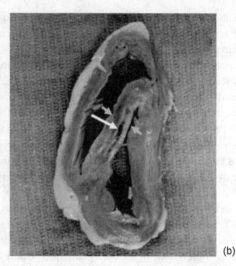

(a)   (b)

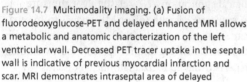

Figure 14.7 Multimodality imaging. (a) Fusion of fluorodeoxyglucose-PET and delayed enhanced MRI allows a metabolic and anatomic characterization of the left ventricular wall. Decreased PET tracer uptake in the septal wall is indicative of previous myocardial infarction and scar. MRI demonstrates intraseptal area of delayed enhancement (white arrow) with right and left ventricular rim of surviving myocardium (black arrows). (b) Corresponding pathological specimen confirms an area of intraseptal myocardial scar (white arrow) enclosed in layers of surviving myocardium along the right and left ventricular endocardium (gray arrows).

This would facilitate a true anatomic guidance for substrate modification.

Fusion or Multimodality Imaging: The current image integration software only allows the integration of a single data set. However, the fusion of multiple imaging modalities will allow a more comprehensive scar characterization. For ventricular tachycardia ablations, individual combination of PET, CT, and MRI will allow a metabolic and morphological evaluation of the scar, its border zone, and the remaining left ventricular cavity.

Imaging of Ablation Lesions

The procedural success of ablations depends on the correct placement of RF lesions and the continuity of linear ablation lines. Gaps can result from insufficient power delivery (catheter contact and stability, coagulum formation, temperature or power limitation) or inadvertent placement of the catheter tip too far away from the previous ablation site. As MRI and CT has the ability to visualize myocardial scar, it has been has also been evaluated for direct visualization of ablation lesions.

Magnetic Resonance Imaging

Delayed enhanced MRI was first evaluated in ventricular lesions. Lardo *et al.* described the ability to

visualize RF ablations in the RV apex of six mongrel dogs after about 2 minutes with an increase in signal intensity over the first 12 ± 2.1 minutes [90].

Further animal studies demonstrated a characteristic four-stage enhancement pattern for ventricular ablation lesions [91]. After gadolinium injection ablation lesions could consistently be visualized as a contrast-void (phase 1). After a protracted period of progressive peripheral enhancement (phase 2) complete delayed enhancement was achieved after 98 ± 21 minutes (phase 3: "very" delayed enhancement"). The lesions remain visible during a prolonged washout-period of >12 hours (phase 4). The different kinetics compared to myocardial infarction is likely due to a complete loss of the cellular architecture and total disruption of the vascular system. Enhancement, therefore, relies solely on a diffusion process starting from the lesion periphery. Lesion size measured during the first three phases of contrast enhancement correlated well with the histopathological lesion size [91].

Improvement in imaging protocols has recently allowed the visualization of atrial ablation lesions.

Peters *et al.* reported delayed enhancement in 23 patients after atrial fibrillation ablation. Using high-resolution free-breathing MR protocols

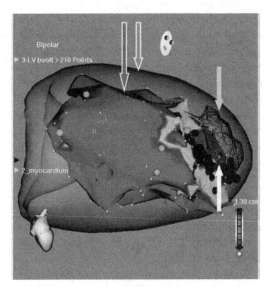

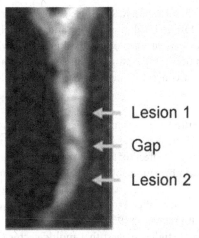

Figure 14.9 Magnetic resonance imaging of left atrial ablation lesion. Transmural ablation lesions are visualized after transmural ablation with a high-resolution coil using delayed enhanced MR imaging. Two single-ablation lesions can be seen as areas of increased enhancement 30 minutes after contrast injection. The spatial resolution is sufficient to visualize a 2–3 mm gap of nonablated myocardium between the ablation lesions and could be used to guide additional ablation lesions.

Figure 14.8 Integration of 3D left ventricular anatomy and scar reconstruction. Left ventricular endocardial voltage map (purple arrow) in right anterior oblique view demonstrates normal voltages normal voltages (purple; >1.5 mV) and antero-apical area of scar (red; <1.5 mV). PET-CT derived left ventricular anatomy (green arrow) is registered to the endocardial voltage map. Myocardial scar is reconstructed from fluorodeoxyglucose-PET and registered/embedded into the PET/CT shell (mesh display; gray arrow). This allowed the correct prediction of the left ventricular scar location prior to the detailed voltage map. The catheter tip icon, which is updated in real-time and represents the actual catheter locations, is seen within the apical scar (white arrow).

ablated areas could be well visualized with a signal-to-noise ratio of 22 vs 15 and 12 for nonablated areas and blood, respectively ($p <$ 0.5). Despite an attempt of complete circular ablation lesions only 62% of patients demonstrated >90% circumferential enhancement. Delayed enhancement thickness appears to decrease over time and is inversely related to the time between the procedure and the MRI scan [92].

In a follow-up study, Wylie *et al.* reported a left atrial scar volume 8.1 ± 3.7 mL. A linear relation existed between the amount of left atrial scarring and the decrease of left atrial ejection fraction [39].

In a case report, Reddy *et al.* demonstrated the ability to register the delayed enhanced scar with a 3D mapping system to facilitate further repeat ablation procedures [93].

High-resolution animal studies have demonstrated the feasibility of delineating single ablation lesions and gaps in the left atrial wall (Figure 14.9). This raises the possibility of performing periprocedural and postprocedural MRIs to assess the extent of the ablation procedure and localize gaps, which require further RF applications.

Given the recent reports of nephrogenic systemic fibrosis after gadolinium exposure [67] several studies have shown that heat-induced biophysical changes in the T_1 and T_2 relaxation parameters alone (interstitial edema, hyperemia, conformational changes, methemoglobin, and tissue coagulation) enable non-contrast-enhanced visualization of ablation lesions.

Lardo *et al.* showed that acute ablation lesions can be detected in T2-weighted images as areas of increased signal intensity in the RV apex in dogs about 2 minutes after ablation [90]. In further studies our laboratory found that ventricular lesions can be reliably visualized using T_1 or T_2 weighted sequences during a total follow-up time of 12 hours [94]. Ablation lesions appeared as areas of increased signal intensity and lesion size correlated well between MRI and necropsy (T_2: $r = 0.87$; $p < 0.05$ and T_1:

$r = 0.83, p < 0.05$). MRI was also able to accurately assess intralesional morphology and accurately assess the existence and location of necrotic cavities, which occur during high power settings. This may enable a concept of noninvasive "MRI histology" [94].

Computed Tomography

Using electrobeam CT Okada *et al.* was able to visualize indirect effects of RF in 77 patients undergoing an atrial fibrillation ablation. Following circumferential ablation they reported left atrial edema of 4.8 ± 1.3 mm after 24–48 hours, which resolved at 1-month follow-up [95].

Recent studies suggest that multidetector CT is also able to directly visualize ablation lesions due to the different diffusion patterns of contrast material. In six canines right and left ventricular ablation lesions appeared as areas of significantly decreased signal intensity when compared to remote myocardium (106.7 ± 25.9 and 171.2 ± 15.5 Hounsfield Units, respectively). MDCT derived lesion area (normalized for myocardial area) compared well with those measured by postmortem exam ($2.16\% \pm 1.09\%$ vs $2.24\% \pm 1.64\%$, respectively $- p = $ NS) [96]. Further work is on-going, which aims to minimize radiation doses and reduce administration of nephrotoxic contrast material.

Real-Time Guidance

An emerging field of significant clinical interest in EP is the field of real-time imaging. It would allow to eliminate registration errors inherent to current image integration systems. Real-time imaging displays the true catheter position in relation to the actual cardiac anatomy and may allow the direct visualization of ablation lesions as well as the early detection of procedural complications.

Real-Time Magnetic Resonance Imaging

Real-time MRI has the additional advantage of eliminating ionizing radiation. However, its environment is challenging in regard to safety (catheter heating), EP data quality (electromagnetic signal interference), and imaging quality (signal distortion).

Recently, the development of a custom-made, nonferromagnetic recording system and EP catheters has been reported. Using either "passive"

or "active" catheters Nazarian *et al.* were able to navigate to the right atrium, His-bundle and right ventricle in 10 dogs using a fast gradient recall echo sequence with a temporal resolution of ~5 frames per second. Employing serial low- and high-pass RF filters intracardiac signals could be adequately interpreted even during scan sequences. Average times of catheter positioning to right atrial, His bundle, and right ventricular target sites were 169.5 ± 102.5, 447.1 ± 363.5, and 127.3 ± 53.7 seconds, respectively. In two human studies, catheters could be successfully visualized at the cavo-tricuspid isthmus and intracardiac signals recorded during the MRI scanning. Standard imaging sequences resulted in a temperature rise of $<2°C$ as measured in a normal saline-filled phantom [97].

Further technical development is required to enable a wide clinical application of real-time MRI. Currently, exact knowledge of the catheter location is necessary to prescribe the correct imaging planes. Real-time catheter tracking technology is being developed to enable a rapid and continuous visualization of the ablation catheter during navigation. Development of a clinical grade, steerable, MRI-compatible catheters is challenging without use of ferro-magnetic materials. Carbon tips are currently being evaluated and appear promising for electrical recording and RF delivery. New imaging protocols that allow a high spatial and temporal resolution are being developed to improve visualization. Of further interest is the assessment of myocardial heating using photon resonance frequency shift thermography. In a canine model a cutoff of $13°C$ allowed a more accurate delineation of ablation lesions that the use of delayed enhancement [98].

Real-Time Guided CT

With rapid technical improvements real-time imaging with MDCT has become increasingly possible. In animal studies the location of electrophysiological catheters could be identified with submillimeter resolution in relation to the surrounding anatomy. Catheter shaft and tip were well visualized over a wide range of imaging parameters including ultra-low settings of 80 kV, 15 mA (Figure 14.10). Using custom-made software the catheters could be alternatively displayed in either a "fluoroscopy-like" projection view or as 2D or 3D volume rendered images.

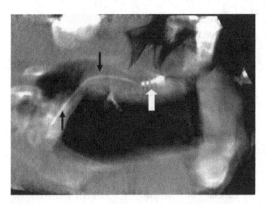

Figure 14.10 Real-time CT guidance of radiofrequency ablations. Catheter shaft is visible within oblique volume reconstruction of swine thorax using a slab thickness of 1.5 cm along inferior vena cava and right atrium (black arrows). Individual metal components of quadro-polar ablation tip of can be seen as areas of high signal density along the anterior wall of the right ventricle (white arrow).

In swine catheter navigation to all four cardiac chambers as well as real-time guided transseptal puncture were possible. Accuracy assessed by anatomically targeted ablation at the pulmonary ostia was 2.6 ± 0.7 mm. Precision defined as the distance between repeat independent navigations and ablations to the identical, predefined lateral RA site was 2.2 ± 0.4 mm. Additionally, linear ablation lesions in the RV and LV demonstrated a maximum deviation of 2.8 ± 0.6 mm [99].

Decreasing tube voltage (140–80 kV) and current (50–30 mA) resulted in a ~10-fold and ~2-fold reduction of the radiation exposure, respectively. The animal exposure for right atrial ablation was 0.26 cGy. Dose rates rapidly decreased with distance to 60 μGy/minute (physician's hands) and 30 μGy/minute (thyroid gland) and were similar to standard fluoroscopy with low CT parameters [100]. Currently, human pilot studies are evaluating its applicability in clinical practice.

References

1. Gallagher JJ, Svenson RH, Kasell JH, *et al.* Catheter technique for closed-chest ablation of the atrioventricular conduction system. *N Engl J Med.* 1982;306(4):194–200.
2. Scheinman MM, Morady F, Hess DS, Gonzalez R. Catheter-induced ablation of the atrioventricular junction to control refractory supraventricular arrhythmias. *JAMA.* 1982;248(7):851–855.
3. Budde T, Breithardt G, Borggrefe M, Podczeck A, Langwasser J. Initial experiences with high-frequency electric ablation of the AV conduction system in the human. *Z Kardiol.* 1987;76(4):204–210.
4. Haissaguerre M, Jais P, Shah DC, *et al.* Spontaneous initiation of atrial fibrillation by ectopic beats originating in the pulmonary veins. *N Engl J Med.* 1998;339(10):659–666.
5. Chen SA, Hsieh MH, Tai CT, *et al.* Initiation of atrial fibrillation by ectopic beats originating from the pulmonary veins: electrophysiological characteristics, pharmacological responses, and effects of radiofrequency ablation. *Circulation.* 1999;100(18):1879–1886.
6. Haissaguerre M, Jais P, Shah DC, *et al.* Electrophysiological end point for catheter ablation of atrial fibrillation initiated from multiple pulmonary venous foci. *Circulation.* 2000;101(12):1409–1417.
7. Pappone C, Rosanio S, Oreto G, *et al.* Circumferential radiofrequency ablation of pulmonary vein ostia: a new anatomic approach for curing atrial fibrillation. *Circulation.* 2000;102(21):2619–2628.
8. Gepstein L, Hayam G, Ben Haim SA. A novel method for nonfluoroscopic catheter-based electroanatomical mapping of the heart. In vitro and in vivo accuracy results. *Circulation.* 1997;95(6):1611–1622.
9. Wongcharoen W, Tsao HM, Wu MH, *et al.* Morphologic characteristics of the left atrial appendage, roof, and septum: implications for the ablation of atrial fibrillation. *J Cardiovasc Electrophysiol.* 2006;17(9):951–956.
10. Chiang SJ, Tsao HM, Wu MH, *et al.* Anatomic characteristics of the left atrial isthmus in patients with atrial fibrillation: lessons from computed tomographic images. *J Cardiovasc Electrophysiol.* 2006;17(12):1274–1278.
11. Kato R, Lickfett L, Meininger G, *et al.* Pulmonary vein anatomy in patients undergoing catheter ablation of atrial fibrillation: lessons learned by use of magnetic resonance imaging. *Circulation.* 2003;107(15):2004–2010.
12. Lickfett L, Kato R, Tandri H, *et al.* Characterization of a new pulmonary vein variant using magnetic resonance angiography: incidence, imaging, and interventional implications of the "right top pulmonary vein". *J Cardiovasc Electrophysiol.* 2004;15(5):538–543.
13. Lickfett L, Dickfeld T, Kato R, *et al.* Changes of pulmonary vein orifice size and location throughout the cardiac cycle: dynamic analysis using magnetic resonance cine imaging. *J Cardiovasc Electrophysiol.* 2005;16(6):582–588.
14. Noseworthy PA, Malchano ZJ, Ahmed J, Holmvang G, Ruskin JN, Reddy VY. The impact of respiration on left atrial and pulmonary venous anatomy: implications for image-guided intervention. *HeartRhythm.* 2005;2(11):1173–1178.

15. Dong J, Calkins H, Solomon SB, *et al.* Integrated electroanatomic mapping with three-dimensional computed tomographic images for real-time guided ablations. *Circulation.* 2006;113(2):186–194.

16. Richmond L, Rajappan K, Voth E, *et al.* Validation of computed tomography image integration into the En-Site NavX mapping system to perform catheter ablation of atrial fibrillation. *J Cardiovasc Electrophysiol.* 2008;19(8):821–827.

17. Packer DL, Keelan P, Munger TM, *et al.* Clinical presentation, investigation, and management of pulmonary vein stenosis complicating ablation for atrial fibrillation. *Circulation.* 2005;111(5):546–554.

18. Pappone C, Oral H, Santinelli V, *et al.* Atrio-esophageal fistula as a complication of percutaneous transcatheter ablation of atrial fibrillation. *Circulation.* 2004;109(22):2724–2726.

19. Kottkamp H, Hugl B, Krauss B, *et al.* Electromagnetic versus fluoroscopic mapping of the inferior isthmus for ablation of typical atrial flutter: a prospective randomized study. *Circulation.* 2000;102(17):2082–2086.

20. Estner HL, Deisenhofer I, Luik A, *et al.* Electrical isolation of pulmonary veins in patients with atrial fibrillation: reduction of fluoroscopy exposure and procedure duration by the use of a non-fluoroscopic navigation system (NavX). *Europace.* 2006;8(8):583–587.

21. Dickfeld T, Calkins H, Zviman M, *et al.* Anatomic stereotactic catheter ablation on three-dimensional magnetic resonance images in real time. *Circulation.* 2003;108(19):2407–2413.

22. Solomon SB, Dickfeld T, Calkins H. Real-time cardiac catheter navigation on three-dimensional CT images. *J Interv Card Electrophysiol.* 2003;8(1):27–36.

23. Brooks AG, Wilson L, Kuklik P, *et al.* Image integration using NavX Fusion: initial experience and validation. *HeartRhythm.* 2008;5(4):526–535.

24. Dong J, Dickfeld T, Dalal D, *et al.* Initial experience in the use of integrated electroanatomic mapping with three-dimensional MR/CT images to guide catheter ablation of atrial fibrillation. *J Cardiovasc Electrophysiol.* 2006;17(5):459–466.

25. Heist EK, Refaat M, Danik SB, Holmvang G, Ruskin JN, Mansour M. Analysis of the left atrial appendage by magnetic resonance angiography in patients with atrial fibrillation. *HeartRhythm.* 2006;3(11):1313–1318.

26. Dong J, Dalal D, Scherr D, *et al.* Impact of heart rhythm status on registration accuracy of the left atrium for catheter ablation of atrial fibrillation. *J Cardiovasc Electrophysiol.* 2007;18(12):1269–1276.

27. Kistler PM, Rajappan K, Jahngir M, *et al.* The impact of CT image integration into an electroanatomic mapping system on clinical outcomes of catheter ablation of atrial fibrillation. *J Cardiovasc Electrophysiol.* 2006;17(10):1093–1101.

28. Martinek M, Nesser HJ, Aichinger J, Boehm G, Purerfellner H. Impact of integration of multislice computed tomography imaging into three-dimensional electroanatomic mapping on clinical outcomes, safety, and efficacy using radiofrequency ablation for atrial fibrillation. *Pacing Clin Electrophysiol.* 2007;30(10):1215–1223.

29. Cappato R, Calkins H, Chen SA, *et al.* Worldwide survey on the methods, efficacy, and safety of catheter ablation for human atrial fibrillation. *Circulation.* 2005;111(9):1100–1105.

30. Calkins H, Brugada J, Packer DL, *et al.* HRS/EHRA/ECAS expert consensus statement on catheter and surgical ablation of atrial fibrillation: recommendations for personnel, policy, procedures and follow-up. A report of the Heart Rhythm Society (HRS) Task Force on Catheter and Surgical Ablation of Atrial Fibrillation developed in partnership with the European Heart Rhythm Association (EHRA) and the European Cardiac Arrhythmia Society (ECAS); in collaboration with the American College of Cardiology (ACC), American Heart Association (AHA), and the Society of Thoracic Surgeons (STS). Endorsed and approved by the governing bodies of the American College of Cardiology, the American Heart Association, the European Cardiac Arrhythmia Society, the European Heart Rhythm Association, the Society of Thoracic Surgeons, and the Heart Rhythm Society. *Europace.* 2007;9(6):335–379.

31. Lickfett L, Hackenbroch M, Lewalter T, *et al.* Cerebral diffusion-weighted magnetic resonance imaging: a tool to monitor the thrombogenicity of left atrial catheter ablation. *J Cardiovasc Electrophysiol.* 2006;17(1):1–7.

32. Cummings JE, Schweikert RA, Saliba WI, *et al.* Assessment of temperature, proximity, and course of the esophagus during radiofrequency ablation within the left atrium. *Circulation.* 2005;112(4):459–464.

33. Lemola K, Sneider M, Desjardins B, *et al.* Computed tomographic analysis of the anatomy of the left atrium and the esophagus: implications for left atrial catheter ablation. *Circulation.* 2004;110(24):3655–3660.

34. Good E, Oral H, Lemola K, *et al.* Movement of the esophagus during left atrial catheter ablation for atrial fibrillation. *J Am Coll Cardiol.* 2005;46(11):2107–2110.

35. Cummings JE, Schweikert RA, Saliba WI, *et al.* Brief communication: atrial-esophageal fistulas after radiofrequency ablation. *Ann Intern Med.* 2006;144(8):572–574.

36. Lemola K, Sneider M, Desjardins B, *et al.* Effects of left atrial ablation of atrial fibrillation on size of the left atrium and pulmonary veins. *HeartRhythm.* 2004;1(5):576–581.

37. Verma A, Kilicaslan F, Adams JR, *et al*. Extensive ablation during pulmonary vein antrum isolation has no adverse impact on left atrial function: an echocardiography and cine computed tomography analysis. *J Cardiovasc Electrophysiol.* 2006;17(7):741–746.

38. Tsao HM, Wu MH, Huang BH, *et al*. Morphologic remodeling of pulmonary veins and left atrium after catheter ablation of atrial fibrillation: insight from long-term follow-up of three-dimensional magnetic resonance imaging. *J Cardiovasc Electrophysiol.* 2005;16(1):7–12.

39. Wylie JV, Jr, Peters DC, Essebag V, Manning WJ, Josephson ME, Hauser TH. Left atrial function and scar after catheter ablation of atrial fibrillation. *HeartRhythm.* 2008;5(5):656–662.

40. McCullough PA, Philbin EF, Spertus JA, Kaatz S, Sandberg KR, Weaver WD. Confirmation of a heart failure epidemic: findings from the resource utilization among congestive heart failure (REACH) study. *J Am Coll Cardiol.* 2002;39(1):60–69.

41. Redfield MM. Heart failure–an epidemic of uncertain proportions. *N Engl J Med.* 2002;347(18):1442–1444.

42. Bardy GH, Lee KL, Mark DB, *et al*. Amiodarone or an implantable cardioverter-defibrillator for congestive heart failure. *N Engl J Med.* 2005;352(3):225–237.

43. Moss AJ, Zareba W, Hall WJ, *et al*. Prophylactic implantation of a defibrillator in patients with myocardial infarction and reduced ejection fraction. *N Engl J Med.* 2002;346(12):877–883.

44. Marchlinski FE, Callans DJ, Gottlieb CD, Zado E. Linear ablation lesions for control of unmappable ventricular tachycardia in patients with ischemic and nonischemic cardiomyopathy. *Circulation.* 2000;101(11):1288–1296.

45. Morady F, Harvey M, Kalbfleisch SJ, El-Atassi R, Calkins H, Langberg JJ. Radiofrequency catheter ablation of ventricular tachycardia in patients with coronary artery disease. *Circulation.* 1993;87(2):363–372.

46. Stevenson WG, Khan H, Sager P, *et al*. Identification of reentry circuit sites during catheter mapping and radiofrequency ablation of ventricular tachycardia late after myocardial infarction. *Circulation.* 1993;88(4 Pt 1):1647–1670.

47. Reddy VY, Reynolds MR, Neuzil P, *et al*. Prophylactic catheter ablation for the prevention of defibrillator therapy. *N Engl J Med.* 2007;357(26):2657–2665.

48. Hunold P, Schlosser T, Vogt FM, *et al*. Myocardial late enhancement in contrast-enhanced cardiac MRI: distinction between infarction scar and non-infarction-related disease. *AJR Am J Roentgenol.* 2005;184(5):1420–1426.

49. de Bakker JM, van Capelle FJ, Janse MJ, *et al*. Reentry as a cause of ventricular tachycardia in patients with chronic ischemic heart disease: electrophysiologic and anatomic correlation. *Circulation.* 1988;77(3):589–606.

50. de Bakker JM, van Capelle FJ, Janse MJ, *et al*. Slow conduction in the infarcted human heart. "Zigzag" course of activation. *Circulation.* 1993;88(3):915–926.

51. Verma A, Marrouche NF, Schweikert RA, *et al*. Relationship between successful ablation sites and the scar border zone defined by substrate mapping for ventricular tachycardia post-myocardial infarction. *J Cardiovasc Electrophysiol.* 2005;16(5):465–471.

52. Ashikaga H, Sasano T, Dong J, *et al*. Magnetic resonance-based anatomical analysis of scar-related ventricular tachycardia: implications for catheter ablation. *Circ Res.* 2007;101(9):939–947.

53. Oza S, Wilber DJ. Substrate-based endocardial ablation of postinfarction ventricular tachycardia. *HeartRhythm.* 2006;3(5):607–609.

54. Gepstein L, Goldin A, Lessick J, *et al*. Electromechanical characterization of chronic myocardial infarction in the canine coronary occlusion model. *Circulation.* 1998;98(19):2055–2064.

55. Callans DJ, Ren JF, Michele J, Marchlinski FE, Dillon SM. Electroanatomic left ventricular mapping in the porcine model of healed anterior myocardial infarction. Correlation with intracardiac echocardiography and pathological analysis. *Circulation.* 1999;100(16):1744–1750.

56. Kornowski R, Hong MK, Gepstein L, *et al*. Preliminary animal and clinical experiences using an electromechanical endocardial mapping procedure to distinguish infarcted from healthy myocardium. *Circulation.* 1998;98(11):1116–1124.

57. Kim RJ, Fieno DS, Parrish TB, *et al*. Relationship of MRI delayed contrast enhancement to irreversible injury, infarct age, and contractile function. *Circulation.* 1999;100(19):1992–2002.

58. Lima JA, Judd RM, Bazille A, Schulman SP, Atalar E, Zerhouni EA. Regional heterogeneity of human myocardial infarcts demonstrated by contrast-enhanced MRI. Potential mechanisms. *Circulation.* 1995;92(5):1117–1125.

59. Rogers WJ, Jr, Kramer CM, Geskin G, *et al*. Early contrast-enhanced MRI predicts late functional recovery after reperfused myocardial infarction. *Circulation.* 1999;99(6):744–750.

60. Rehwald WG, Fieno DS, Chen EL, Kim RJ, Judd RM. Myocardial magnetic resonance imaging contrast agent concentrations after reversible and irreversible ischemic injury. *Circulation.* 2002;105(2):224–229.

61. Kwong RY, Chan AK, Brown KA, *et al*. Impact of unrecognized myocardial scar detected by cardiac magnetic resonance imaging on event-free survival in patients presenting with signs or symptoms of coronary artery disease. *Circulation.* 2006;113(23):2733–2743.

62. Bello D, Fieno DS, Kim RJ, *et al.* Infarct morphology identifies patients with substrate for sustained ventricular tachycardia. *J Am Coll Cardiol.* 2005;45(7):1104–1108.

63. Nazarian S, Bluemke DA, Lardo AC, *et al.* Magnetic resonance assessment of the substrate for inducible ventricular tachycardia in nonischemic cardiomyopathy. *Circulation.* 2005;112(18):2821–2825.

64. Yan AT, Shayne AJ, Brown KA, *et al.* Characterization of the peri-infarct zone by contrast-enhanced cardiac magnetic resonance imaging is a powerful predictor of post-myocardial infarction mortality. *Circulation.* 2006;114(1):32–39.

65. Schmidt A, Azevedo CF, Cheng A, *et al.* Infarct tissue heterogeneity by magnetic resonance imaging identifies enhanced cardiac arrhythmia susceptibility in patients with left ventricular dysfunction. *Circulation.* 2007;115(15):2006–2014.

66. Faris OP, Shein M. Food and drug administration perspective: magnetic resonance imaging of pacemaker and implantable cardioverter-defibrillator patients. *Circulation.* 2006;114(12):1232–1233.

67. Marckmann P, Skov L, Rossen K, *et al.* Nephrogenic systemic fibrosis: suspected causative role of gadodiamide used for contrast-enhanced magnetic resonance imaging. *J Am Soc Nephrol.* 2006;17(9):2359–2362.

68. Francone M, Carbone I, Danti M, *et al.* ECG-gated multi-detector row spiral CT in the assessment of myocardial infarction: correlation with non-invasive angiographic findings. *Eur Radiol.* 2006;16(1):15–24.

69. Nieman K, Cury RC, Ferencik M, *et al.* Differentiation of recent and chronic myocardial infarction by cardiac computed tomography. *Am J Cardiol.* 2006;98(3):303–308.

70. Lessick J, Mutlak D, Rispler S, *et al.* Comparison of multidetector computed tomography versus echocardiography for assessing regional left ventricular function. *Am J Cardiol.* 2005;96(7):1011–1015.

71. Gerber BL, Belge B, Legros GJ, *et al.* Characterization of acute and chronic myocardial infarcts by multidetector computed tomography: comparison with contrast-enhanced magnetic resonance. *Circulation.* 2006;113(6):823–833.

72. Mahnken AH, Koos R, Katoh M, *et al.* Assessment of myocardial viability in reperfused acute myocardial infarction using 16-slice computed tomography in comparison to magnetic resonance imaging. *J Am Coll Cardiol.* 2005;45(12):2042–2047.

73. Nieman K, Shapiro MD, Ferencik M, *et al.* Reperfused myocardial infarction: contrast-enhanced 64-Section CT in comparison to MR imaging. *Radiology.* 2008;247(1):49–56.

74. Margonato A, Mailhac A, Bonetti F, *et al.* Exercise-induced ischemic arrhythmias in patients with previous myocardial infarction: role of perfusion and tissue viability. *J Am Coll Cardiol.* 1996;27(3):593–598.

75. Krause BJ, Poeppel TD, Reinhardt M, *et al.* Myocardial perfusion/metabolism mismatch and ventricular arrhythmias in the chronic post infarction state. *Nuklearmedizin.* 2005;44(3):69–75.

76. Sasano T, Abraham MR, Chang KC, *et al.* Abnormal sympathetic innervation of viable myocardium and the substrate of ventricular tachycardia after myocardial infarction. *J Am Coll Cardiol.* 2008;51(23):2266–2275.

77. Fallavollita JA, Luisi AJ, Jr, Michalek SM, *et al.* Prediction of arrhythmic events with positron emission tomography: PAREPET study design and methods. *Contemp Clin Trials.* 2006;27(4):374–388.

78. Brunken R, Tillisch J, Schwaiger M, *et al.* Regional perfusion, glucose metabolism, and wall motion in patients with chronic electrocardiographic Q wave infarctions: evidence for persistence of viable tissue in some infarct regions by positron emission tomography. *Circulation.* 1986;73(5):951–963.

79. Maes A, Flameng W, Nuyts J, *et al.* Histological alterations in chronically hypoperfused myocardium. Correlation with PET findings. *Circulation.* 1994;90(2):735–745.

80. Tamaki N, Kawamoto M, Tadamura E, *et al.* Prediction of reversible ischemia after revascularization. Perfusion and metabolic studies with positron emission tomography. *Circulation.* 1995;91(6):1697–1705.

81. Yoshida K, Gould KL. Quantitative relation of myocardial infarct size and myocardial viability by positron emission tomography to left ventricular ejection fraction and 3-year mortality with and without revascularization. *J Am Coll Cardiol.* 1993;22(4):984–997.

82. Chareonthaitawee P, Schaefers K, Baker CS, *et al.* Assessment of infarct size by positron emission tomography and [18F]2-fluoro-2-deoxy-D-glucose: a new absolute threshold technique. *Eur J Nucl Med Mol Imaging.* 2002;29(2):203–215.

83. Higuchi T, Nekolla SG, Jankaukas A, *et al.* Characterization of normal and infarcted rat myocardium using a combination of small-animal PET and clinical MRI. *J Nucl Med.* 2007;48(2):288–294.

84. Berry JJ, Hoffman JM, Steenbergen C, *et al.* Human pathologic correlation with PET in ischemic and nonischemic cardiomyopathy. *J Nucl Med.* 1993;34(1):39–47.

85. Kuhl HP, Beek AM, Van Der Weerdt AP, *et al.* Myocardial viability in chronic ischemic heart disease: comparison of contrast-enhanced magnetic resonance imaging with (18)F-fluorodeoxyglucose positron emission tomography. *J Am Coll Cardiol.* 2003;41(8):1341–1348.

86. Koch KC, vom DJ, Wenderdel M, *et al.* Myocardial viability assessment by endocardial electroanatomic mapping: comparison with metabolic imaging and functional recovery after coronary revascularization. *J Am Coll Cardiol.* 2001;38(1):91–98.

87. Botker HE, Lassen JF, Hermansen F, *et al.* Electromechanical mapping for detection of myocardial viability in patients with ischemic cardiomyopathy. *Circulation.* 2001;103(12):1631–1637.

88. Dickfeld T, Lei P, Dilsizian V, *et al.* Integration of three-dimensional scar maps for ventricular tachycardia ablation with positron emission tomography-computed tomography. *J Am Coll Cardiol Img.* 2008;1: 73–82.

89. Shekhar R, Walimbe V, Raja S, *et al.* Automated 3-dimensional elastic registration of whole-body PET and CT from separate or combined scanners. *J Nucl Med.* 2005;46(9):1488–1496.

90. Lardo AC, McVeigh ER, Jumrussirikul P, *et al.* Visualization and temporal/spatial characterization of cardiac radiofrequency ablation lesions using magnetic resonance imaging. *Circulation.* 2000;102(6):698–705.

91. Dickfeld T, Kato R, Zviman M, *et al.* Characterization of radiofrequency ablation lesions with gadolinium-enhanced cardiovascular magnetic resonance imaging. *J Am Coll Cardiol.* 2006;47(2):370–378.

92. Peters DC, Wylie JV, Hauser TH, *et al.* Detection of pulmonary vein and left atrial scar after catheter ablation with three-dimensional navigator-gated delayed enhancement MR imaging: initial experience. *Radiology.* 2007;243(3):690–695.

93. Reddy VY, Schmidt EJ, Holmvang G, Fung M. Arrhythmia recurrence after atrial fibrillation ablation: can magnetic resonance imaging identify gaps in atrial ablation lines? *J Cardiovasc Electrophysiol.* 2008;19(4):434–437.

94. Dickfeld T, Kato R, Zviman M, *et al.* Characterization of acute and subacute radiofrequency ablation lesions with nonenhanced magnetic resonance imaging. *HeartRhythm.* 2007;4(2):208–214.

95. Okada T, Yamada T, Murakami Y, *et al.* Prevalence and severity of left atrial edema detected by electron beam tomography early after pulmonary vein ablation. *J Am Coll Cardiol.* 2007;49(13):1436–1442.

96. Cordeiro M, Silva C, Zviman M, *et al.* Characterization of cardiac radiofrequency ablation lesions using contrast-enhanced multidetector computed tomography imaging. *Circulation.* 2006;114(18):2619.

97. Nazarian S, Kolandaivelu A, Zviman MM, *et al.* Feasibility of real-time magnetic resonance imaging for catheter guidance in electrophysiology studies. *Circulation* 2008;118(3):223–229.

98. Kolandaivelu A, Zviman M, Castro V, Ranjan R, Berger R, Halperin H. Non-invasive monitoring of tissue heating during cardiac RF ablation is possible using MRI thermography. *HeartRhythm.* 2008;5(5S):S99.

99. Dickfeld T, Engelhardt M, Read K, *et al.* Real-time computed tomography (RT-CT) for guidance of catheter navigation, transseptal puncture and anatomically targeted radiofrequency ablation. *Circulation.* 2007;116:II-489.

100. Dickfeld T, Hodefi D, Read K, *et al.* Real-time CT guided ablation procedures: radiation exposure, safety and feasibility [Abstract]. *HeartRhythm.* 2008;5(5S):S272.

CHAPTER 15

Structural and Molecular Imaging of Vulnerable Plaques

Farouc A. Jaffer[1] *& Jagat Narula*[2]

[1] Massachusetts General Hospital, Harvard Medical School, Boston, MA, USA
[2] University of California, Irvine, CA, USA

Structural and molecular imaging of atherosclerosis offers an exciting opportunity to detect and follow high-risk coronary lesions that are likely to produce acute coronary events. Such high-risk lesions, or vulnerable plaques, induce thrombotic occlusions of the coronary artery, typically in the proximal portions [1–4]. Rupture of an inflamed, thin fibrous capped, lipid-rich atherosclerotic plaque is responsible for acute coronary occlusions in up to three-fourths of subjects. Plaque erosion, characterized by selective endothelial loss and hyaluranon-rich lesion which is generally less intensely inflamed, is the next most common substrate underlying thrombotic occlusion of subjects that died of an acute coronary event [2]. Plaque rupture is associated with traditional cardiac risk factors (smoking, dyslipidemia, hypertension, diabetes mellitus, family history), whereas plaque erosion is generally associated with smoking and is commonly observed in women or younger subjects. Histopathological examination has demonstrated that disrupted plaques are nearly always large and occupy at least 50% of vascular area in cross section [1–3]. Such plaques also harbor large necrotic cores comprising a substantial portion of the plaque volume. These necrotic cores are surrounded by neo-vascular growth which is associated with intraplaque hypoxia-induced adventitial vasa vasorum proliferation and often results in plaque hemorrhage. Overlying these necrotic cores are markedly attenuated fibrous cap (<65 µm thickness) that are intensely inflamed from infiltrating macrophages.

Imaging strategies to identify rupture-prone coronary arterial plaques therefore have two strategic and complementary pathways: structural imaging aimed at the detection of thin-capped, voluminous plaques and necrotic cores [1,3,4] and molecular imaging employed to detect plaque inflammation, apoptosis, and neoangiogenesis [5–8]. For structural imaging, major noninvasive approaches have targeted (1) coronary vessel wall positive remodeling by CT and MRI and (2) coronary plaque lipid by CT (low Hounsfield units or HU) and possibly MRI. For molecular imaging, clinical strategies have included imaging of the extent of monocyte–macrophage infiltration and their apoptosis in carotid arteries, with more recent efforts in developing targeted coronary arterial-based imaging strategies.

Structural Imaging of High-Risk Plaques

Imaging of Positive Remodeling and Lipid-Rich Atheromata

Coronary plaques that rupture typically occupy >50% of the total cross-sectional vascular area; and in many cases more than 75% of the vascular area; these plaques are routinely associated with positive, or expansive vessel wall remodeling (Figure 15.1) [1–4]. In spite of substantial plaque bulk, only about one and a half of such plaques

Cardiac CT, PET and MR, 2nd edition. Edited by Vasken Dilsizian and Gerry Pohost. © 2010 Blackwell Publishing Ltd.

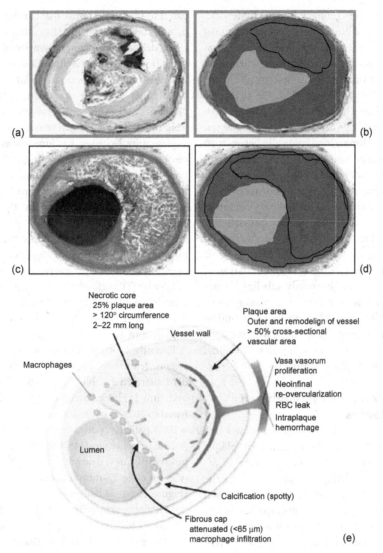

Figure 15.1 The ultrastructure of high-risk plaques. Respective histopathological assessment and schematic representation of a (a and b) ruptured coronary plaque and (c–d) a high-risk plaque that is prone to disruption. In contradistinction to stable atherosclerotic plaques that are collagen- and smooth-muscle-cell-rich, rupture-prone plaques are usually large and contain a necrotic core housed by an attenuated and inflamed fibrous cap. If rupture of the fibrous cap occurs, typically at areas of high wall stress, the highly thrombogenic necrotic core is exposed to luminal blood and provokes thrombosis. Notably, ruptured plaques responsible for acute myocardial infarction are usually significantly voluminous, but may not always produce luminal obstruction. Consequently these plaques may not be detected by perfusion-based imaging stress tests or luminal angiography alone, motivating the need for direct plaque imaging methods. The lumen and cross-sectional vessel area are outlined in (b) and (d); the plaque necrotic core

has been colored red, the non-necrotic plaque area colored blue, and the lumen colored green. Disrupted plaques almost always occupy >50% of the cross-sectional vessel area (red + blue area divided by red + blue + green area), and in up to half of subjects they may comprise >75% of the cross-sectional area. Disrupted plaques and pre-existing high-risk plaques usually demonstrate large necrotic cores (a–d). Necrotic cores usually occupy more than 25% of the plaque area (red area divided by red + blue area) and commonly extend >120° in circumference involvement of the vessel. Coronary plaque necrotic cores average 9 mm in circumferential length (range 2–22 mm). The risk of plaque rupture appears to increase in plaques of larger areas and in those housing larger necrotic cores. Although vulnerable plaques are usually large with substantial necrotic cores, they often first expand outwards and may not induce a significant luminal stenosis. This process of positive

critically narrow the coronary lumen. If stenotic, such plaques should induce the classic syndrome of exertional angina and the corresponding stress test should reveal inducible ischemia. Such patients will ideally receive optimal medical therapy and coronary revascularization if indicated. On the other hand, many subjects harbor coronary plaques with large volumes and large necrotic cores that have not yet induced flow limitations (typically between 30 and 70% luminal stenoses). Despite the greater likelihood of major acute coronary events, such patients may remain asymptomatic, may perform normally on stress tests, and may be erroneously reassured of low-risk status. Such asymptomatic patients may present with acute coronary syndromes including unstable angina, acute myocardial infarction, or sudden cardiac death, as the first manifestation of their undiagnosed (or previously subclinical) but high-risk condition. Therefore, an imaging technique that is able to precisely identify large, nonflow limiting coronary plaques associated with substantial lipid-rich enclosures and expansive remodeling, should be of intense clinical import.

Structural Coronary CT Imaging of High-risk Plaques

CT angiography, predominantly employed for the assessment of luminal narrowing by plaque encroachment, has the added advantage of simultaneously visualizing the plaque itself, the extent of necrotic core, and the type of segmental remodeling [9]. A study of patients experiencing an acute coronary syndrome (ACS) compared to those with stable angina has showed remarkably different plaque characteristics. Specifically, CT angiography of ACS patients showed greater prevalence of positive remodeling (PR) of the vessel wall, defined as an external vessel wall diameter >110% greater com-

pared to the normal proximal (or distal vessel segment), and of noncalcified low attenuation plaques (LAP, defined as a plaque intensity of less than 30 HU) (Figure 15.2). Of note, spotty calcification was also more commonly associated with culprit ACS lesions. These features demonstrated a high predictive ability to identify culprit lesions responsible for ACS [9]. Plaque characterization by CT angiography, however, has limitations. Inadequate resolution limits precise definition of the vascular boundary, and the corresponding measurement of the extent of PR may be over- or underestimated. Similarly, as LAP is defined by the HU intensity, various imaging/technical parameters can influence plaque HU measurements, and various investigators have therefore suggested different HU thresholds to define plaque types. A comparison of IVUS with CT angiography demonstrated that most echo-lucent plaques on IVUS (indicating lipid-rich plaques) had values of <30 HU on coronary CT angiography [10].

Recently, a prospective study of two CT angiographic features of high-risk plaques, PR and LAP, demonstrated an ability to predict plaque rupture over time [11]. In a coronary CTA study that evaluated >10,000 coronary arterial segments from >1000 patients, patients with both PR and low-attenuation plaques (45 out of 1059 two-feature positive plaques) demonstrated a *22%* incidence of ACS over the 27-month average follow-up period (Figure 15.3). In contradistinction, patients without PR plaques and without LAP (two-feature negative group, 820 out of 1059 patients) had only a *0.5%* incidence of ACS (40-fold less than the two-feature positive group above). Predictors of plaque rupture included a greater degree of positive remodeling and larger plaque area. Notably, patients without evidence of coronary atherosclerosis plaques did

---

Figure 15.1 (*Continued*) or outward remodeling in contrast does not typify stable plaques with small or absent lipid cores, and in contrast their relatively fibrotic composition may produce constrictive/negative remodeling or segmental shrinkage (luminal stenosis). Consequently the fundamental hypothesis underlying vulnerable plaque imaging is that high-risk structural and molecular features exist prior to plaque disruption. Exemplary lesions include large plaques (red + blue) area possessing a large necrotic core (red, with abundant cholesterol crystals ghosted as residual clefts on histology),

covered by a significantly thinned and inflamed fibrous cap. Structural-based clinical detection of high-risk plaques thus should focus on demonstration of large plaque and necrotic core volumes and the expansive remodeling of the plaque carrying vascular segment. These morphological characteristics of plaque vulnerability are shown in the schematic representation (e). Additional molecular and cellular characteristics of vulnerability shown in the scheme are described below. (Reproduced from [2], with permission.).

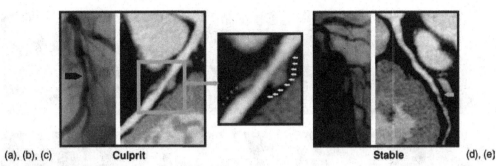

(a), (b), (c)   Culprit   **Stable   (d), (e)**

Figure 15.2 Structural characteristics of a culprit coronary artery lesion defined by computed tomography angiography (CTA). Invasive X-ray (a) and noninvasive CTA (b) demonstrates that this culprit lesion responsible for unstable angina may not be significantly flow-limiting. Magnification image of the culprit lesion on CTA (c) shows high-risk plaque features of positive remodeling (yellow arrows), and low attenuation plaque (red arrowheads). In contrast, a stable angina-producing lesion (d and e) in another patient severely narrows the lumen as seen by invasive X-ray (d) and CT (e) angiography, is not positively remodeled and shows intermediate rather than low attenuation plaque (green arrow). Intravascular ultrasound assessment further revealed that IVUS-defined soft plaques had a low attenuation signal (<30 HU), and fibrous plaques (noncalcified) had an intermediate attenuation (30–150 HU). (Reproduced from [2], with permission.)

not experience any adverse events. This important study may allow exploration of a noninvasive approach to identify subjects with high-risk plaques before experiencing an associated myocardial infarction [12].

Structural MRI of High-risk Coronary Arterial Plaques

In larger vessels such as the carotid arteries, MRI may identify key anatomical and functional markers of high-risk carotid plaques [13]. In particular,

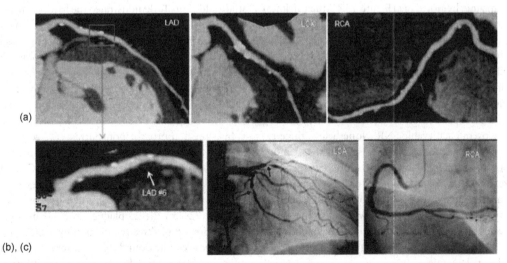

(a)

(b), (c)

Figure 15.3 CT angiography of a high-risk coronary atheroma producing an acute coronary syndrome (ACS) 6 months later. (a) Curved multiplanar reformation images of the left anterior descending artery (LAD), left circumflex artery (LCX), and right coronary artery (RCA). (b) Magnified lesion in the LAD (LAD #6) on baseline CTA demonstrated positive remodeling (outward growth of the plaque), low attenuation (HU < 30), and spotty calcification. (c) The patient presented with an ACS 6 months after the initial CTA. Invasive coronary angiography demonstrated that LAD #6 was the culprit lesion. The presence of both positive remodeling (PR) and low attenuation plaques (LAP) on CTA increased the ACS event rate by more than 50-fold compared to subjects without PR and without LAP during a 27-month mean follow-up period. LCA, left coronary artery. (Reproduced from [2], with permission.)

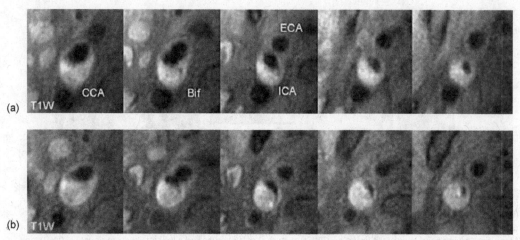

Figure 15.4 Carotid plaque MRI-detected intraplaque hemorrhage is associated with rapid plaque progression on follow-up MRI. T_1 weighted (T1W) images at 1.5T of a patient with a moderate carotid atherosclerotic lesion are shown at (a) baseline and (b) 18 months later. Each column shows matched cross-sectional locations in the carotid artery at baseline and 18 months later. At baseline, hyperintense signal on T1W images demonstrated intraplaque hemorrhage throughout the lesion. On follow-up serial imaging, the lumen area markedly diminished and the plaque area substantially increased. A 4-element phased-array carotid coil was utilized to optimize the signal-to-noise ratio. Bif, bifurcation; CCA, common carotid artery; ECA, external carotid artery; ICA, internal carotid artery; T1W, T1-weighted. (Reproduced from Takaya *et al*. [14], with permission.)

multicontrast MRI protocols can visualize intraplaque hemorrhage (Figure 15.4), the thickness or thinness of the fibrous cap, and the lipid-rich necrotic core; each of these parameters has been associated with plaque progression and/or future ipsilateral stroke in prospective cohorts [14,15]. MRI of coronary atherosclerosis imaging poses a greater challenge due to higher-resolution requirements and multiple sources of motion artifact, limiting the overall achievable SNR. Nonetheless, three recent strategies for coronary vessel wall MRI demonstrate the potential for MRI to illuminate high-risk features of coronary plaques. In the first approach, cardiac-gated black-blood coronary MRI sequences (typically inversion recovery with fat suppression) have been developed to allow imaging of coronary vessel wall positive remodeling [16,17], a feature of high-risk plaques.

In a second approach, delayed-enhancement contrast MRI (via intravenous injection of 0.2 mmol/kg of gadolinium-DTPA) revealed selective enhancement of coronary plaques [18]. Multislice coronary CT angiography and invasive coronary angiography served as "gold standards" for the presence of atherosclerosis (Figure 15.5). A recent study additionally demonstrated the MRI temporal characteristics of delayed enhancement of coronary plaques in patients with acute myocardial infarction [19]. The mechanism of augmented gadolinium uptake into coronary atheroma has yet to be precisely elucidated, but may be related to augmented endothelial permeability, neovessels, or inflammatory cells [20].

In a third approach, noncontrast T_1 weighted MRI of stenotic coronary lesions (>70% narrowing) was performed, and correlated with MSCT and IVUS [21]. Compared to coronary plaques with low T_1 weighted signal, high-intensity coronary plaques (72% of the 25 plaques studied) demonstrated greater positive remodeling by MSCT and IVUS, reduced ultrasound signal, lower Hounsfield units on MSCT, and higher spotty calcification rates. In addition, high-intensity plaques were six times more likely to be associated with slow-flow following interventional treatment of the imaged plaque. These findings suggest that T_1 weighted MRI may identify high-risk coronary plaques undergoing PCI. Further studies will be needed to

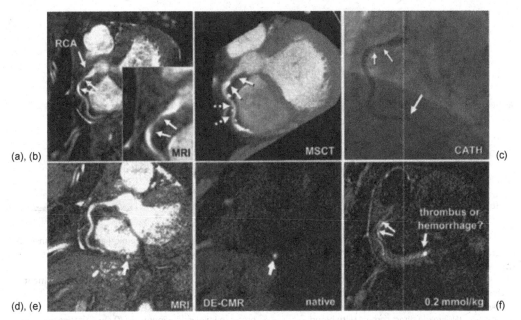

Figure 15.5 Coronary MRI shows delayed enhancement of a focal proximal RCA lesion. (a) Coronary MR angiogram (1.5T, free-breathing, ECG-gated steady-state free precession (SSFP) pulse sequence, with magnified inset) and (b) correlative multislice computed tomography (MSCT) (b) show a proximal RCA focal plaque (white arrows), with MSCT revealing a mixed calcified and noncalcified plaque. The corresponding invasive X-ray angiogram (c) shows an expected moderately stenotic proximal RCA lesion, without any information on the vessel wall itself. (e) On a precontrast delayed-enhancement cardiovascular magnetic resonance (DE-CMR) vessel wall scan, a "hot spot" is visible in a distal RCA plaque (arrow), indicating plaque hemorrhage or thrombus. (d) The hot spot is also seen on the reformatted matched section of the initial coronary MRA image. Interestingly the corresponding X-ray angiogram (c) shows a subtotal occlusion at after the posterior descending artery takeoff, suggesting recent plaque complication. On the DE-CMR image (f) the proximal RCA stenosis (solid white arrows) demonstrates enhanced signal, as does the midsection of the RCA where the matched MSCT (b) reveals a mixed calcified/noncalcified plaque (dashed white arrows). CATH = invasive X-ray coronary angiography. Reproduced from Yeon et al. [18], with permission.)

determine whether high-intensity plaque signal on T_1 weighted imaging predicts future acute myocardial infarction.

Imaging of Plaque Vascularity and Adventitial Vasa Vasorum

Neovessel proliferation in evolving atheromata are high-risk indicators of vulnerable plaques due to their potential to induce intraplaque hemorrhage and to enhance inflammation. Recently, microbubble contrast-enhanced intravascular ultrasound has been employed to image vascularity of the plaques [22]. The stringent resolution requirements for coronary vaso vasorum imaging will require new approaches for CTA or MRI, perhaps through molecular imaging, discussed subsequently.

Molecular Imaging of High-Risk Plaques

Molecular imaging incorporates the radiological, chemical, biological, and engineering sciences to illuminate specific molecules and cells in living subjects. Through the application of efficient imaging agents paired with appropriate imaging hardware systems, molecular imaging can visualize mechanisms of atherosclerosis disease initiation, progression, and complication in vivo [5–8]. Excitingly, molecular imaging approaches now exist from bench-to-bedside, enabling the visualization of cardinal biological processes in human atherosclerosis such as inflammation and apoptosis.

The last several years have witnessed substantial progress in clinical molecular imaging of larger

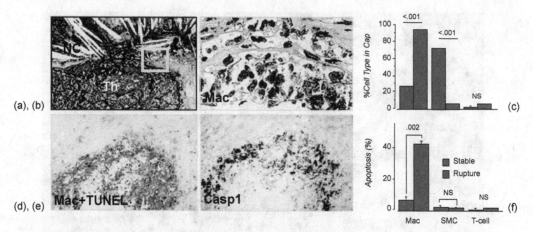

Figure 15.6 Molecular imaging targets that characterize vulnerable plaques include macrophages and their associated inflammatory proteases, and cellular apoptosis. (a) High-risk plaques often harbor intense zones of macrophage infiltration within the fibrous cap. Following plaque rupture (yellow square), the highly thrombogenic necrotic core (NC) made direct contact with blood coagulation factors and platelets, leading to a thrombotic occlusion (Th). (b) Magnified view of the area in yellow square reveals abundant immunostained macrophages. (c) Quantitative immunohistochemical analyses demonstrate that macrophages predominate in ruptured plaques, whereas smooth cells predominate in stable atherosclerotic lesions. (d) Plaque apoptosis is augmented in also lesional macrophages with (e) upregulated expression of caspase-1 (CASP1, brown staining), a protease involved in apoptosis. (f) Quantitative analyses reveal that apoptosis is largely a feature of macrophages in ruptured plaques. (Reproduced from [2], with permission.)

atherosclerotic arteries (carotids, aorta) via MRI, PET, and single photon emission computed tomography (SPECT)-based approaches [5–8]. In upcoming years, as more efficient imaging agents translate into the clinic, substantial progress in anticipated in clinical coronary molecular imaging.

Imaging of Plaque Inflammation

Macrophages are the key inflammatory cell in atherosclerosis. Macrophages identify high-risk plaques [23] and are a well-established target for molecular imaging (Figure 15.6). Following molecular imaging approaches have demonstrated clinical utility for atherosclerosis: ultrasmall superparamagnetic iron oxide (USPIO) nanoparticle enhanced MRI, and 18-fluorine-fluorodeoxygluocose (^{18}F-FDG) positron emission tomography (PET) imaging.

18-Fluorine-fluorodexoyglucose (^{18}F-FDG) PET Imaging of Plaque Metabolic Activity/Macrophages

In 2002, Rudd *et al.* prospectively demonstrated that ^{18}F-FDG PET identified macrophage-rich carotid atherosclerotic lesions (Figure 15.7) [24]. Subse-quent PET/histology correlative atheroma studies demonstrated a more precise relationship between the in vivo ^{18}F-FDG PET signal in human carotid plaques and the density of plaque macrophages ($r > 0.7$) [25]. Vascular studies utilizing ^{18}F-FDG PET have revealed augmented plaque metabolism/inflammation in 30% of statin-naïve patients [26] and in metabolic syndrome patients [27]. ^{18}F-FDG PET studies of drug efficacy have provided insights into the inflammation-modulating effects of statins (Figure 15.8) [28] and homocysteine therapy [29].

As ^{18}F-FDG PET atherosclerosis imaging possesses good reproducibility (interclass coefficients > 0.75 [31]), ^{18}F-FDG PET may be well suited to assess the anti-inflammatory atherosclerosis effects of new pharmacotherapies. Advantages of ^{18}F-FDG PET for molecular imaging include the widespread availability of ^{18}F-FDG through commercial distributors (now tested in thousands of patients with atherosclerosis) thereby eliminating the need for a cyclotron, as well as very high inherent molecular sensitivity, and the availability of integrate CT-PET scanners to optimize co-registration and reliability. Disadvantages of ^{18}F-FDG PET include the lack

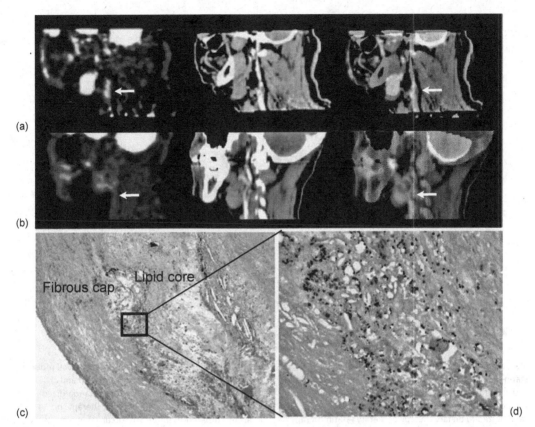

Figure 15.7 Molecular imaging of macrophage metabolism/inflammation in human carotid plaques: ^{18}F-fluorodeoxyglucose (^{18}FDG)-based PET imaging. Matched (a) ^{18}FDG-PET (left), contrast-enhanced CT (middle), and co-registered PET/CT (right) images of a symptomatic patient who carotid atherosclerosis. Focal signal is present on PET image within a right carotid plaque (arrow), as registered by the CT angiogram and seen on the fusion image. (b) In an asymptomatic patient injected with ^{18}FDG, the patient's carotid plaque shows weaker signal. (c) A resected carotid plaque of a symptomatic patient was incubated with tritiated deoxyglucose, an analog of ^{18}FDG enabling microautoradiography. Autoradiographic images show colocalization of tritiated deoxygluycose (silver grains) with immunostained plaque macrophages (d, anti-CD68 antibody, ×200) in the fibrous cap and lipid core. (Adapted from Rudd et al. [24].

of precise reporting on macrophage-based inflammation, as ^{18}F-FDG can report on other plaque cells such as endothelial cells [32] and lymphocytes [33]. Newer macrophage-specific PET tracers [34] may overcome this limitation. In addition, significant radiation exposure occurs during 18F-FDG PET imaging (>5–10 mSv), particularly if combined with CT and if multiple imaging sessions are required.

Magnetic Nanoparticle-Enhanced MRI of Plaque Macrophages

Clinical magnetic nanoparticles (MNP) contain a 3-nm ultrasmall superparamagnetic iron oxide (USPIO) core encased by uncrosslinked dextran, resulting a full particle size of ~30 nm. USPIO particles induce strong T_2-weighted contrast, or signal loss in the presence of a magnetic field [35]. USPIOs show significant promise in excluding cancer metastases [36] and more recently, in identifying macrophages in carotid atherosclerosis (Figure 15.9) [37–39]. In addition a recent study demonstrates the ability of molecular MRI to distinguish the in vivo anti-inflammatory effects of high-dose statin therapy versus low-dose statin therapy for carotid plaque inflammation [39]. An advantage of molecular MRI is the ability to also acquire high-resolution (submillimeter) anatomical imaging of plaque composition (discussed above) without ionizing radiation.

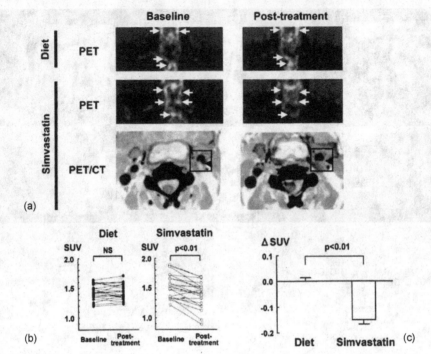

(a)

(b)

(c)

Figure 15.8 Serial PET molecular imaging of statin-mediated reductions in carotid plaque metabolic activity/inflammation. Cancer patients with incidental atherosclerosis detected on [18]FDG staging scans were randomized to dietary therapy or dietary+statin therapy (simvastatin) for 3 months. Patients underwent ^{18}F-FDG PET imaging of carotid arteries followed-by contrast-enhanced carotid CTA. (a) In control patients, the carotid plaque ^{18}F-FDG signal was similar after 3 months.

In contrast, patients receiving simvastatin showed reduced ^{18}F-FDG plaque signal after just 3 months. (b and c) Statin-treated patients showed reduced standardized uptake values (SUVs) after 3 months of therapy; no significant differences in the SUV occurred in control patients. ΔSUV = change in the SUV following treatment. Bar = 1 standard deviation. (Adapted from Tahara et al. [28 and Trivedi et al. [30], with permission.)

Figure 15.9 Clinical molecular MRI of carotid arterial plaque inflammatory macrophages with ultrasmall superparamagnetic iron oxide (USPIO) nanoparticles. (a) Pre- and (b) post-USPIO axial MRI above the left carotid artery bifurcation. The patient was intravenously injected with USPIO 36 hours prior to imaging. On T_2^* weighted MRI, USPIO particles induce signal loss within the plaque (yellow arrow) compared to the baseline image. (c) Plaque histology revealed a thin fibrous cap (black arrowhead) overlying a large lipid core (white arrowhead). (d) High-power double Perls and MAC387 stains for USPIO and macrophages, respectively, demonstrated that USPIO (blue) colocalized with plaque macrophages in the fibrous cap (brown; 40× magnification). (Reproduced from Trivedi et al. [43], with permission.)

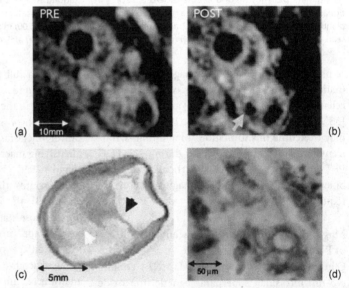

Challenges of molecular MRI include its lower inherent molecular sensitivity compared to nuclear and optical approaches, although this limitation is partially overcome by very high relaxivity compounds such as USPIO and other nanoparticle constructs [40]. Positive contrast sequences for that render USPIO contrast bright may improve image assessment [41], particularly in low signal-to-noise regions.

Imaging of Plaque Apoptosis Burden

Apoptosis, a high-risk feature of plaques associated with rupture [23], has been preliminary imaged in four clinical subjects with carotid atherosclerosis [42], using technetium-99m labeled annexin A5, a ligand that binds to phopsphatidylserine residues exposed on apoptotic (and necrotic) cells. Recently, plaque lymphocytes in 23 patients with carotid atherosclerosis have been imaged utilizing noninvasive SPECT imaging [44].

Molecular Imaging Strategies for Coronary Plaques

The last several years have witnessed tremendous growth in high-sensitivity molecular imaging approaches for atherosclerosis utilizing MRI, nuclear, ultrasound, and optical strategies (reviewed in references [5–8]). Many of these imaging agents show promise for clinical translation. Below we briefly highlight three promising translatable strategies with high applicability to imaging of coronary arterial inflammation, a key unmet need for clinical molecular imaging of high-risk plaques.

^{18}F-FDG PET Imaging of Coronary Plaque Metabolism/Inflammation

In a recent retrospective study, augmented *coronary* plaque metabolism/inflammation was imaged employing a low-carbohydrate, high-fat diet to suppress myocardial background suppression [45]. Patients were culled from a cohort of patients that underwent ^{18}F-FDG PET/CT imaging for cancer staging and had a cardiac catheterization within 3 months of the PET scan (typically for preoperative cancer resection risk assessment). PET studies were not obtained with respiratory or cardiac gating. Myocardial suppression of ^{18}F-FDG was deemed good (average SUV 2.8) or adequate (average SUV 5.0) in 63% of the 32 patients studied. Fusion images with anatomical CT scans (nongated, non intravenous contrast) showed that augmented coronary ^{18}F-FDG signal in 15 of the 20 patients with adequate or good myocardial suppression (Figure 15.10). Correlation with invasive

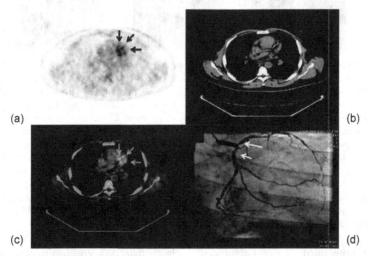

(a) (b) (c) (d)

Figure 15.10 Molecular imaging of coronary macrophage metabolism/inflammation by ^{18}F-FDG PET. Patients received a high-fat, low carbohydrate cocktail to suppress ^{18}F-FDG myocardial uptake, allowing detection of coronary arterial-based ^{18}F-FDG signal. Representative images of (a) ^{18}F-FDG PET, (b) ungated, noncontrast CT, (c) fusion PET/CT image with arrows highlighting enhanced ^{18}F-FDG signal over the left anterior descending (LAD) artery, and (d) invasive X-ray angiography demonstrating ostial LAD and circumflex lesions. (Reproduced from Wykrzykowska *et al.* [45], with permission.)

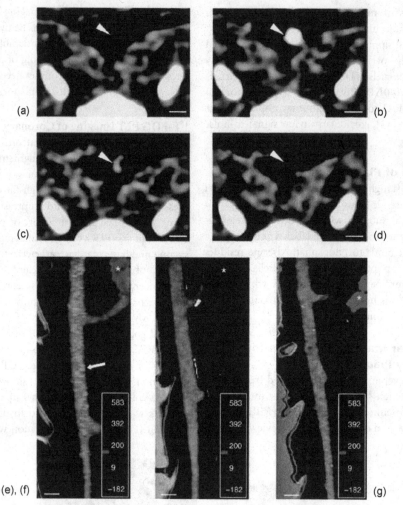

Figure 15.11 CT molecular imaging of inflammatory plaque macrophages in coronary-sized vessels. Specialized macrophage-targeted iodinated nanoparticles (N1177) were tested atherosclerotic and control rabbits (250 mg iodine/kg, intravenous injection). In addition, the same animals were also injected (in a separate imaging study 1 week prior) with a conventional iodinated angiographic contrast agent (iopamidol, 250 mg iodine/kg). Vascular CT images were obtained preinjection, during infusion, and then 2 hours after injection of either N1177 or iopamidol. (a–c) Axial CT images of an atherosclerotic aorta (a) Baseline imaging pre-agent injection revealed minimal luminal and vessel wall signal. (b) During infusion, N1177 provides a vascular angiogram, similar to conventional iodine. (c) N1177 induces late enhancement of atheroma at 2 hours postinjection (arrow), in contradistinction to (d) conventional iodine. (e–g) Fusion images of 2-hour delayed aortic CT image (pseudocolored red) and the initial CTA obtained during agent infusion. (e) N1177-injected rabbits showed strong late-enhanced plaque signal (red) throughout the aorta. In contrast, minimal signal was present in control animals receiving N1177 (f) and in atherosclerotic rabbits injected with conventional iodine (g). White asterisk, spleen. Scale bar, 5 mm. (Reproduced from Hyafil *et al.* [46], with permission.)

angiography demonstrated a near-significant ($p = 0.07$) relationship between ^{18}F-FDG uptake and the presence of coronary stenoses on angiography. This foundational study may offer a non-invasive clinical approach to coronary high-risk plaque detection, and future gains are anticipated with the incorporation of more potent myocardial suppression methods and the use of cardiac-gated, contrast-enhanced CT angiography to determine whether PR and/or LAP correlates with augmented

^{18}F-FDG signal. Challenges of this method include volume averaging, but prospective studies are clearly indicated.

Noninvasive CT of Plaque Macrophages

Crystalline-iodinated nanoparticles (N1177) can now visualize plaque macrophages in coronary-sized vessels in atherosclerotic rabbits (Figure 15.11) [46]. Detection of plaque macrophages further enhances the powerful capabilities of coronary CT, potentially enabling a one-stop shop option to image the coronary lumen (angiography), calcified and noncalcified plaque, and plaque inflammation. Challenges for N1177 nanoparticle-enhanced coronary CT imaging include exposure to radiation(double dose in the current pre- and postinjection protocols). Excitingly, a subcutaneous form of the agent is already in Phase I clinical trials for cancer imaging [47].

Near-infrared Fluorescence Sensing of Plaque Protease Activity

Augmented protease activity, a hallmark of inflamed vulnerable plaques, has been imaged in coronary-sized vessels via a novel intravascular NIRF catheter coupled with a high-sensitivity protease-activatable imaging agent (Prosense750) [48]. Intriguingly, plaque protease activity in rabbits was detected in real-time through blood, without the need for flushing, affirming the favorable optical transmission properties of the NIR window. A scintigraphic analog of the Prosense750 agent has previously completed clinical trials [49]. In the future, noninvasive fluorescence mediated tomography [50] may develop into a clinical inflammation imaging modality, especially for the larger, more superficial carotid arteries.

Conclusions

Developing accurate plaque imaging strategies is a critical step in predicting and ultimately preventing plaque rupture and myocardial infarction. Imaging strategies utilizing CT, nuclear scintigraphy, and MRI, as well as ultrasound and NIRF imaging are driving structural and molecular imaging of high-risk coronary plaques into the clinical arena. Promising imaging strategies are spurring prospective patient registries to determine their predictive ability to predict coronary events, a mandatory step before widespread application to the at-risk population. Ultimately high-risk plaque imaging is positioned to diagnose and offer risk stratification for high-risk patients, and to guide the systemic and local management of vulnerable plaques.

References

1. Narula J, Strauss HW. The popcorn plaques. *Nat Med.* 2007;13:532–534.
2. Narula J. Who gets the heart attack? Noninvasive imaging of unstable plaques. *J Nucl Cardiol.* 2009;16(6):860–868.
3. Shapiro E, Bush D, Motoyama S, Virmani R, Narula J. Imaging atherosclerotic plaques vulnerable to rupture. In: Volume Editors: Budoff MJ, Aschebach S, Narula J. Series Editor: Braunwald E. *Atlas of Computed Tomography.* Philadelphia: Current Medicine, 2007.
4. Narula J, Garg P, Achenbach S, Motoyama S, Virmani R, Strauss HW. Arithmetic of vulnerable plaques for noninvasive imaging. *Nat Clin Pract Cardiovasc Med.* 2008; 5 Suppl. 2: S2–S10.
5. Jaffer FA, Weissleder R. Molecular imaging in the clinical arena. *JAMA.* 2005;293:855–862.
6. Jaffer FA, Libby P, Weissleder R. Molecular and cellular imaging of atherosclerosis: emerging applications. *J Am Coll Cardiol.* 2006;47:1328–1338.
7. Jaffer FA, Libby P, Weissleder R. Molecular imaging of cardiovascular disease. *Circulation.* 2007;116:1052–1061.
8. Sanz J, Fayad ZA. Imaging of atherosclerotic cardiovascular disease. *Nature.* 2008;451:953–957.
9. Motoyama S, Kondo T, Sarai M, et al. Multislice computed tomographic characteristics of coronary lesions in acute coronary syndromes. *J Am Coll Cardiol.* 2007;50: 319–326.
10. Motoyama S, Kondo T, Anno H, et al. Atherosclerotic plaque characterization by 0.5-mm-slice multislice computed tomographic imaging. *Circ J.* 2007;71:363–366.
11. Motoyama S, Sarai M, Harigaya H, et al. Computed tomographic angiography characteristics of atherosclerotic plaques subsequently resulting in acute coronary syndrome. *J Am Coll Cardiol.* 2009;54:49–57.
12. Braunwald E. Noninvasive detection of vulnerable coronary plaques: locking the barn door before the horse is stolen. *J Am Coll Cardiol.* 2009;54:58–59.
13. Chu B, Ferguson MS, Chen H, et al. Cardiac magnetic resonance features of the disruption-prone and the disrupted carotid plaque. *JACC Cardiovasc Imaging.* 2009; 2:883–896.
14. Takaya N, Yuan C, Chu B, et al. Presence of intraplaque hemorrhage stimulates progression of carotid

atherosclerotic plaques: a high-resolution magnetic resonance imaging study. *Circulation*. 2005;111:2768–2775.

15. Altaf N, Daniels L, Morgan PS, *et al.* Detection of intraplaque hemorrhage by magnetic resonance imaging in symptomatic patients with mild to moderate carotid stenosis predicts recurrent neurological events. *J Vasc Surg.* 2008;47:337–342.

16. Kim WY, Stuber M, Bornert P, Kissinger KV, Manning WJ, Botnar RM. Three-dimensional black-blood cardiac magnetic resonance coronary vessel wall imaging detects positive arterial remodeling in patients with nonsignificant coronary artery disease. *Circulation.* 2002; 106:296–299.

17. Miao C, Chen S, Macedo R, *et al.* Positive remodeling of the coronary arteries detected by magnetic resonance imaging in an asymptomatic population: MESA (multiethnic study of atherosclerosis). *J Am Coll Cardiol.* 2009; 53:1708–1715.

18. Yeon SB, Sabir A, Clouse M, *et al.* Delayed-enhancement cardiovascular magnetic resonance coronary artery wall imaging: comparison with multislice computed tomography and quantitative coronary angiography. *J Am Coll Cardiol.* 2007;50:441–447.

19. Ibrahim T, Makowski MR, Jankauskas A, *et al.* Serial contrast-enhanced cardiac magnetic resonance imaging demonstrates regression of hyperenhancement within the coronary artery wall in patients after acute myocardial infarction. *JACC Cardiovasc Imaging.* 2009;2:580–588.

20. Kerwin WS, O'Brien KD, Ferguson MS, Polissar N, Hatsukami TS, Yuan C. Inflammation in carotid atherosclerotic plaque: a dynamic contrast-enhanced MR imaging study. *Radiology.* 2006;241:459–468.

21. Kawasaki T, Koga S, Koga N, *et al.* Characterization of hyperintense plaque with noncontrast T(1)-weighted cardiac magnetic resonance coronary plaque imaging: comparison with multislice computed tomography and intravascular ultrasound. *JACC Cardiovasc Imaging.* 2009;2:720–728.

22. Vavuranakis M, Kakadiaris IA, O'Malley SM, *et al.* A new method for assessment of plaque vulnerability based on vasa vasorum imaging, by using contrast-enhanced intravascular ultrasound and differential image analysis. *Int J Cardiol.* 2008;130:23–29.

23. Naghavi M, Libby P, Falk E, *et al.* From vulnerable plaque to vulnerable patient: a call for new definitions and risk assessment strategies: Part I. *Circulation.* 2003; 108:1664–1672.

24. Rudd JH, Warburton EA, Fryer TD, *et al.* Imaging atherosclerotic plaque inflammation with [18F]-fluorodeoxyglucose positron emission tomography. *Circulation.* 2002;105:2708–2711.

25. Tawakol A, Migrino RQ, Bashian GG, *et al.* In vivo 18F-fluorodeoxyglucose positron emission tomography imaging provides a noninvasive measure of carotid plaque inflammation in patients. *J Am Coll Cardiol.* 2006; 48:1818–1824.

26. Tahara N, Kai H, Nakaura H, *et al.* The prevalence of inflammation in carotid atherosclerosis: analysis with fluorodeoxyglucose-positron emission tomography. *Eur Heart J.* 2007;28:2243–2248.

27. Tahara N, Kai H, Yamagishi S, *et al.* Vascular inflammation evaluated by [18F]-fluorodeoxyglucose positron emission tomography is associated with the metabolic syndrome. *J Am Coll Cardiol.* 2007;49:1533–1539.

28. Tahara N, Kai H, Ishibashi M, *et al.* Simvastatin attenuates plaque inflammation: evaluation by fluorodeoxyglucose positron emission tomography. *J Am Coll Cardiol.* 2006;48:1825–1831.

29. Potter K, Lenzo N, Eikelboom JW, Arnolda LF, Beer C, Hankey GJ. Effect of long-term homocysteine reduction with B vitamins on arterial wall inflammation assessed by fluorodeoxyglucose positron emission tomography: a randomised double-blind, placebo-controlled trial. *Cerebrovasc Dis.* 2009;27:259–265.

30. Trivedi RA, Mallawarachi C, U-King-Im J, *et al.* Identifying inflamed carotid plaques using in vivo USPIO-enhanced MR imaging to label plaque macrophages. *Arterioscler Thromb Vasc Biol.* 2006;26:1601–1606.

31. Rudd JH, Myers KS, Bansilal S, *et al.* (18)Fluorodeoxyglucose positron emission tomography imaging of atherosclerotic plaque inflammation is highly reproducible: implications for atherosclerosis therapy trials. *J Am Coll Cardiol.* 2007;50:892–896.

32. Maschauer S, Prante O, Hoffmann M, Deichen JT, Kuwert T. Characterization of 18F-FDG uptake in human endothelial cells in vitro. *J Nucl Med.* 2004;45:455–460.

33. Ishimori T, Saga T, Mamede M, *et al.* Increased (18)F-FDG uptake in a model of inflammation: concanavalin A-mediated lymphocyte activation. *J Nucl Med.* 2002;43: 658–663.

34. Fujimura Y, Hwang PM, Trout Iii H, *et al.* Increased peripheral benzodiazepine receptors in arterial plaque of patients with atherosclerosis: an autoradiographic study with [(3)H]PK 11195. *Atherosclerosis,* 2008;201(1):108–111. Epub 2008 Mar 14.

35. Weissleder R, Elizondo G, Wittenberg J, Rabito CA, Bengele HH, Josephson L. Ultrasmall superparamagnetic iron oxide: characterization of a new class of contrast agents for MR imaging. Radiology. 1990;175:489–493.

36. Harisinghani MG, Barentsz J, Hahn PF, *et al.* Noninvasive detection of clinically occult lymph-node metastases in prostate cancer. *N Engl J Med.* 2003;348:2491–2499.

37. Kooi ME, Cappendijk VC, Cleutjens KB, *et al.* Accumulation of ultrasmall superparamagnetic particles of iron oxide in human atherosclerotic plaques can be detected by

in vivo magnetic resonance imaging. *Circulation.* 2003; 107:2453–2458.

38. Trivedi RA, U-King-Im J, Graves MJ, *et al.* In vivo detection of macrophages in human carotid atheroma: temporal dependence of ultrasmall superparamagnetic particles of iron oxide-enhanced MRI. *Stroke.* 2004;35: 1631–1635.

39. Tang TY, Howarth SP, Miller SR, *et al.* The ATHEROMA (Atorvastatin Therapy: Effects on Reduction of Macrophage Activity) Study. Evaluation using ultrasmall superparamagnetic iron oxide-enhanced magnetic resonance imaging in carotid disease. *J Am Coll Cardiol.* 2009;53:2039–2050.

40. Cormode DP, Skajaa T, Fayad ZA, Mulder WJ. Nanotechnology in medical imaging: probe design and applications. *Arterioscler Thromb Vasc Biol.* 2009;29:992–1000.

41. Korosoglou G, Weiss RG, Kedziorek DA, *et al.* Noninvasive detection of macrophage-rich atherosclerotic plaque in hyperlipidemic rabbits using "positive contrast" magnetic resonance imaging. *J Am Coll Cardiol.* 2008;52: 483–491.

42. Kietselaer BL, Reutelingsperger CP, Heidendal GA, *et al.* Noninvasive detection of plaque instability with use of radiolabeled annexin A5 in patients with carotid-artery atherosclerosis. *N Engl J Med.* 2004;350:1472–1473.

43. Trivedi RA, U-King-Im JM, Graves MJ, Kirkpatrick PJ, Gillard JH. Noninvasive imaging of carotid plaque inflammation. *Neurology.* 2004;63:187–188.

44. Annovazzi A, Bonanno E, Arca M, *et al.* 99mTc-interleukin-2 scintigraphy for the in vivo imaging of vulnerable atherosclerotic plaques. *Eur J Nucl Med Mol Imaging.* 2006;33:117–126.

45. Wykrzykowska J, Lehman S, Williams G, *et al.* Imaging of inflamed and vulnerable plaque in coronary arteries with 18F-FDG PET/CT in patients with suppression of myocardial uptake using a low-carbohydrate, high-fat preparation. *J Nucl Med.* 2009;50:563–568.

46. Hyafil F, Cornily JC, Feig JE, *et al. Nat Med.* 2007; 13:636–641.

47. Available at: http://www.nanoscanimaging.com/clinical_trials.cfm. Accessed August 4, 2009.

48. Jaffer FA, Vinegoni C, John MC, *et al.* Real-time catheter molecular sensing of inflammation in proteolytically active atherosclerosis. *Circulation.* 2008;118:1802–1809.

49. Callahan RJ, Bogdanov A, Jr., Fischman AJ, Brady TJ, Weissleder R. Preclinical evaluation and phase I clinical trial of a 99mTc-labeled synthetic polymer used in blood pool imaging. *AJR Am J Roentgenol.* 1998;171:137–143.

50. Ntziachristos V, Tung CH, Bremer C, Weissleder R. Fluorescence molecular tomography resolves protease activity in vivo. *Nat Med.* 2002;8:757–760.

Index

Note: Italicized page numbers refer to figures and tables.